Contents

Preface to the fourth edition

How to use this book

Even if you are an experienced research worker or technologist, please **READ CHAPTER 1 BEFORE ATTEMPTING TO CARRY OUT ANY PRACTICAL INSTRUCTIONS**, and look at the list of *Conventions and abbreviations* on page xi. Otherwise, go directly to any subject that interests you, by way of the *Contents* list or the *Index*. There are many cross-references to numbered sections of other chapters. Nobody reads this kind of book from beginning to end.

The purpose of this book is to teach the chemical, physical and biological principles of fixation, staining and histochemistry. I urge the reader always to determine the reason for every step in a method before doing it. The theoretical explanations and practical instructions are, therefore, closely integrated. This is to encourage an intelligent approach to microtechnique, in which the user reviews the rationale of each new technique rather than trying to follow to the letter a list of poorly understood technical instructions. There is a reason for each instruction, and the printed procedural details may not apply equally to all tissues. Adaptations and adjustments are often necessary, and are likely to be successful when they are justified by knowledge and understanding.

The reader requires some knowledge of chemistry (descriptive rather than mathematical) and biology (structure of cells and tissues) to use this book effectively. The particular hazards of histological processing (mainly toxicity and fire) are noted as they arise, but this is not a textbook of laboratory safety, and the warnings do not cover every risk. Note that in some institutions, the use of certain chemicals may be forbidden because of real or (more frequently) suspected hazards. It is necessary to comply with such prohibitions even if you do not agree with them. Local regulations must also be followed for disposing of solvents and other chemicals, and of materials of human or other biological origin.

Readers, especially graduate students and others involved in research, are urged to follow up the references provided for the methods they are using. A textbook cannot provide all the information, and there is often controversy, especially concerning mechanisms of fixation and staining.

What's new in the fourth edition?

As with the third edition (1999) I have tried to include newer procedures that seem likely to become 'standard' methods in research, diagnostic pathology, or the preparation of teaching materials. Deletions have been necessary to compensate for the new material, but overall there is more that needs to be said than there was 8 years ago.

To avoid increasing the size of the book, I have removed the questions that in earlier editions were at the ends of the chapters. These were used in a Histochemistry course at the University of Western Ontario, but otherwise only two people have told me that they looked at these end of chapter exercises. I will be happy to email to any interested reader a PDF file containing all the questions and answers sections from the third edition.

Methods for fixing and processing tissues continue to become more numerous and more diverse, and the first four chapters of this edition contain descriptions of various newer reagents and techniques. Ordinary staining with dyes is carried out as much as ever, and several methods, not all of them new, have been added to Chapters 6, 7 and 8. The reader will also find enough theoretical and practical information to make up combinations of staining procedures appropriate to the needs of the moment. The thoughtful use of dyes in this way is encouraged as an alternative to trying out several published procedures in the hope of finding one that is suitable.

Chapter 9 (nucleic acids) now includes discussion of *in situ* hybridization and methods for detecting apoptotic cells. Throughout the book, the scope of applications is wider than in earlier editions. Histological and histochemical methods for animal tissues still predominate, but now there is some discussion, with instructions, of the fixing, processing and staining of plants and microorganisms. All chapters have been updated. Although some references have been deleted, the size of the Bibliography has increased by about 12%, to more than 1300 items.

J.A. Kiernan
London, Ontario, Canada, August 2007

Acknowledgements

Thanks are due to many people who have given advice and criticism over the years. Among present and former colleagues at the University of Western Ontario, I thank Drs K. Baines, R. C. Buck, M. G. Cherian, B. A. Flumerfelt, P. Haase, E. A. Heinicke, P. K. Lala, D. G. Montemurro, C. C. Naus and N. Rajakumar. I have also learned much from Dr R. W. Horobin (Sheffield), Dr Sarah Pixley (Cincinnati) and the late Dr P. E. Reid (Vancouver). Discussions over the Internet have taught me about histological practice in many parts of the world. For sharing their wisdom I thank many people, some of whom I have never met, including Russ Allison, Gayle Callis, Freida Carson, Jim Elsam, Tony Henwood, Bryan Hewlett, Ian Montgomery, Phil Oshel, Bob Richmond, Barry Rittman, Ron Stead and many others. Comments and questions from students have also prompted corrections and clarification in several places. Finally, I thank Dr Jonathan Ray of Scion Publishing for his guidance during the preparation of the fourth edition.

J. A. KIERNAN
London, Ontario, Canada

Conventions and abbreviations

Conventions

It is important that the reader be familiar with the conventions listed here before attempting to follow the instructions for any practical procedure.

[ ] Square brackets:

(a) Enclose a complex, such as $[Ag(NH_3)_2]^+$ or $[PdCl_4]^{2-}$.

(b) Indicate 'concentration of' in molar terms. Thus, $[Ca^{2+}]^3$ = the cube of the molar concentration of calcium ions.

Accuracy. Unless otherwise stated, solids should be weighed and liquids measured to an accuracy of ±5%. With quantities less than 10 mg or 1.0 ml, an accuracy of ±10% is usually acceptable.

Alcohol. Unqualified, this word is used for methanol, ethanol, isopropanol, or industrial methylated spirit (which is treated as 95% v/v). When the use of a specific alcohol is necessary, this is stated. 'Absolute' refers to commercially obtained '100%' ethanol, which really contains nearly 1% water and may also contain traces of benzene. Absolute ethanol is hygroscopic and should be kept in securely capped bottles. In an ordinary covered staining tank, ethanol does not remain acceptably 'absolute' for more than about 5 days.

When diluting alcohols for any purpose, use distilled or deionized water.

Concentrations expressed as percentages. The symbol % is used in various ways:

(a) For solids in solution, % = grams of solid dissolved in 100 ml of the final solution.

(b) For liquids diluted with other liquids, % = number of millilitres of the principal component present in 100 ml of the mixture, the balance being made up by the diluent (usually water). '70% ethanol' means 70 ml of absolute ethanol (or 74 ml of 95% ethanol) made up to 100 ml with water.

(c) For gases (e.g. formaldehyde), % = grams of the gas contained in 100 ml of solution.

(d) Where doubt may arise, the symbol v/v, w/v, or w/w is appended to the % sign. For dilution of common acids and ammonia, see Chapter 20.

Formalin. This word refers to the commercially obtained solution containing 37% w/w (40% w/v) of formaldehyde in water. The shortened form 'formal' is used in the names of mixtures such as formal–saline and formal–calcium. The term 'formol' is found in some books, but this is wrong because the ending -ol suggests, incorrectly, that formaldehyde is an alcohol.

Safety precautions. The precautions necessary in any laboratory, especially for prevention of fire, should be observed at all times. Some reagents used in histology and histochemistry have their special hazards. These are mentioned as they arise in the text.

- *Concentrated mineral acids* (especially sulphuric) must be diluted by adding acid to water (not water to acid) slowly with stirring.

- *Acids* should be carefully diluted and neutralized before discarding.

- *Formaldehyde and hydrochloric acid* should not be thrown down a sink together: their vapours can react together in the air to form bis-chloromethyl ether, a carcinogen. Each substance should be flushed down the drain separately, with copious running tap water.

- *Concentrated nitric acid must not be allowed to come into contact with organic liquids, especially alcohol:* the strongly exothermic reaction may result in an explosion.

Salts–water of crystallization. The crystalline forms of salts are shown in instructions for mixing solutions. If the form stated is not available, it will be necessary to calculate the equivalent amount of the alternative material. This is simply done by substitution in the formula:

$$\frac{W_1}{M_1} = \frac{W_2}{M_2}$$

where W = weight, M = molecular weight, and subscripts 1 and 2 refer to the prescribed and the alternative compounds respectively.

For example, 125 mg of cupric sulphate ($CuSO_4$) is prescribed, but only the hydrated salt, $CuSO_4.5H_2O$, is available. Molecular weights are 223.14 and 249.68 respectively. Then:

$$\frac{125}{223.14} = \frac{W_2}{249.68}$$

$$W_2 = \frac{125 \times 249.68}{223.14}$$

$$= 139.9$$

It will therefore be necessary to use 139.9 (i.e. 140) mg of $CuSO_4.5H_2O$ in place of 125 mg of the anhydrous salt.

Solutions. If a solvent is not named (e.g. '1% silver nitrate'), it is assumed to be water. See also **Water**, below.

Structural formulae. Aromatic rings are shown as Kekulé formulae, with alternating double bonds. Thus benzene is:

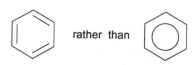

The second designation indicates the equivalence of all the bonds in the ring, but with Kekulé formulae it is easier to understand structural changes associated with the formation of coloured compounds (Chapter 5).

A few deviations from standard chemical notation (e.g. in formulae for lipids) are explained where they arise.

Temperature. Unless otherwise stated, all procedures are carried out at room temperature, which is assumed to be 15–25°C. The other commonly used temperatures are 37°C and about 60°C. A histological laboratory should have ovens or incubators maintained at these temperatures. If an oven containing melted paraffin wax is used as a 60°C incubator, make sure that any aqueous or alcoholic solutions put in it are covered. Water or alcohol vapour may otherwise contaminate the wax. For most staining purposes, a water bath is preferable to an oven.

Water. When 'water' is prescribed in practical instructions, it means distilled or deionized water. When water from the public supply may be used, it is specifically mentioned as 'tap water'.

Abbreviations

Specialized abbreviations are explained as they are introduced in the text. The following are used in several places.

α, β   (a) Used to indicate the configuration at position Cl in glycosides (Chapter 11).

(b) In aliphatic compounds the α carbon atom is adjacent to the carbon atom bearing the principal functional group (i.e. α is carbon number 2). The use of numbers and Greek letters is shown below for *n*-hexanol:

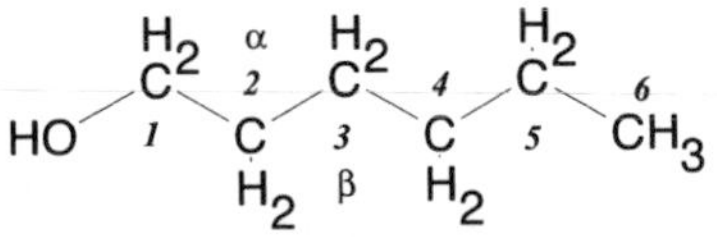

$$HO \underset{1}{\overset{H_2}{C}} \underset{\beta}{\overset{\alpha}{\underset{3}{C}}} \underset{2}{\overset{H_2}{C}} \underset{\beta}{\overset{4}{\underset{H_2}{C}}} \underset{5}{\overset{H_2}{C}} \underset{6}{CH_3}$$

(c) In glycerol and its derivatives, the middle carbon atom is designated as β and the carbons on either side as α and α'.

(d) In derivatives of naphthalene, to indicate the position of a substituent relative to the site of fusion of the rings:

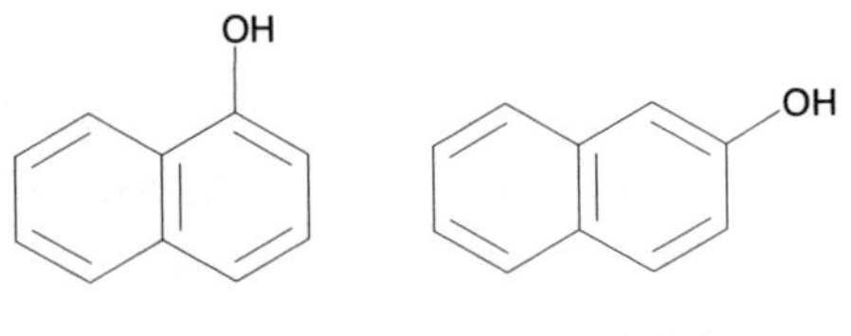

α-naphthol   β-naphthol
(= 1-naphthol)   (= 2-naphthol)

Δ   Symbol used to indicate double bonds in lipids (Chapter 12).

ε   Indicates carbon number 6 or a substituent on this atom, as in the case of the amino group at the end of the side-chain of lysine.

μg   Microgram (10^{-6} g or 10^{-3} mg).

μm	Micrometer (10^{-6} m or 10^{-3} mm); also sometimes called a 'micron'.
Ar	An aryl radical (in formulae).
ATP	Adenosine triphosphate.
ATPase	Adenosine triphosphatase.
bis-	Twice (in names of compounds).
BP	British Pharmacopoeia; boiling point.
BSS	Balanced salt solution (Chapter 23).
°C	Degrees Celsius (Centigrade).
CI	Colour Index (Chapter 5).
cis-	Indicates a geometrical isomer in which two substituents lie on the same side of the molecule.
CNS	Central nervous system.
cyt.	Cytochrome (with identifying letter, *a*, *b*, *c*, etc.).
D-	Indicates a compound, usually a sugar, of the D-series. The compound itself is not necessarily dextrorotatory.
DAB	3,3'-Diaminobenzidine.
dansyl	The 5-(dimethylamino)-1-naphthalenesulphonyl radical.
DMP	2,2-Dimethoxypropane.
DNA	Deoxyribonucleic acid.
DNase	Deoxyribonuclease.
DOPA	β-3,4,-dihydroxyphenylalanine.
DPX	A resinous mounting medium. The initials stand for its three components, distrene-80 (a polystyrene, MW 80 000), a plasticizer, and xylene (Chapter 4).
E_o, E_o'	Symbols for oxidation–reduction potentials (Chapter 16).
EC	Enzyme Commission (Chapter 14).
EDTA	Ethylenediamine tetraacetic acid. Also known as versene, sequestrene, edetic acid, and (ethylenedinitrilo)-tetraacetic acid. Usually used as its disodium salt, Na_2EDTA.
Fab	Part of the immunoglobulin molecule (Chapter 19).
FAD	Flavin adenine dinucleotide (Chapter 16).
Fc	Part of the immunoglobulin molecule (Chapter 19).
FMN	Flavin mononucleotide (Chapter 16).
H & E	Haemalum and eosin (Chapter 6).
H-acid	8-amino-1-naphthol-3,6-disulphonic acid.
H-chain	Part of the immunoglobulin molecule (Chapter 19).
HRP	Horseradish peroxidase.
IgG	Immunoglobulin G.

L-	Indicates a compound (usually a sugar or an amino acid) of the L-series. The compound itself is not necessarily laevorotatory.
M	(as in 0. 1 M) Molar (moles per litre).
m-	*meta-* (in names of benzene derivatives, substituents at positions 1 and 3).
MW	Molecular weight.
mole	The molecular weight, expressed in grams.
N	(as in 0. 1 N) Normal (gram-equivalents per litre; Chapter 20).
N–	Indicates bonding to a nitrogen atom in names of some compounds.
n-	Normal, indicating an unbranched chain, as in *n*-butanol.
NAD$^+$	Nicotinamide adenine dinucleotide.
NADP$^+$	Nicotinamide adenine dinucleotide phosphate
NANA	N-acetylneuraminic acid.
nm	nanometre (10^{-9} m or 10^{-3} μm).
O–	Indicates bonding to an oxygen atom in names of some compounds.
o-	*ortho-* (in names of benzene derivatives, substituents at positions 1 and 2).
p-	*para-* (in names of benzene derivatives, substituents at positions 1 and 4).
PAS	Periodic acid–Schiff (method; Chapter 11).
PBS	Phosphate-buffered saline (Chapter 23).
pg	picogram (10^{-12} g).
pH	The logarithm (to base 10) of the reciprocal of the molar concentration of hydrogen ions.
PMA	Phosphomolybdic acid.
PNS	Peripheral nervous system.
PTA	Phosphotungstic acid.
PVA	Polyvinyl alcohol.
PVP	Polyvinylpyrollidone (also called povidone).
R, R'	Indicate alkyl or aryl radicals, in formulae.
RNA	Ribonucleic acid.
RNase	Ribonuclease.
SG	Specific gravity (also density, in g/cm^3).
t-	Tertiary, as in *t*-butanol: $(CH_3)_3COH$.
trans-	Indicates a geometrical isomer in which two substituents lie on opposite sides of the molecule.
TRIS	Tris(hydroxymethyl)aminomethane.
USP	United States Pharmacopoeia.

v/v   Volume/volume (a 1% v/v solution = 1 ml diluted to 100 ml).

w/v   Weight/volume (a 1% w/v solution = 1 g dissolved to make 100 ml).

w/w   Weight/weight (100 g of 37% w/w hydrochloric acid contains 37 g of HCl and 63 g of water; see also Chapter 20).

1 | Introduction to microtechnique

Many theoretical explanations and practical instructions are contained in this book. The present chapter concerns aspects of the making of microscopical preparations that are fundamental to all the techniques described in the later chapters. It cannot be over-emphasized that unless the student or technician understands the rationale of all that is to be done, he will not do it properly. **Chapter 4 and Section 1.6 of this chapter contain some of the practical information relevant to the manipulations discussed in all parts of the book.**

With an ordinary microscope it is possible to see only limited structural detail in a living or freshly removed part of a large organism. More information can be obtained with special techniques, including **video-enhanced contrast** microscopy (Allen, 1987; Breuer *et al.*, 1988), with which otherwise inconspicuous features can be emphasized, and **infrared microscopy** (Dodt and Zieglandberger, 1998), which can show the shapes of individual cells at the surface of an organ. For the resolution of finer structure within and around cells it is necessary to study **fixed specimens**. These are pieces of animal or plant material that have been structurally stabilized, usually by a chemical treatment. Fixation, which is reviewed in Chapter 2, arrests post-mortem decay and also gives a harder consistency to many tissues. Fixation introduces structural and chemical artifacts, but these are fairly well understood and for most purposes they outweigh the technical difficulties and artifacts encountered in the examination of unfixed material. Some naturally hard materials require softening treatments after fixation (Chapter 3); bone, for example, can be decalcified.

1.1. Thickness and contrast

In order to be examined with a microscope, a specimen must be sufficiently thin to be transparent and must possess sufficient contrast to permit the resolution of structural detail. Thinness may be an intrinsic property of the object to be examined. Thus, small animals and plants, films, smears of cells, tissue cultures, macerated or teased tissues, and spread-out sheets of epithelium or connective tissue are all thin enough to mount on slides directly. In the study of histology, histopathology and histochemistry, one is more often concerned with the internal structure of larger, solid specimens. These must be cut into thin slices or **sections** in order to make them suitable for microscopical examination. (Methods also exist for examination of surfaces: notably scanning electron microscopy, and atomic force microscopy. Preparative methods for such techniques are outside the scope of this book.)

Freehand sections, cut with a razor, are rarely used in animal histology but are still sometimes employed for botanical material. Though some expertise is necessary, sectioning in this way has the advantage of requiring little in the way of time or special equipment. In a recent variant of the freehand technique, sections of animal tissues are obtained by fixing a specimen with cyanoacrylate glue to either a glass slide or a cellulose acetate sheet, and then shaving it off with an inclined razor blade (Troyer *et al.*, 2002; Dobkin and Troyer, 2003). When sections of human or animal tissues are needed in a hurry, **frozen sections** are commonly used. A traditional **freezing microtome** is used for fixed material, especially when rather thick sections are needed. The **cryostat**, a microtome mounted in a freezing cabinet, may be used for cutting thin (5–10 μm) sections of either fixed or unfixed tissue. The operation of a cryostat demands more skill than the use of a freezing microtome. Another advantage of cutting frozen sections, aside from speed, is the preservation of some lipid constituents, which are dissolved out during the course of dehydration and embedding in paraffin or plastic. A **vibrating microtome** (Vibratome) can cut thick (50–100 μm) sections of unfixed, unfrozen specimens. The blade of this instrument passes with a sawing motion through a block of tissue immersed in an isotonic saline solution. The cutting process is much slower than with other types of microtome, so it is not feasible to prepare large numbers of sections. Vibratome sections of fixed material are similar to thick frozen sections, but they do not contain holes or other artifacts associated with ice crystal formation.

When the preservation of lipids or of heat-labile substances such as enzymes is not important, the specimens are **dehydrated**, **cleared** (which means, in this context, equilibrated with a solvent that is miscible with paraffin), **infiltrated** with molten paraffin wax, and finally, **embedded** (blocked out) in solidified wax. **Paraffin sections** are most commonly cut on a rotary microtome, though a rocking microtome or a sledge microtome may also be used. The sections come off the knife in ribbons, and with sufficient skill it is possible to obtain serial sections as little as 4 μm thick through the whole block of tissue. **Polyester wax** (Steedman, 1960), which is miscible with 95% alcohol, is handled in much the same way as paraffin. Cutting is difficult, but the lower melting point (about 40°C, compared with 55–60°C for most paraffin waxes) is an advantage for some tissues and histochemical methods. Large specimens are embedded in **cellulose nitrate**; the material manufactured for the purpose is more commonly called **nitrocellulose**, **celloidin** or **low-viscosity nitrocellulose (LVN)**. Celloidin sections, 50–200 μm thick, are usually cut on a sledge microtome. Various **synthetic resins** (plastics) are also used as embedding media for light microscopy, though their main application is in the cutting of extremely thin sections for examination in the electron microscope. Resin-embedded tissue is usually sectioned with an ultramicrotome, using a glass or diamond knife. Sections 0.5–1.0 μm thick, suitably stained for optical examination, are valuable for comparison with the much thinner sections used in ultrastructural studies. The light microscope provides greater resolution of detail in plastic-embedded sections than in paraffin sections, but the latter are more easily stained in contrasting colours. Larger resin-embedded objects are sectioned with a heavy-duty paraffin microtome and a tungsten carbide knife.

The optical contrast in a thin specimen is determined partly by its intrinsic properties but largely by the way in which it is processed. If the specimen is not stained, contrast will be greatest when the mounting medium has a refractive index substantially different from that of the specimen. The visibility of a transparent specimen can be increased, at the expense of resolution, by defocusing the condenser of the microscope and by reducing the size of the substage diaphragm. Differences in refractile properties are emphasized in the **phase contrast** and the **differential interference contrast** (Nomarski) microscopes. These instruments are valuable for the study of living cells, such as those grown in tissue culture. With **video-enhanced contrast** otherwise inconspicuous features are enhanced by manipulation of electronically acquired images (see Shotton, 1993; Diaspro, 2002).

In **confocal microscopy**, the field is scanned, usually by a laser, to provide images of optical sections through thick specimens (see Diaspro, 2002; Hoppert, 2003). The images are derived from fluorescence or (less frequently) from reflected light. Optical sections are obtained by placing a pinhole in the light path between the objective and the detector. With a small enough pinhole, only the light emitted from an extremely thin layer within the specimen will reach the detector. With larger pinholes the thickness of the optical section increases. Images in different planes are recorded electronically, and synthesized to provide either three-dimensional pictures or flat pictures of selected objects that are too thick or tortuous to be seen in a single focal plane. Images from a confocal microscope are stored as files on a computer disk, and the contrast and other features can be manipulated prior to the production of a physical picture (see Wingate, 2002).

In histology, the natural refractility of a tissue is usually deliberately suppressed by the use of a **mounting medium** with a refractive index close to that of the anhydrous material constituting the section (approximately 1.53). Almost all the contrast is produced artificially by **staining**.

Fluorescence is the property exhibited by substances that absorb light of short wavelength such as ultraviolet or blue and emit light of longer wavelength, such as green, yellow, or red. The phenomenon can be observed with a **fluorescence microscope** in which arrangements are made for the emitted (long wavelength) light to reach the eye while the exciting (short wavelength) light does not. Fluorescing materials therefore appear as bright objects on a dark background. The fluorescence microscope can be used to observe **autofluorescence** due to substances naturally present and **secondary fluorescence** produced by appropriate chemical treatment of the specimen. The fluorescence of living cells arises from mitochondria and lysosomes (Andersson *et al.*, 1998). Autofluorescence is due to

Table 1.1. Some methods for suppressing autofluorescence

Method	Reference
Before applying a fluorochrome or fluorescently labelled protein: Immerse slides in 0.2% aqueous osmium tetroxide for 5 min. Wash in gently running tap water for 2 h	Ornstein *et al.* (1957) Stoddart and Kiernan (1973)
Stain the sections with 0.05% Chicago blue 6B* in PBS with 1% DMSO for 15 min.	Cowen *et al.* (1985)
Expose the slides sections, mounted on slides, to a mixture of visible and near-UV light from a set of fluorescent tubes, for 12 to 48 h. The irradiation causes fading of the unwanted autofluorescence.	Neumann and Gabel (2002)
After carrying out a fluorescent immunohistochemical method: Stain the slides with Sudan black B (Section 12.5.4).	Schnell *et al.* (1999) Baschong *et al.* (2001)

* This dye (C.I. 24410, Direct blue 1) is also known as pontamine sky blue 6B and Niagara blue 6B. Benzo blue BB (see Section 5.9.4.8) is very similar to Chicago blue 6B. Either dye should reduce autofluorescence.

various endogenous compounds, including flavoproteins, lipofuscin pigment, and elastin. Fluorescent compounds are also formed in tissues by chemical reactions between some fixatives and proteins (Collins and Goldsmith, 1981). See Section 1.4 for a brief introduction to fixation, and Chapter 2 for more information. Fixative-induced secondary fluorescence is often called autofluorescence. Any intrinsic fluorescence of a tissue is likely to interfere with the interpretation of secondary fluorescence. Various physical and chemical treatments can be used to suppress unwanted autofluorescence and fixative-induced fluorescence before or even after applying fluorescent reagents to sections, smears or cell cultures (see Kiernan, 2002a). Some of these are summarized in *Table 1.1*. These tricks for suppressing autofluorescence work in different ways, and some can interfere with techniques used to generate desirable secondary fluorescence. The references in the table should be consulted before applying the treatments to sections or cells used for diagnosis or research.

1.2. Staining and histochemistry

The histologist stains sections in order to see structural details. The histochemist, on the other hand, seeks to determine the locations of known substances within the structural framework. The disciplines of histology and histochemistry overlap to a large extent, but one consequence of the two approaches is that the staining techniques used primarily for morphological purposes are sometimes poorly understood in chemical terms. It is desirable to demonstrate structural components by 'staining' for substances they are known to contain, but many valuable empirically derived histological techniques are not based on well understood chemical principles.

1.3. Some physical considerations

The intelligent handling of microscopical preparations requires familiarity with the physical properties of several materials that are used in almost all techniques. All too often, the beginner will ruin a beautifully stained section by forgetting that two solvents are immiscible, or by leaving the slides overnight in a liquid which dissolves the coloured product. The following remarks relate mainly to sections mounted on slides, but they apply also to blocks of tissue, smears, films, whole mounts, and free-floating sections.

Water is completely miscible with the common alcohols (methanol, ethanol, isopropanol, methylated ethyl alcohol). Water is immiscible with xylene, benzene, chloroform, and other non-polar solvents. These non-polar liquids, which are called **clearing agents**, are miscible with the alcohols in the absence of water. Melted paraffin wax and the resinous mounting media (Canada balsam, Xam, Permount, DPX, etc.) are miscible with the clearing agents but not with the alcohols or with water. One resinous mounting medium, euparal, is notable for being miscible with absolute alcohol as well as with xylene. Because of these properties of the common solvents, **a specimen must be passed through a series of liquids** during the course of embedding, staining, and mounting for examination.

For example, a piece of tissue removed from an aqueous fixative, such as a formaldehyde solution, must pass through a **dehydrating agent** (such as alcohol) and a **clearing agent** (such as chloroform) before it can be infiltrated with paraffin wax. Ribbons of paraffin sections are floated on warm water, which removes wrinkles, and mounted on glass slides. A thin layer of a suitable **adhesive** (Chapter 4) may be interposed between the slide and the sections, but this is not always necessary. The slides must then be **dried** thoroughly in warm air before being placed in a **clearing agent**, usually xylene, to dissolve and remove the wax. The slides now bear sections of tissue that are equilibrated with the clearing agent. Passage through **alcohol** (or any other solvent miscible with both xylene and water) must precede immersion of the slides in water. Sudden changes are avoided if possible, so a series of graded mixtures of alcohol with water is used. Most staining solutions and histochemical reagents are aqueous solutions. If a permanent mount in a resinous medium is required, the slides carrying the stained sections must be **dehydrated**, without unintentionally removing the stain, in alcohol or a similar solvent, **cleared** (usually in xylene), and, finally, **mounted** by applying the resinous medium and a coverslip.

Several **synthetic resins** are used as embedding media. In most procedures the specimen is first infiltrated with a mixture of monomer and a catalyst at room temperature, and then moved to an oven (60°C) to initiate polymerization. Most monomers are miscible with ethanol or other organic solvents. Some of the polymers are similarly soluble; others can only be removed from the sections by reagents that break covalent bonds in the matrix of resin.

Resinous mounting media contain clearing agents, so a newly mounted preparation does not become completely transparent for a few hours. The resin has to permeate the section and the solvent has to evaporate at the edges of the coverslip. When these events have taken place, the specimen will be equilibrated with the mounting medium and should have almost the same refractive index as the latter. Consequently, most of the observed contrast will be due to the staining method.

Frozen sections of fixed tissues are collected into water or an aqueous solution. They may be affixed to slides and dried in the air either before or after staining. The frozen section on the slide is, therefore, at first equilibrated with water and must be dehydrated and cleared before mounting in a resinous medium. **Cryostat sections** (fixed or unfixed tissue) are usually collected onto slides or coverslips from the microtome knife; they may then be rapidly thawed and air dried (can cause artifacts if unfixed) or immersed immediately in a fixative. If the products of a staining method would dissolve in organic solvents, as is the case with the Sudan dyes and with the end-products of some histochemical reactions, it is necessary to use a **water-miscible mounting medium**. Several such media are available (e.g. glycerol jelly, fructose syrup, Apathy's, Farrant's, polyvinylpyrrolidone), but they usually do not suppress the intrinsic refractility of the specimen as completely as do the non-polar resins.

Nitrocellulose sections require special handling owing to the properties of the embedding medium. Cellulose nitrate is soluble in a mixture of equal volumes of ethanol and diethyl ether, commonly called ether–alcohol. It also dissolves in absolute methanol and in cellosolve (2-ethoxyethanol). Nitrocellulose can be hardened by treating with 70% ethanol, chloroform, or phenol. Absolute ethanol makes this embedding medium swell, but does not dissolve it. Aqueous solutions can penetrate freely through a nitrocellulose matrix, so it is not necessary to remove the latter in before staining the contained section of tissue. Molten paraffin wax can also permeate nitrocellulose without dissolving it. Specimens that are expected to be difficult to section can be infiltrated with nitrocellulose, cleared, and then infiltrated with and embedded in wax. This procedure is known as **double embedding**.

Many of the dyes used in histology can be removed from stained sections by alcohol–water mixtures. This property is useful for the extraction of excess dye, a process known as **differentiation** or **destaining**, but it can also be a nuisance. A stained preparation must be completely dehydrated as well as adequately differentiated.

Consequently, the timing and rate of passage through graded alcohols is often critical. It is one of the arts of histological technique to obtain the correct degree of differentiation.

Consistency in the preparative procedure is necessary when objects are to be counted or measured in sections. The different fixatives and embedding media are associated with different amounts of shrinkage and with qualitative differences in the appearances of stained cells and their nuclei (Boon *et al.*, 1994).

1.4. Properties of tissues

Freshly removed cells and tissues, especially those of animals, are chemically and physically unstable. The treatments to which they are exposed in preparation for microscopy would damage them severely if they were not stabilized in some way. This stabilization is usually accomplished by **fixation**, which is discussed in Chapter 2. For some purposes, especially in enzyme histochemistry, it is necessary to use sections of unfixed tissues. As already stated, such sections may be cut with a cryostat or a vibrating microtome. Unfixed sections are stable when dried onto glass slides or coverslips but become labile again when wetted with aqueous liquids that do not produce fixation. Many histological staining methods do not work properly on unfixed tissues.

Most methods of fixation make the tissues harder than they were in the living state. Provided that it is not excessive, **hardening** is advantageous because it renders the tissues easier to cut into sections. However, some tissues such as bone are too hard to cut even before they have been fixed. These have to be softened after fixation but before dehydration, clearing, and embedding. Calcified tissues are softened by dissolving out the inorganic salts that make them hard, a procedure known as **decalcification** (Chapter 3). Other hard substances such as cartilage, chitin and wood require different treatments. Exceptionally robust microtomes, equipped with massive chisel-like tungsten carbide knives, are used to cut sections of undecalcified bones and teeth and other hard materials, including metal implants.

Even initially soft specimens sometimes become unduly hard by the time they are embedded in wax. These can be softened by cutting sections to expose the interior of the tissue at the face of the block and then immersing for a few hours in water. Although the solid wax is present in all the interstices of the tissue, materials such as collagen can still imbibe some water and be made much softer. Various proprietary 'softening agents' are marketed for the same purpose, but they are, in my experience, no better than plain water. Another important factor in microtomy is the hardness of the embedding mass relative to that of the tissue. This is determined by the composition of the former and by the ambient temperature. Obviously, the proper use of the microtome is also necessary if satisfactory sections are to be cut.

1.5. Books and journals

There is a profusion of books, large and small, that give directions in practical microtechnique. Some of the more modern ones also briefly explain the rationales of the different methods described. Bradbury (1973), Culling (1974), Humason (1979), Drury and Wallington (1980), Clark (1981), Bancroft and Cook (1984); Culling *et al.* (1985), Sanderson (1994), Carson (1997), Presnell and Schreibman (1997) and Bancroft and Gamble (2002) can all be recommended, but there are many others equally valuable. These books are concerned principally with human and other animal tissues. For botanical microtechnique, see Berlyn and Miksche (1976) and Ruzin (1999).

The works of Gatenby and Beams (1950) and Gray (1954) were comprehensive in their day, and they contain numerous older recipes and useful technical hints. James (1976) and Slayter and Slayter (1992) provide full accounts of the light microscope and its operation.

For histochemistry the major treatise is the three-volume work of Pearse (1980, 1985) and Pearse and Stoward (1991). Other important books are Barka and Anderson (1963), Ganter and Jollès (1969,1970; in French), Gabe (1976), Lillie and Fullmer (1976) and Sumner (1988). In these works it is usually assumed that the reader is familiar with the chemical principles underlying the explanations of how the methods work. Hayat (1993) presents detailed reviews of many modern preparative and histochemical histochemical techniques, for light and electron microscopy. The chemical and physical principles of microtechnique and histo-chemistry are discussed critically and at length by Baker (1958), Horobin (1982, 1988) and Lyon (1991).

Some journals are devoted largely to the publication of papers on methodology. The major ones are *Biotechnic and Histochemistry* (formerly *Stain Technology*), the *Journal of Histochemistry and Cytochemistry, Histochemistry and Cell Biology* (originally *Histochemie* and later *Histochemistry*), the *Journal of Molecular Histology* (formerly *Histochemical Journal*), *Acta Histochemica*, the *Journal of Histotechnology*, and the *Journal of Microscopy* (formerly *Journal of the Royal Microscopical Society*). Relevant papers appear in other journals too, but by scanning the ones listed above it is not difficult to keep up with the major advances in the field.

1.6. On carrying out instructions

THIS IS IMPORTANT. READ THIS SECTION BEFORE ATTEMPTING TO PERFORM ANY OF THE TECHNIQUES DESCRIBED IN LATER CHAPTERS. See also *'Conventions and abbreviations'* for methods used to express concentrations of solutions, for the correct interpretation of such terms as 'alcohol' and 'water', and for guidance on precision of measurement of weight, volume, and temperature.

In this and other texts, practical schedules are given for many techniques. The number of methods described in this book is relatively small, so it is possible to be quite explicit. The methods should all work properly if the instructions are followed exactly. There are, however, some general rules applicable to nearly all staining methods. These will therefore be given now, in order to avoid tedious repetition in the following chapters.

1.6.1.
De-waxing and hydration of paraffin sections

Place the slides (usually 8–12 of them) in a glass or stainless steel rack and immerse in a rectangular glass tank containing about 400 ml of xylene or another wax solvent. This is the most useful size of tank for most purposes. Smaller ones are available, but when they are used their contents must be renewed more often. A 'commercial' or 'technical' grade of xylene (mixed isomers) is satisfactory. Proprietary solvents are available as alternatives to xylene. They should never be used in research work unless the exact composition is revealed, which is not usually the case. Agitate the rack, up and down and laterally, three or four times over the course of 2–3 min. If for some reason it is inconvenient to agitate the slides, they should be left to stand in the xylene for at least 5 min. A single slide is de-waxed by moving it slowly back and forth in a tank of xylene for 1 min. Individual slides should be held with stainless steel forceps.

Lift the rack (or individual slide) out of the xylene, shake it four or five times and touch it onto bibulous paper (three or four thicknesses of paper towel, or filter paper) and place in a second tank of xylene. Agitate as described above, but this time 1 min is long enough. The purpose of this second bath of xylene is to remove the wax-laden xylene from the initial bath, thereby reducing the chance of precipitation of wax upon the sections when they are passed into alcohol, in which wax is insoluble. The removal of excess fluid by shaking and blotting is very important and must be done every time a rack or slide is passed from one tank to another. If it is not done, the useful life of each tank of xylene or alcohol will be greatly shortened. **The instruction 'drain slides' refers to this shaking-off of easily removed excess liquid.**

After the second bath of xylene, drain the rack of slides and place it in a tank containing about 400 ml of absolute ethyl, isopropyl or methyl alcohol. Agitate at intervals of 10–20 s for 30 s to 2 min. Drain the slides, transfer to 95% alcohol and agitate in this for about 1 min. Drain slides and transfer to 70% alcohol. Agitate for at least 1 min. For an individual slide, it is sufficient to move it about with forceps for about 20 s in each change of alcohol. If the slides have to be left for several hours, or even for a few days, they should be immersed in 70% alcohol. This will prevent the growth of fungi and bacteria on the sections but will not make them come off the slides or become unduly brittle. If some sections do detach from the slides during de-waxing or hydration, more will certainly be lost in later processing. If attachment of the sections appears to be precarious, a protective film of cellulose nitrate (nitrocellulose) should be applied, as described in Chapter 4.

Hydration of the sections is completed by lifting the rack (or individual slide) out of the 70% alcohol, draining it, and immersing in water. Agitation for at least 30 s is necessary for removal of the alcohol. Without agitation, this takes 2–3 min. A second rinse in water is desirable if all traces of alcohol are to be removed.

It is possible to use small volumes of xylene and alcohol by carrying out the above operations in coplin jars (which usually hold up to five slides) or rectangular staining dishes (for 10–12 slides). The xylenes and alcohols are poured into these vessels and the slides agitated continuously with forceps. To change the liquid, pour it out (without losing the slides) and replace it with the next one in the series. Working in this way, each lot of xylene or alcohol should be used only once. When tanks holding 400 ml are used, the liquids can be used repeatedly. They should all be renewed when traces of white sludge (precipitated wax) appear in the absolute ethanol. This commonly occurs after 10–12 racks of slides have been de-waxed and hydrated. In order to minimize evaporation, contamination by water vapour and the risk of fire, all tanks containing alcohol or xylene should have their lids on when not in use. Solvents should be used only in a well ventilated room, well away from any source of ignition.

**1.6.2.
Staining**

An instruction such as 'stain for 5 min' means that the sections must be in intimate contact with the dye solution for the length of time stated. Slides (alone, or in racks, coplin jars or staining dishes, as convenient) are immersed in the solution, agitated for about 10 s, and then left undisturbed. Free-floating frozen sections are transferred to cavity-blocks, watch-glasses, or the wells of a haemagglutination tray or an ice-cube tray containing the staining solution. Folds and creases in such sections must be straightened out if uniform penetration of the dye is to occur. The best instrument for handling frozen sections is a glass hook or 'hockey stick', fashioned by drawing out a piece of glass rod in the flame of a Bunsen burner. A glass hook is easier to keep clean than a paintbrush. Cryostat sections are collected onto slides or coverslips and are then handled in the same way as mounted, hydrated paraffin sections. Plastic-embedded sections are similarly treated; it is sometimes necessary to treat with a solvent to remove or permeabilize the resin. Nitrocellulose sections, if not affixed to slides, are manipulated in the same way as frozen sections.

In some techniques of enzyme histochemistry, immunocytochemistry and nucleic acid hybridization, only one drop of a scarce or costly reagent can be applied to each section. This is done with the slide lying horizontally. The slide bearing the section, covered by the drop, is placed on wet filter paper in a closed petri dish: the drop will not evaporate if the air above is saturated with water vapour. Special slides with slightly raised corners are available for applying small drops: with such slides, a coverslip is applied to the preparation, and a thin film of the reagent is present between the top of the section and the underside of the coverslip. Horizontal slides are also used in staining methods for blood films. In this case the reagents are not expensive, so the slides are placed, film upwards, on a pair of glass rods over a sink. The staining solution is poured on to flood the slides and later washed off by a stream of water or of a suitable buffer.

Sections of tissue take up only minute quantities of dyes and other substances, so there is no need for the volume of a staining solution or histochemical reagent to be any greater than that required to cover the sections. Exceptions to this general rule are rare and are mentioned in the instructions for the methods concerned.

1.6.3. Washing and rinsing

The excess of unbound dye or other reagent is removed from the stained sections by washing or rinsing, usually with water. A 'wash' is a more prolonged and vigorous treatment than a 'rinse'. Agitation of slides for 1 min or more in each of three changes of water constitutes an adequate wash. When tap water is suitable, the slides are placed for about 3 min in a tank through which the water is running quickly enough to produce obvious turbulence. A rack of slides should be lifted out of the running tap water and then replaced every 20–30 s in order to ensure that all the slides are thoroughly washed. A rinse, rather than a wash, is prescribed when excessive exposure to water would remove some of the dye specifically bound to the sections. Rinsing is done in the same way as washing, but the slides are agitated continuously and the total time of exposure to water is only about 15 s.

With unmounted sections, it is more difficult to control the process of washing. The sections are carried through three successive baths (50 ml beakers are convenient) of water and are kept in constant motion for 20–40 s in each. Free-floating sections should not be allowed to fold or to crumple into little balls. Stains that are easily extracted by water should not be applied to unmounted sections.

In some staining techniques, the washing or rinsing is called **differentiation** or destaining, and is a crucial part of the procedure. As a general rule, an acidic wash removes cationic dyes (Chapter 5) from tissues and prevents the loss of anionic dyes. A neutral or alkaline wash extracts anionic but not cationic dyes.

1.6.4. Dehydration and clearing

For stains or histochemical end-products insoluble in water and alcohol, dehydration is a simple matter. The slides are agitated continuously for about 1 min in each of the following: 70% alcohol, 95% alcohol; two changes of absolute ethanol, methanol, or isopropanol. There is no objection to taking them straight into 100% alcohol (in which case, three or four changes will be needed), but the use of lower alcohols will protect the more expensive anhydrous liquids from excessive contamination with water. **Slides must be drained** (Section 1.6.1) as they are transferred from one tank to the next. Clearing is accomplished by passing the slides from absolute alcohol into xylene (two changes, 1 min with agitation in each). They may remain in the last change of xylene for several days if mounting in a resinous medium cannot be carried out immediately. Used as described, the alcohols and xylenes, in 400 ml tanks, can be used repeatedly for about 12 racks of slides. The contents of all the tanks must be renewed when the first xylene becomes faintly turbid.

Many dyes are extracted by alcohol, especially if water is also present. When this is the case, and the intention is not to differentiate the stain, the instruction will be to 'dehydrate rapidly'. For **rapid dehydration**, drain off as much water as possible and then transfer the slides directly to absolute alcohol. Agitate very vigorously for 5–10 s in each of three tanks of this liquid, draining between changes, and then clear in xylene as described above. The alcohol used for rapid dehydration should be renewed after processing five racks of slides. It is not possible to dehydrate free-floating sections rapidly. These should be mounted onto slides after washing, allowed to dry in the air, and then passed quickly through absolute alcohol into xylene.

Instead of dehydrating rapidly in alcohol, slides bearing stained sections may be washed in water and then allowed to dry by evaporation (at least 2 h, preferably overnight) and then moved into xylene. Air-dried sections that have not been cleared or mounted are sometimes used for fluorescence microscopy but are not suitable for examination in ordinary transmitted light. Do not apply a non-aqueous mounting directly to an air-dried slide without first using a clearing agent; trapped air will appear as black, granular dirt that conceals the structure of the section.

1.6.5.
Staining through paraffin: an irrational method

The preceding paragraphs have emphasized the importance of passing specimens and sections only between mutually miscible liquids. It is sometimes possible and even advantageous to break this golden rule. Hydrophobic embedding media do not enter all the components of an infiltrated tissue, and aqueous reagents can penetrate from the cut surface of a section, especially through widely distributed hydrophilic substances such as cellulose in plant (Bronner, 1975) and collagen in animal (Horobin and Tomlinson, 1976) tissues. Useful staining of sections can consequently be obtained if dyes are applied before removing the wax from sections (Sakai, 1973; Graham and Joshi, 1995, 1996). The only use of a solvent other than water is to remove the wax from the air-dried stained sections before coverslipping.

If staining in the presence of paraffin is to succeed, the wax must not have been melted or even softened by heat after mounting the sections on the slide, and not surprisingly the staining times are longer than for sections that have been conventionally dewaxed and hydrated (Kiernan, 1996b). With some plant tissues there is improved structural preservation of the sections if the paraffin is not removed before staining (Graham and Joshi, 1995, 1996; Xi and Burnett, 1997). Staining through paraffin saves solvents and labour but not time. Not all staining methods will work in the presence of wax; in particular, it is not possible to obtain the expected colours from some mixtures of dyes that penetrate the tissue at different rates (Kiernan, 1996; see also Chapter 8).

1.6.6.
Mechanization

All the technical instructions in this book are for manual processing of tissue blocks and staining of sections. In busy laboratories, however, programmable machines are used for these tasks, especially when large numbers of slides are to be stained by a routine method such as haemalum and eosin (Chapter 6). Some suitable schedules for mechanized processing and staining are given by Carson (1997) and Allison (2002).

1.7. Whole mounts and free cells

Thin specimens of epithelium can be obtained by pressing the surface of an organ on a gelatin-coated slide and carefully peeling it off. The separation of an epithelium from its underlying connective tissue may be enhanced by first soaking the fresh material in a solution of a proteolytic enzyme (collagenase, trypsin), or in other reagents including EDTA and dithiothreitol (Epstein *et al.*, 1979). If a cut surface of an organ is placed against a slide, it leaves an **impression smear** consisting of detached cells. This old technique is occasionally used as a quick alternative to cutting a section (Matyas *et al.*, 1995), but only crude micro-anatomical detail is retained in such preparations. Impressions can be useful when staining for the presence of intracellular bacteria or viral inclusion bodies; for this purpose it is not necessary to preserve the architecture of the tissue.

The isolation of dead cells without changing their shapes is called **maceration**. Tissues can be macerated by any of a variety of methods, including:

(a) Prolonged immersion in a dilute solution of any fixative agent that does not form covalent chemical bonds with proteins.

(b) The method of Goodrich (1942). In this, the forces that hold the cells to their basal lamina and to one another are reduced by soaking in boric acid, which probably works by combining with the carbohydrates of the outside surfaces of cells, displacing calcium and other ions that are involved in intercellular adhesion (Williams and Atalla, 1981). Goodrich's medium for maceration also contains iodine, which kills the cells and preserves their shapes, but does not cause chemical cross-linking. Boric acid fails to loosen cells if the tissue has been fixed in glutaraldehyde (Chapter 2), which stabilizes the structure by forming strong bonds between protein molecules (Vial and Porter, 1975).

(c) Storing fragments of tissue at −70°C in ethylene glycol and pushing them through a fine sieve (Sinicropi *et al.*, 1989).

(d) Placing fixed specimens in acetone in an ultrasonic glassware cleaner (Low and McClugage, 1994).

(e) Incubation of freshly removed fragments in calcium- and magnesium-free buffered saline containing a proteolytic enzyme such as trypsin or collagenase. This is not maceration because it releases living cells, which can be cultured. Their original shapes are not maintained: dissociated cells usually assume spherical forms in suspension and a variety of unnatural shapes when growing on a flat surface, though cilia and other appendages may persist (Kleene and Gesteland, 1983). Suspensions of living cells may be deposited on slides and then fixed and stained (Chapter 7).

1.8. Understanding the methods

There is a reason for everything that is done in making a microscopical preparation. Before trying out a technique for the first time, the student should read about and understand the underlying physics and chemistry. He should then read through all the practical instructions and make sure that he understands the purpose of every stage of the procedure.

Some technical methods can be learned only by practice. These include cutting sections, mounting sections onto slides, and applying coverslips to sections. In this book, no attempt is made to teach these skills, which must be acquired under the guidance of more experienced colleagues. There are excellent descriptions of these procedures in Krajian and Gradwohl (1952), Gray (1954), Berlyn and Miksche (1976), Gabe (1976), Brown (1978), Culling *et al.* (1985), Sanderson (1994), Carson (1997), Bancroft and Gamble (2002) and many other books, but there is no substitute for practice in the laboratory. Success in microtechnique requires the integration of craftsmanship with intelligent appreciation of scientific principles.

2 | Fixation

It is not sufficient for the histologist that a specimen be transparent and that it possess adequate optical contrast. The cells and extracellular materials must be preserved in such a way that there has been as little alteration as possible to the structure and chemical composition of the living tissue. Such preservation is the object of fixation. Without being spatially displaced, the structural proteins and other constituents of the tissue must be rendered insoluble in all the reagents to which they will subsequently be exposed. 'Perfect' fixation is, of course, theoretically and practically impossible to attain. Biological material may be fixed in many ways and some of these are now discussed.

2.1. Physical methods of fixation

2.1.1.
Heat

The simplest physical method is the application of heat. This results in the coagulation of proteins and the melting of lipids. The resemblance to the living state is not very close after such treatment, but the method is often used in diagnostic microbiology. The shapes and staining properties of bacteria are preserved well enough to permit identification. Heating of large specimens can be accomplished by immersion in boiling saline (usually also containing formaldehyde), but nowadays it is usually done in a **microwave oven**. When microwave radiation is the sole fixative agent and the temperature is brought to about 80°C the stained sections contain deformed, shrunken nuclei and coarsely coagulated cytoplasm (Bernhard, 1974). The current practice is to bring the temperature to 55°C with the specimen already immersed in a chemical fixative solution (see Kok and Boon, 1992; Lemire, 2000). Externally applied heat acts first on the superficial layers of an object, but heat delivered by microwaves is absorbed by water and lipids at all depths within a specimen. Microwaves can accelerate some chemical reactions to a greater degree than externally applied heat if the radiation is selectively absorbed by the reacting molecules (Hayes, 2002). All the effects of microwave radiation on tissue fixation are attributable to heating (Feirabend et al., 1993; Ruijgrok et al., 1993), which promotes diffusion of fixative into the block and, in the case of formaldehyde solutions, accelerates the chemical reactions of cross-linking of proteins (Hopwood et al., 1988). For example, Kahveci et al. (1997) obtained in less than 20 min fixation superior to that obtained after 48 h in formaldehyde at room temperature.

Before using it in a histology laboratory a domestic microwave oven must be carefully tested and standardized, because (a) the spatial distribution of energy varies from one oven to another, and (b) there is a short delay, also variable, between switching on and the delivery of the microwave radiation. Objects to be fixed are placed in a square or rectangular container, always in the same place, on the floor of the oven. They are irradiated until the temperature of the fluid is 55°C. (A round container is unsuitable because internal reflection concentrates the microwaves at its centre, which is then heated excessively.) These considerations also apply to other uses of microwave ovens, such as acceleration of staining (Leonard and Shepardson, 1994; Churukian, 1997) and treatments applied to sections to unmask antigens (Chapter 19). Special microwave ovens for laboratory use are available. These provide for precise control of the irradiation of specimens, but they are very expensive. For more information about microwave-assisted fixation, see Boon (1990), Kok and Boon (1992), Login and Dvorak (1993) and Schichnes *et al.* (2005).

2.1.2. **Freezing**

Animal tissues are sometimes processed by the techniques known as freeze-drying and freeze-substitution, though only the former is purely physical in nature.

A specimen must be frozen in such a way as to minimize the formation of ice crystals, which can replace the architecture of any tissue with a meaningless array of cell-sized holes. This artifact is usually seen in large specimens that have been frozen slowly. In preparation for freeze-drying, freeze-substitution or the cutting of sections with a cryostat, the piece of tissue, which should be no more than 2 mm thick, is either frozen as quickly as possible or cryoprotected prior to freezing more slowly. Suitable quick freezing techniques include (a) immersion in isopentane cooled to its freezing point (−170°C) by liquid nitrogen, and (b) placing on a metal block that has already been brought to the temperature of liquid nitrogen (−196°C), solid carbon dioxide (dry ice and acetone mixture, −75°C) or even liquid helium (−268°C). For more information on rapid freezing techniques, see Pearse (1980), Bald (1983) and Lemke *et al.* (1994).

It is often not feasible to obtain ideal conditions for rapid freezing, but damage due to ice can be greatly reduced by **cryoprotection**, in which the specimen is first equilibrated with a solution of a cryoprotective compound in physiological saline or buffer. Suitable cryoprotective agents are dimethylsulphoxide (DMSO), glycerol, propylene glycol and sucrose, at 10–20% concentrations (see Terracio and Schwabe, 1981). DMSO is the best understood agent for cryoprotection (Ashwood-Smith, 1971), but the way in which it works is still not properly understood (see Pearse, 1980). Sucrose is the cryoprotectant most commonly used for fixed tissues. It is usually used as a 15–30% solution in water or a neutral buffer, but electron microscope and X-ray diffraction studies indicate that the concentration should be at least 60% to prevent ice crystal formation (Lepault *et al.*, 1997). Gum–sucrose, an aqueous solution of sucrose (30%) and gum acacia (1%) was introduced by Holt *et al.* (1960) to improve the retention of enzymes prior to cutting frozen sections; since about 1970 it has been usual to omit the gum. Cryoprotection with 15% propylene glycol in sea water was recommended by Campbell *et al.* (1991) prior to freeze-substitution of marine invertebrate embryos in ethanol. Pieces of fixed tissue are stored in a cryoprotective solution for at least 12 h, at 4°C, before freezing.

For **freeze-drying**, the frozen specimen is transferred to an evacuated chamber and maintained at about −40°C until all the ice has sublimed and has been condensed in a vapour trap maintained at an even lower temperature. Alternatively, the water vapour may be absorbed into phosphorus pentoxide. A freeze-dried specimen may be infiltrated with paraffin wax and sectioned in the usual way, but the sections cannot be flattened on water. Freeze-drying does not insolubilize proteins, so it is not, strictly speaking, a method of fixation. Indeed, proteolytic enzymes remain active in unfixed freeze-dried tissue (Mori *et al.*, 1992) and can cause structural deterioration in sections (Goodwin and Grizzle, 1994). However, water-soluble substances of low molecular weight are not lost. A freeze-dried block may be treated with gaseous formaldehyde, thus combining the advantages of freeze-drying and chemical cross-linking of proteins.

In **freeze-substitution** the frozen specimen is dehydrated by leaving it in a liquid dehydrating agent, usually ethanol or acetone, at a temperature below −49°C. The physics of the process have been reviewed by Hippe-Sanwald (1993). The organic liquid dissolves the ice but does not, at the low temperature, coagulate proteins. When dehydration is complete, the temperature is raised to 4°C for a few hours, to allow coagulant fixation by the alcohol or acetone to take place. The block is then cleared and embedded in paraffin. Alternatively, *n*-butanol, which is miscible with wax, can be used for simultaneous freeze-substitution and clearing. Sections prepared by the latter method are preferred to cryostat sections for some techniques of enzyme histochemistry (Klaushofer and von Mayersbach, 1979).

2.2. Chemical methods of fixation

Liquid fixatives are used for most histological and histochemical purposes. These substances affect the tissues both physically and chemically. The principal physical changes produced are shrinkage or swelling, and many of the fixatives in common use are mixtures of different agents, formulated to balance these two undesirable effects. Most fixatives harden tissues. Moderate hardening is desirable for sectioning with a freezing microtome, or if embedding is to be in cellulose nitrate or plastic, but it can lead to difficulty in cutting wax-embedded material. Dehydration and infiltration with paraffin always produce some further shrinkage and hardening, whatever the state of the tissue when it came out of the fixative. The volume of a fixed, paraffin-embedded specimen is commonly 60–70% of what it was in life. Another important property of a chemical fixative is its rate of penetration. This rate determines the duration of fixation and the maximum permissible size of the specimen. These physical aspects of fixatives are reviewed by Baker (1958). Many chemical reactions are involved in fixation, and some of these will now be described. The chemistry of fixation has been reviewed by Baker (1958), Pearse (1980), Hayat (1981), Horobin (1982), Bullock (1984) and Lyon (1991).

2.3. General properties of fixatives

The structure of an animal tissue is determined largely by the configuration of its contained proteins. The main contributors to structure are the **lipoproteins**, which are major components of the plasmalemmae and membranous organelles of cells, **cytoskeletal fibrous proteins**, the **fibrous glycoproteins** of such extracellular elements as collagen and basement membranes, and the **globular proteins**, which are dissolved in the cytoplasm and extracellular fluid. In some tissues, extracellular **mucosubstances** (e.g. chondroitin sulphates) also contribute substantially to the local architecture. Plant tissues are held together by the **cellulose** and other carbohydrates of the cell walls. All these substances must be stabilized by fixation. The nucleic acids and their associated nucleoproteins should also be preserved, as should the macromolecular carbohydrates (mucosubstances: comprising glycoproteins, proteoglycans, and at least one polysaccharide, glycogen) and, if their histochemical demonstration is required, the lipids. Fortunately, most fixatives render insoluble the proteins, nucleic acids and mucosubstances, though some may be more completely preserved than others by particular agents. Many fixatives do not directly affect lipids, whose preservation depends largely on the avoidance of agents that dissolve them.

**2.3.1.
Physical
considerations**

The **rate of penetration** will dictate the maximum size of a block to be fixed by immersion. Rapidly penetrating fixatives will usually fix in 24 h a specimen whose smallest dimension is 5 mm. For slowly penetrating fixatives the thickness of the block should not exceed 2 mm. The duration of fixation should not exceed 24 h except in the case of formaldehyde, which penetrates quickly but takes a week to cause full stabilization of histological structure. There are many circumstances, however, in which incomplete formaldehyde fixation is desirable. Distortion due to slow penetration can be offset by perfusion of the fixative through blood vessels or by injection into thin-walled cavities. **Shrinkage and swelling** are not necessarily detrimental to the quality of fixation, but must be allowed for in quantitative work. The overall change in size is easily determined by measuring appropriate dimensions of the fresh specimen and of the stained, mounted sections. It must not be assumed that all components of an organ or tissue will shrink or swell equally. Empty spaces due to unequal shrinkage of cells or larger regions of tissues are common artifacts, especially in paraffin sections. The consequences of **hardening** due to fixation have already been mentioned. When a specimen contains materials of widely varying hardness (e.g. glands and muscle), the embedding procedure should be chosen to suit the hardest component. For such specimens, either double-embedding or resin embedding (Chapter 4) is often preferable to simple paraffin processing.

**2.3.2.
Coagulants and
non-coagulants**

Fixatives that coagulate proteins can destroy or distort cytoplasmic organelles such as mitochondria, lysosomes and secretory granules, but they do not seriously disturb the supporting extracellular materials, which are already partly solid before being fixed. It is thought that coagulant fixatives produce a sponge-like proteinaceous reticulum that is easily permeated, after dehydration and clearing, by the large hydrophobic molecules of melted paraffin wax (Baker, 1958). Coagulant fixation usually allows easy sectioning of wax-embedded animal and plant tissue.

Non-coagulant fixatives act mainly by cross-linking the structural macromolecules of a tissue. Cross-linking of proteins converts the cytoplasm into an insoluble gel in which the organelles are well preserved. Such a gel may be less easily penetrated by paraffin than coagulated cytoplasm. In animal tissues, where the major structural macromolecules are proteins within and outside cells, artifactual shrinkage spaces and cracks are seen in paraffin sections of specimens fixed by non-coagulant agents. These artifacts result from different shrinkage of cellular and extracellular components of the fixed tissue, especially during passage through organic solvents and infiltration with molten wax (Leong, 1994). Embedding in cellulose nitrate or a synthetic resin causes less distortion within fixed tissues than does paraffin. These embedding media are discussed in Chapter 4.

Whether coagulant or non-coagulant, a fixative may also be designated as **additive** or **non-additive**. An additive fixative has molecules or ions that combine chemically with proteins, cellulose or other structural macromolecules. All cross-linking fixatives are additive, as are some coagulants. A non-additive fixative such as alcohol or acetic acid causes changes in the tissue but is removed by washing or other later procedures.

Many fixative mixtures contain both coagulant and non-coagulant compounds and combine the advantages of both. For light microscopy it is necessary to settle for either a mixture that gives adequate cytoplasmic fixation (due mainly to non-coagulant insolubilization of protein) or one that provides superior structural preservation on a larger scale (for which coagulation is necessary). In electron microscopy the cytoplasmic disruption due to coagulant fixation is unacceptable, and non-coagulant agents must be used. Fortunately the plastics used as embedding media for electron microscopy cause much less distortion of the delicate architecture of tissues than does paraffin wax. The latter is still needed, however, for the larger specimens examined with the light microscope.

The nuclei of cells are deliberately stained in most histological preparations, especially of animal tissue. A fixative mixture should therefore contain a substance that either coagulates the chromatin or renders it resistant to extraction by water and other solvents (see *Table 2.1*). Sharply defined interphase nuclei, with patterns of darkly stained chromatin characteristic of each cell type, are considered desirable for most purposes, but it should be remembered that their appearances are artifacts of coagulant fixation. The chromosomes of dividing cells are likewise shown to best advantage after fixation in agents that coagulate nucleoproteins and nucleic acids. The mitotic chromosomes become shorter and thicker than in life, and features such as centromeres and transverse banding patterns are exaggerated.

Most fixatives do not react chemically with macromolecular carbohydrates and lipids, though these substances are often protected from extraction as a consequence of the insolubilization of associated proteins.

2.3.3.
Effects on staining

Another important consideration is the effect of fixation on the subsequent reactivity of the tissues with dyes or histochemical reagents. For example, a glance at *Table 2.1* will show that osmium tetroxide should not be used to fix specimens intended for the staining of tissues with anionic (acid) dyes. The fixatives that interfere with staining are those that react chemically with the amino or carboxyl groups of proteins.

2.4. Individual fixative agents

2.4.1.
Simple organic coagulants

This group includes liquids such as **acetone**, **ethanol**, and **methanol** that displace water from proteinaceous materials, thereby breaking hydrogen bonds and disturbing the tertiary structure of proteins and other macromolecules. Soluble proteins of cytoplasm are coagulated and made insoluble in water (denatured). Membrane-bound organelles such as mitochondria are destroyed. Nucleic acids are not precipitated, but they are not extracted from the tissue because they remain closely associated with proteins. At low temperatures (below −5°C) ethanol precipitates many proteins without causing them to become permanently insoluble in water. Precipitated protein that has not been denatured retains enzymatic and other biological properties, and remains soluble in water. Alcohols, acetone, and other such solvents extract much lipid from tissues (Schwarz and Futerman, 1997). Carbohydrate-containing components, however, are largely unaffected. Ethanol and methanol make hepatic glycogen insoluble, but acetone does not do this.

Advantages are claimed for methanol over ethanol in non-aqueous fixatives. The former causes less hardening of animal tissues than the latter, and may provide superior preservation of both cellular integrity (Puchtler *et al.*, 1970) and antigenic determinants (Zbaeren *et al.*, 2004). The differences may be due to methanol being a more polar (less hydrophobic) liquid than ethanol. Alcohols act properly as fixatives only when very little water is present; objects must be immersed in a large (20×) excess of the fixative, and must then be transferred to 100% alcohol. Exposure to more than about 10% water during or after fixation results in excessive shrinkage and hardening of the tissue during subsequent processing and infiltration with paraffin (Puchtler *et al.*, 1968, 1970).

Trichloroacetic acid (TCA; CCl_3COOH) is widely used by biochemists to precipitate proteins from solutions. The coagulation is probably due to electrostatic interaction of trichloroacetate anions with positively charged groups ($-NH_3^+$, etc.) of proteins. The highly non-polar Cl_3C- group enables the TCA molecule to penetrate into hydrophobic domains within proteins. The consequent combination of hydrophobic interaction and ionic attraction by the same ion is probably responsible for breaking the hydrogen bonds that hold the protein molecules in their normal conformations. TCA extracts nucleic acids, but only at higher concentrations and temperatures than those used in histological fixation (Chapter 9).

Methanol, ethanol and acetone are used alone for fixing films, smears of cells, and previously unfixed cryostat sections. They are not suitable for blocks of animal tissue (unless very small) because they cause considerable shrinkage and hardening. Brief fixation below 5°C is compatible with some techniques of enzyme histochemistry (Chapter 14), because some proteins are precipitated without being denatured. TCA is a component of fixative mixtures, but is seldom used alone. Simple coagulants distort protein molecules without changing the sequences of their amino acids. Short antigenic sequences (epitopes) that are normally buried in the interior of large protein molecules can thereby be made more accessible to large antibody molecules, which are the reagents used in immunohistochemical methods (Chapter 19). Plant specimens may be fixed in 50–70% alcohol for anatomical study, which requires preservation principally of the cell walls.

2.4.2. Mercuric chloride

Solutions of mercuric chloride contain molecules Cl–Hg–Cl and hardly any free

$$HgCl_2 \ + \ H_2O \ \rightleftharpoons \ HO-Hg-Cl \ + \ H^+ \ + \ Cl^-$$

Hg^{2+} ions. With water there is slight formation of a hydroxo complex:
but this hydrolysis is reversed in acid solutions. In the presence of chloride ions, as

$$HgCl_2 \ + \ 2Cl^- \ \longrightarrow \ [HgCl_4]^{2-}$$

from added sodium chloride, a complex anion is produced:
The chemistry of fixation by mercuric chloride is poorly understood, but some inferences can be drawn from known reactions of the compound (see Whitmore, 1921;

$$HgCl_2 \ + \ 2NH_4^+ \ \rightleftharpoons \ Hg(NH_3)_2Cl_2(s) \ + \ 2H^+$$

McAuliffe, 1977). Thus, with ammonium salts or amines:
Similar mercury–nitrogen bonds are formed with amides and amino acids. Cross-linking of two nitrogens by mercury can also occur. Thus, addition of mercury and cross-linking may account for the insolubilization of proteins by mercuric chloride. However, the carbon–nitrogen bonds are unstable in the presence of halide ions:

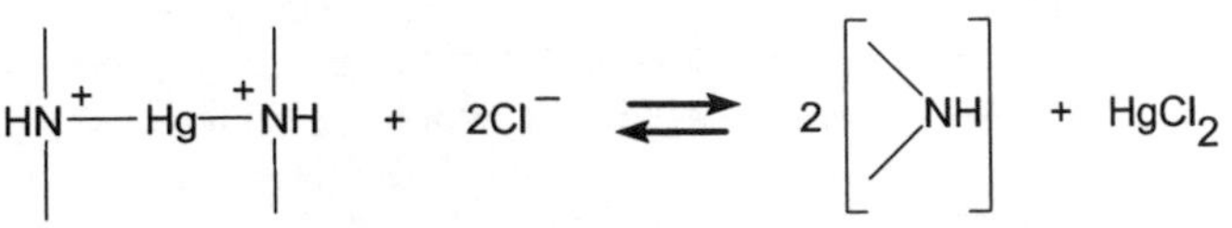

Acids or thiosulphate ions have effects similar to that of halide.

Bonds much more stable than those to nitrogen are formed with the sulphydryl group of cysteine:

$$HgCl_2 + HS\text{—}\boxed{PROTEIN} \longrightarrow Cl\text{—}Hg\text{—}S\text{—}\boxed{PROTEIN} + H^+ + Cl^-$$

This reaction certainly occurs during fixation, but its significance in stabilizing structure is not known. Mercury adds to unsaturated linkages of lipids, but this addition is probably not important in fixation, except in relation to the plasmal reaction (Chapter 12).

Fixative mixtures containing mercuric chloride provide excellent structural stabilization of animal cells and extracellular structures because the protein coagulation is on a scale too small to be visible by light microscopy. Mercuric chloride is also notable for enhancing the brightness of subsequent staining with dyes; the reason for this is not known. A crystalline precipitate (of uncertain chemical composition but probably mostly mercurous chloride, Hg_2Cl_2) forms within mercury-fixed tissues and must be removed, before the sections are stained, by treatment with a solution of iodine followed by sodium thiosulphate (Chapter 4). Another important practical point is that $HgCl_2$ penetrates rapidly through the tissue and causes hardening. The latter effect becomes excessive if the time of fixation is unduly prolonged.

In old texts of histological technique, $HgCl_2$ is usually called 'corrosive sublimate' or simply 'sublimate'. It is a very poisonous substance, and for this reason its use in laboratories is often avoided.

2.4.3.
Zinc salts

Zinc chloride was first used in a fixative more than a century ago. Fish (1895) recommended an aqueous solution containing 0.7% $ZnCl_2$, 4.9% NaCl and 0.1% formaldehyde. The fixative action of the zinc ion due to protein coagulation, recalling the traditional therapeutic use of zinc salts as astringents and antiseptics. Zinc salts have become popular in more recent years, sometimes as the sole active ingredient (Beckstead, 1994, zinc chloride and acetate) but more often in formaldehyde-containing mixtures similar to that of Fish. Zinc sulphate, which forms less acidic solutions than the chloride, is probably the salt of choice (Dapson, 1993). Zinc–formaldehyde mixtures are claimed to give adequate structural preservation and affinity for stains, while preserving the antigenic properties of tissue components. Masking of antigenic determinants, which commonly occurs with formaldehyde as the sole fixative agent, is not usually seen after fixatives that contain zinc salts or other coagulants (Mugnaini and Dahl, 1983; Dapson, 1993; Lynn et al., 1994; Arnold et al., 1996). Beckstead's fixative, with zinc ions as the only active ingredient, has become popular for immunohistochemistry (Hicks et al., 2006). It produces more shrinkage, especially of cytoplasm, than formaldehyde-based fixatives.

Zinc salts are cheaper and less toxic than mercury compounds, and $ZnCl_2$ has been substituted for $HgCl_2$ in mixtures such as Zenker's fluid (Barszcz, 1976; Churukian et al., 2000). The fixative action of zinc is attributed by Dapson (1993) to the formation of coordinate bonds to amino acid side-chains and to nucleic acids, perhaps stabilizing the folded states of these macromolecules before they react with the formaldehyde also present in the fixing solution.

Zinc sulphate is insoluble in alcohol; the acetate and chloride are somewhat and very alcohol-soluble respectively. Zinc-fixed specimens must not be transferred into a phosphate-buffered solution because zinc phosphate is insoluble. Water or 50% alcohol should be used to wash out excess fixative.

2.4.4.
Picric acid

Picric acid is trinitrophenol. It is a much stronger acid than unsubstituted phenol in aqueous solution, owing to the electron-withdrawing effect of the three nitro groups on the hydroxyl group:

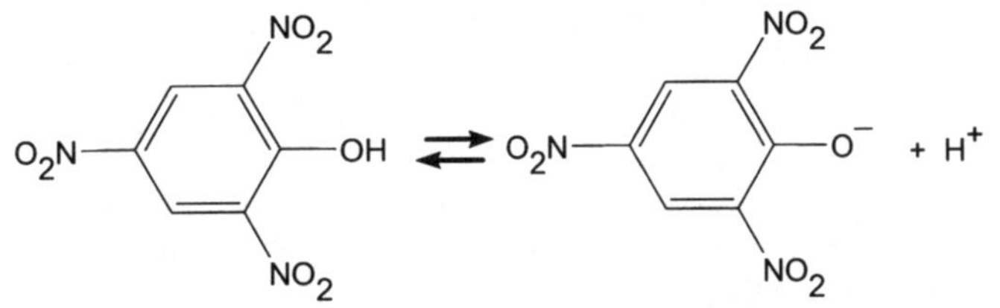

Trinitrophenol is a bright yellow solid, and is also used as a stain (Chapters 5 and 8). It is dangerously explosive when dry and is therefore stored under water. Stock bottles should be inspected from time to time and water added as necessary to give a layer about 2 cm deep on top of the powder.

A near-saturated aqueous solution of picric acid (pH 1.5–2.0) causes coagulation by forming salts (picrates) with the basic groups of proteins. Precipitation does not occur in a neutral solution, and neutralization allows precipitated proteins to redissolve. Tissues fixed in mixtures containing picric acid are usually transferred directly to 70% alcohol, supposedly to coagulate the precipitated protein. When other fixatives (e.g. formaldehyde) are mixed with picric acid, it is unlikely that any proteins in the fixed tissue are still soluble in water yet coagulable by alcohol.

The low pH of a picric acid solution brings about hydrolysis of nucleic acids. Fixatives containing picric acid are avoided for quantitative histochemical studies of DNA and RNA. (Fixation for several days at room temperature does not suppress the staining of these substances for qualitative purposes.) Blocks fixed in picric acid are passed through several changes of 70% alcohol to remove as much as possible of the yellow colour. According to Luna (1968), prolonged contact with picric acid, even in solid paraffin wax, may cause structural deterioration and poor staining. When tissues are sectioned less than a month after fixing, persistence of picric acid does not matter. It is easily washed out of the sections by a dilute (e.g. 0.13% = one-tenth of saturated) aqueous solution of lithium carbonate (Li_2CO_3).

Like mercuric chloride, picric acid in a fixative mixture predisposes the tissue to bright staining with dyes.

2.4.5.
Acetic acid

Acetic acid does not fix proteins, but it coagulates nucleic acids. The mechanism by which this change is brought about is obscure. Like the rapid penetration and production of swelling (*Table 2.1*), it is a property of the undissociated acid, and not of the acetate ion. These properties are shared by other carboxylic acids that are miscible with both water and oils (Zirkle, 1933). Acetic acid is included in fixative mixtures to preserve chromosomes, to precipitate the chromatin of interphase nuclei, and to oppose the shrinking actions of other agents such as ethanol and picric acid.

2.4.6.
Chromium compounds

The compounds of chromium used in fixation are chromium trioxide and potassium dichromate. These contain the metal in its highest oxidation state, +6 (see Cotton et al., 1999). Chromium trioxide dissolves in water to form the deep red-orange 'chromic acid', which is completely ionized. The anions are $HCrO_4^-$ (hydrogen chromate) and $Cr_2O_7^{2-}$ (dichromate):

$$CrO_3 + H_2O \longrightarrow H^+ + HCrO_4^-$$

$$2HCrO_4^- \longrightarrow Cr_2O_7^{2-} + H_2O$$

The position of the equilibrium of the second reaction is influenced by hydrogen ions, so that a high [H+] (low pH) favours the formation of $HCrO_4^-$ (red), whereas $Cr_2O_7^{2-}$ (orange) predominates in moderately acidic solutions. If a dichromate solution is made alkaline (low [H+], high [OH−], high pH) the yellow chromate ion is generated:

$$Cr_2O_7^{2-} + 2OH^- \longrightarrow 2CrO_4^{2-} + H_2O$$

The strength of these Cr(VI) anions as oxidizing agents varies inversely with the pH (Waters, 1958). Acidic solutions oxidize many organic compounds, with concomitant reduction of Cr(VI) to Cr(III). The latter occurs as the chromic (Cr^{3+}) cation.

Strongly acid (pH <3.5) solutions of chromium trioxide or potassium dichromate coagulate proteins and chromatin. A reticulated texture is produced in the cytoplasm, and the chromosomes of dividing cells are well preserved, as is the mitotic spindle. DNA is partly hydrolyzed by chromic acid so that it gives a positive reaction in histochemical tests for aldehydes. Any strong acid will do this to DNA; the reaction is discussed in Chapter 9.

A change in the fixative properties of the dichromate ion occurs when the pH is higher than 3.5. The less acid solutions insolubilize proteins without coagulation. Chromium is bound by proteins, DNA and RNA (Cupo and Wetterhahn, 1985; Wedrychowski et al., 1985). The proteins become insoluble, but nucleic acids do not (Table 2.1). Alkaline solutions containing Cr(VI) (chromates) are not used as fixatives.

The chemistry of fixation of proteins by dichromate is poorly understood. Zirkle (1928) and Casselman (1955) suggested that reduction of Cr(VI) by components of the tissue was followed by the formation of coordination compounds of Cr(III) with oxygen and nitrogen atoms of structural macromolecules. Similar reduction is a prerequisite of binding of chromium in cell nuclei (Kortenkamp et al., 1991). The chromic ion is notable for its ability to form six coordinate bonds with a great variety of ligands. The complexes are formed and broken much more slowly than are similar bonds with most other metals (Cotton et al., 1999). They have such forms as:

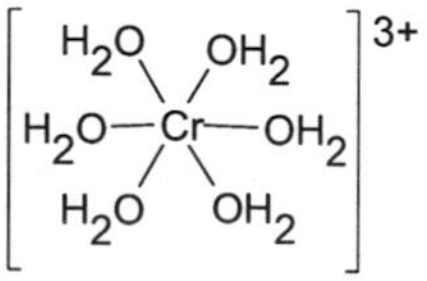

hydrated chromic ion

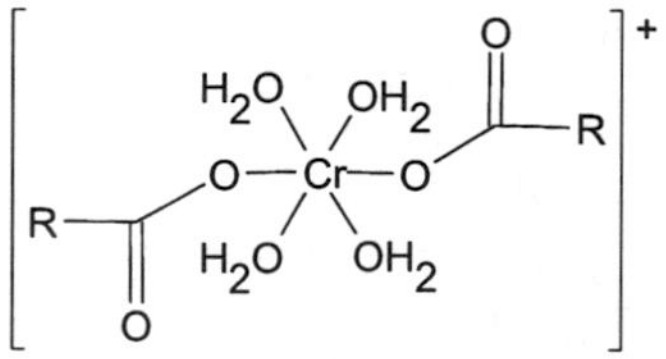

complex with two carboxylic acid anions and four water molecules

Chromic salts are used in chrome tanning (Gustavson, 1956), which is one of the industrial methods for conversion of collagen into leather, and in the hardening of gelatin for photographic emulsions (Burness and Pouradier, 1977; Pouradier, 1977). Gelatin is collagen that has been altered by prolonged boiling in water. Chrome-hardened gelatin is insoluble in water. Both processes are comparable to fixation, and it is known that the greatest numbers of coordinate bonds are formed between chromium atoms and the carboxyl groups of amino acids of collagen:

$$2 \;\boxed{\text{PROTEIN}} \!-\! \underset{\underset{O}{\|}}{C}\!-\!O^- \;+\; [Cr(H_2O)_6]^{3+} \longrightarrow$$

$$\boxed{\text{PROTEIN}} \!-\! \underset{\underset{O}{\|}}{C}\!-\!O\!-\!\underset{\underset{H_2O}{\overset{H_2O \;\; OH_2}{\big\backslash \!\!\!\overset{+}{}\!\!\!\big/}}}{Cr}\!-\!O\!-\!\underset{\underset{O}{\|}}{C}\!-\! \boxed{\text{PROTEIN}} \;+\; 2H_2O$$

The pH of a chrome tanning solution is critical, because excessive acidity inhibits the formation of Cr(III) complexes, whereas neutrality favours the formation of large ions in which water molecules are cross-linked through chromium. Macromolecular complex ions cannot permeate the collagenous matrix (Britton, 1956; Thorstensen, 1969; Heidemann, 1988).

It might be expected that chromic salts would have the same fixative properties as dichromates, but this is not so (Kiernan, 1985). Solutions of chromic sulphate or acetate are destructive to animal tissues, whatever the pH. However, chromic ions do contribute significantly to the properties of a few excellent fixative mixtures. I have suggested (Kiernan, 1985) that the formation of Cr(III) complexes occurs too slowly to be useful for primary fixation, but that cross-links are formed after primary stabilization by other agents such as formaldehyde. The protein–chromium–protein linkages protect the fixed tissue from further damage during the course of embedding in paraffin. Immersion of glutaraldehyde-fixed tissue in a solution containing chromic ions imparts increased electron opacity to membranes, cytoplasmic granules and various extracellular materials, and is helpful for examining the ultrastructure of bone, as an alternative to post-osmication (Liem and Jansen, 1984).

Oxidation by the dichromate ion is exploited in the chromaffin reaction, whereby catecholamines (adrenaline and noradrenaline) are transformed into brown compounds (Chapter 17). Gelatin can be hardened by oxidation in an alkaline medium (Tull, 1972), but there is no reason to believe that oxidation contributes to the fixation of tissues by chromium compounds. As well as fixing proteins, the dichromate ion can react with phospholipids in such a way as to make them insoluble in non-polar solvents (Chapter 12). This lipid-stabilizing action does not occur with the usual 1 or 2 days of fixation at room temperature.

Material fixed in dichromate must be washed for 12–48 h in running tap water before being transferred to the dehydrating alcohol, in order to avoid the reaction:

$$Cr_2O_7{}^{2-} + 3C_2H_5OH + 2H^+ \longrightarrow 2Cr(OH)_3(s) + 3CH_3CHO + H_2O$$

that would produce an insoluble green precipitate in the tissue. Potassium dichromate is used in mixtures such as Zenker's and Helly's fluids. The first of these contains enough acetic acid to cause the fixative action to be that of a strongly acid solution. Helly's fluid is less acid, and the dichromate in it acts as a non-coagulant fixative. Both these mixtures also contain mercuric chloride, which is a coagulant. Helly's fluid contains formaldehyde too, and is therefore unstable owing to the reaction:

$$Cr_2O_7{}^{2-} + 3HCHO + 2H^+ \longrightarrow 2Cr^{3+} + 3HCOO^- + 4H_2O$$

The reaction proceeds quite slowly, however, because $[H^+]$ in Helly's fluid is not very high. Both the dichromate and the formaldehyde have time to act upon the tissue before they are themselves respectively changed into chromic and formate ions.

2.4.7. Osmium tetroxide

This substance, sometimes wrongly called 'osmic acid', is a non-ionic solid, OsO_4, which is volatile at room temperature. The vapour is irritating and can cause corneal opacities. OsO_4 is soluble (without ionization) in water but much more soluble in non-polar organic solvents. It is somewhat unstable in solution, being reduced by traces of organic matter to the dioxide, $OsO_2.2H_2O$. This reduction is also brought about by alcohols, but not by carbonyl compounds such as formaldehyde, glutaraldehyde, and acetone, provided that these substances are pure. Osmium tetroxide is one of the oldest chemical fixatives, having been used for this purpose since 1865 (Maxwell, 1988).

OsO_4 is toxic, but it is not an environmental hazard because it is so quickly reduced (Smith *et al.*, 1978). However, it is wasteful to throw used solutions of this expensive substance down the sink. They should be stored and then chemically processed to recover the osmium (for methods, see Jacobs and Liggett, 1971 or Kiernan, 1978). Care is necessary when handling OsO_4 because the vapour from an aqueous solution is intensely irritating to the respiratory system and can also attack the cornea of the eye. According to Griffith (1967) there has been one fatal instance of human poisoning by osmium tetroxide; this was due to an accident in a factory and occurred over 100 years ago.

Although OsO_4 can react in the test-tube with proteins (especially sulphydryl groups) and carbohydrates (Bahr, 1954), it extracts quite large amounts of these substances from tissues during the course of fixation. Protein solutions are gelated but not coagulated by OsO_4, and some cross-linking occurs. The molecular size is increased, indicating cross-linking (Hopwood, 1969b) but the chemical reactions producing this change are not yet understood (Nielson and Griffith, 1979; Hopwood, 1996). The best understood fixative action is with the unsaturated linkages of lipids (see Adams *et al.*, 1967; Schroder, 1980). A cyclic ester is first formed, by addition:

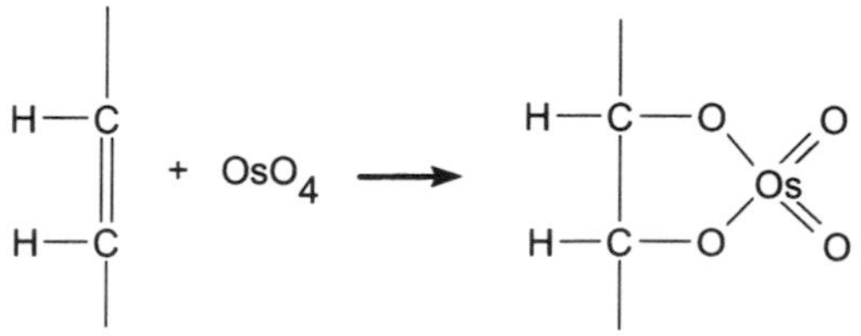

In this reaction, oxidation occurs at the carbon atoms (2 electrons lost), while the osmium is reduced, by gaining 2 electrons, so that its oxidation number changes from +8 to +6.

When two unsaturated linkages are suitably positioned they may be cross-linked (Wigglesworth, 1957). Chemical studies by Korn (1967) indicate that a diester is formed by the reaction:

$$\underset{\substack{HC \\ \| \\ HC}}{} \;+\; 2OsO_4 \;+\; \underset{\substack{HC \\ \| \\ HC}}{} \;\longrightarrow\; \underset{\substack{HC-O \qquad O-CH \\ \diagdown Os \diagup \\ HC-O \qquad O-CH}}{\overset{O \atop \|}{}} \;+\; OsO_3$$

The oxide OsO_3 is unstable and disproportionates:

$$2OsO_3 \;\longrightarrow\; OsO_2(s) \;+\; OsO_4$$

The osmium (VI) addition compounds and diesters are colourless or brown and may be soluble in organic solvents. The precipitated osmium dioxide is black and insoluble. Blackening of tissue fixed or stained with osmium tetroxide is increased in some circumstances with passage through alcohol, which may effect a reaction of the type:

$$\underset{\substack{H-C-O \\ \\ H-C-O}}{\overset{O \atop \diagup}{Os}\overset{O}{\diagdown}} \;+\; C_2H_5OH \;+\; 2H_2O \;\longrightarrow\; \underset{\substack{HC-OH \\ \\ HC-OH}}{} \;+\; OsO_2.2H_2O(s) \;+\; CH_3CHO$$

Any unreacted OsO_4 that has not been washed out of the tissue is similarly reduced:

$$OsO_4 \;+\; 2C_2H_5OH \;\longrightarrow\; OsO_2.2H_2O \;+\; 2CH_3CHO$$

Ordered arrays of lipid molecules are present predominantly in biological membranes, and OsO_4 is most valuable as a fixative for these structures, which are rendered insoluble, black and electron dense. Although individual membranes cannot be resolved with the light microscope, it is possible to see structures that are largely composed of membranous material, such as mitochondria and the myelin sheaths of nerve fibres. Solution of OsO_4 in non-polar substances, followed by its reduction, causes blackening of the contents of fat cells.

Treatment with OsO_4 largely abolishes the affinity of tissue proteins for anionic (acid) dyes, and normally acidophilic elements become stainable by cationic (basic) dyes. This change, which is in need of investigation, may be due to oxidation of terminal and side-chain amino groups of proteins with concomitant formation of carboxyl groups. By analogy with other oxidative deaminations the reaction would be expected to occur in three stages:

$$\boxed{PROTEIN}\underset{H_2}{-C-NH_2} \quad \overset{OsO_4}{\underset{oxidation}{\longrightarrow}} \quad \boxed{PROTEIN}\underset{H}{-C=NH}$$

$$\text{(acidophilic)} \qquad\qquad\qquad\qquad\qquad \text{unstable imine}$$

$$\boxed{PROTEIN}\underset{H}{-C=NH} \;+\; H_2O \quad \underset{hydrolysis}{\longrightarrow} \quad \boxed{PROTEIN}\underset{H}{-C=O} \;+\; NH_3$$

$$\boxed{PROTEIN}\underset{H}{-C=O} \quad \underset{oxidation}{\longrightarrow} \quad \boxed{PROTEIN}\underset{OH}{-C=O}$$

$$\text{(? by } OsO_4 \text{ or } O_2\text{)}$$

The product of reduction of OsO_4 is probably not $OsO_2.2H_2O$ because, if it were, proteins would be blackened. A soluble osmate, $[OsO_2(OH)_4]^{2-}$, or osmiamate, $[OsO_3N]^-$, may be the principal by-product of the reaction.

Osmium tetroxide penetrates blocks of tissue to a depth of only 0.5–1.0 mm, so its use as a fixative is limited to small blocks. By stabilizing membranes and gelating dissolved proteins, OsO_4 provides lifelike fixation of the internal structures of cells. The absence of morphological artifact has been demonstrated by microscopic observation of living cells during the course of fixation by OsO_4 (Strangeways and Canti, 1927; Policard, Bessis and Bricka, 1952). Unfortunately, however, pieces of osmium-fixed tissue have a crumbly consistency which is made worse by embedding in wax, and leads to the formation of cracks and shrinkage spaces. Osmium tetroxide may be used as a secondary fixative (**post-fixation**) after formaldehyde or glutaraldehyde, as in electron microscopy, and it may be used to stain frozen sections for unsaturated lipids. The vapour above an aqueous solution of OsO_4 is as effective as the solution itself, both as a fixative and as a stain. In several solutions for fixing and post-fixing specimens for electron microscopy, OsO_4 is mixed with other substances (see White *et al.*, 1979; Goldfischer *et al.*, 1981; Hayat, 1981; Emerman and Behrman, 1982; Carrapico *et al.*, 1984; De Bruijn *et al.*, 1984; Neiss, 1984; Scalet *et al.*, 1989), for the purposes of increasing electron-density and reducing the extraction of proteins. Apart from osmium-iodide mixtures (Chapter 18), such solutions are not used as fixatives for light microscopy.

Ruthenium tetroxide is chemically similar to but more reactive than osmium tetroxide (Griffith, 1967). It has little value as a primary fixative because the tissue disintegrates during subsequent processing (Bahr, 1954), but it has been included, with apparent advantage, as one ingredient of a post-osmicating fluid for glutaraldehyde-fixed skin (Vandenbergh *et al.*, 1997).

The uses of osmium tetroxide in the histochemical study of lipids are discussed in Chapter 12.

2.4.8. **Formaldehyde**	Formaldehyde is a gas (BP −21°C) with the structural formula:

It is sold as a solution (**formalin**) containing 37–40% by weight of the gas in water, and as a solid polymer, **paraformaldehyde**, which is $HO(CH_2O)_nH$, n being 6–100. Paraformaldehyde is also seen as the white precipitate that forms in old bottles of formalin. Old, milky solutions can be clarified by heating for 30 min in a Kilner jar in an autoclave (Cares, 1945), but this is seldom done because formalin is not expensive. Although formaldehyde is the simplest of the aldehydes, its chemistry is quite complicated (see Walker, 1964; Pearse, 1980; Fox *et al.*, 1985).

In aqueous solutions formaldehyde is present as methylene hydrate (methylene glycol), the product of the reaction:

$$H_2C{=}O \ + \ H_2O \ \rightleftharpoons \ HOCH_2OH$$

formaldehyde   methylene hydrate

The equilibrium lies far to the right, and hardly any true formaldehyde is present in the solution. It was formerly believed that in the presence of water methylene hydrate was the chemically reactive species (Walker, 1964). The reactions of fixation, which consist mainly of addition to proteins, are currently attributed to formaldehyde itself, which is continuously replenished from the large reserve of methylene hydrate in the solution. Formalin also contains soluble polymers of the form $HO(CH_2O)_nH$ (where $n = 2$–8), known as lower polyoxymethylene glycols. Continued addition of methylene hydrate molecules occurs spontaneously, and this is the reason for the precipitation of paraformaldehyde in formalin that has been stored for a long time. Formalin also contains methanol (about 10% v/v), which is added as a stabilizer to inhibit polymerization. Methanol does this by forming with formaldehyde a hemiacetal (methylal), which is more stable than methylene hydrate.

$$H_2C\!=\!O \;+\; HOCH_3 \longrightarrow H_2C\!\!\begin{array}{c} OH \\ \diagdown \\ O\!-\!CH_3 \end{array}$$

methylal

The polymers are hydrolyzed when formalin is diluted with an excess of water. Thus, for trioxymethylene, $HO(CH_2O)_3H$,

$$HO\!-\!\underset{H_2}{C}\!-\!O\!-\!\underset{H_2}{C}\!-\!O\!-\!\underset{H_2}{C}\!-\!OH \;+\; 2H_2O \longrightarrow 3\,HO\!-\!\underset{H_2}{C}\!-\!OH$$

trioxymethylene   methylene hydrate

The equilibrium is displaced to the right because of the high concentration of water, but the reaction is very slow (taking some weeks for completion) between pH 2 and 5, as in non-neutralized formalin. The depolymerization occurs quite rapidly, however, in neutral media. If formalin is to be used as a fixative in simple aqueous solution it should be diluted several days in advance, but when buffered to approximate neutrality it may be used immediately. Neutrality may also be achieved by keeping some marble chips (calcium carbonate) in the bottom of the bottle of diluted formalin.

Formalin deteriorates during storage as the result of a Cannizzaro reaction:

$$2HCHO \;+\; H_2O \longrightarrow CH_3OH \;+\; HCOOH$$

The pH of the solution falls, though very slowly, as more formic acid is produced (Fox et al., 1985). With other aldehydes, Cannizzaro reactions are significant only in alkaline media. Oxidation of formaldehyde by atmospheric oxygen (which would also generate formic acid) is exceedingly slow, and is not a significant cause of deterioration.

Formaldehyde solutions for use as fixatives are also made by depolymerizing paraformaldehyde. This substance dissolves very slowly in water but more quickly in near-neutral buffer solutions. A solution made in this way does not contain methanol or formic acid, and is often preferred to diluted formalin as a fixative for histochemistry and electron microscopy. Paraformaldehyde can also be depolymerized by heating. Small specimens, including those of freeze-dried tissues, are sometimes fixed by exposure to the vapour, which is gaseous formaldehyde, at 50–80°C.

The content of formaldehyde in a fixative is best denoted by stating the percentage by weight of the gas rather than the amount of formalin used in preparing the mixture. Thus, '4% formaldehyde' is preferred to '10% formalin' (for the same solution), though the latter designation is in common use. It is a common but incorrect practice to state that tissues were fixed in '4% paraformaldehyde'. The correct designation is '4% formaldehyde, from paraformaldehyde'. (The weight of formaldehyde may be assumed to equal the weight of the polymer used to prepare the solution.)

Formaldehyde reacts with several parts of protein molecules (see Walker, 1964; Hopwood, 1969a; Pearse, 1980, for more information). The formaldehyde molecule adds to many functional groups to form hemiacetals and related adducts. For example, with primary amines (N-terminal amino acids and lysine side-chains):

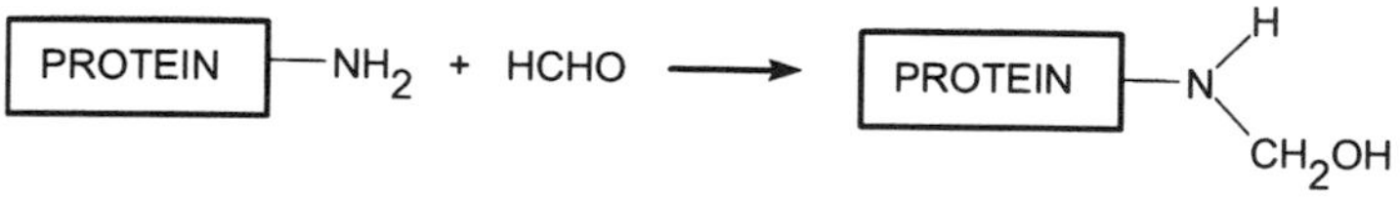

With guanidyl groups of arginine side-chains:

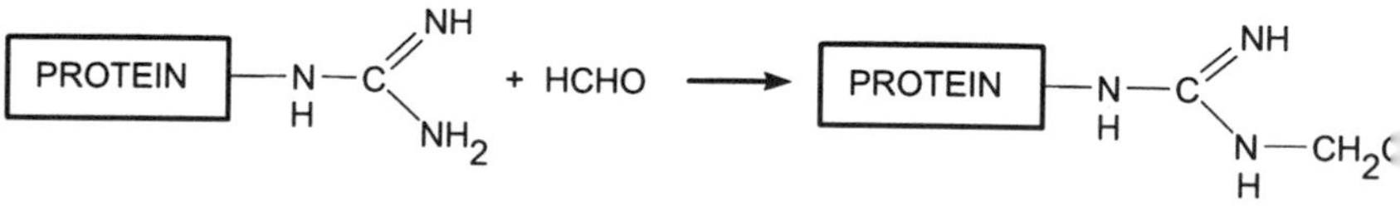

With sulphydryl groups of cysteine:

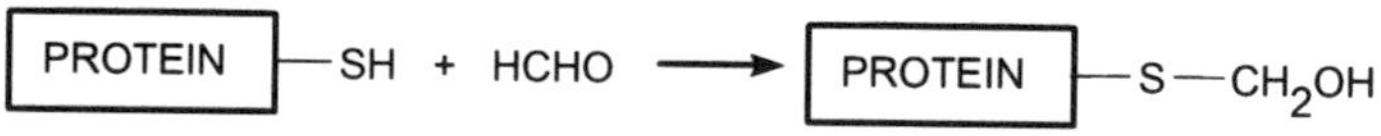

With aliphatic hydroxyl groups (serine, threonine):

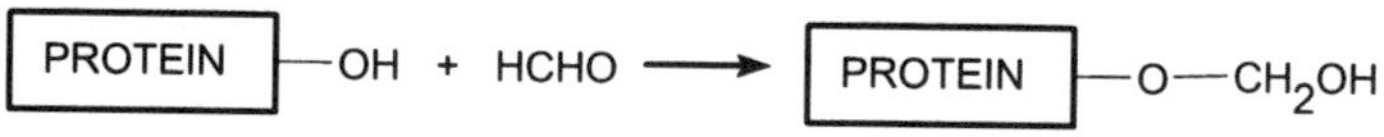

With amide nitrogen (at accessible peptide linkages):

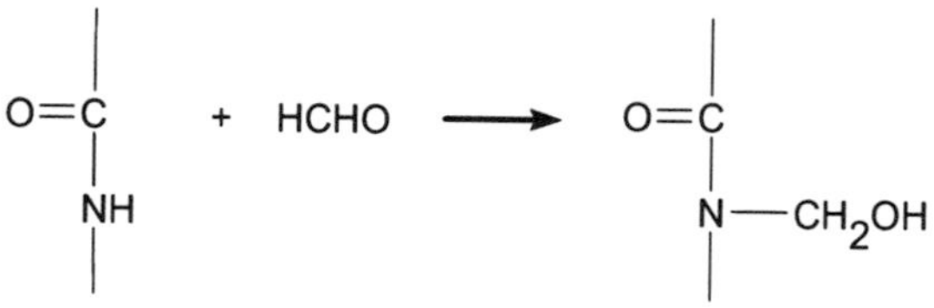

The simple addition of formaldehyde to $-NH_2$, $-NHC(NH)NH_2$, and $-SH$ groups of proteins inhibits many enzymes, thereby preventing autolysis, but does not structurally stabilize the tissue. Most of the added hydroxymethylene ($-CH_2OH$) groups are removed when an object briefly fixed in formaldehyde is washed for several hours in water or alcohol (Helander, 1994), with regeneration of the functional groups of the proteins. While they are bound to protein, however, the hydroxymethylene groups are capable of further reaction with suitably positioned functional groups on the same or other protein molecules:

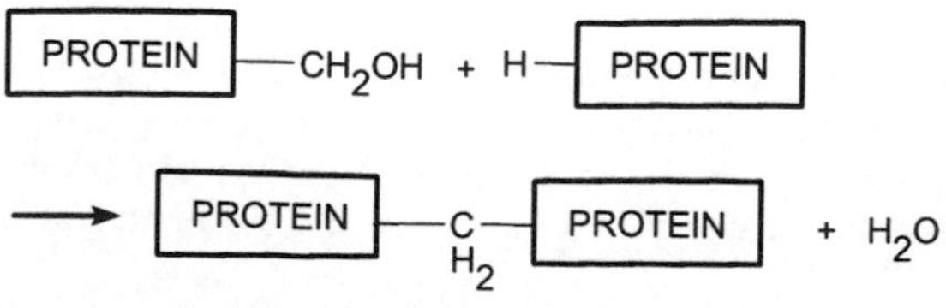

Thus, different protein molecules can be joined together by chemically stable methylene bridges. The secondary structures of polypeptide chains are also stabilized in proteins that have reacted with formaldehyde (Mason and O'Leary, 1991). Formaldehyde is used in the tanning of collagen to produce leather. Investigations of this industrial process (see Gustavson, 1956) have led to the conclusion that although cross-links of many kinds are possible, the great majority are formed between ε-amino groups of lysine and the amide nitrogen atoms of peptide linkages:

$$O=C \quad\quad\quad\quad\quad\quad\quad\quad\quad C=O$$
$$HC - (CH_3)_4 - NH_2 \;+\; HCHO \;+\; H - N$$
$$NH$$

$$\xrightarrow{\quad\quad} \quad O=C \quad\quad\quad\quad\quad\quad C=O$$
$$HC - (CH_3)_4 - \underset{H}{N} - CH_2 - N$$
$$NH \quad\quad\quad + \; H_2O$$

The formation of methylene bridges in this reaction is probably largely responsible for the cross-linking of protein molecules that constitutes fixation and structural stabilization of tissues by formaldehyde. Many ε-amino groups will not be close to peptide linkages and will therefore be able to form only the unstable hemiacetal-like adducts. Thus, the histochemical reactivity of primary amines (including the binding of anionic dyes) will be only slightly depressed in the fixed tissue. After prolonged storage (e.g. 6 months to 10 years) in formalin, the free $-NHCH_2OH$ groups may be oxidized by the atmosphere to the more stable $-NHCOOH$. This change may account for the eventual loss of stainability by anionic dyes that occurs in old, stored specimens. The quantity of [^{14}C]formaldehyde bound by animal tissue reaches a plateau in 24–50 h, with half the maximum amount being bound in 3–5 h (Helander, 1994, 1999). Bound ^{14}C can be removed from these tissues by washing in water: half is removed in less than 24 h, and 90% after 4 weeks of washing (Helander, 1994). Loss of formaldehyde with prolonged washing is presumably due to hydrolysis of covalent links to protein, but these results do not determine the proportion of tightly bound formaldehyde-derived carbon that exists as methylene cross-links.

Cross-linking of protein molecules by formaldehyde is much slower than the chemical reactions of other fixative agents. It is usually stated (e.g. Pearse, 1980; Kiernan, 2000) that fixation requires 1–2 weeks for completion at room temperature. For histochemical purposes, tissues are commonly fixed for 12–24 h at 4°C, but many non-histochemical methods, especially for the nervous system, work better after complete fixation. Sufficient hardening for the cutting of frozen sections is usually attained after 24 h. Very long periods of storage in formaldehyde solutions result in excessive hardening, loss of stainability of nuclei, and (with acidic solutions) deposition of brown **'formalin pigment'**. This is a haematin formed by acid degradation of haemoglobin. It can be removed by treating the sections with an alcoholic solution of picric acid or with any of a variety of oxidizing agents or alkalis (see Lillie and Fullmer, 1976). The 'pigment' does not form if the formaldehyde solution has been buffered to approximate neutrality.

Formaldehyde preserves most lipids, especially if the fixing solution contains calcium ions which, for ill-understood reasons, reduce the solubilities of some phospholipids in water. The only chemical reactions of formaldehyde with lipids under ordinary conditions of fixation are (1) addition to the amino groups of phosphatidyl ethanolamines, which is probably reversible by washing in water, and (2) prevention of the histochemical reactivity of plasmalogens (Chapter 12) owing to oxidation, probably to a glycol, of the ethylenic linkage next to the ether group. The latter reaction may be brought about by atmospheric oxygen rather than by formaldehyde. With prolonged fixation in formaldehyde solutions (3 months to 2 years), other double bonds are attacked, and several products are formed, all of which are more soluble in water than the original lipids (Jones, 1972).

Formaldehyde does not react significantly with carbohydrates. All the common mucosubstances can be demonstrated after fixation with formaldehyde, though appreciable quantities of glycogen and proteoglycans are lost. Dissolution of the latter can be greatly reduced by certain cationic additives (Section 2.4.11).

A neutral, buffered aqueous solution (pH 7.2–7.4) containing 2–5% of formaldehyde, is the most generally useful (though not the best) fixative for most histological and histochemical purposes. When histochemical methods are not to be used, mixtures such as Bouin's fluid and SUSA (Section 2.5.3) are preferable to formaldehyde because (a) they protect the tissue against damaging effects of embedding in wax, and (b) staining with almost all dyes is brighter than after formaldehyde alone.

The speed and quality of fixation with neutral formaldehyde solution can be improved by addition of an aliphatic amine such as cyclohexylamine or lysine (Luther and Bloch, 1989), or of phenol (Hopwood and Slidders, 1989). These compounds react with formaldehyde and their presence probably results in the formation of polymeric cross-links of variable length within the tissue, providing fixation comparable to that obtainable with glutaraldehyde (Sections 2.4.8 and 2.4.9(g)). Hopwood et al. (1989) recommend primary fixation in 4% formaldehyde containing 2% phenol at pH 7.0, followed by secondary fixation at pH 5.5. Many stains and immunohistochemical methods worked well after such treatment, and reasonable preservation for electron microscopy was also obtained.

2.4.9. Glutaraldehyde

Glutaraldehyde,

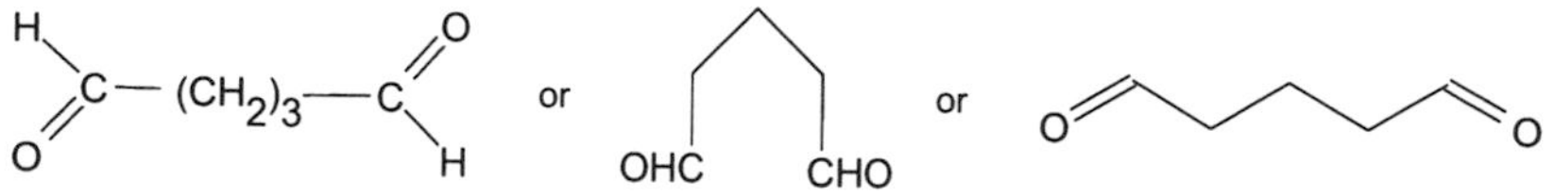

is the most widely used bifunctional aldehyde fixative. Glutaraldehyde polymerizes in aqueous solution. The polymers, which are of a different type from those present in solutions of formaldehyde, are formed by aldol condensation. This reaction yields a product in which an olefinic double bond (C=C) is conjugated with the carbonyl (C=O) double bond of the aldehyde group (Monsan, Puzo and Marzarguil, 1975):

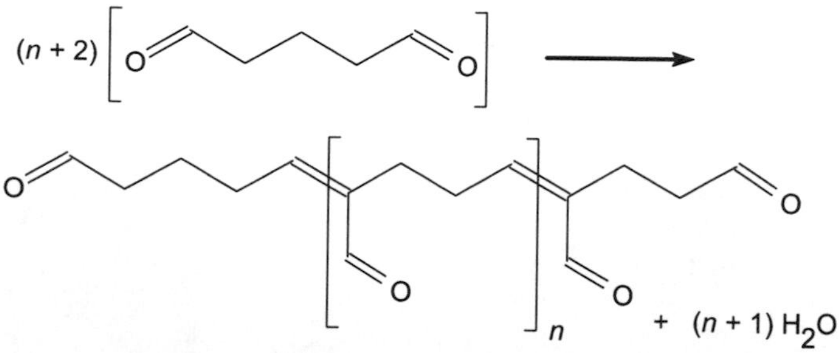

Dimers ($n = 0$) and trimers ($n = 1$) are the most abundant polymers in solutions of glutaraldehyde. The value of n increases with the age of the solution and with rise in pH. Solid polymers are precipitated from alkaline solutions. Glutaraldehyde is bought as a concentrated (usually 25%, sometimes 50%) aqueous solution at pH 3, which is kept in a refrigerator. Glutaraldehyde is unsuitable for use as a fixative if excessive polymerization has occurred. The condition of the solution can be checked spectrophotometrically, and Prento (1995) has shown that solutions are usable for up to 8 h after dilution with a neutral buffer.

Both types of aldehyde group in a low polymer of glutaraldehyde can react with amino groups of proteins, to form imines (compounds with C=N bonds; see also Chapter 10):

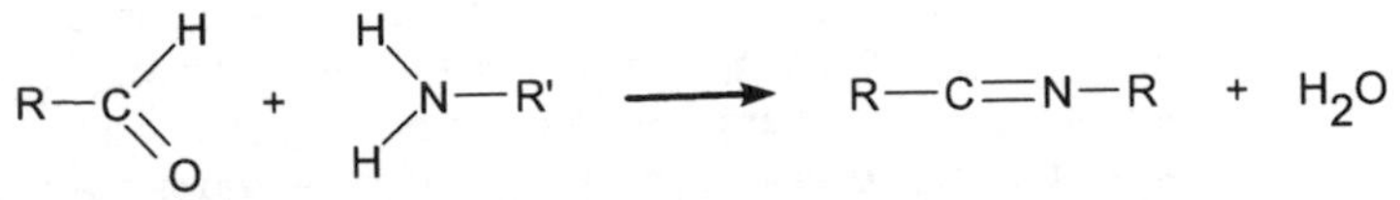

$$R-C{\overset{H}{\underset{O}{}}} \quad + \quad {\overset{H}{\underset{H}{}}}N-R' \quad \longrightarrow \quad R-C{=}N-R \quad + \quad H_2O$$

The imines that form from the terminal aldehyde groups of poly(glutaraldehyde) are, like most aliphatic imines, unstable. However, aldehyde groups within the repeating units of the polymer can form imines that are stable, owing to conjugation of their C=N bonds with the C=C bonds of the polymer. Consequently, the only significant reaction of poly(glutaraldehyde) with amino groups of protein is:

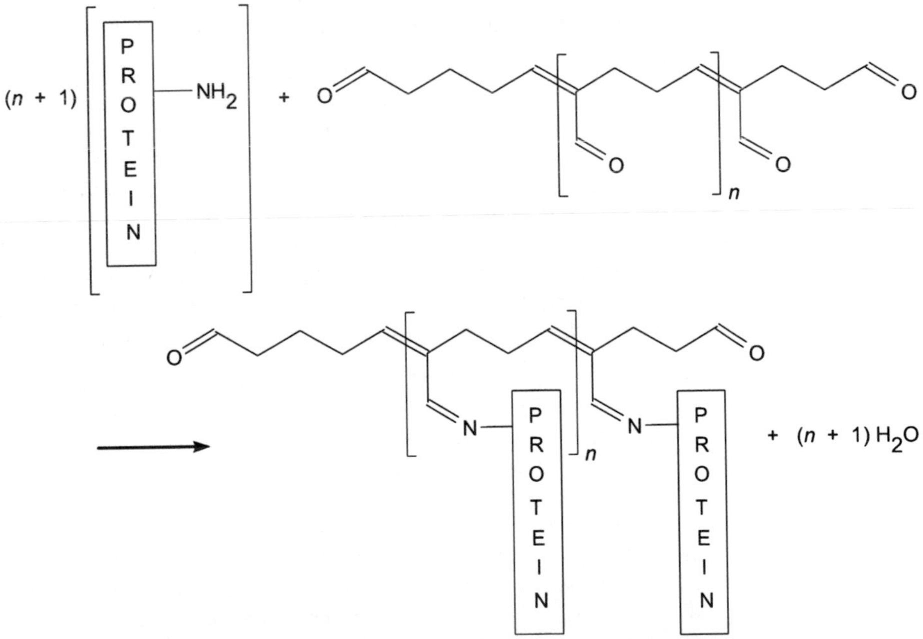

Like formaldehyde, glutaraldehyde probably also combines with reactive groups of proteins other than the ε-amino of lysine, but the reactions have not been studied in the context of histological fixation.

Mid-chain aldehyde groups of the poly(glutaraldehyde) molecule are the only ones involved in fixation (Monsan *et al.*, 1975), so the terminal aldehyde groups remain free, as do any mid-chain groups that have not combined with reactive side-chains of proteins. Consequently, **glutaraldehyde-fixed tissues are full of artificially** introduced aldehyde groups, which react with many histochemical reagents. This phenomenon must be taken into account when sections of glutaraldehyde-fixed material are to be treated by the Feulgen or periodic acid–Schiff procedures, in which the detection of DNA or of carbohydrate-containing substances is made possible by the chemical production of aldehydes. Free aldehyde groups can also bind, non-specifically, any reagents that are proteins, including enzymes and antibodies. Furthermore, the reducing properties of the aldehyde group can lead to false-positive results in autoradiography. **Aldehyde groups introduced by the fixative must be irreversibly chemically blocked before any of the above methods can be used.** Suitable blocking procedures are described in Chapter 10.

Glutaraldehyde penetrates tissues slowly, so it should be perfused through the vascular system if possible. Cross-linking of proteins occurs much more rapidly than with formaldehyde: fixation and is complete after only a few hours (see Kiernan, 2000). Tissues fixed in glutaraldehyde are more strongly stabilized by cross-linking than those fixed in formaldehyde, and this is probably the reason why ultrastructural features are so well preserved by the former substance. However, glutaraldehyde causes more difficulty than formaldehyde with the sectioning of paraffin-embedded material.

The activities of some enzymes are preserved after brief fixation in glutaraldehyde, but formaldehyde usually causes less inhibition, probably because it forms fewer cross-links between protein molecules. Cross-linking interferes chemically with the antigenicity of proteins, and also retards the passage of large antibody molecules into sections of fixed tissue. Consequently, glutaraldehyde should be avoided if possible when immunohistochemical staining methods are to be used.

A solution containing glutaraldehyde and formaldehyde, buffered to pH 7.2–7.4 (Karnovsky, 1965), is the most widely used fixative for electron microscopy. The mixture produces much more chemical modification of proteins than either of the aldehydes acting alone (Kirkeby and Moe, 1986), and can even cause insolubilization of free amines and amino acid ions (Conger *et al.*, 1978). If fixed material is to be examined immunohistochemically, pure glutaraldehyde causes less masking of antigens than a mixture with formaldehyde (Mrini *et al.*, 1995). Aldehyde fixatives do not add electron-opacity to tissues, so post-fixation in osmium tetroxide and contrast-staining with salts of other heavy metals are usually practised when ultrathin sections are to be examined by electron microscopy.

2.4.10.
Other aldehydes

Several other aldehydes have been used as fixatives. A few examples follow. **Chloral hydrate**, $Cl_3C–CH(OH)_2$, is the stable hydrated derivative of trichloroacetaldehyde. It is included in several older fixatives, especially for nervous tissue. Its reactions with tissues have not been critically examined. **Acrolein**, $H_2C{=}CH–CHO$, is a very toxic unsaturated aldehyde occasionally used as a fixative for electron microscopy. Reaction occurs with its olefinic as well as with its aldehyde group, with resultant cross-linking of proteins. The actions of acrolein on tissues closely resemble those of glutaraldehyde. **Hydroxyadipaldehyde**, $OHC–CH(OH)–(CH_2)_3–CHO$, and **crotonaldehyde**, $H_3C–CH{=}CH–CHO$, were introduced as fixatives for electron microscopy by Sabatini, Bensch and Barrnett (1963), at the same time as glutaraldehyde. They cause less inhibition of enzymes than glutaraldehyde or acrolein, but this is associated with inferior ultrastructural preservation.

Glyoxal, also known as ethanedial or oxalaldehyde ($OHC–CHO$) is another bifunctional aldehyde. The pure substance is a liquid (MP 15°C, BP 50.4°C) but the article of commerce, comparable to formalin, is a 30–40% aqueous solution that contains polymers and various hydrated forms of glyoxal:

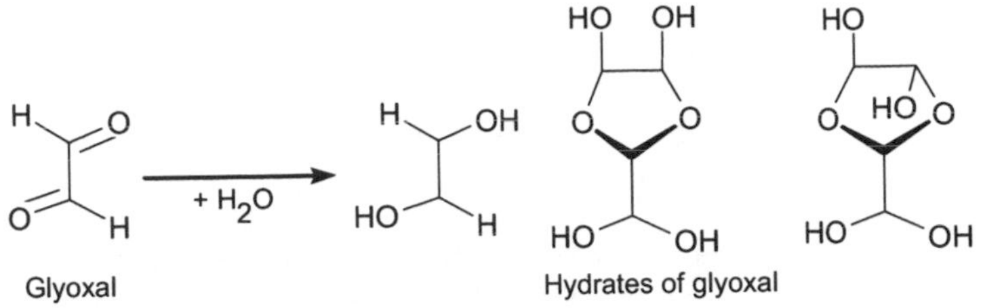

Glyoxal   Hydrates of glyoxal

The hydrate shown at the right-hand end of the above equation is the most abundant component of aqueous glyoxal solutions. Like formaldehyde, glyoxal reacts with itself in a Cannizzaro reaction, generating glycolic (2-hydroxyacetic) acid:

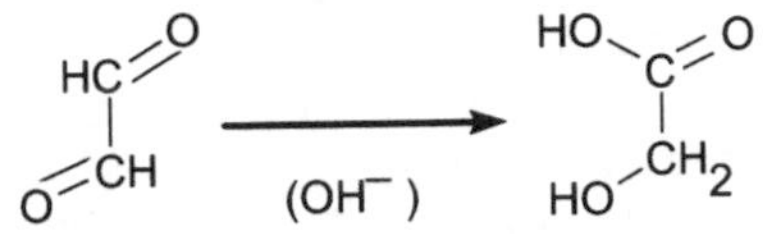

This reaction occurs rapidly in neutral or alkaline solutions (Mattioda et al., 1983), and probably accounts for the failure of early attempts to use this aldehyde as a fixative. Fixative solutions containing glyoxal must be buffered to approximately pH 4.0 and must also contain a small percentage of alcohol, which catalyses the reactions with proteins (Dapson et al., 2006). Unfortunately, glyoxal is available for fixation only as solutions whose exact compositions are trade secrets; there appear to be no published formulations of proven efficacy.

Owing to its many industrial uses (see Mattioda et al., 1983) the reactions of glyoxal with proteins and other macromolecules are quite well understood. They are similar to the reactions of formaldehyde, but occur more rapidly. Tissues are adequately fixed after 1 h of contact with glyoxal. Larger specimens require immersion for up to 9 h, to allow penetration of the tissue by the fixative. Cross-linking has been shown to occur when proteins react in solution with glyoxal (Glomb and Monnier, 1995) but in tissues fixed at pH 4 the principal reaction is addition to amino groups (N-termini and lysine side-chains), the –SH group of cysteine and the guanidino side-chain of arginine (Dapson et al., 2006). In the reaction with arginine, an imidazole ring is formed and the positive charge is lost:

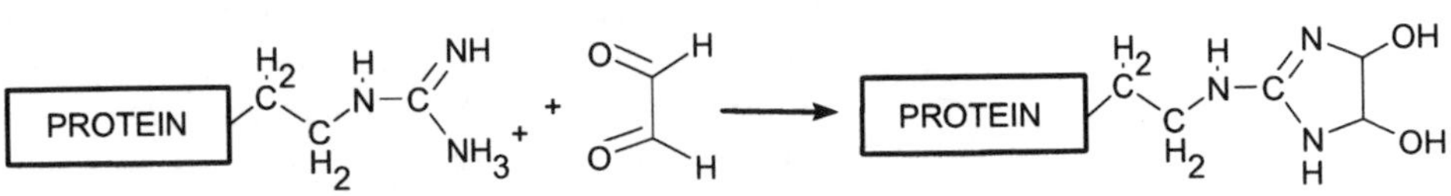

As a consequence of this reaction, arginine-rich structures (Chapter 10) lose their affinity for anionic dyes. Some immunohistochemical reactions are inhibited, but antigenicity can usually be retrieved (Chapter 19) by heating the sections in a slightly alkaline buffer, which brings about hydrolysis of the imidazole ring and restores the guanidino group (Dapson et al., 2006).

2.4.11.
Other fixative reagents

The major individual fixatives have now been described, but many other substances have also been used, some in mixtures that are now obsolete or at least out of fashion, and others in more recent years for special purposes. These minor fixative agents include:

(a) **Mineral acids**, that serve as coagulants. Examples are H_2SO_4 and HNO_3. Hardly any fixatives in modern use contain them.

(b) Several **metal ions and complexes** that cause precipitation of proteins have been included in fixative solutions. Examples are Cd^{2+}, Co^{2+}, Cu^{2+}, $[PtCl_6]^{2-}$, Pb^{2+}, $[UO_2]^{2+}$, Zn^{2+}. See Gray (1954) for many earlier mixtures, and Osterberg (1974) for a review of the chemistry of reactions of metal ions with proteins.

(c) **Iodine** is one of the oldest reagents used in microtechnique. The element is almost insoluble in water but it dissolves easily in the presence of potassium iodide, owing to formation of the complex triiodide ion:

$$I_2 \ + \ I^- \longrightarrow I_3^-$$

A 1% solution of iodine in 2% potassium iodide is known as Gram's iodine. Lugol's iodine contains 6% iodine in 4% KI. An early use of such a solution was as a primary fixative that also imparted colour to cytoplasm in animal (Arnold, 1898) and plant (Gardiner, 1898) tissues. It has also been used to fix invertebrate blood cells (Goodrich, 1919) and protozoa (Jerome et al., 1993). Iodine vapour has been tried as a fixative for unfixed sections of animal tissue, but found to be useless (Frederik et al., 1984). There are also a few fixative mixtures that contain iodine together with chromium compounds (Lenoir, 1926; Waterman, 1934). Waterman's fixative compares favourably with more commonly used mixtures (Kiernan, 1985).

Iodine diffuses rapidly through hydrophilic and hydrophobic domains of a tissue and is loosely bound by proteins, which it colors brown (Baker, 1958). It reacts irreversibly with unsaturated linkages of lipids and with the aromatic rings of tyrosine and histidine (Wolff and Covelli, 1969).

(d) **Organic protein coagulants** include p-toluenesulphonic acid (Malm, 1962) and tannic acid (Chaplin, 1985). The latter is commonly added to aldehyde fixatives for electron microscopy to promote protein retention and to enhance the binding of heavy metals used as contrast stains (Afzelius, 1992). Post-fixation of aldehyde-fixed tissues in tannic acid allows adequate contrast for electron microscopy without using osmium as one of the contrast-inducing metals (Phend et al., 1995). Tannic acid has also been shown to increase the retention of extracellular glycosaminoglycans in animal tissues (Levanon and Stein, 1995).

(e) **Cationic surfactants** (detergents) such as cetylpyridinium chloride and **cationic dyes** form insoluble salt-like complexes with polyanions, especially with proteoglycans. (Williams and Jackson, 1956). Dyes used for this purpose include alcian blue (Shea, 1971), and a coloured inorganic compound, ruthenium ammine (Nuehring et al., 1991). These also confer electron-opacity. Other dyes that insolubilize proteoglycans include acridine orange (Brandes and Reale, 1990) and safranine O. The latter has been shown to reduce the loss of intercellular matrix proteoglycan from about 50% to about 3% (Kiraly et al., 1996a). **Uncharged surfactants**, notably saponin and various synthetic esters, are applied to tissues and to cells in suspension, either before fixation or along with a fixative, to make the surface membranes permeable to macromolecules. The membranes are irreversibly changed, and this allows outward diffusion of cytosolic proteins (including the haemoglobin of erythrocytes; see Chapter 7) and the inward diffusion of antibodies used as reagents in immunohistochemistry (Chapter 19).

(f) **Bifunctional organic compounds other than aldehydes**. These can combine with and cross-link amino, hydroxyl, carboxyl and sulphydryl groups. Examples are: cyanuric chloride, diethyl pyrocarbonate, and various carbodiimides, imido esters and quinones, (Pearse and Polak, 1975; Bu'Lock et al., 1982; Robinson, 1987; Panula et al., 1988; Rubbi et al., 1994). Compounds of this kind are occasionally advantageous for immobilizing antigens whose immunoreactivity is blocked by more conventional fixatives. An acidic solution of a trifunctional diazonium salt, hexazotized pararosaniline, was used by De Jong *et al.* (1991) and Schrijver *et al.* (2000) to fix cryostat sections of lymphoid tissue, and was said to be superior to acetone for preserving cellular structure and antigenicity. This solution does not cross-link proteins, however, and its protective action on cryostat sections appears to be due only to its low pH (Kiernan, 2004).

(g) **Sodium periodate with lysine and formaldehyde** (McLean and Nakane, 1974). With this combination, introduced for immunohistochemical studies, the idea is that the periodate ion oxidizes carbohydrate side-chains of glycoproteins to aldehydes (Chapter 11), which then combine with the two amino groups of lysine (Chapter 10). Thus, glycoprotein molecules, especially those on the surfaces of cells, should be cross-linked. However, Hixson *et al.* (1981) showed that the lysine in the mixture reacted immediately with the formaldehyde, forming polymeric products, and that glycoproteins were cross-linked after treatment with periodate alone. They suggested that periodate-generated aldehyde groups combined with the amino groups of nearby protein molecules, and that the formaldehyde-lysine compounds formed longer cross-links than did formaldehyde alone, thus favouring the permeation of the tissue by large antibody molecules. The production of longer cross-links by combining an amine or a phenol with formaldehyde was discussed in the last part of Section 2.4.8.

2.4.12. Chemically inactive ingredients

In addition to one or more of the components discussed above, an aqueous fixative mixture commonly includes 'indifferent' substances that influence its osmotic pressure and its pH.

The most rapidly penetrating component of an aqueous fixative is water, so the central parts of a specimen are likely to be bathed in a hypotonic medium before they are fixed. This would lead to swelling or rupture of cells and disorganization of their surrounding connective tissue. To prevent such damage, unreactive salts with small, rapidly diffusing ions (e.g. sodium chloride or sulphate) are incorporated into the fixative mixture. Sucrose is also used to raise the osmotic pressure, but its molecules are fairly large, so it should probably be employed only in fixatives for vascular perfusion or for immersion of very small specimens. Another osmoprotective solute is betaine, $(CH_3)_2N^+CH_2COO^-$, even at a low concentration (22 mM) that hardly raises the osmotic pressure (Swan, 1999). This zwitterionic compound may enter cells more rapidly than other components of the fixative and become concentrated in the cytoplasm.

Most histologists and electron microscopists agree that the best results are obtained when the osmotic pressure due to the chemically inactive components of a fixative is slightly higher than that of the extracellular fluid (Schook, 1980; Hayat, 1981). The additional osmotic effect of the chemically active ingredients is not taken into account, because the osmotic properties of cell membranes are changed by contact with such substances.

Hydrophilic polymers, notably polyethylene glycol, are used to prevent diffusion of soluble enzymes in cryostat sections of unfixed tissues (see Chayen and Bitensky, 1991; see also Chapter 14). Scott (1974) showed that such polymers could also limit diffusion of fragments of hydrolyzed DNA, and likened this action to fixation. Certain proprietary solutions, sold as primary fixatives and storage media for use in histopathology, contain polyethylene glycol and alcohol (Boon and Kok, 1991). In my hands, a similar solution of disclosed composition (3.5% polyethylene glycol, MW 300 in 50% ethanol; called 'Leiden fixative' by Sanderson, 1994) gave poor structural preservation of mouse tissues that were subsequently processed into paraffin. A similar solution, Saccomanno's fluid, is 2% polyethylene glycol, MW 1300–1600, in 50% ethanol. This is used for cells collected for clinical diagnostic purposes, and is sometimes called a transport medium rather than a fixative.

Non-aqueous fixatives coagulate the tissue as they penetrate, so for these the control of osmotic pressure is unnecessary. The solvent penetrates more rapidly than any dissolved ingredients, however. For example, the centre of a large specimen immersed in an alcoholic solution of picric acid will be fixed primarily by the alcohol alone.

The pH of a fixative must be appropriate for the chemical reactions of fixation. Formaldehyde, glutaraldehyde, and OsO_4 are all fully active at and around neutrality, so their solutions may, with advantage, be buffered to approximately the same pH as the extracellular fluid. This is pH 7.2–7.6 for mammals. The prevention of an abrupt change in pH during fixation probably minimizes fine structural disturbance within dying cells. Some of that disruption may be due to spontaneous acidification by metabolites such as carbon dioxide and lactic acid. Buffering is of greatest value in the case of formaldehyde, which penetrates quickly but reacts with proteins much more slowly than other fixatives.

Most fixatives other than the three mentioned in the preceding paragraph are active only when their solutions are considerably more acid than the extracellular fluid. The correct pH is produced when the fixative mixture is made and a buffer is not needed. Glyoxal is used at pH 4 (Section 2.4.10). In the design of new fixatives, care must be taken to avoid irrational combinations. For example, the advantages of mixing acetic acid with formaldehyde or osmium tetroxide would be lost if the mixture were then buffered to pH 7.4. The effect of pH on the type of fixation produced by the dichromate ion has already been described.

Solutions of indifferent salts, buffers, and sucrose are often used to wash fixed specimens, especially in processing for electron microscopy. Completely fixed tissues are, however, no longer responsive to changes in the osmotic pressures of the solutions in which they are immersed. Plain water is satisfactory for washing all specimens intended for ordinary histological or cytological examination with the light microscope. Isotonic buffers are recommended, however, for washing specimens that have received only partial fixation for any reason. Incomplete aldehyde fixation commonly precedes application of histochemical methods for enzymes, immunohistochemistry, or processing for electron microscopy. Paljarvi *et al.* (1979) found that tissues were still susceptible to damage by osmotic stress after fixation for 24 h in buffered 4% formaldehyde. 3% glutaraldehyde used for the same length of time conferred complete stabilization.

**2.4.13.
Summary of
some properties
of individual
fixatives**

The more important effects of the major fixative agents upon tissues are presented briefly in *Table 2.1*.

2.5. Choice of fixative

A fixative is chosen according to the structural or chemical components of the tissue that are to be demonstrated. Often a mixture of different agents is employed in order to offset undesirable effects of individual substances and to obtain more than one type of chemical fixation. A few commonly used liquids will now be described. Fixatives for some specialized purposes are described in other chapters.

Table 2.1. Properties of individual fixative agents

	Ethanol, methanol, acetone	Acetic acid	Trichloro-acetic acid	Picric acid	Formaldehyde	Glutaraldehyde	Glyoxal	Mercuric chloride	Zinc salts	pH <3.5 (CrO_3)	Dichromate ion: pH > 3.5 ($K_2Cr_2O_7$)	Osmium tetroxide
Usual concentration (%) alone or in mixtures	35–100	5–35	2–5	0.5–5	2–10	0.25–4	?	3–6	0.1–3	0.2–0.8	1–5	0.5–2
Penetration	Fast	Fast	Fast	Slow	Fast	Slow	Fast	Quite fast	Quite fast	Slow	Quite fast	Slow
Change in volume of tissue	↓+++	↑+++	↑++	↓+	Nil	Nil	Nil	↓+	↓+	↓+	Nil	Nil
Hardening	++	Nil	Nil (?)	+	++	++	+ (?)	++	++ (?)	++	+	+
Fixative effect on proteins	Non-additive, coagulant	Some extraction	Non-additive, coagulant	Additive, coagulant	Additive, non-coagulant	Additive, non-coagulant	Additive, non-coagulant	Additive, coagulant	Additive, coagulant	Additive, coagulant	Additive, non-coagulant	Oxidation
Action on nucleic acids	Nil	Precipitation	Some extraction	Partial hydrolysis	Slight extraction	Slight extraction	Nil (?)	Coagulation	Coagulation (?)	Coagulation; some hydrolysis	Some extraction	Slight extraction
Effects on carbohydrates	Nil	Nil	Nil	Nil	Nil	Cross-linking	Cross-linking	Nil	Nil	Oxidation	Nil	Some oxidation (?)
Effects on lipids	Much extraction	Nil	Nil	Nil	Slow chemical changes	Similar to formaldehyde	?	Plasmal reaction	?	Oxidation of double bonds	Slowly insolubilized	Addition to double bonds
Effects on enzyme activities	Some preserved if kept cold	Inhibition (?)	Inhibition	Inhibition	Some preserved (short time; cold)	Most are inhibited	?	Inhibition	Inhibition (?)	Inhibition	Inhibition	Inhibition
Effects on organelles (especially mitochondria)	Destroyed	Destroyed	Preserved	Distorted	Preserved	Well preserved	?	Preserved	?	Considerable distortion	Very little distortion	Well preserved
Staining with: Anionic dyes	Satisfactory	Poor	Satisfactory	Good	Satisfactory	Satisfactory	Satisfactory	Good	Good	Satisfactory	Good	Acidophilia is changed to basophilia
Cationic dyes	Satisfactory	Good	Good	Satisfactory	Satisfactory	Satisfactory	Good	Good	Good	Satisfactory	Satisfactory	Satisfactory
Value as sole fixative agent	Only for smears, sections, or tiny blocks	Nil	Quite good but not used	Poor; never used alone	Useful	Seldom used alone	Used in trade-secret mixtures	Poor	Quite good	Poor	Poor	Specialized uses only

Arrows indicate increase (↑) or decrease (↓). Plus signs show relative magnitude of effect. ? Indicates uncertainty.

2.5.1.
Non-aqueous
fixatives

The following mixtures are used for general histology and for the preservation of nucleic acids and macromolecular carbohydrates. They are usually mixed no more than a few hours before using, because of slow chemical reactions between ingredients. An exception is Gendre's fluid (Section 2.5.3), which may improve with age.

Clarke's fluid

Absolute ethanol:	3 volumes
Glacial acetic acid:	1 volume

Mix just before using. Ethyl acetate (fruity odour) is formed with storage for more than a month, but may not detract from the quality of fixation.

This is one of the oldest fixatives, and is notable for excellent results with subsequent paraffin embedding. In comparisons of fixatives for light microscopy, this crude old mixture always gets a high score for micro-anatomical preservation (see Baker, 1958; Kiernan, 1985). Fixed specimens are moved into 95% or 100% alcohol.

Carnoy's fluid

Absolute ethanol:	60 ml
Chloroform:	30 ml
Glacial acetic acid:	10 ml

It is usual to mix just before using, but according to Puchtler *et al.* (1968) the mixture is stable and can be kept in stock.

Like Clarke's, this is a rapidly penetrating fixative that coagulates protein and nucleic acids and extracts lipids. Many carbohydrate components are preserved. Blocks of tissue up to 5 mm thick are fixed for 6–8 h and then moved into 95% or 100% alcohol. Fixation in Carnoy for more than 18 h can result in hydrolysis of nucleic acids, with loss of RNA. This effect can be suppressed by using 5 ml instead of 10 ml of acetic acid. The low-acetic fixative is called **modified Carnoy** (James and Tas, 1984). Substitution of methanol for ethanol in the original Carnoy formula gives **methacarn** (Puchtler *et al.*, 1970), which provides superior preservation of intracytoplasmic fibrillary structures.

Alcohol–formalin–acetic mixtures
A typical member of this group is **AFA** or **FAA**.

Ethanol (95–100%):	85 ml
Formalin (37–40% HCHO):	10 ml
Glacial acetic acid:	5 ml

Mix before using.

This is one of many similar mixtures. The amount of acetic acid or formalin may be varied, and methanol is sometimes used instead of ethanol. Penetration is rapid. Specimens are fixed for 4–48 h. Smears or whole mounts on slides are fixed for 10–30 min. The formaldehyde probably does not contribute much to fixation when the duration is short. As with Carnoy, AFA preserves general morphology, nucleic acids and carbohydrates well, and most lipids are extracted. After fixation the specimens are transferred to 95% alcohol, and then processed for embedding in wax. FAA suppresses immunostaining of antigens to a greater extent than neutral buffered formaldehyde, but the antigenicity can be restored by antigen retrieval procedures (Zhang *et al.*, 1998).

Some alcohol–formalin–acetic fixatives contain more water than the usual AFA or FAA mixtures. An example is **Davidson's fixative**, which is sometimes called Hartmann's fixative. It has been used for smears of cells and for solid specimens:

Formalin (37%):	40 ml
Alcohol:	60 ml
Glacial acetic acid:	20 ml
Tap water:	60 ml

Mix before using. Some workers add a drop of eosin staining solution to impart a pale pink colour to the liquid. Eosin used in this way stains the tissue slightly, and can be helpful for seeing and handling very small specimens.

Specimens are fixed by immersion for less than 24 h, transferred to 70% alcohol, and then processed for paraffin embedding. It appears that neither William McKay Davidson (a British haematologist) nor William H. Hartmann (an American pathologist) published this mixture. It first published use may have been in studies of the human sex chromatin (Moore *et al.*, 1953).

2.5.2. Aqueous aldehyde solutions

Formal–saline
This is a simple aqueous formaldehyde fixative. It contains nothing to neutralize the acidity derived from commercial formalin, and its acidity increases with storage.

Formalin (37–40% HCHO):	100 ml
Sodium chloride (NaCl):	9.0 g
Water:	to make 1000 ml

The solution should be made up at least a day before using, to allow time for depolymerization of formaldehyde polymers. It can then be kept for several months. Specimens of animal tissues should not remain in it for more than about a week, or 'formalin pigment' (Section 2.4.2) may be deposited. Marble chips ($CaCO_3$) are often put in the bottom of a bottle of formal–saline to oppose acidification.

Neutral buffered formalin
Fixatives with this name vary in composition, but all contain approximately 4% w/v formaldehyde in water that has been buffered to pH 7.2–7.4. A sodium phosphate buffer is most frequently used, but others (cacodylate, barbitone, *s*-collidine) are sometimes preferred in fixatives for electron microscopy. Three phosphate-buffered mixtures are described here.

The first is a solution of formaldehyde in a 0.075 M phosphate buffer, introduced by R.D. Lillie, after whom it is sometimes named.

| Sodium phosphate, monobasic ($NaH_2PO_4.H_2O$): | 4.0 g |
| Sodium phosphate, dibasic (Na_2HPO_4): | 6.5 g |

Either dissolve in 750 ml of water, add 100ml of formalin (37–40% HCHO), and make up to 1000 ml with water.
Or dissolve in water to 1000 ml, heat to 60–70°C (in fume hood), add 40 g of paraformaldehyde powder, stir well, cool and filter.

Can be kept for several months. The pH is 7.2–7.4.

Some batches of paraformaldehyde are unsuitable because they dissolve too slowly. The concentration of formaldehyde is not critical, and may range from 2.5% to 10%. The mixture made from formalin is used when the presence of traces of methanol and formate can be tolerated (as in most histological work). Paraformaldehyde is commonly used when the fixative is for electron microscopy, enzyme histochemistry or immunohistochemistry.

The second mixture (Carson *et al.*, 1973) has an osmotic pressure closer to that of mammalian extracellular fluids, is slightly easier to make, and is said to be satisfactory for either light or electron microscopy:

Formaldehyde, 37–40%:	100 ml
Water:	900 ml
Sodium phosphate, monobasic ($NaH_2PO_4.H_2O$):	18.6 g
Sodium hydroxide (NaOH):	4.2 g

Can be kept for several months. The pH is 7.2–7.4.

The third is made as required from 0.1 M sodium phosphate buffer or phosphate-buffered saline (PBS), one or both of which are usually stocked in a histological or immunohistochemical laboratory. The fixative will be somewhat hypertonic if it is made from the PBS mixture described in Chapter 20.

Either 0.1 M sodium phosphate buffer (pH 7.2–7.4):	900 ml
Or Phosphate-buffered saline (PBS):	900 ml
And Formalin (37–40% HCHO):	100 ml

Can be kept for several months. Adjust the pH to 7.2–7.4 if necessary.

With any of these mixtures, fix for 12–24 h at 4°C to preserve enzymes and labile antigens. For general histology fix overnight or longer at room temperature. It is advantageous to fix for at least one week at room temperature, and this is necessary if traditional neurological staining methods are to be carried out. If graded alcohols are not used for dehydration, wash the fixed specimens in water for 30 min to remove the buffer salts, which are not soluble in organic solvents. The adverse effects of formaldehyde on subsequent immunostaining can often be reversed by antigen retrieval procedures, described in Chapter 19.

Formaldehyde with glutaraldehyde

For reasons given in Section 2.4.9 the stock solution of glutaraldehyde (25% or 50%) must be of an 'EM grade' designated by the supplier as a suitable fixative for electron microscopy, and it should be used before the expiry date shown on the label.

The addition of 10 ml of 25% aqueous glutaraldehyde to 90 ml of neutral buffered formaldehyde gives a solution similar to Karnovsky's (1965) fixative that preserves many intracytoplasmic structures such as mitochondria. These organelles may be further stabilized for paraffin embedding by post-fixing small pieces of the tissue in osmium tetroxide (1% aqueous, 6 h) or potassium dichromate (3% aqueous, 7 days).

Formal–calcium

Formalin (37–40% HCHO):	100 ml
Calcium acetate ($(CH_3COO)_2Ca.H_2O$:	20 g
Water:	to make 1000 ml

The acetate ions neutralize acidity derived from formalin, provide some buffering, and raise the osmotic pressure. The calcium ions insolubilize phospholipids prior to cutting frozen sections. Specimens are fixed for 1–3 days. (See also Chapter 12.)

Zinc–formalin

Formalin (37–40% HCHO):	100 ml
Zinc sulphate ($ZnSO_4.7H_2O$):	10 g
Water:	to make 1000 ml

(See Herman *et al.*, 1988.) Adjust the pH, if desired, by adding drops of 1.0 M HCl or 1.0 M NaOH. Mugnaini and Dahl (1983) adjusted to pH 4.0 or 6.5.

Small animals may be fixed by vascular perfusion (Section 2.6) for 1 h. Solid specimens are fixed in 6–8 h but may remain in zinc–formalin for up to one week. Immerse in a cryoprotectant (Section 2.1.2) before cutting frozen or cryostat sections. Alternatively, wash in water (not phosphate buffer) for 30 min to remove zinc salts, then process for paraffin or plastic embedding (Chapter 4).

2.5.3
Other aqueous fixatives for general histology

Bouin's fluid

Saturated aqueous picric acid:	750 ml
Formalin (37–40% HCHO):	250 ml
Glacial acetic acid:	50 ml

Keeps indefinitely.

Bouin's fluid preserves morphological features, especially of nuclei and connective tissue, well. Erythrocytes are lysed. This fixative is valuable for general histological work, because physical distortion of tissues is minimal, paraffin sections are easy to cut, and staining methods using multiple dyes usually give bright, well separated colours. Cytoplasmic organelles are poorly preserved. Specimens are usually fixed for 24 h, then transferred to 70% or 95% alcohol. Material stored in Bouin for several months is still usable, but the acidic solution extracts RNA and partly hydrolyses DNA, so that nuclei give a positive histochemical reaction for aldehyde groups (Chapter 9).

Gendre's fluid (alcoholic Bouin)

Saturated alcoholic picric acid:	800 ml
Formalin (40% HCHO):	150 ml
Glacial acetic acid:	50 ml

(The alcoholic picric acid solution is made up in 90–95% ethanol or industrial methylated spirit.)

This mixture can be kept indefinitely, but its chemical composition changes considerably. The concentrations of ethanol and formaldehyde decline, and there is concomitant improvement of the fixative properties, at least for some invertebrate tissues (Gregory, Greenway and Lord, 1980). Gregory (1980) recommends an **'artificially aged alcoholic Bouin'** with the following composition:

Picric acid:	0.5 g
Formalin (40% HCHO):	15 ml
Ethanol:	25 ml
Glacial acetic acid:	5 ml
Ethyl acetate:	25 ml
Water:	to make 100 ml

These non-aqueous fixatives are similar to Bouin, but they also immobilize some water-soluble carbohydrates (glycogen; mast cell granules of some species) that dissolve in aqueous fixatives. Specimens are fixed overnight (12 h) and then washed in several changes of 95% alcohol. **Caution.** Do not allow these fixatives to evaporate (Section 2.4.4).

Heidenhain's SUSA

The nickname SUSA is from the German *Sublimat* ($HgCl_2$) and *Säure* (acid), but the literature contains many references to 'Susa's fixative'!

Mercuric chloride ($HgCl_2$):	45 g
Sodium chloride (NaCl):	5 g
Trichloroacetic acid:	20 g
Glacial acetic acid:	40 ml
Formalin (40% HCHO):	200 ml
Water:	to make 1000 ml

Keeps indefinitely.

Pieces of tissues are fixed for no more than 24 h and traditionally are transferred directly to 95% alcohol, supposedly to avoid swelling. My experience is that no harm follows washing in water after fixation in SUSA. Stains for nuclei, cytoplasm, and connective tissue all work brightly after this fixative, as do some histochemical methods for carbohydrates. **Mercurial deposits must be removed (Chapter 4) prior to staining. Caution.** Toxic hazard (mercuric chloride); trichloroacetic acid is strongly corrosive before dilution.

Zenker's and Helly's fluids

Helly and Zenker contain mercuric chloride and potassium dichromate. These fixatives are excellent for morphological work, but are not compatible with many histochemical techniques. **It is important to wash out all the dichromate (running tap water overnight) before dehydrating the specimens in alcohol, and to remove mercury deposits (Chapter 4) before staining. Caution.** Toxic hazard (especially mercuric chloride). These fixatives must be disposed of as toxic waste.

Zinc chloride ($ZnCl_2$) may be substituted for mercuric chloride in the stock Zenker solution and in the working Zenker fixative (Barszcz, 1976). Structural integrity may be slightly inferior to that attainable with $HgCl_2$, and iodine–thiosulphate treatment of the sections is not needed. Unlike the mercury compound, zinc salts do not protect intracellular iron deposits against some of the loss that occurs with acid decalcification of bone marrow core biopsies (DePalma, 1996).

Stock Zenker solution:

Mercuric chloride ($HgCl_2$):	50 g
Potassium dichromate ($K_2Cr_2O_7$):	25 g
Sodium sulphate ($Na_2SO_4.10H_2O$):	10 g
Water:	to make 1000 ml

Keeps indefinitely. This solution, named **Zenker without acetic** by Baker (1958) is an excellent fixative without added acetic acid (Zenker's fluid) or formaldehyde (Helly's fluid).

Working Zenker's fixative

Immediately before use, mix 5 ml of glacial acetic acid with 100 ml of the stock solution.

This mixture is stable indefinitely. Because of the low pH at which the dichromate is used, nuclear morphology is clearly displayed by all staining methods, but cytoplasmic proteins are rather coarsely coagulated, and most organelles are not preserved.

For embryonic tissues, structural preservation by Zenker (6 h) can be improved by post-fixing for 7 days in neutral, buffered formaldehyde (Howard *et al.*, 1989). It is possible the buffer arrests the damaging effect of acidity on cytoplasm. The formaldehyde may reduce residual Cr(VI) in the tissue to Cr(III), which could be expected to cause additional cross-linking of proteins (Section 2.4.5) and protect against damage that might be incurred during dehydration, clearing and embedding.

Working Helly's fixative

This fixative is similar to Zenker's except that the glacial acetic acid is replaced by 5 ml of formalin (37–40% formaldehyde).

Helly's fluid is used mainly to fix cytoplasmic elements such as mitochondria and granules, as in endocrine organs and haemopoietic tissue. The non-coagulant components (formaldehyde, dichromate at neutral pH) offset the coagulant action of the mercuric chloride so that organelles are not destroyed by coarse coagulation of the cytoplasm. The mixture goes green and murky on standing, owing to reduction of dichromate to chromic salts by formaldehyde. Fixation should not be for more than 12–24 h.

**2.5.4.
Traditional
cytological
fixatives**

Although intracellular structures are best studied with the electron microscope, most of the components of the nucleus and cytoplasm were discovered long before that instrument was invented. Different fixatives must be used for the examination of chromosomes, intracellular cytoskeletal filaments or cytoplasmic organelles with the light microscope. The nucleoprotein and DNA of chromosomes are rendered insoluble by either acetic acid or chromic acid (pH <3.5). The latter also preserves proteinaceous filaments of the mitotic spindle, but it largely destroys the cytoplasm. Neutral dichromate (pH > 3.5) is included in solutions for the fixation of organelles. Osmium tetroxide is a common component of both types of cytological fixative because insoluble osmium compounds are reliably deposited at all sites of unsaturated lipids, which are present in all the membranes of cells.

Cell fixatives for light microscopy are made up from stock aqueous solutions of chromium trioxide (5%), potassium dichromate (5%) and osmium tetroxide (2%). The pieces of tissue must be tiny (1 mm or less in thickness). Fixation for 6–18 h is followed by thorough washing in water to remove unbound chemicals. Very clean glass (not plastic) containers must be used for all solutions containing osmium tetroxide. **See Chapter 12 (Section 12.6.1) for notes on the safe handling and disposal of osmium tetroxide.**

Altmann's fixative

2% osmium tetroxide:	5.0 ml
5% potassium dichromate:	5.0 ml

Mix before using, though it keeps for a year or longer in a clean, tightly capped bottle. This cytoplasmic fixative can also be used to post-fix material that was fixed in a buffered glutaraldehyde or a formaldehyde–glutaraldehyde mixture.

Flemming's strong fluid

2% osmium tetroxide:	2.0 ml
5% chromium trioxide:	1.5 ml
Glacial acetic acid:	0.5 ml
Water:	to make 10 ml

Mix before using, but it is stable for several days. This fixative is for mitotic and meiotic nuclei.

Mann's fixative

2% osmium tetroxide:	5 ml
Water:	5 ml
Saturated solution of mercuric chloride ($HgCl_2$, about 7%), in 0.75% aqueous sodium chloride:	10 ml

Mix before using, but it is stable for several days. This fixative is for cytoplasmic organelles, including the Golgi apparatus.

**2.5.5.
Fixatives for
immuno-
histochemistry**

These three mixtures are used principally for specimens to be examined by immunohistochemical methods. Their possible mechanisms of action have been discussed earlier in this chapter.

Buffered formaldehyde with picrate

Paraformaldehyde:	20 g
Picric acid (saturated aqueous solution, filtered):	150 ml

Heat to 60°C. Add 2–5 drops of 1.0 M (4%) aqueous sodium hydroxide, if necessary, to dissolve the paraformaldehyde. Filter, cool, and make up to 1000 ml with the following phosphate buffer:

Sodium phosphate, monobasic ($NaH_2PO_4.H_2O$):   3.31 g
Sodium phosphate, dibasic (Na_2HPO_4):   17.89 g
Water: to make 1000 ml

The pH is 7.3. This fixative (Stefanini et al., 1967) is stable for at least 12 months at room temperature. Picrate does not precipitate proteins in neutral solution, and the reasons why it improves the preservation of structure and antigenicity (Accini et al., 1974) are not known. Structural preservation in paraffin sections of brain and kidney is superior to that obtained with ordinary neutral buffered formaldehyde or Bouin (Kiernan, 1985). After fixation for 8–24 h the specimens are washed in water and moved into 70% alcohol.

This mixture is sometimes cited as 'Zamboni's fixative', but the short report of Zamboni and De Martino (1967) did not state the concentrations of the ingredients, and contained a confusing statement suggesting similarity to Bouin's fluid.

Periodate–lysine–paraformaldehyde
See Section 2.4.11(g) for discussion of this fixative, which is prepared as follows. A 0.1 M solution of dibasic sodium phosphate and a 0.1 M sodium phosphate buffer, pH 7.4 are needed (Chapter 20). A stock 8% solution of formaldehyde should also be available. It is made by heating 750 ml of water to 60–70°C, then adding 80 g of paraformaldehyde followed by a few drops of 1.0 M (4%) sodium hydroxide, and making up to 1000 ml with water when the solution is transparent. The working solution is prepared as follows:

Lysine monohydrochloride: 1.83 g
Water: 50 ml

(This is a 0.2 M solution; adjust the weight of lysine if a form other than the monohydrochloride is used.)

Add 0.1 M Na_2HPO_4 until pH is 7.4
Add 0.1 M sodium phosphate buffer, pH 7.4 to bring volume to 100 ml.
Add in order:
8% paraformaldehyde solution (see above):   33 ml
Finally, add either sodium metaperiodate ($NalO_4$):   284 mg
or sodium paraperiodate, $Na_3H_2IO_6$:   391 mg

(The pH of the final mixture is not adjusted when it falls following addition of the sodium periodate.)

Beckstead's fixative
(See Beckstead, 1994.) A more detailed account of the preparation of the solution was given by Beckstead (1995), along with some variants. The only active fixative ingredient is the Zn^{2+} ion.

Tris(hydroxymethyl)aminomethane
(also known as TRIS, THAM, tromethamine):   12.1 g
Water: 900 ml
1.0 M hydrochloric acid: 81.5 ml
Water: to make 1000 ml

At this stage the pH should be 7.4. Adjust if necessary before adding the following salts.

Calcium acetate [$(CH_3COO)_2Ca$]:   0.5 g
Zinc acetate [$(CH_3COO)_2Zn.2H_2O$]:   5.0 g
Zinc chloride ($ZnCl_2$):   5.0 g

The final pH of the solution is 6.8. It must not rise above 7.0 or a precipitate will form.

Pieces of tissue 2–3 mm thick are immersed for 24 h, washed in 50% or 70% alcohol, dehydrated, cleared and embedded in paraffin. Alternatively, cut frozen sections.

2.5.6.
Secret mixtures

Some suppliers of laboratory chemicals provide fixative solutions that have trade-names. Commonly the composition is not disclosed, and there is simply a statement that it 'contains zinc' or is 'formaldehyde-free'. Ready-made solutions are convenient for laboratories with plenty of money to spend, but liquids of unknown composition have no place in any kind of scientific work. Fixation is the step that has the greatest effect on the final appearance of a microscopical preparation. Consequently, the use of an unknown fixative is unwise even for 'routine' histopathological specimens.

2.6. Methods of fixation

Slides bearing films, smears, or cryostat sections of unfixed material are immersed in buffered formalin, cold (0–4°C) acetone, or absolute ethanol or methanol, either before or after the application of blood stains (Chapter 7) or histochemical methods for enzymes (Chapters 14–16), according to the requirements of the particular techniques. Methanol probably provides better fixation of nuclei and cytoplasm than other organic liquids (Puchtler et al., 1970). Solid specimens are fixed by **immersion** in at least ten times their own volumes of the appropriate solution (20× for non-aqueous fixatives), or by **perfusion** of the fixative through the vascular system. The latter technique has the advantage of ensuring that the fixing agent is rapidly brought into contact with all parts of all organs. Usually a whole animal is perfused (*Fig. 2.1*), but it is also feasible to cannulate and perfuse the

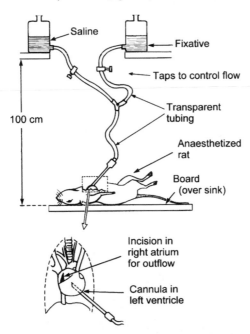

Figure 2.1. Fixation of an anaesthetized small mammal by perfusion from the left ventricle to the right atrium. The saline is run through first, until the effluent fluid is clear. The fixative (usually a formaldehyde or glutaraldehyde solution) is then perfused until the whole body of the animal is hard and inflexible. About 100 ml of fixative is required for a 200–300 g rat, and the whole procedure takes about 15 min. According to Thorball and Tranum-Jensen (1983), it takes 5–10 min to saturate all the glutaraldehyde-binding sites in the tissues of a well perfused rat. Formaldehyde reacts much more slowly, so fixation is continued by immersion of removed organs.

vasculature of a single organ. Fixation of material removed from a perfused animal is usually continued by immersion in the same fluid.

Perfusion fixation is usually carried out at room temperature, though some investigators prefer either a cool (4°C) or a warm (37°C) solution. In an attempt to keep tissues oxygenated for as long as possible, Rostgaard et al. (1993) included in their fixative an oxygen-carrying fluorocarbon compound that has been used as an experimental blood substitute.

Small or thin pieces may be fixed by leaving them for 2–24 h in the **vapour** above an aqueous solution of osmium tetroxide, and freeze-dried blocks are fixed in the vapour of formaldehyde or glutaraldehyde. The latter procedures were commonly used in histochemical studies of monoamines (Chapter 17) in the 1960s and 1970s.

Another method for small pieces is **phase partition fixation**, in which the fixative agent is dissolved in a liquid that does not mix with water. A solution of glutaraldehyde in heptane (McAuliffe and Nettleton, 1984) is suitable. When the specimen is immersed, the glutaraldehyde passes from the non-aqueous phase (heptane) into the specimen's aqueous phase (water, of extra- and intracellular fluids). The ionic compositions of fluids in the specimen are not disturbed by dilution with an unnatural aqueous solvent, as they are with conventional immersion or perfusion, and the solvent extracts less protein and free amino acids than an aqueous fixative (Mays et al., 1984). Phase partition fixation in formaldehyde or glutaraldehyde is acceptable for light or electron microscopy (Nettleton and McAuliffe, 1986). In a variant of this method, Sims and Horne (1994) perfused small animals with solutions of osmium tetroxide in a fluorocarbon.

3 | Decalcification and other treatments for hard tissues

When the hard mineral components are the sole objects of interest, a thin section of a dry piece of bone or tooth can be prepared by grinding (see Culling, 1974; Dickson, 1984). This is a skilled and time-consuming procedure that wastes most of the piece being ground, but it provides preparations in which the mineral crystals are clearly visible (see Sanderson, 1997). Hard specimens cannot be sectioned with an ordinary microtome, but they can be softened after fixation, usually by removing the substances responsible for the hardness of the tissue. Decalcification is the chemical dissolution of insoluble calcium salts with a suitable acid or chelating agent. Other approaches are available for softening hard materials that contain silica, or which owe their hardness to compact organic materials.

Tissues such as bone, dentine, horn and wood can be embedded in plastic (Chapter 4) and cut with a particularly rugged microtome, equipped with a chisel-shaped knife of hardened steel. This is the technology of choice in laboratories that specialize in such fields as bone maturation and wood anatomy. Techniques for bone and teeth are thoroughly discussed by Callis (2002) and An and Martin (2004), and methods for hard plant tissues are described in Berlyn and Miksche (1976) and Ruzin (1999).

3.1. Decalcification by acids

The principal mineral component of the calcified tissues of vertebrate animals is a hydroxyapatite formally designated as $Ca_{10}(PO_4)_6(OH)_2$. Like other 'insoluble' salts this exists, when wet, in equilibrium with its saturated solution, which contains very low concentrations of calcium, phosphate, and hydroxide ions:

$$Ca_{10}(PO_4)_6(OH)_2 \rightleftharpoons 10Ca^{2+} + 6PO_4^{3-} + 2OH^-$$

Continuous removal of calcium, phosphate, or hydroxide ions from the solution will prevent the system from reaching equilibrium. The reaction will therefore proceed from left to right until all the hydroxyapatite has dissolved. If the liquid surrounding the specimen has a high concentration of hydrogen ions, the reaction:

$$H^+ + OH^- \rightleftharpoons H_2O$$

will be driven from left to right, removing the hydroxide ions liberated as a result of dissolution of the hydroxyapatite. Any strong acid could serve as a source of hydrogen ions, but those that form sparingly soluble calcium salts (e.g. sulphuric acid) are, for obvious reasons, unsuitable. Hydrochloric, nitric and formic acids are the ones most often used. The overall reactions of these acids with hydroxyapatite are respectively:

$$Ca_{10}(PO_4)_6(OH)_2 + 20H^+ + 20Cl^- \longrightarrow 10Ca^{2+} + 20Cl^- + 6H_3PO_4 + 2H_2O$$

$$Ca_{10}(PO_4)_6(OH)_2 + 20H^+ + 20NO_3^- \longrightarrow 10Ca^{2+} + 20NO_3^- + 6H_3PO_4 + 2H_2O$$

$$Ca_{10}(PO_4)_6(OH)_2 + 20HCOOH \longrightarrow 10Ca^{2+} + 20HCOO^- + 6H_3PO_4 + 2H_2O$$

The calcium from the tissue ends up as calcium ions dissolved in the decalcifying fluid. If the latter is changed frequently the completion of decalcification can be recognized when extracted calcium ions are no longer detectable by a simple chemical test.

The crystal lattice of the hydroxyapatite of bones and teeth incorporates small numbers of carbonate ions in addition to the more abundant phosphates and hydroxides. The mineralized tissue contains, in effect, a small percentage of calcium carbonate. This is dissolved by acids:

$$CaCO_3 + 2H^+ \longrightarrow Ca^{2+} + H_2O + CO_2(g)$$

Minute bubbles of carbon dioxide are formed within and on the surfaces of specimens being decalcified in acids, but they do not usually produce signs of damage visible under the microscope.

Most enzymes are put out of action by acid decalcifying agents, but the structure of the tissue is only slightly disrupted provided that fixation has been adequate. Immunohistochemical staining is often poor after decalcification at low pH, and weaker acids such as acetic (Henzen-Longmans et al., 1985) or ascorbic, pH about 2.5, (Merchan-Perez et al., 1999) are preferred for most antigens.

Decalcification by acids can result in hydrolysis of nucleic acids. RNA is broken into soluble fragments, with resulting reduction or loss of cytoplasmic staining by cationic dyes. The purine and pyrimidine bases are removed from the sugar-phosphate backbone of DNA; this occurs less completely than in a deliberate Feulgen hydrolysis (Chapter 9), but nevertheless interferes with the interpretation of densitometric measurements of histochemically stained sections or with in situ hybridization (Alers et al., 1999). In a comparison of decalcifying solutions Shibata et al. (2000) found that hybridization of labelled probes with mRNA in dental tissues was severely impaired by mineral acids but was satisfactory after solutions containing formic acid.

3.2. Decalcification by chelating agents

A chelating agent is an organic compound or ion that is able to combine with a metal ion to form a compound known as a metal chelate. In the chelate, the metal atom is covalently bound as part of a 5- or 6-membered ring. Chelates are stable compounds and do not readily decompose to liberate metal ions. Consequently, the reaction of a metal ion with a chelating agent, although reversible, proceeds almost to completion if the chelating agent is present in excess.

Ethylenediamine tetraacetic acid (EDTA) forms ordinary salts (four are possible) with sodium and other alkali metals, but the ethylenediamine tetraacetate ions combine with most other metal ions to form stable, soluble chelates. If a piece of calcified tissue is immersed in liquid containing EDTA anions, free calcium ions will be removed from the solution by chelation. Hydroxyapatite will therefore dissolve because it will be unable to attain equilibrium with a saturated solution.

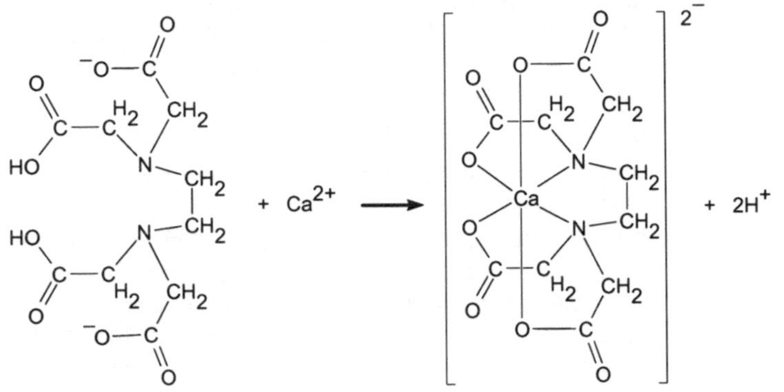

$[EDTA]^{2-}$

As in a solution of the disodium salt of EDTA

$[CaEDTA]^{2-}$

The bonds to the Ca atom are of equal length and mutually at right angles, directed as if to the vertices of a regular octahedron.

For a full account of the chemistry of chelation, see Chaberek and Martell (1959). The chelation of metal ions by dye molecules is described in Chapter 5. of this book. Decalcification by EDTA differs from decalcification by acids in that hydrogen ions play no part in the chemical reaction involved. The chelating agent is used on the alkaline side of neutrality, so the deleterious effects of acids on labile substances such as nucleic acids and enzymes are avoided. Strongly alkaline solutions are not used, however, because they extract proteoglycans from the extracellular matrix of the tissue (Ippolito et al., 1981). The main disadvantage of EDTA is that it acts more slowly than the acids.

Note that EDTA has many names, including versene, sequestrene, edetic acid, eth-ylene-*bis*(iminodiacetic acid) and (ethylenedinitrilo)tetraacetic acid, with corresponding names for the sodium salts. In a solution of any of the salts the number of ionized carboxyl groups available for chelation increases with the pH. A 1% solution of Na_2EDTA has a pH of 5.3 whereas with Na_3EDTA the pH is 9.3 and with Na_4EDTA it is 11.3.

3.3. Decalcification in practice

Specimens that are to be decalcified must be properly fixed and no longer responsive to changes in osmotic pressure. Usually the fixative must be thoroughly washed out of the tissue with water prior to decalcification in order to avoid undesirable chemical reactions. For example, residual sodium phosphates from a buffered formaldehyde fixative would oppose the action of an acid decalcifier. Dichromate ions would be reduced by formic acid, and mercury or zinc would form a chelate with EDTA. The volume of decalcifying fluid should be at least 20 times that of the specimen. An acid mixture is changed every 24–48 h; an EDTA solution every 3–5 days. If the ammonium oxalate test (Section 3.3.3) is to be used, the anticipated last change of decalcifier should have only about five times the volume of the specimen, so that any calcium in the liquid will be present at higher concentration than in a larger volume.

Teeth present various difficulties not encountered with bone. The enamel consists almost entirely of calcium salts, with a tenuous framework of protein that usually collapses after decalcification. The fixative should be one that strongly cross-links protein molecules; glutaraldehyde is suitable. The pulp can shrink, tearing the odontoblast processes, which pass from the pulp into the dentine. This artifact is also reduced by glutaraldehyde fixation (van Wyk, 1993).

3.3.1.
Acid decalcifiers

Formic acid, at pH 1.5 to 3.5 is the decalcifier of choice for most purposes. Several mixtures similar to the one below have been described. Some of them also contain formaldehyde, in an attempt to offset the consequences of inadequate primary fixation. Other organic acids used for decalcification include acetic and citric, which are slow, and lactic, which is nearly as fast as formic (Eggert and Germain, 1979). Adequately fixed specimens (several days in formaldehyde; shorter times in more rapidly acting fixatives) can be decalcified in 1.0 M hydrochloric or nitric acid (Chapter 20). These mineral acids (pH = 0) remove calcified deposits more quickly than formic acid (see Sanderson, 1994). De Castro's fluid is one of many older decalcifying fluids that contain a mineral acid. Ascorbic acid is suitable only for delicate objects containing only thin layers of bone.

An acid decalcifier typically takes 4–5 days to soften a 5 mm cube of cancellous bone (Culling, 1974). Nilsson *et al.* (1991) perfused rats with a fixative, followed by an acid decalcifier for 6 h. This was as effective as immersing fixed tissues for 72 h in the same liquid. A more generally applicable way to reduce the time consists of heating to 55°C in a microwave oven. This is said to produce a 10-fold acceleration of the reaction (Kok and Boon, 1992). Thus, a piece of bone requiring 30 h to decalcify at room temperature can be ready to dehydrate and embed after as little as 3 h in at 55°C.

When decalcification is complete (Section 3.3.3) the specimen should be washed in several changes of water or 70% alcohol.

Buffered formic acid (Clark, 1954)

Formic acid (90%):	250 ml
Water:	750 ml
Sodium formate (HCOONa):	34 g

Alternatively, a solution with the same composition can be made by dissolving 19.8g of sodium hydroxide in 729 ml water and adding 271 ml of 90% formic acid.

This solution keeps indefinitely. Its pH is 2.0, and it produces only minimal suppression of the stainability of nucleic acids. Ippolito *et al.* (1981) found that formic acid at pH 2.0 extracted less proteoglycan from cartilage than 5 other decalcifying agents tested.

De Castro's fluid

Absolute ethanol:	300 ml
Chloral hydrate:	50 g
Water:	670 ml
Concentrated nitric acid (70% HNO_3):	30 ml

Mix in order stated. Keeps indefinitely.

Caution. The nitric acid must be added last. Concentrated HNO_3 reacts explosively with concentrated ethanol.

De Castro's fluid is traditionally used in conjunction with neurological staining methods. It is strongly acidic and decalcifies rapidly. The alcohol and chloral hydrate in the mixture are supposed to prevent swelling of the tissue, presumably by increasing the osmotic pressure of the fluid. This may be unimportant when adequately fixed specimens are being decalcified. However, de Castro's mixture was formerly used as a simultaneous fixing and decalcifying agent. In this circumstance the osmotic effects, as well as the fixative properties of all three ingredients, assumed greater significance.

Ascorbic acid in saline (Merchan-Perez et al., 1999)

Ascorbic acid:	1.0 g
Sodium chloride:	0.85 g
Water:	100 ml

This solution is prepared immediately before use and is used only once. It is suitable for small specimens, notably the inner ears of small animals, with which Merchan-Perez et al. (1999) found immunohistochemical staining for various antigens to be superior to that seen after decalcification in EDTA.

3.3.2.
Chelation with
EDTA

Decalcification with EDTA proceeds much more slowly than with acids, several weeks occasionally being required, but this is not injurious to the tissues. EDTA is frequently used when the sections are to be stained with immunohistochemical methods, and is able to unmask some antigens (Hosoya et al., 2005; see also Chapter 19). After decalcification with EDTA some histochemical methods for enzymes can subsequently be performed upon frozen sections. An EDTA solution is made up immediately before using and is used only once.

Disodium EDTA solution

This solution is recommended for routine decalcification.

Either 5 or 10 g of disodium ethylenediamine tetraacetate, $[CH_2N(CH_2COOH)CH_2COONa]_2.2H_2O$, is dissolved in 100 ml of water, and 4% NaOH is added until the pH is between 7 and 8.

Ammonium EDTA solution

This solution is recommended for specimens containing dense bone. Sanderson et al. (1995) found that it took 6 days to decalcify material that required 18 days in other EDTA mixtures.

Ethylenediamine tetraacetic acid $[CH_2N(CH_2COOH)_2]_2$:	14 g
(Note that this is EDTA acid, not one of its salts.)	
Ammonium hydroxide (ammonia solution, 28–30%, SG 0.9):	9 ml
Water:	76 ml

Stir until dissolved, then add more ammonium hydroxide until the pH is 7.1.

The specimen is put in a perforated plastic casette in the jar containing the EDTA solution, and left on a magnetic stirrer to keep the liquid in gentle motion while decalcification proceeds. An EDTA solution should be changed every third or fourth day. When decalcified, the specimens should be washed in water before dehydration, because the EDTA salts are insoluble in alcohol. (Alcohol-soluble salts of EDTA are available, but according to Eggert et al. (1981) they have no special advantages as histological decalcifying agents.)

3.3.3.
End-point of
decalcification

If the specimen is large enough, extends beyond the region of interest and contains calcified tissue throughout, it may be trimmed with a razor blade or scalpel at intervals during decalcification. When it can be cut easily, it will also be soft enough to be sectioned on a microtome. Sometimes the specimen is too small to be trimmed, or the calcified material is isolated in the middle of the block. An otherwise unwanted piece of bone of approximately the same size can then be processed alongside the specimen. When this piece of bone is fully softened the specimen for histological study should also be decalcified. Specimens should never be tested by poking needles into them; the holes will persist in the sections.

A more exact test for completeness of decalcification makes use of the fact that calcium oxalate, though soluble in mineral acids, is insoluble in water and in aqueous solutions of alkalis.

$$Ca^{2+} + C_2O_4^{2-} + H_2O \longrightarrow CaC_2O_4 \cdot H_2O(s)$$

The test is conducted as follows:

(1) Add drops of strong ammonia solution (ammonium hydroxide, SG 0.9) to about 5 ml of used decalcifying fluid until the mixture becomes alkaline to litmus paper (pH > 7).
(2) Add 5 ml of a saturated aqueous solution of ammonium oxalate (approximately 3% $(NH_4)_2C_2O_4 \cdot H_2O$; can be kept on the shelf for years) and leave to stand for 30 min.

If no white precipitate has formed after this time, the fluid contains no calcium ions. This test can also be used to determine the end-point of decalcification by EDTA, even though solutions of the latter do not contain free calcium ions (Eggert and Germain, 1979). The $[CaEDTA]^{2-}$ anion presumably dissociates as the highly insoluble oxalate is formed. Rosen (1981) recommends adjusting EDTA solutions to pH 3.2–3.6 for maximum sensitivity of the oxalate test.

If an X-ray machine is available, the presence or absence of calcified deposits in a specimen can be demonstrated by radiography. Control specimens known to contain and not to contain calcified material should be X-rayed alongside the specimen being tested in order to assess the amount of radio-opacity due to soft tissues.

It is particularly important to determine the end-point of decalcification when 1.0 M nitric or hydrochloric acid is used, because excessive exposure to these solutions will cause hydrolysis of proteins and macromolecular carbohydrates as well as nucleic acids, with consequent structural damage.

3.4. Softening of non-calcareous materials

Cartilage in vertebrates and **chitin** in arthropods are composed largely of macromolecular carbohydrates, but they often also contain insoluble calcium salts. These materials can be softened to some extent by demineralization in acids or chelating agents. The hard external layer of insect cuticle can be softened with an alkaline hypochlorite solution and removed by careful dissection (Haas, 1992).

Wood is cellulose, reinforced by lignin (Chapter 10), and often contains deposits of silica (SiO_2). Crystals of silica can cause sectioning difficulties with other tissues, including leaves of some grasses. Hydrofluoric acid (HF), which dissolves silica, is sometimes used as a softening agent for hard plant tissues. The concentration may range from 15% to 60% depending on the hardness, applied for 12–36 h (see Ruzin, 1999). If calcium silicate is also present, the solution should also include a little sulphuric acid (Tomasi and Rovasio, 1997). *Extreme caution* is needed when using concentrated hydrofluoric acid: protection of the eyes, hands (nitrile or natural rubber gloves) and body (natural rubber or neoprene apron) and an adequate fume hood. Calcium carbonate or hydroxide powder should be to hand for neutral-izing spills. Calcium fluoride is insoluble and not hazardous. Many institutions require specific training of personnel who are to use HF.

Carlquist (1982) preferred a solution containing ethylenediamine. Its mechanism of action is uncertain. The original author used 4% ethylenediamine, prior to desili-cifying very hard woods with 24% HF (Kukachka, 1977; this publication gives detailed instructions and is freely available on the internet).

Ethylenediamine solution for softening wood (Carlquist, 1982)

Ethylenediamine [$H_2N(CH_2)_2NH_2$]:	10 ml
Water:	to make 100 ml

Caution. Ethylenediamine is a caustic alkali. Keep stoppered to reduce absorption of atmospheric CO_2.

Put boiled or alcohol-fixed wood in the ethylenediamine solution for 3 days. Dehydrate and clear in *t*-butanol (Chapter 4) and embed in paraffin wax. Berlyn and Miksche (1976), Carlquist (1982) and Ruzin (1999) provide many other use-ful practical instructions for processing hard plant tissues.

3.5. Softening specimens already embedded in wax

Incomplete dehydration or clearing is one cause of excessive hardening of normal-ly soft tissues embedded in paraffin, but specimens are sometimes unexpectedly difficult to cut for no discernible reason. Hard material encountered at the time of sectioning can be softened by cutting sections of the trimmed wax block until the tissue is entered, and then immersing the face of the block in water for 15 to 30 min. Water enters the exposed tissue, and often softens it for a depth of up to 500 µm into the block.

Softening agents containing ethanol, glycerol and phenol are preferred to water by many workers, and were found to be superior to plain water in a comparative study by Wynnchuk (1992). A suitable mixture was **Horne's softening agent**, with the following composition:

95% Ethanol:	476 ml
Glycerol:	160 ml
Acetone:	40 ml
Liquid phenol (this is an 80% aqueous solution):	40 ml

For some other softening agents that are easily made in the laboratory, see Sanderson (1994). If the water or softening mixture is cold (0–4°C) it will harden the wax, which also facilitates sectioning.

4 Processing and mounting

This chapter contains some practical instructions for the processing of specimens and the handling of sections and slides. The procedures described are used in nearly all the staining and histochemical techniques presented elsewhere in the book. Much of the underlying theory has already been explained in Chapter 1.

4.1. Processing

For a brief review of dehydration, clearing and embedding, see Wynnchuk (1993). Comprehensive accounts are given by Gabe (1976), Humason (1979), Culling *et al.* (1985), Sanderson (1994), Presnell and Schreibman (1997), Bancroft and Gamble (2002) and Allison (2002). The properties of several of the solvents used in these procedures are summarized in *Table 4.1*.

4.1.1.
Gelatin embedding

Prolonged infiltration with gelatin, followed by drying, gives a hard block from which thin (2 µm) sections may be cut. This classical technique (see Gabe, 1976) has been replaced by the use of synthetic resins (Section 4.1.5), which are easier to use. In modern procedures, the gelatin does not penetrate the minute interstices of a specimen in the same way as paraffin or nitrocellulose. It surrounds the block of tissue and fills in the larger cavities and cracks. This amount of support permits the cutting of frozen sections of objects that would otherwise disperse into fragments when placed into water.

(1) Wash formaldehyde-fixed specimens in a large excess of water for 30–60 min. (If fixation has been brief, as for enzyme histochemistry, use a suitable buffered saline instead of water.)

(2) Infiltrate with the following solution (which has to be melted before use) for 1–2 h at 37°C, with occasional turning of the specimen.

Gelatin powder:	30 g
Glycerol:	30 ml
Water:	140 ml
Thymol (as a bacteriostatic):	1 small crystal

Keeps for a few weeks at 4°C. (For enzyme histochemistry, use freshly dissolved 10% gelatin in buffered saline, for 30 min.)

(3) Orient the specimen in the gelatin in a small petri dish, and place in refrigerator until set: about 1 h.

(4) Cut out a square block, leaving about 3 mm of gelatin around the specimen, and place the block in 4% neutral, buffered formaldehyde (Chapter 2) at 4°C overnight. This will make the gelatin insoluble. For enzyme histochemistry, the treatment with formalin should be much shorter. 2 h at 4°C is recommended.

(5) Cut frozen sections in the usual way, and mount onto slides. Albumen or chrome-gelatin may be used as an adhesive. Dry by draining, and then place the slides on a hotplate (45–50°C) for 10–15 min, or until gelatin begins to soften. (For enzyme histochemistry, omit the heating.)

The gelatin embedding mass, which cannot be removed, is coloured quite strongly by anionic dyes, but this does not interfere with the interpretation of the appearance of the stained section.

Other water-miscible embedding masses are agar and polyacrylamide (Hausen and Dreyer, 1981). The latter is suitable only for specimens to be cut with a cryostat. Neither is as easy to use as gelatin. There are also water-soluble waxes, but they are used only for specialized purposes.

4.1.2.
Dehydration,
clearing, and
paraffin
embedding

As explained in Chapter 1, a specimen can be embedded only after it has been fixed and then equilibrated with a solvent that is miscible with wax. This is typically accomplished by replacing the water in the specimen, first with alcohol and then with a paraffin solvent (clearing agent) such as xylene. Another approach is chemical dehydration (Section 4.1.2.4).

Most paraffin waxes for histology melt at 52–58°C. The melting point can be varied by mixing different waxes; a higher melting point gives a harder block. The properties of paraffin wax are said to be improved by adding extra ingredients. These include beeswax or crepe rubber to promote ribboning of sections, and dimethylsulphoxide (DMSO) to accelerate the penetration of the tissue. Most laboratories buy mixtures that are sold specially for embedding. In these, the paraffin is mixed with a synthetic polymer (sometimes polyisobutylene, but its identity is seldom disclosed by the manufacturer). Wax should be kept about 2°C above its melting point; higher temperatures (above 60°C) are said to degrade the secret additives. The virtues and vices of different waxes and the effects of some added substances were discussed at length by Steedman (1960). More recent studies, which included scanning electron microscopy of the effects of sectioning on the crystalline structures of more than 200 different wax formulations (Allison, 1978, 1979) indicated that known and secret additives hardly altered the properties from those of plain paraffin.

Prolonged immersion in molten wax, especially if the temperature is too high, may cause excessive hardening of the tissue. Gabe (1976) maintained that hardening occurred only if the specimens had not been completely dehydrated. I agree with Gabe; the effects of insufficient infiltration are much more serious than those of

Table 4.1. Properties of solvents used in histology

Name	Refractive index (at 20°C)	Boiling point (°C)	Fire hazard[a]	Remarks
GROUP 1. Dehydrating agents. Miscible with water and with clearing agents (Group 2), but not miscible with melted paraffin wax or with resinous mounting media.				
Acetone	1.36	56	++	The 'absolute' liquids usually contain
Ethanol (ethyl alcohol)	1.36	78	+	about 1% by volume of water, but
Isopropanol (isopropyl alcohol; propan-2-ol)	1.38	80	+	this can usually be ignored. Ethanol and isopropanol are preferred to the
Methanol (methyl alcohol)	1.33	65	+	more volatile solvents for most purposes.
GROUP 2. Clearing agents. Miscible with dehydrating agents (Group 1), melted paraffin wax, and resinous mounting media. Not miscible with water. Tissues become transparent only when the refractive index of the clearing agent is higher than 1.47. Replacement of an 'oily' clearing agent (boiling point above 150°C) by wax is notably slower with a more volatile liquid.				
Amyl acetate (isoamyl acetate)	1.40	142	+	Strong odour of 'pear drops.'
Benzene	1.50	80	+	Avoid inhalation of vapour.
n-Butanol (n-butyl alcohol; butan-1-ol)	1.40	118	+	Partly miscible with water. May be used for dehydration of blotted sections. Less extraction of dyes than with ethanol. Irritating vapour.
Carbon tetrachloride	1.46	77		Toxic vapour.
Chloroform	1.45	61		SG 1.49. Cleared specimens do not sink. Often used mixed with benzene.
Cedarwood oil	1.51	260 (approx.)		Only partly miscible with methanol. Does not harden tissues.
Benzyl benzoate	1.57	323		Almost odourless. Confers transparency.
DL-Limonene	1.47	176		Contained in some proprietary products.
Methyl benzoate (oil of niobe)	1.51	200		Unpleasant odour. Confers transparency.
Methyl siacylate (oil of wintergreen)	1.54	223		Penetrating odour; not unpleasant. Useful for transparent whole-mounts.
Terpineol (mixed isomers; synthetic oil of lilac)	1.48	200 (approx.)		Miscible with ethanol containing up to 15% water. Does not harden tissue.
Toluene	1.50	111	+	Avoid inhalation of vapour.
1,1,1-Trichloroethane (methyl chloroform)	1.44	74		Irritating vapour. Sometimes used as substitute for xylene or toluene.
Xylene (mixed isomers)	1.50	140 (approx.)	+	The most commonly used clearing agent for blocks and sections. Avoid inhalation of vapour.
GROUP 3. Solvents for combined dehydration and clearing. Miscible with water and with melted paraffin wax. Not necessarily miscible with resinous mounting media.				
Acetic acid (glacial acetic acid)	1.37	118		Freezes at 16.6°C. Used in fixatives and for acidifying stains etc. Rarely used for dehydration and clearing.
t-Butanol (tertiary butyl alcohol; 2-methyl-propan-2-ol)	1.39	83	+	Freezes at 26°C. Much used for processing plant specimens.
Dioxane (1,4-dioxane; diethylene oxide)	1.42	101	+	Toxic vapour. Explosive peroxides form in old bottles. Test before using.[b]
Dimethyl sulphoxide	1.48	189		Melting point 18.5°C. Supercools easily.
Tetrahydrofuran (THF) (tetramethylene oxide)	1.41	66	++	Toxic vapour. Explosive peroxides form in old bottles. Test before using.[b]
GROUP 4. Miscellaneous liquids.				
Water	1.33	100		Ethylene glycol, glycerol and propylene glycol are
Ethylene glycol	1.43	198		miscible with water and with dehydrants (Group 1)
Glycerol (glycerin)	1.47	290		but not with clearing agents (Group 2).
Propylene glycol	1.43	188		

Table 4.1. Continued

Name	Refractive index (at 20°C)	Boiling point (°C)	Fire hazard[a]	Remarks
Phenol	1.54 (at 41°C)	182		Melts at 43°C. Soluble in water and in dehydrants, and in even the most hydrophobic clearing agents.[c] Caustic and toxic. Avoid skin contact.
Ether (diethyl ether)	1.35	35	++	Explosive peroxides form in old bottles. Test before using.[b] Used in histology as mixture with ethanol, which dissolves nitrocellulose.
Propylene oxide		34	++	Partly miscible with water; fully with alcohols. Used in epoxy resin embedding.
Acetonitrile	1.35	82	+	Mixes with water and most solvents in Groups 1, 2 and 3 and with epoxy monomers, but not with paraffin. Poisonous.
Ligroin (low boiling)		60–120	++	Ligroin and petroleum ether are sometimes used as
Petroleum ether (mainly hexanes)	1.37 (*n*-hexane)	60 (approx.)	++	clearing agents for paraffin blocks or sections. They are only partly miscible mwith alcohols.
Mineral oil (liquid paraffin, liquid petrolatum)	1.48	360 (minimum)		Not miscible with methanol or ethanol; slight miscibility with isopropanol.
Isopentane (2-methyl butane)	1.42	28	++	Freezes at −160°C. Used in rapid freezing procedures.
Liquid nitrogen		−196		Used in rapid freezing procedures.

* + Indicates the liquid is flammable and should not be used near a naked flame. ++ Indicates the liquid is dangerously flammable. When these liquids are in use, all flames must be extinguished and no smoking allowed anywhere in the room. No symbol in this column means the liquid, if flammable, is not volatile enough to constitute a serious hazard. Water, chloroform, trichloroethylene and carbon tetrachloride are the only volatile liquids in the list whose vapours are non-flammable.

** Test for peroxides: Add 10 ml of the liquid to 1 ml of freshly prepared 10% aqueous potassium iodide. Insert stopper and leave in a dark place for 1 hour, shaking occasionally. If peroxides are present, a brown colour (iodine) develops. Peroxides should be neutralized (by adding some solid ferrous sulphate) before disposing of the solvent.

*** If absolute alcohol is not available, phenol (about 10%) may be added to a clearing agent such as benzene, toluene or xylene. Do not confuse pure (solid) phenol with 'liquefied phenol,' which is an 80–90% solution in water. Phenol may also soften some tissues and facilitate the penetration of the embedding medium.

unnecessarily long exposure to hot paraffin. If the cutting properties of a wax-embedded tissue are unsatisfactory, the block should be melted and the specimen rehydrated and processed again into paraffin. Goss *et al.* (1992) showed that rehydration and re-embedding of routinely processed specimens caused a remarkable inprovement in the histological appearances of lymphoid tissues. This observation indicates that routine procedures for dehydration and clearing may often be inadequate.

Some automated tissue processors provide for intermittent increases of atmospheric pressure, supposedly to force solvents or melted wax into the specimens. External pressure increases the flow (bulk diffusion) of fluids through pores that are more than 0.05 μm wide. Permeation of smaller spaces occurs by mechanisms other than bulk diffusion, and is not affected by pressure. Increased temperature greatly accelerates movement of fluid into the smallest pores (below 2 nm) that exist within and between macromolecules (see Nelson, 2000). Reduced atmospheric pressure, optimistically called **vacuum embedding**, is available with manual and automatic tissue processing equipment. The boiling point of the clearing agent is lowered, accelerating its removal by evaporation while the specimens are being infiltrated with molten wax. Low pressure also helps to remove entrapped air from specimens. One would expect to see damage from the expansion of air bubbles and boiling of solvents; surprisingly, such artifacts are seldom encountered. Probably the solvent vapour dissolves in the wax before microscopic bubbles can form. The more viscous ('oily') clearing agents (Section 4.1.2.1 and *Table 4.1*) have boiling points so high that reduced pressure is unlikely to accelerate their removal from the tissue and replacement by wax. Some oily clearing agents have odours that are evident when the blocks are being sectioned. Retention of one of these liquids within the solidified wax and the embedded specimen may facilitate the cutting of the thin (2–4 μm) sections that are needed for the study of small (0.2–1.0 μm) intracellular objects such as lysosomes, secretory granules and mitochondria (Gabe, 1976).

Heating in wax has been shown to affect the staining properties of tissues. Allison and Bryant (1998) obtained markedly different results with stains for connective tissue after embedding in a wax that melted at 45°C instead of the usual 52–58°C. They suggested that temperature influenced the subsequent permeability of tissues to dye molecules of different sizes.

Safety note. Flammable liquids should not be poured down the sink. They should be collected in metal solvent drums for eventual safe disposal. Chlorinated solvents (with 'chloro' anywhere in the name) are not flammable. For disposal, chlorinated solvents should not be mixed with flammable solvents because incineration generates toxic gases.

4.1.2.1. Standard slow procedure
This 'slow procedure' is suitable for pieces of tissue 3–5 mm thick. The times for washing, dehydration, clearing, and infiltration should be longer for larger specimens.

The starting point given below is water. If alcoholic fixatives have been used, the earlier stages of dehydration are omitted. Throughout the procedure, the volume of liquid should be 10–20 times that of the specimen. The 'alcohol' may be ethanol, methanol, industrial methylated spirit (up to 95%), or isopropanol. The 'oily clearing agent' is one of the more viscous and less volatile liquids from Group 2 of *Table 4.1*: amyl acetate, benzyl benzoate, cedarwood oil, methyl salicylate or terpineol. My favourite is terpineol.

Pass the specimen through:

(1) (Delicate specimens only; most solid pieces can go directly to Step 2.) Two hours in each of 15%, 25%, and 50% alcohol
(2) 70% alcohol: 2 h (or overnight)
(3) 95% alcohol: 2 h
(4) 100% alcohol (1): 2 h
(5) 100% alcohol (2): 1 h
(6) An oily clearing agent (1): 2–24 h
(7) An oily clearing agent (2): 2–24 h
(8) Benzene or toluene 15–30 min
     (to remove oily material from surface of specimen):
(9) Wax (1): 1 h
(10) Wax (2): 1 h
(11) Wax (3): 1 h
(12) Wax (4): 1 h
     The infiltration with wax may be carried out in the oven or in a vacuum-embedding chamber. The latter has the advantages of accelerating removal of volatile solvents and extracting air bubbles.
(13) Block out in wax in a suitable mould.

Delicate specimens are those that contain much water, and include many plant and invertebrate tissues. Other methods for dehydrating delicate specimens are described in Sections 4.1.2.4 to 4.1.2.8. Alcohols are used only once. New solvents must be used for Step 7, but once-used solvent is permissible for Step 6. The first two lots of wax must be discarded after they have been used to infiltrate specimens cleared in non-volatile solvents. The wax from the third or fourth change may be used once again for changes 9 and 10 with subsequent specimens.

4.1.2.2. Standard fast procedure

Viscous clearing agents are not used in this 4- or 5-h procedure, which is based on recommendations of Culling *et al.* (1985) and Sanderson (1994). The prescribed times are for pieces of tissue no more than 3 mm thick. If difficulties are encountered when cutting sections of some tissues, use the more reliable slow method next time. Studies of extraction of [³H]water indicate that dehydration occurs 10–20 times more quickly if the specimens are agitated than if they are left motionless in the solvent (Helander, 1987).

If wax is not adequately removed from paraffin sections, birefringent crystal-like bodies are seen in the tissue, within nuclei. See Nedzel (1951) for further information concerning this interesting artifact.

Pass the specimen through:

(1) (Delicate specimens only; most solid pieces can go directly to step 2.) Thirty min in each of 15%, 25%, and 50% alcohol
(2) 70% alcohol: 30 min (longer if convenient)
(3) 100% alcohol (1):   30 min
(4) 100% alcohol (2):   30 min
(5) 100% alcohol (3):   30 min
(6) Xylene or toluene (1):   15 min
(7) Xylene or toluene (2):   15 min
(8) Wax (1):   30 min
(9) Wax (2):   30 min
(10) Wax (3):   30 min
(Infiltration with wax may be carried out in an oven or a vacuum-embedding chamber.)

Tissue processing machines are available that use microwave heating to accelerate processing and infiltration. Artifacts from inadequate dehydration and excessive heat or vacuum are described and illustrated by Bosch *et al.* (1996).

4.1.2.3. Other clearing agents: xylene substitutes

Alternative clearing agents include benzene, chloroform, or a mixture of chloroform with benzene or toluene (equal volumes). Benzene is avoided in most laboratories (it being a greater fire and toxicity hazard than toluene and xylene). Chloroform, although not flammable, is toxic to the human liver, and produces a variety of other undesirable effects when administered to rats and mice. D-Limonene (an oil extracted from orange peel) and the synthetic DL-limonene (inactive limonene, or dipentene), are sold under several trade-names as 'xylene substitutes'. They penetrate more slowly than xylene, however, and are not miscible with all resinous mounting media (Silverman, 1999). Both limonenes can be recognized by their strong citrus odour. Odourless 'xylene substitutes' are probably mixtures of aliphatic hydrocarbons similar to petroleum ether and ligroin (*Table 4.1*). Mineral oil was recommended by Buesa (2000), following dehydration in an ethanol-isopropanol mixture. These alcohols have only slight solubility (less than 1%) in mineral oil.

4.1.2.4. Automated processing

In early tissue processing machines, a basket of specimens, each in a labelled casette, was moved through a series of solvents and two changes of melted wax. Modern processors hold the casettes in a single container (often called a retort), and the processing fluids are pumped in and out in sequence. There are optional provisions for agitation in solvents and for raised temperature and reduced atmospheric pressure during infiltration with wax. The time at each stage can be set appropriately for the types and sizes of the specimens. Usually a tissue processor is programmed to work overnight, so that the specimens will be infiltrated and ready for blocking out at the start of the working day. A shorter schedule (4–5 h) is suitable for small specimens (least dimension less than 2 mm). The information in *Table 4.2* is based on Allison (2002). For more information see Culling *et al.* (1985) and Carson (1997).

Table 4.2. Schedules for fixed, washed specimens in tissue processing machines

Overnight schedule

Liquid	Temperature	Time
Alcohol (50%)	Room temperature	1 h with agitation
Alcohol (70%)	Room temperature	1 h with agitation
Alcohol (90%)	Room temperature	1 h with agitation
Alcohol (100%)	Room temperature	1 h with agitation
Alcohol (100%)	Room temperature	1 h with agitation
Alcohol (100%)	Room temperature	1 h with agitation
Xylene	Room temperature	1 h with agitation
Xylene	Room temperature	1 h with agitation
Xylene	45°C	1 h with agitation
Paraffin wax	60°C	1 h with vacuum
Paraffin wax	60°C	1 h with vacuum
Paraffin wax	60°C	1 h with vacuum

Rapid schedule for small specimens

Liquid	Temperature	Time
Alcohol (50%)	Room temperature	15 min with agitation
Alcohol (70%)	Room temperature	15 min with agitation
Alcohol (90%)	Room temperature	15 min with agitation
Alcohol (100%)	Room temperature	20 min with agitation
Alcohol (100%)	Room temperature	20 min with agitation
Alcohol (100%)	Room temperature	30 min with agitation
Xylene	Room temperature	15 min with agitation
Xylene	Room temperature	20 min with agitation
Xylene	45°C	30 min with agitation
Paraffin wax	60°C	30 min with vacuum
Paraffin wax	60°C	30 min with vacuum
Paraffin wax	60°C	30 min with vacuum

Each fluid used in a tissue processing machine must be replaced before it is exhausted by undue contamination with the fluid that precedes it in the cycle. Usually the last liquid of a group is replaced with new stock and the preceding liquids are moved back along the processing cycle, with the oldest being discarded. For example, the last of three changes of 100% alcohol is moved into the second place; the first container of 100% alcohol becomes the last change of 95% alcohol, etc. For a processor that is run once a day, Allison (2002) recommends changing the fluids weekly.

4.1.2.5. Methods using only one solvent

Some liquids (Group 3 in *Table 4.1*) are miscible with water and with melted wax, and can therefore be used as combined dehydrating and clearing agents. These solvents are usually rather expensive, but processing is quicker when they are used. It is important that the tissue be adequately fixed and no longer susceptible to changes in osmotic pressure, or the specimens may be distorted by the sudden move from water to the solvent.

(1) Move fixed specimens from water or 70% alcohol into dioxane, tetrahydrofuran or *t*-butanol. Leave for 1–2 h (longer for larger pieces).
(2) Transfer to three more changes of the same solvent, each for 1–2 h. (Only two changes are needed if the procedure was started from 70% alcohol.)
(3) Wax (1): 30 min
(4) Wax (2): 30 min
(5) Wax (3): 30 min
(Infiltration with wax may be carried out in an oven or a vacuum-embedding chamber.)

See *Table 4.1* for safety notes on dioxane and tetrahydrofuran, and remember that *t*-butanol is solid below 26°C.

4.1.2.6. Dehydrating delicate specimens

Specimens that are composed mostly of water, such as parts of plants, many invertebrate animals, some hollow organs, and even the softer solid ones can easily be crushed when being cut or picked up with forceps. Extensive damage is often not evident until stained sections are examined with the microscope. Such specimens are also liable to collapse and distortion if they are not dehydrated gradually. The use of several dilute alcohols (Step 1 of each of the preceding methods) suffices for most such specimens. The following procedure (Berlyn and Miksche, 1976) though slow, is even more gentle:

(1) Place fixed and washed specimens in 5% (v/v) glycerol in water. Allow approximately 10 ml for each specimen, and mark the fluid level on the side of the container.
(2) After about 4 h, put the open container in a vessel with reduced atmospheric pressure (maintained by a water pump or similar source of suction), and wait for most of the water to evaporate. The later stages of evaporation can be hastened by including a dessicant such as silica gel or anhydrous calcium chloride in the container.
(3) When the fluid level indicates that 95% of the volume has been lost, the specimens are dehydrated and equilibrated with glycerol.
(4) Remove most of the glycerol, then pass the specimens through two changes of 100% alcohol, followed by a mixture of equal volumes of alcohol and chloroform (about 4 h for each change).
(5) Clear in chloroform (2 changes, each 2–4 h). The specimens will not become transparent, and they will not sink.
(6) Infiltrate with melted wax (3 changes, each 45 min) and make blocks in the usual way.

A viscous, non-volatile clearing agent (such as cedarwood oil or methyl salicylate; see *Table 2.1*) may be substituted for chloroform, or the chloroform may be mixed with an equal volume of benzene or toluene, to give a liquid in which the specimens can sink.

4.1.2.7. Chemical dehydration

Instead of replacing the water in a specimen with alcohol, dioxane, or the like, it is possible to use a reagent that reacts chemically with water to give liquid products that are miscible with the clearing agent. 2,2-Dimethoxypropane (DMP) is such a reagent. It is a ketal and is hydrolyzed by water in the presence of an acid as catalyst, to yield methanol and acetone:

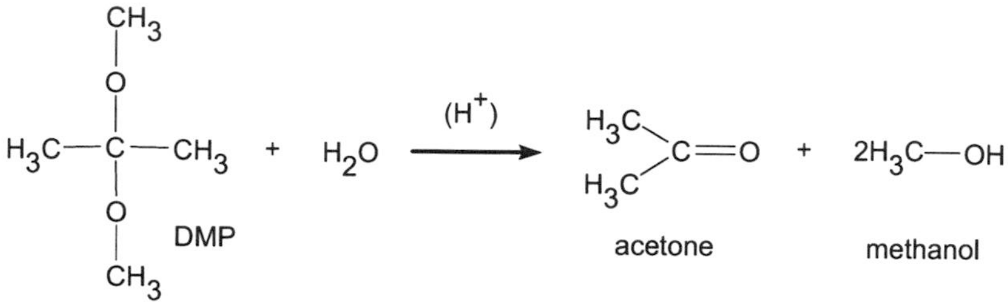

If a reasonable excess of DMP is provided, almost all the water in a specimen will react (Erley, 1957). The hydrolysis is a strongly endothermic reaction, so it is advisable to warm the specimen and the acidified DMP to about 30°C to minimize the risk of formation of ice within the specimen while it is being penetrated by the reagent (Prento, 1978). When dehydration is complete, the specimen is equilibrated with a mixture of DMP, methanol, and acetone. DMP itself is immiscible with water but it is fully miscible with most organic solvents and with paraffin wax, and it extracts most lipids from the tissue (Beckmann and Dierichs, 1982). Acetone and methanol do not mix with melted paraffin however, so the specimens must be cleared before infiltration.

Several practical procedures for chemical dehydration with DMP have been described. The following method (based on my experiences) is suitable for fixed pieces of tissue 1–5 mm thick. Much larger objects can be dehydrated by increasing the time for Step 3 to 12–24 h.

(1) Add 0.02 ml (1 tiny drop) of concentrated hydrochloric acid to 50 ml of 2,2-dimethoxypropane (DMP) and stir thoroughly. 5–10 ml is needed for each specimen. (Any left-over acidified DMP can be kept, but it evaporates quickly if not covered.)

(2) Warm the acidified DMP and the specimen (which may be in water or 70% alcohol) to 25–35°C. This is conveniently done by standing the vials on top of an oven or hotplate.

(3) Place each specimen in 5–10 ml of the warm acidified DMP. Leave for 30–60 min, with agitation at 15 min intervals.

(4) Clear in benzene, toluene or xylene (15 ml per specimen) for 15–60 min, with occasional agitation. Larger specimens will take longer. Only one change of the clearing agent is needed. More viscous clearing agents such as terpineol, benzyl benzoate may also be used, as may a 1:1 mixture of DMP with mineral oil, followed by 2 changes of pure mineral oil (Moller and Moller, 1994).

(5) Infiltrate with molten wax (3 changes, each 45 min), and make blocks in the usual way.

DMP is not a viscous liquid. Its rather slow penetration is probably due to immiscibility with water. Specimens more than about 6 mm thick cannot be dehydrated with DMP by the method given above, but overnight immersion in a single change of the reagent (10 times the volume of the specimen) will completely dehydrate pieces of tissue 2 cm thick (Conway and Kiernan, 1999). According to Zuniga *et al.*

(1994), sponges and corals processed through DMP and methyl salicylate exhibit structural preservation superior to that attained by dehydration through graded alcohols. Although DMP is more expensive than the commonly used alcohols, its use can save money because of the much smaller volume needed (Conway and Kiernan, 1999).

4.1.2.8. Microwave oven methods

Microwave irradiation can deliver heat uniformly to water, organic solvents and melted wax. The heating accelerates the penetration of these liquids, and the time from the end of fixation to blocking out can be less than 2 h. In the fastest microwave procedures, specimens are transferred directly from isopropanol into wax, despite the immiscibility of the two liquids, and the solvent is removed by boiling under reduced pressure (see Kok and Boon, 1992). These procedures require a special laboratory microwave oven in which the temperature and evacuation can be precisely controlled. Otherwise, excessive heating introduces a variety of artifacts, and unduly rapid boiling of the solvent makes clefts and holes in the tissue (Bosch *et al.*, 1996). Microwave heating can also lead to uneven penetration of solvents and paraffin, which move move unduly rapidly through porous tissue components such as plant cell walls; for an illustrated account and practical recommendations, see Schichnes *et al.* (2005). The capabilities of modern laboratory microwave ovens are reviewed by Galvez (2006).

4.1.3.
Nitrocellulose
embedding

Cellulose nitrates are products of reaction of cellulose with nitric acid. They are not nitro compounds, but the word nitrocellulose has been in widespread use for many years. Types of nitrocellulose suitable for use in histology are sold under such names as celloidin, Parlodion, Necolloidin, and low-viscosity nitrocellulose (LVN). Stock solutions of nitrocellulose are made up well in advance (or bought ready-made) and are stored in tightly screw-capped bottles. They are dangerously flammable. Those required are: 8%, 4%, and 2% nitrocellulose, dissolved in a mixture of equal volumes of ethanol and diethyl ether. The times given below are for specimens approximately 15 mm thick. They may be halved for specimens 5 mm thick. The volume of liquid should be 5–10 times that of the specimen.

The tissue is equilibrated with absolute ethanol and then transferred to a securely stoppered glass tube, in:

(1) Ether–alcohol mixture: Overnight
(2) 2% nitrocellulose: 1 week
(3) 4% nitrocellulose: 1 week
(4) 8% nitrocellulose: 1 week

(For low viscosity nitrocellulose the instructions are different. See below.)

Orient the infiltrated specimen in a suitable mould, which must have a removable cover and be at least three times as deep as the specimen. Mark the level of the surface of the 8% nitrocellulose solution on the outside of this container. Leave covered for 12 h or until free of bubbles, then remove the lid and place the mould in a desiccator, with the lid partly open, in a fume hood. Leave until the depth has halved as a result of slow evaporation of the solvent. This takes 2–10 days. Put some chloroform in the bottom of the desiccator, close the lid, and leave for a further 48 h. The nitrocellulose is hardened by the action of the chloroform vapour. Cut out a block containing the specimen and glue it with 4% nitrocellulose to a wooden block. Store the block in 70% ethanol, which causes further hardening of the embedding medium. Hardened nitrocellulose blocks must not be allowed to dry out.

For **low viscosity nitrocellulose (LVN)**, use 5%, 10%, and 20% solutions of LVN in ether–alcohol containing 0.5% of castor oil. The times of infiltration given above may be halved, and evaporation is allowed to proceed only until a hard crust has formed. Culling (1974) gives a full account of the use of LVN.

Other embedding media that can be concentrated by evaporation of their solvents include polystyrene (Frangioni and Borgioli, 1979) and fully polymerized methyl methacrylate (Gorbsky and Borisy, 1986), but these are not often used.

4.1.4. Double embedding

4.1.4.1. Nitrocellulose and paraffin

Hardened nitrocellulose can itself be infiltrated with melted wax in the procedure known as double embedding. This should be used for specimens that contain both hard and soft tissues. Some published methods probably do not introduce enough nitrocellulose into the specimen to make much difference to the hardness of the softer tissues. The following procedure (Kiernan, 1998; based on Pfühl's method as cited by Gabe, 1976) is slow, but it allows thorough infiltration with nitrocellulose, which is then hardened by chloroform and by the action of the phenol dissolved in the clearing agent.

Nitrocellulose solutions

2% and 4% nitrocellulose (celloidin, Parlodion, LVN) in *either* ether–alcohol (50:50) *or* absolute methanol.

These solutions are stable indefinitely. Evaporative losses can be made good by topping up with the solvent.

Caution. Dangerously flammable.

Phenolic toluene (clearing agent)

Weigh out 100 (±10) g of solid phenol into a beaker. Stand it in an oven at 60°C until all melted, then pour it into 800 ml of toluene in a 1 l bottle. Add toluene to make 1000–1100 ml. (The original method called for benzene. Toluene is a safer substitute.)

Keeps for 10 years in a dark cupboard. Light brown discoloration does not matter; discard when dark brown.

Procedure

(1)	Dehydrate specimens into methanol:	4 to 8 h.
(2)	2% nitrocellulose:	1 to 4 days.
(3)	4% nitrocellulose:	2 to 8 days (twice as long as step 2)
(4)	Wipe off excess nitrocellulose, and transfer to chloroform:	1 to 2 days
(5)	Clear in phenolic toluene:	12 to 24 h
(6)	Infiltrate with wax (4 changes, each 2 h) and make blocks in the usual way.	

4.1.4.2. Agar and paraffin

Specimens too small to be easily seen with the unaided eye, such as oocytes, early embryos and small aquatic organisms, can be embedded in paraffin if they are carried in a larger object. Agar, a mixture of neutral and sulphated polysaccharides extracted from certain marine algae, provides suitable support. Agar sets at about 40°C but has to be heated to 70°C to be melted. The original technique of Chatton (1923) was improved by Samuel (1944), whose method is summarized here. Suspended cells or protozoans can also be embedded in agar before processing into paraffin.

Solutions required

A. **1.3% Agar**
    Dissolve 1.3 g of agar in 95 ml of water (requires heating to near boiling). When cool add 5 ml of formalin (which is 40% formaldehyde, see Chapter 2). Store in a large test-tube.

B. **0.65% Agar**

As for Solution A, but with 0.65 g of agar.

Both solutions can be kept indefinitely as gels at room temperature. For use, melt the agar by standing the tubes in boiling water, then transfer to a water bath at 40°C. The solutions remain liquid at this temperature; they solidify quite quickly at room temperature.

Procedure

(1) Make a layer of 1.3% agar (Solution A) on a glass slide and allow it to solidify.
(2) Using a Pasteur pipette transfer the fixed and washed specimen to the slide. Draw off excess water with a piece of filter paper.
(3) Place a drop of 0.65% agar (Solution B) over the specimen and allow it to solidify.
(4) Make a layer of 1.3% agar (Solution A) over the whole preparation and allow it to solidify.
(5) Cut from the slide a piece of agar that includes the whole drop of 0.65% agar containing the specimen. If the enclosing layers of 1.3% agar begin to separate, seal them together by touching with a hot (60–80°C) metal rod.
(6) Transfer the agar sandwich to 15% alcohol.
(7) Complete the dehydration, clear and embed in paraffin wax (see the parts of Section 4.1.2 that relate to delicate specimens. See also *Notes 1* and *2* below.

Notes

(1) Samuel (1944) dehydrated in an apparatus that added 100% alcohol dropwise, with stirring, so that the transition from 10 ml of 15% to about 100 ml of 90% alcohol occurred overnight.
(2) A few drops of an alcoholic eosin solution added to the final dehydrating alcohol stains the specimen more strongly than the agar. When in the clearing agent, the agar sandwich can be examined on a microscope slide and cut with a flat facet for correct orientation when blocking out into wax.
(3) **Agarose**, which is a neutral polysaccharide (not stained by cationic or anionic dyes), may be substituted for agar.
(4) A slab of 2% aqueous agarose, 30 × 20 × 15 mm, dehydrated, cleared and embedded in paraffin, is used to prepare tissue **microarrays**. Multiple cores, 0.6 to 2 mm in diameter are collected from paraffin blocks and inserted into holes in the agarose-paraffin block. When the block is heated to allow fusion of the inserted cores with the paraffin of the recipient block, the embedded agarose limits movement of the tissue fragments (Yan *et al.*, 2007). A microarrray can contain up to 300 items, which are identified from their noted X–Y coordinates in the composite block.
(5) In the original technique (Chatton, 1923) small organisms were simply placed in a drop of agar (1.2% in water), which was then allowed to set before processing.

4.1.5.
Embedding in plastic

Synthetic resins ('plastics') are the only acceptable embedding media for electron microscopy. The principles involved in their use are simple: the specimen is infiltrated with a reactive monomer (small molecules), which is then polymerized to form the plastic (large molecules or a cross-linked matrix). Resins are harder than wax or nitrocellulose, making possible the cutting of the ultrathin sections needed for transmission electron microscopy. It is also possible to cut sections at 0.5–3.0 μm for light microscopy. Much more fine detail is visible than in sections of wax-embedded material, which cannot usually be sectioned below 4 μm. Specimens for electron microscopy, which are less than 1 mm across, are cut with glass or diamond knives. Larger specimens for light microscopy must be cut with a steel knife or with a special long glass knife (known as a Ralph knife), and the plastic should not be as hard as it is for cutting ultrathin sections. The desired hardness is attained by mixing the monomer with either wax or a wax-like plasticizer. This is more conveniently done with methacrylate resins than with the epoxy resins favoured by electron microscopists.

Methacrylates are esters with the general formula $H_2C=C(CH_3)COOR$, in which the $C=O$ bond is conjugated with the $C=C$ bond. R is methyl in methyl methacrylate, n-butyl in n-butyl methacrylate, or 2-hydroxyethyl in glycol methacrylate. A methacrylate polymerizes thus:

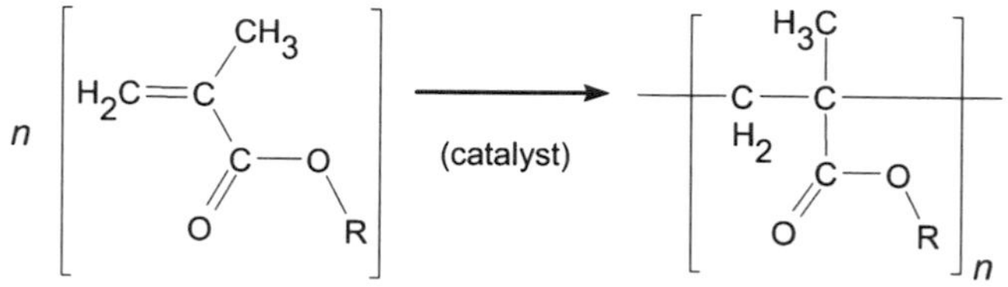

R = CH_3 in methyl methacrylate, n-C_4H_9 in butyl
methacrylate or CH_2CH_2OH in glycol methacrylate

The monomer supplied by the manufacturer contains a stabilizer, often hydroquinone, to retard spontaneous polymerization. The stabilizer can be removed, but an easier way to overcome its action is to add more of the polymerization catalyst (typically benzoyl peroxide) than would otherwise be needed. Butyl methacrylate was the first synthetic resin to be used in histology (Newman et al., 1949).

Two procedures are briefly described below. Techniques for cutting the sections are outside the scope of this book, and the original references should be consulted for technical details.

4.1.5.1. Butyl methacrylate with paraffin

Specimens up to 5 mm thick, fixed in formaldehyde or glutaraldehyde, should be post-fixed in Bouin, which was found by Engen and Wheeler (1978) to improve staining and also the handling properties of the sections.

(1) Dehydrate in graded alcohols.
(2) Transfer from absolute alcohol into two changes of n-butyl methacrylate (each 2 h), and then into the following mixture:
    Butyl methacrylate: 10 ml
    Paraffin wax: 3.5 g
(3) Mix and put in an oven at 60°C, 2–3 h before using. Then add:
    Benzoyl peroxide: 120–460 mg

The optimum amount of catalyst should be determined by trial and error (McMillan et al., 1983). It varies among batches of butyl methacrylate. 200 mg is suggested for the first attempt.

Leave at 50°C for 18–24 h (or longer if necessary, until hard). The container may be a gelatin capsule, a disposable plastic ice-cube holder, or a peel-away embedding mould. Oxygen inhibits polymerization and should be excluded by covering the surface of the liquid with a sheet of plastic or (preferably) by having an atmosphere of nitrogen in the oven.

Allow the polymerized block to cool, then trim it (using a small hacksaw) to within 1–2 mm of the tissue. Place the block in melted paraffin for 30 min, and cast a new block, so that the plastic-embedded specimen is surrounded by wax. Mount this block on the microtome and section at 1–4 µm. (For cutting techniques, see papers cited above.)

The embedding media are removed from the sections with xylene before staining.

4.1.5.2. Glycol methacrylate

Glycol methacrylate (2-hydroxyethyl methacrylate) is miscible with water or alcohol, but its polymer is insoluble in all common solvents, so the sections have to be stained in the presence of the embedding mass. Fixed specimens may be dehydrated in ethanol or in glycol methacrylate. They are then placed in the embedding medium:

Glycol methacrylate:	95 g
Polyethylene glycol 400:	5 g
Benzoyl peroxide:	1.5 g

Two changes, each 1 h, are recommended. The specimens are then transferred to a third change, in embedding blocks, with exclusion of oxygen (see previous method) at 40°C. Polymerization may take as long as 4 days. See Bennett et al. (1976), Murgatroyd (1976), Hayat (1981) and Sanderson (1994) for more information, including alternative embedding mixtures. The polymerized resin is hydrophilic, but cannot be removed. It is penetrated by aqueous stains and other reagents, but longer times are usually needed than for dewaxed paraffin sections. Adaptations of many staining methods for tissues embedded in poly(glycol methacrylate) are given by Litwin (1985).

4.1.6. Embedding in polyethylene glycol

Polyethylene glycols (PEGs) are also known as carbowaxes. They are liquid and solid polymers of the form:

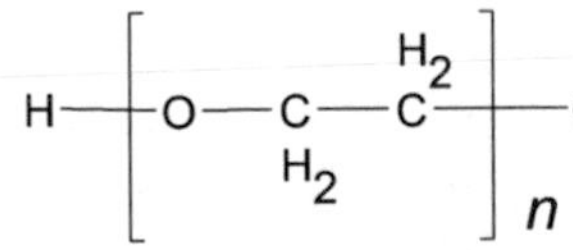

$$H \left[O - \underset{H_2}{\overset{H_2}{C}} - C \right]_n OH$$

(Formula weight of each repeating unit = 44.05)

They are named from the average molecular weights of the polymers. For example, an average macromolecule in PEG-2000 contains 45 or 46 $-OCH_2CH_2-$ units. PEGs with molecular weights 1000–5000 melt at 40–60°C and can be cut on the type of microtome that is used for tissues embedded in paraffin waxes. The abundance of hydroxyl groups makes PEGs strongly hydrophilic, so it is possible to use them for dehydrating as well as for embedding specimens (Blank and McCarthy, 1950).

Avoidance of organic solvents and high temperature are appropriate in preparing tissues for enzyme histochemistry, and PEGs have been used for this purpose (Rohlich, 1956). They have also been used to dehydrate and embed tissues for subsequent immunohistochemistry (Smithson et al., 1983; Gao and Godkin, 1991). PEGs are disliked and generally avoided, however, because (a) they absorb water from the air in humid weather, (b) they are more difficult to section than paraffin wax, (c) the sections cannot usually be flattened by floating on water, and (d) differential shrinkage artifacts can be worse than in paraffin or frozen sections.

It is generally easier to cut and mount cryostat sections than sections of PEG-embedded tissue.

The distortion of polypeptide chains and extraction of lipids that occur during dehydration, clearing and paraffin embedding expose many amino acid sequences that were originally folded into hydrophobic domains. This makes them accessible to large antibody molecules. Consequently paraffin sections allow the immunohistochemical detection of many antigens (see also Chapter 19), but there are others that lose their capacity to combine with antibodies following the same treatments. Klosen *et al.* (1993) determined that this loss of immune reactivity was caused not by dehydration or heating but by infiltration with paraffin. In the light of these findings they developed a procedure in which tissues were dehydrated in ethanol and then slowly infiltrated with PEG-1000 followed by a mixture of PEG-1000 and PEG-1500, in which blocks were made. Dehydration in ethanol averted the uneven shrinkage seen in specimens that were dehydrated in PEG-1000, and it also protected against an unexplained loss of antigen that occurred if alcohol was not used. Several other embedding procedures using PEGs for subsequent immunohistochemistry are described in a book edited by Gao (1993).

4.1.7.
Polyester wax

In the 1980s another alcohol-soluble embedding medium, Steedman's (1960) polyester wax, was rediscovered (Kusakabe *et al.*, 1984) and found to conserve antigens effectively for immunohistochemistry, but the method has not yet become fashionable. When I tried to use a commercially available polyester wax, I encountered great difficulty cutting longitudinal sections of peripheral nerve, a tissue that never gave trouble in paraffin. These difficulties probably could have been overcome with perseverance, but the economics of research seldom permit the dedication of a full-time investigator or technician to an individual procedure, and a service laboratory must use sectioning techniques that are reliable for a wide variety of purposes.

4.2. Keeping sections on slides

4.2.1.
Adhesives for sections

Properly flattened sections will usually stick to grease-free glass slides without the assistance of an adhesive. Thin sections (<7 μm) generally stick better than thicker ones. For most purposes, however, the use of an adhesive is strongly advised. It is essential when the sections are to be exposed to solutions more alkaline than about pH 8. The two adhesives given below are suitable for sections to be stained by almost any techniques. Mayer's albumen has better keeping properties than chrome-gelatin, but the latter is much more efficacious, especially for protection against alkaline reagents. Albumen may be preferable to gelatin if strong acids are used, as in the hydrolysis of nucleic (Chapter 9) or sialic (Chapter 11) acids.

4.2.1.1. Mayer's albumen

Preparation (*three possibilities are available*)
(a)   Collect the whites of one or two eggs into a graduated 250 ml beaker. Add an equal volume of glycerol and mix thoroughly. Filter through cloth and then through cotton wool or coarse filter paper. Filtration is accelerated if carried out in an oven at 55°C. Add a small crystal of thymol to inhibit growth of micro-organisms.
(b)   Make a 5% solution of dried egg-white (commonly called 'albumen, egg' in catalogues) in 0.5% aqueous sodium chloride. It takes a day to dissolve, with occasional stirring. Filter through coarse filter paper and add an equal volume of glycerol to the filtrate. Add a crystal of thymol.
(c)   Buy a ready-made Mayer's albumen solution.

These solutions will keep for several years at room temperature.

Application
Place a *small* drop (1–1.5 mm diameter) on a slide and distribute it evenly over the surface with the tip of a finger. Float out the sections on water, collect onto the slide, drain, and flatten in the usual manner.

Alternatively, do not put Mayer's albumen solution on the slides but add about 20 ml of it to each litre of the water used for floating out the sections.

When the slides have dried, put them in an oven (about 60°C) for 30 min or turn up the temperature of the hotplate used for drying the slides. The heat coagulates the egg albumen. The melting of the wax also promotes closer contact between the sections and the glass. Albumen is lightly stained by most dyes and is most conspicuous around the sites of the edges of the wax ribbon. The layer between the sections and the slide must be extremely thin.

4.2.1.2. Chrome-gelatin

Preparation
Dissolve 1.0 g gelatin powder (a high quality, intended for bacteriological use, gelatin is advised) in 80 ml of warm water and allow to cool. Dissolve 0.1 g chrome alum (chromic potassium sulphate: $CrK(SO_4)_2.12H_2O$) in 20 ml of water.

Mix the two solutions. This mixture quickly becomes infected and should not be used if it is more than 3 days old. The solution cannot be diluted after mixing the two ingredients.

Application
Place a *large* drop (3–5 mm diameter) on a slide, spread it over the surface with a finger, and leave for about 10 min to dry.

Another method is to make a more dilute solution (0.1% gelatin, 0.01% chrome alum), immerse the slides in it, drain, and dry. The staining rack also becomes coated with chrome-gelatin, which accumulates with repeated uses.

Treatment of slides with chrome-gelatin is often called 'subbing'. Subbed slides may be kept for at least 3 months if protected from dust. Float the sections onto the slides, flatten, drain and dry in the usual way.

4.2.1.3. Albumin–glutaraldehyde
This method, developed by Ichikawa and Ajiki (1992), was found to be more effective than treating slides with gelatin, egg-white or polylysine, for preventing section losses with *in situ* hybridization histochemistry. Albumin–glutaraldehyde treatment was also favoured by Nakae and Stoward (1997) for adhesion of unfixed cryostat section for dehydrogenase activity histochemistry; their method is given below.

(1)   Dip slides in a 1% aqueous solution of bovine albumin for 5 min at room temperature.
(2)   Air-dry the slides in an oven at 60°C for 3 h.
(3)   Immerse the slides in 2.5% aqueous glutaraldehyde for 3 min at room temperature.
(4)   Rinse the slides in 3 changes of water, each 10 min.
(5)   Dry at 60°C overnight.

The concentration of glutaraldehyde is probably not critical. Ichikawa and Ajiki (1992) used a 25% solution. These authors specified autoclaved distilled water for Step 4, and used the slides within 2 weeks of coating.

4.2.1.4. Silanized slides

Treatment with a reactive silicon compound chemically changes glass, such that it bears abundant amino groups, which ionize to provide a positively charged surface.

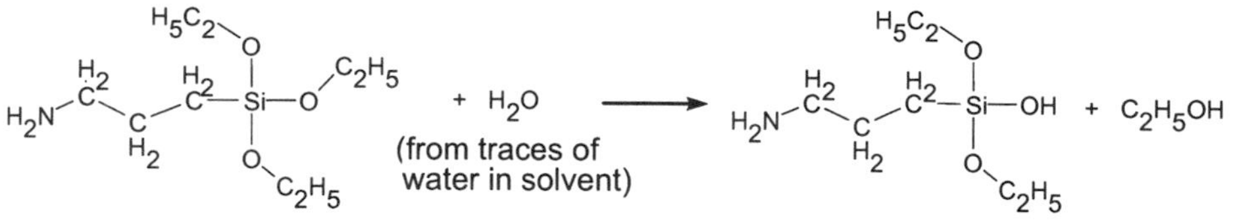

3-aminopropyltriethoxysilane

surface of glass

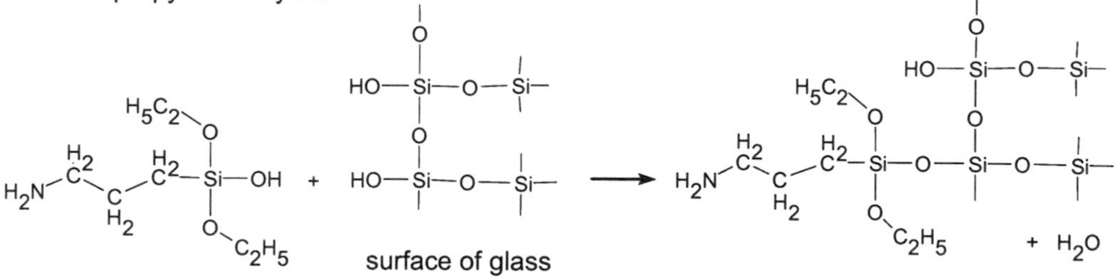

Sections (which contain a preponderance of anionic groups such as carboxyls and sulphate-esters) adhere strongly to such the modified glass. Slides that have been treated in this way (silanized slides) are available commercially, but are expensive. It is easy to make them in the laboratory, however. The only reagents needed are 3-aminopropyltriethoxysilane (a liquid; store at 4°C) and acetone.

(1) Put clean, dry new slides in a glass staining tray that will fit into a small (200 ml) staining tank. A larger (300–400 ml) tank will also be needed. (If the slides were not bought pre-cleaned, they must be thoroughly degreased, washed, rinsed in 95% alcohol, and dried.)

(2) Add 4 ml of 3-aminopropyltriethoxysilane to 200 ml of acetone in the small staining tank. This can be used for hundreds of slides, but the solution is not stable and must be used on the day it is made.

(3) Immerse the slides in the solution for 30–60 s.

(4) Shake off excess liquid and transfer to distilled water in the larger tank. Agitate and leave for about 1 min.

(5) Remove the washed slides and let them stand for 1 h or more (until dry) before packing them in their boxes. Label the boxes so you will know they contain silanized slides.

Other adhesives for sections include starch, various synthetic glues (Edwards and Price, 1982; Jarvinen and Rinne, 1983) and making the glass surface cationic by spraying it with a polylysine solution (Thibodeau et al., 1997) or by staining it with alcian blue (Archimbaud, Islam and Preisler, 1986). A thin film of nitrocellulose (Fink, 1987) or polyvinylformal (formvar; Slater, 1989) promotes adhesion of glycol methacrylate sections. In a comparative study of section adhesion, Marcos et al. (2001) found chrome-gelatin and APES treatment of slides to be equally effective and superior to Mayer's albumen or polylysine.

4.2.2. Coating slides with nitrocellulose

When mounted sections have to be subjected to rough treatment, especially immersion in alkalis or hot acids, it is advisable to supplement the adhesive by encasing the slide in a film of nitrocellulose. This will hold the sections in place if there is failure of the adhesion between tissue and glass. The film should cover the whole slide (both surfaces and all four edges) if it is to be effective. The procedure is as follows:

(1) Take slides to absolute alcohol.
(2) Immerse in ether–alcohol (equal volumes of ethanol and diethyl ether) for 30–60 s.
(3) Immerse in a 0.2–0.4% solution of nitrocellulose in ether–alcohol for 30 s. (The solution is made by diluting one of the stock solutions kept for nitrocellulose embedding. **Caution.** Ether is volatile and dangerously flammable.
(4) Lift out the slides, drain, and allow them to become almost dry. A change in the reflection of light from the glass surface indicates the moment at which to move on to Stage 5. This end-point is easily learned with a little practice.
(5) Place the slides in 70% ethanol for 2 min to harden the film of nitrocellulose.
(6) Carry out the staining procedure. Dehydrate as far as the 95% alcohol stage.
(7) Transfer the slides from 95% alcohol into ether–alcohol, with minimum agitation. Leave in ether–alcohol for 2–3 min to dissolve the nitrocellulose film and complete the dehydration.
(8) Carefully take the slides from ether–alcohol into xylene (1 min) and then into a second change of xylene (at least 1 min). Try not to agitate the slides: this could loosen the sections.
(9) Apply coverslips, using a resinous mounting medium.

4.3. Mounting media

4.3.1.
Resinous media

Resinous mounting media are of three types: natural, semi-synthetic, and wholly synthetic. They are miscible with xylene, but not with alcohol or water. Instructions for making several resinous mounting media are given by Lillie and Fullmer (1976), but it is generally best to buy them ready-made. Unfortunately, many useful media are obtained as products of undisclosed composition. Natural and semi-synthetic mountants are often autofluorescent. Most wholly synthetic media are non-fluorescent, and therefore suitable for use with specimens to be examined by fluorescence microscopy.

4.3.1.1. Canada balsam
This, the traditional natural mounting medium, is the resin of a fir, *Abies balsamea*. 'Natural' Canada balsam, which contains the volatile components of the resin, is a viscous yellow liquid that softens when warmed (Gray, 1954). Dried balsam is a solid, and must be mixed with xylene to give a workable mounting medium. 500 g dry balsam is dissolved in 100 ml xylene. It takes a few days to dissolve.

Unsaturated compounds in the resin make Canada balsam a mild reducing agent. Consequently, preparations stained with dyes fade after months or years in this medium. However, the black colour of cobalt sulphide (a product of some histochemical reactions, which is slowly decolorized by atmospheric oxidation) lasts longer in Canada balsam than in synthetic resins. Acidic components of Canada balsam, notably abietic acid, $C_{19}H_{29}COOH$, may contribute to the deterioration of specimens stained by cationic dyes and the preservation of anionic stains. Other natural resins used in mounting media include **dammar** and **sandarac**. Their effects on stained material are similar to those of Canada balsam. Canada balsam is much more expensive than synthetic mounting media.

4.3.1.2. Synthetic resins
A polystyrene-based medium, **DPX**, is recommended for all purposes except the preservation of cobalt sulphide deposits. It contains polystyrene (MW 80 000, formerly known as distrene-80), a plasticizer (tri-*o*-cresyl phosphate or dibutyl phthalate), and xylene. DPX contains no acids or reducing agents, and is non-fluorescent. The plasticizer modifies the physical properties of the polymer, preventing the

formation of cracks and bubbles under the coverslip. DPX is usually bought, but it can be made in the laboratory (Lillie and Fullmer, 1976):

Add polystyrene beads (25 g) to dibutyl phthalate (5 ml) and xylene (65–75 ml).

Dissolution takes a few days.

The addition of 0.1 ml of 2-mercaptoethanol (foul smell!) to each 10 ml of DPX gives a medium in which the fading of fluorescent dyes is retarded (Franklin and Filion, 1985).

Immunofluorescent preparations are permanent when mounted in DPX and stored in darkness at room temperature (Espada *et al.*, 2005). Unsatisfactory batches of DPX, containing tiny refractile droplets, are occasionally encountered.

Alternative non-fluorescent synthetic media include 'Entellan', 'Cytoseal' and many others that are stated by the manufacturers to contain acrylic polymers, dissolved in toluene or xylene. Other compounds such as plasticizers are probably also present. Many proprietary mounting media are 'semisynthetic', containing polymers of β-pinene, cycloparaffins etc. Most of these, like Canada balsam, have intrinsic fluorescence that is easily seen in areas of the slide where only the mounting medium is present. Such areas are black if the mounting medium is non-fluorescent.

4.3.2.
Aqueous media

Water-miscible media can be bought but are easily made in the laboratory (Kiernan, 1997). Five are listed below. An aqueous mounting medium should be stored in a screw-capped bottle. Care is necessary to ensure that the lid does not become too firmly cemented on.

Aqueous media are often used in conjunction with fluorescence microscopy, and some of the mixtures listed below include substances that retard the fading of fluorochromes. Such additives probably work by combining with oxygen free radicals that form as a result of intense illumination in the fluorescence microscope.

4.3.2.1. Glycerol jelly

Gelatin powder:	10 g
Water:	60 ml
Dissolve by warming, and add:	
Glycerol:	70 ml

Add *either* one drop of saturated aqueous solution of phenol *or* 15 mg of sodium merthiolate as an antibacterial agent. Keeps for a few weeks at 4°C. Discard when turbid or mouldy.

Glycerol jelly must be melted and freed of air bubbles before use. This is conveniently done in a vacuum-embedding chamber. Because of the low refractive index (1.42), many unstained structures remain visible in this medium.

4.3.2.2. Buffered glycerol with an anti-fading agent

This does not solidify, but the coverslip can be held in position by applying a little nail varnish or DPX to its edges. Buffered glycerol is used for fluorescent immunohistochemical preparations (Chapter 19). The high pH provides for optimally efficient fluorescence. The added *p*-phenylenediamine (PPD) (Platt and Michael, 1983) or *n*-propyl gallate (Longin *et al.*, 1993; Battaglia *et al.*, 1994), retards fading.

Buffer:	
Either 0.1 M Sodium phosphate buffer (pH 7.4):	10 ml
or 0.1 M TRIS buffer (pH 9.0):	10 ml

Anti-fading agent:
Either p-phenylenediamine hydrochloride: 100 mg
or n-propyl gallate: 500 mg
Glycerol: 90 ml

Keeps for 3 months in darkness at −20°C.

4.3.2.3. Fructose syrup

This medium is sticky enough to hold a coverslip in position. It is very easy to use, but too acid for preserving cationic dyes. With long storage it will evaporate and crystallize; this can be prevented by scaling the edge of the coverslip with a thin bead of resinous mounting medium.

Fructose (laevulose):   15 g
Water: 5 ml

Put together in a securely capped bottle and leave at 60°C for 1–2 days, until all the sugar has dissolved to form a clear syrup. Keeps for several months.

4.3.2.4. Apathy's medium

Gum arabic (=gum acacia):   50 g
Sucrose: 50 g
Water: 50 ml
Thymol: one small crystal

Dissolve the ingredients, with frequent stirring and occasional heating on a water-bath. The final volume should be approximately 100 ml.

Keeps for a few months at room temperature. Discard if it becomes infected or if the sugar crystallizes.

Apathy's medium has a refractive index (about 1.5) higher than that of glycerol jelly or fructose, so it provides more transparent preparations.

4.3.2.5. Polyvinylpyrollidone (PVP) medium

Polyvinylpyrollidone (MW 10 000):   25 g
Water
(or a phosphate or TRIS buffer, as in Section 4.3.2.2 above): 25 ml

Dissolve the PVP by leaving for several hours on a magnetic stirrer. Then add:

Glycerol: 1.0 ml
Thymol: one small crystal

Usually keeps for 2 to 3 years. Discard if it dries out or looks infected (not transparent).

This mounting medium is less viscous than glycerol jelly or Apathy's and is very easy to handle. The refractive index is 1.46 (Pearse, 1968b), but increases as the water evaporates at the edges of the coverslip until unstained structures are barely visible. Polyvinyl alcohol can be used instead of PVP, and either p-phenylenediamine (10 mg per 100 ml) or n-propyl gallate (600 mg per 100 ml) may be added, if desired, to inhibit fading of fluorescence (Valnes and Brandtzaeg, 1985).

4.4. Treatments before staining

The following treatments are for the eradication of artifacts induced by fixation. The rationales of the methods are explained in Chapter 2.

4.4.1.
Removal of mercury precipitates

Tissues fixed in mixtures containing mercuric chloride contain randomly distributed black particles. The nature of this deposit is not known, but is generally assumed to be mercurous chloride (Hg_2Cl_2), possibly with some metallic mercury. The precipitate does not disturb the structure of the tissue and it is easily removed by the following method. **Sections of all mercuric chloride-fixed specimens must be subjected to this procedure before staining.**

Solutions required
(a) **Alcoholic iodine**
      Iodine (I_2):   2.5 g
      70% ethanol: 500 ml
      Keeps indefinitely and can be reused many times. (See also *Note* below.)
(b) **Sodium thiosulphate solution**
      Sodium thiosulphate ($Na_2S_2O_3.5H_2O$):   15 g
      Dissolve in water and make up to: 250 ml
      Keeps indefinitely. May be re-used three or four times.

Procedure
(1) Take sections to 70% ethanol.
(2) Immerse in alcoholic iodine (solution A) for approximately 3 min. With continuous agitation, 1 min is sufficient.
(3) Rinse in water.
(4) Immerse in 5% sodium thiosulphate (solution B) until the yellow staining due to iodine has all been removed. This usually takes about 30 s.
(5) Wash in running tap water for 2 min, then rinse in distilled water.

Note
Alternatively a 1% solution of iodine in 2% aqueous potassium iodide (Gram's iodine) may be used. This stains the sections deep brown and the decolorization at stage 4 takes longer than after 0.5% alcoholic iodine.

4.4.2.
Removal of picric acid

The yellow colour of picric acid (from Bouin's and similar fixatives) seldom interferes with staining, but it can be removed by immersing the hydrated slides for about 30 s in a dilute alkali. Lithium carbonate is traditional:

      Lithium carbonate (Li_2CO_3):   1 g
      Water: 500 ml

Alternatively, keep a stock of saturated aqueous lithium carbonate (about 1% w/v) and dilute it fivefold for this purpose.

The 0.2% Li_2CO_3 may be used directly, or diluted a further 10–20 times with water. The more dilute solutions take longer to work but are less likely to dislodge the sections.

4.4.3.
Removal of 'formalin pigment'

The dark, crystalline deposits of 'acid haematin' that form after fixation of blood-rich tissues in formaldehyde at pH <6.0 are removed by immersion of the hydrated sections for 5 min in a saturated (about 8%) solution of picric acid in 95% alcohol. **Caution.** See Chapter 2, Section 2.4.4 for notes on safe storage of picric acid. If there is dry yellow incrustation around the cap or stopper, wash it off with running tap water before opening the bottle.

Formalin pigment can also be removed by alkali (e.g. 0.01% potassium hydroxide in 80% alcohol, 10 min), but alkaline liquids can detach sections from slides. After either treatment, the sections are rinsed in three changes of water.

4.4.4.
Removal of osmium dioxide

Black deposits are present in tissues that have been fixed or post-fixed in osmium tetroxide. The dark colour can be removed from sections by immersion in 1 or 2% aqueous hydrogen peroxide for 2–30 min. The solution should be freshly diluted from a stock bottle of 30% ('100 volumes available oxygen') H_2O_2. Alternatively, make a 3% w/v solution of urea hydrogen peroxide, which is a stable solid containing about 35% H_2O_2 (w/w). **Caution.** The concentrated H_2O_2 solution is injurious to skin and clothing; so is solid urea hydrogen peroxide. The diluted solution is harmless.

When the sections are decolorized, they *must be washed thoroughly* to remove the OsO_4 formed by oxidation of the black material: 30 min in running tap water for mounted sections; 10 changes of 50 ml water, each 1–2 min with agitation, for free-floating sections.

4.4.5.
Blocking free aldehyde groups

The following procedure will prevent non-specific histochemical reactions and binding of proteins by the free aldehyde groups introduced by fixation with glutaraldehyde. (For rationale, see Chapter 10.)

Sodium borohydride solution

Sodium phosphate, dibasic (disodium hydrogen phosphate; Na_2HPO_4):	1 g
Water:	100 ml
Dissolve, then add:	
Sodium borohydride ($NaBH_4$):	50 mg

This solution must be fresh. **Caution.** Large volumes of hydrogen (fire or explosion hazard) are evolved if borohydride solutions are acidified, so do not acidify. Wash down sink with copious running water after use.

Procedure

Immerse hydrated sections in the borohydride solution for 10 min, with gentle agitation every 2 min to shake off bubbles. Wash in 4 changes of water.

Note

The solution is alkaline, and therefore likely to cause losses of mounted sections. Coating with nitrocellulose (Section 4.2.2) is often needed.

5 | Dyes

Many compounds are coloured but not all of them are dyes. A dye is a coloured compound that can be bound by a substrate. In histological staining dyes are used to impart colours to the various components of tissues. Sometimes the colouring process has a high degree of chemical specificity, so that the dye can be used as a histochemical reagent. In many other histochemical techniques the reagents are colourless, but coloured substances are formed by reactions involving components of the tissue. Often these end-products are insoluble compounds chemically related to dyestuffs.

An important work of reference for biologists who use dyes is *Conn's Biological Stains* (9th edn by Lillie, 1977, and 10th edn by Horobin and Kiernan, 2002), which includes descriptions of many dyes and much other information. The 9th edn of *Conn's* is still useful because it includes many dyes that were omitted from the 10th edn to make room for more recently introduced compounds. Textbooks of dye chemistry include Abrahart (1968), Allen (1971), Bird and Boston (1975), Gordon and Gregory (1983), Waring and Hallas (1990), Shore (2002a), Hunger (2003) and Zollinger (2003). Larger treatises include Venkataraman (1952–1978) and the *Colour Index* (Section 5.6).

5.1 General structure of dye molecules

A dye molecule is traditionally described as having two parts. These are the **chromogen**, which is the coloured part, and the **auxochrome**, which is the part of the molecule that attaches to the substrate. The **chromophore** is the arrangement of atoms within the chromogen that is responsible for the absorption of light in the visible part of the spectrum. The word 'auxochrome' is used here as it is by dye chemists and histologists. Organic chemists use the same word to mean an atom or group of atoms that changes the wavelength at which a chromophore absorbs maximally. The auxochrome, which is a side-chain attached to the chromogen, may be (1) an ionizable group, (2) a group that reacts to form a covalent bond with a substrate, or (3) an arrangement of atoms that forms coordinate bonds with a metal ('mordant') ion. Many dyes contain more than one auxochrome and most contain additional radicals that modify the colour of the complete compound. The colour is also influenced by the number and types of auxochromic groups. The ionic charge of an auxochrome is balanced by an oppositely charged ion, most commonly H^+, Na^+, or Cl^-. Dyes that have affinity for hydrophobic materials generally lack ionized side-chains.

A **fluorochrome** absorbs ultraviolet, violet, blue or green light and emits light of longer wavelength. Fluorochromes that absorb in the ultraviolet are not or scarcely coloured. These compounds are used in fluorescence microscopy. Some compounds become fluorescent only after they have united with components of tissues.

5.2. Colour and chromophores

Compounds are coloured because their molecules absorb quanta of electromagnetic radiation in the visible part of the spectrum. The energy absorbed by the molecule causes changes in the energy levels of electrons involved in covalent bonding and the lone pairs of electrons associated with some atoms. With organic compounds such as dyes the absorption of visible light is largely attributable to the electrons associated with combinations of atoms known as chromophores. Chromophores are arrangements of the following atomic linkages:

$$C=C \quad C=O \quad C=S \quad C=N \quad N=N \quad N=O \quad C-NO_2$$

The double bonds always alternate with single bonds to form what are known as **conjugated systems**. The bonding electrons are able to move from one atom to another along a conjugated system, with the effect of exchanging the positions of the atomic linkages formally designated as double and single bonds. This phenomenon is known as **resonance**. Benzene is a resonance hybrid of the extreme structures:

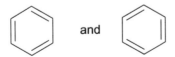

and

Intermediate forms cannot be represented by simple structural formulae. The equivalence of the bonds in a ring such as that of benzene confers a stability that would not otherwise be expected in a cyclic unsaturated compound. Rings stabilized by resonance are said to display **aromatic** character. The conjugated chromophoric system of a dye usually includes double bonds embodied in the formal structure of one or more aromatic rings. The resonance of the bonds in such rings commonly permits the existence of both aromatic and non-aromatic configurations in different rings within the same dye molecule.

The following chromophoric systems are those most frequently encountered in biological stains:

(a)   The **nitro** group:

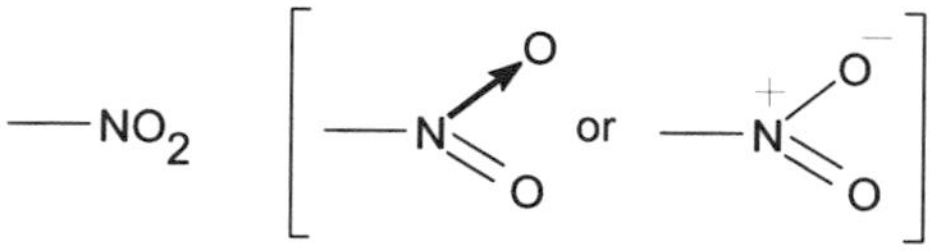

The single (dative) and double bonds between N and O are equivalent because of resonance.

(b)   The **nitroso** group:

$$-N=O$$

(c)   The **indamine** group:

$$-N=$$

This always forms part of a larger chromophoric system.

(d)   The **azo** group:

$$-N=N-$$

This will be discussed at some length later (Section 5.9.3).

(e)   The **quinonoid** configuration:

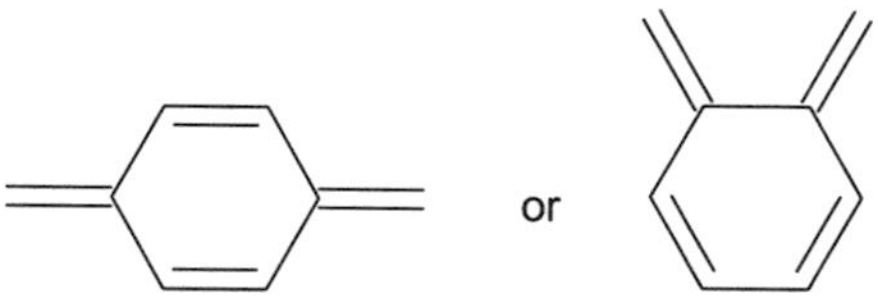

Note that the quinonoid ring is not aromatic. In dyes, resonance often exists among quinonoid and aromatic rings in the same molecule.

Often, the common chromophores (a)–(e) shown above occur in combination. Thus, the **quinone-imine** configuration is present in many dyes, such as the triphenylmethanes, the azines, the oxazines and the thiazines:

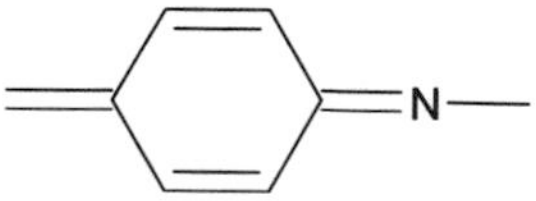

A few other chromophoric systems will be mentioned in connection with certain dyes.

5.3. Auxochromic groups

The auxochrome or 'colligator' (Gurr, 1971) is traditionally held to be responsible for attaching the chromogen to the substrate. Other factors are also involved in the binding of dyes; they will be discussed later.

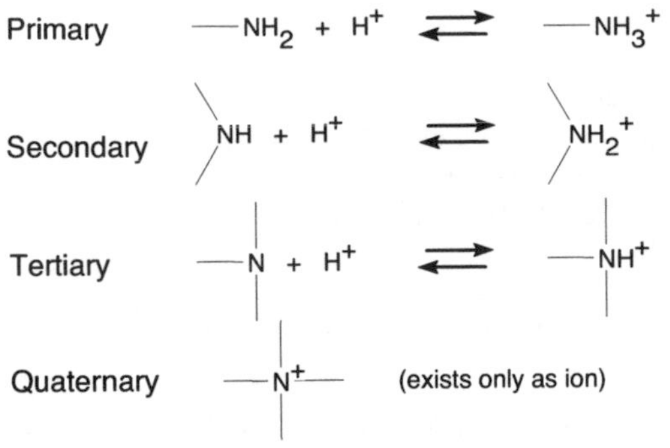

Primary $—NH_2 + H^+$ ⇌ $—NH_3^+$

Secondary $\diagdown NH + H^+$ ⇌ $\diagdown NH_2^+$

Tertiary $—N + H^+$ ⇌ $—NH^+$

Quaternary $—N^+—$ (exists only as ion)

The **basic** auxochromes are amines, which can be protonated to form anions:
A dye with a net positive charge is called a **basic** or (preferably) a **cationic dye**. On treatment with strong alkali, the free bases (typically unionized amines) of such dyes will be liberated. Acid solutions will favour the formation of cations. The coloured ions of such dyes are usually balanced by chloride or sulphate ions.

The **acid** auxochromes are derived from sulphonic or carboxylic acids or from phenolic hydroxyl groups:

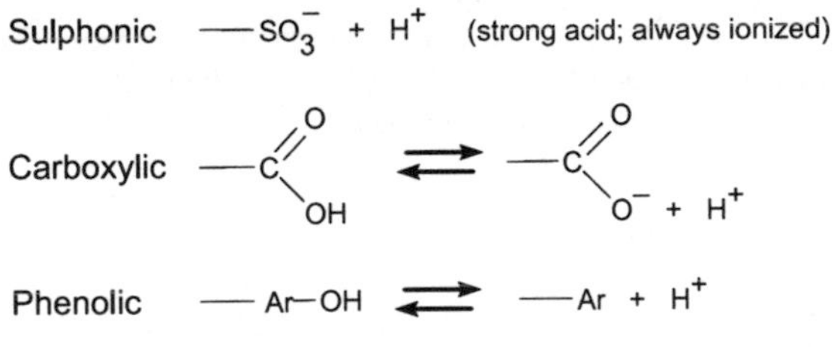

Sulphonic $—SO_3^- + H^+$ (strong acid; always ionized)

Carboxylic $—C\diagup^O_{OH}$ ⇌ $—C\diagup^O_{O^-} + H^+$

Phenolic $— Ar—OH$ ⇌ $—Ar + H^+$

(Ar = aromatic ring)

They occur in **acid (anionic)** dyes, which may be encountered as the free acids or phenols, or as salts, usually of sodium. Sulphonic acids are strong, meaning that they are always ionized and exist as sulphonate ions even at low pH. Carboxylic acids are weak acids, being only partly ionized in aqueous media. Most phenols are even weaker acids. Consequently, dyes with carboxylic acid or phenolic auxochromes cannot exist as anions in the presence of high concentrations of hydrogen ions, because the equilibrium:

$Dye—OH$ ⇌ $Dye—O^- + H^+$

will be pushed over to the left.

From the foregoing paragraphs it will be seen that the pH of the solution will have profound effects on the colouring abilities of anionic and cationic dyes.

Reactive auxochromes are able to combine with hydroxyl and amino groups of the substrate to form covalent bonds. Important reactive auxochromes include the halogenated triazinyl groups, such as **dichlorotriazinyl**:

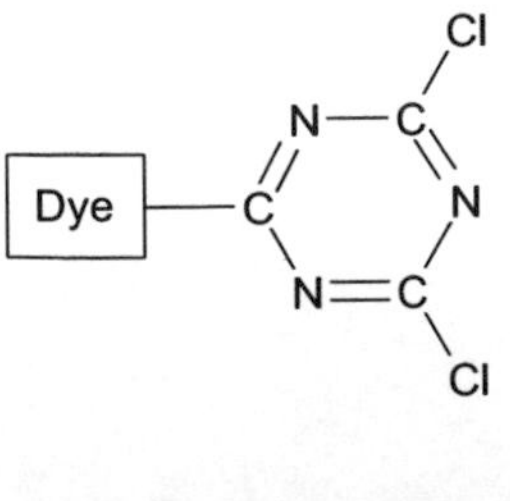

which is derived from cyanuric chloride. These auxochromes are usually attached to a nitrogen atom of the chromogen. In the **monochlorotriazinyl** group, one of the chlorine atoms in the above formula is replaced by an alkyl or an amino group. The chlorine atoms confer high chemical reactivity, similar to that of the acyl halides. Condensation with hydroxyl or amino groups of the substrate, with elimination of HCl, occurs most readily in alkaline conditions:

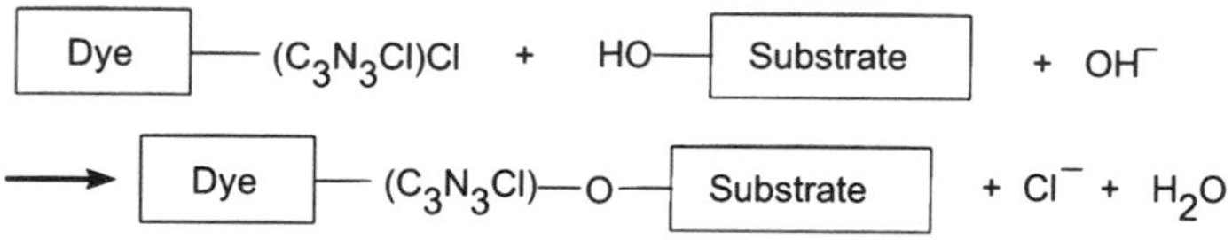

The dichlorotriazinyl group is more reactive than monochlorotriazinyl, and will combine with –OH or –NH$_2$ at room temperature. Other reactive auxochromes used in textile dyeing include pyrimidines and vinyl sulphones, which also react in alkaline conditions.

Dyes and other compounds with reactive auxochromes are not often used to stain tissues but they are used extensively in the preparation of labelled macromolecules for use in nucleic acid hybridization (Chapter 9) and immunohistochemistry (Chapter 19). The principal reactive auxochromic groups for these applications are isothiocyanates, dichlorotriazinyls, sulphonyl chlorides and succinimide esters, used because they combine with amino groups.

5.4. Fluorescent compounds

The chemical features that enable an organic compound to fluoresce are less easily defined than those responsible for colour. In order to be fluorescent, a molecule must contain a system of conjugated double bonds in its hydrocarbon skeleton. The double bonds may include those of aromatic rings; indeed, cyclic conjugated systems are associated with stronger fluorescence than are linear ones. Strongly fluorescent compounds, which are the ones of interest in microscopy, usually have rigidly coplanar molecules. Thus, fluorene, in which planarity is stabilized by a methylene bridge, is more strongly fluorescent than biphenyl in which the two phenyl radicals are free to rotate about the single bond that joins them:

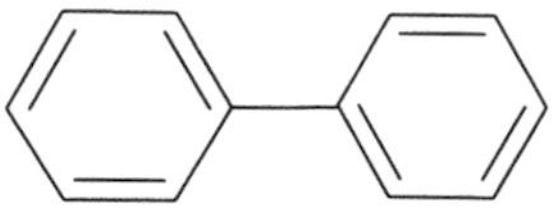

biphenyl 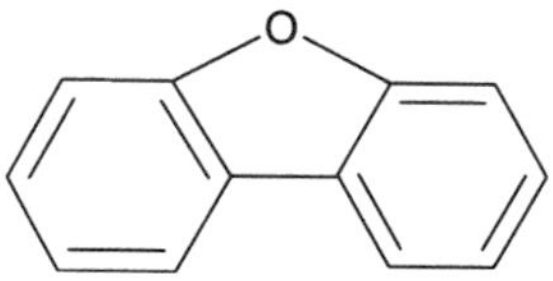   fluorene

Compounds with coplanar fused ring systems are more strongly fluorescent when the rings are all joined side to side than when there is a bend in the structure. Anthracene therefore fluoresces more brightly than phenanthrene in response to the same level of exciting illumination. That is, anthracene has the higher **fluorescence efficiency** of the two compounds:

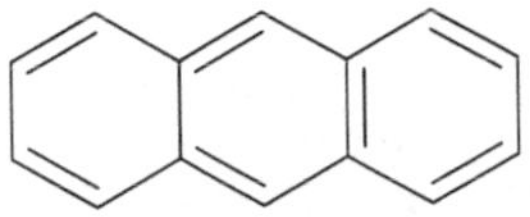

anthracene

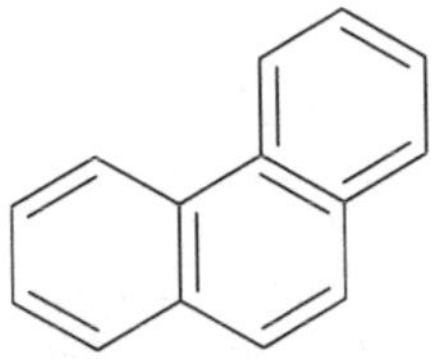

phenanthrene

Fluorescence is also affected by substituents on the conjugated hydrocarbon skeleton of the molecule. When a single substituent is present the fluorescence efficiency is usually increased by $-OH$, $-OCH_3$, $-F$, $-CN$, $-NH_2$, $-NHCH_3$, and $-N(CH_3)_2$, and reduced by $>C=O$, $-COOH$, $-Cl$, $-Br$, $-NO_2$ or $-SO_3H$. Alkyl sidechains generally have no effect unless they sterically hinder the assumption of a planar configuration. The above generalizations do not always apply when more than one substituent is present. Salicylic acid (o-hydroxybenzoic acid), for example, is fluorescent despite its carboxyl group. With heterocyclic compounds, including many dyes, the situation is complex and not fully understood. The fluorescent properties of such substances cannot be predicted by simple inspection of their structural formulae. Juarranz *et al.* (1986) found that fluorescence of dyes correlated with the number of conjugated bonds in the molecule. A dye was most likely to be fluorescent if this number was in the range 28–30.

The fluorescence of a compound can be influenced by other substances with which it is mixed and by the pH of an aqueous solvent or histological mounting medium. For a more detailed but still introductory account of the fluorescence of organic compounds, see Bridges (1968).

5.5. **Combination of dyes with substrates**

The binding of dyes to textiles has been studied for many years (see Giles, 1975; Hunger, 2003; Zollinger, 2003). In the coloration of textiles most of the dissolved dye is moved into the material being dyed. Exhaustion of the dyebath is commonly achieved by heating and addition of inorganic salts. In contrast, the histologist uses a large excess of the staining solution, usually at room temperature, and the amount of dye taken up by the smeared cells or sections of tissue is a negligible proportion of that present in the vessel. Staining is said to be **progressive** when a dye solution is allowed to act slowly until the desired effect is obtained. In **regressive** staining, an object is deliberately overstained, and then placed in a liquid (often water, alcohol, or acidified alcohol) that slowly removes the dye until the latter is left behind only in the components in which colour is wanted. This process of controlled removal of a dye is known as **differentiation** or **destaining**. The success of both the progressive and the regressive modes of staining depends on the fact that dyes attach more strongly to some components of cells or tissues than to others.

The interactions between dyes and tissues have been reviewed in great detail by Horobin (1982, 2002), Prento (2001) and Dapson (2005a). The occurrence or non-occurrence of staining by a dye is determined partly by thermodynamic principles that apply to all dyes and substrates (see Goldstein, 1963; Goldstein and Horobin, 1974), and partly by formation of chemical bonds that vary with the different types of dye and substrate.

**5.5.1.
General physical
considerations**

Physical prerequisites for the dyeing of textile fibres or tissues include:

(a) **Size of the dye particles.** An approximate indication of the particle size is given by the molecular weight of the dye. However, most dye molecules have a strong tendency to stick together and form **aggregates**. Aggregation, which is a reversible process, occurs most readily with the larger dye molecules, in concentrated solutions, and at low temperatures. Large particles diffuse in and out of a fibre or a component of a tissue more slowly than small ones.

(b) **Porosity of the substrate.** Dye molecules or aggregates diffuse through submicroscopic spaces or pores within the substrate. These channels cannot usually be directly observed by electron microscopy, but their properties can be determined by studying the rates of permeation of molecules of known size. Thus, it is found that much of the volume of cotton (cellulose) fibres consists of pores about 3 nm in diameter. In sections of fixed biological specimens, the refractive index is an indicator of porosity (Goldstein, 1964). Cellulose is observed to be more permeable than most of the other substances that contribute to the structure of plant and animal tissues.

(c) **Interfacial effect.** This is a consequence of the lowering of the surface tension of water by many solutes, including most dyes: the dye has a higher concentration at a surface than in the bulk of the solution. When a dye solution permeates a porous substrate, the solute becomes concentrated at the interface between the solution and the walls of the pores. In cotton fibres, for example, dyes are concentrated some 50–60 times, without the formation of any chemical bonds.

**5.5.2
Electrovalent
attraction**

The most easily understood mode of dyeing is that whereby there is electrostatic attraction of oppositely charged ionized groups in the dye and substrate. For example:

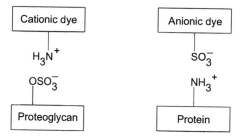

The electrovalent bonds are readily disrupted by acids or by high concentrations of electrolytes, which may therefore be included in the staining mixture to retard or limit the extent of dyeing.

In histological staining, cationic and anionic dyes are used at low pH. This enhances the protonation of the basic auxochromes of cationic dyes:

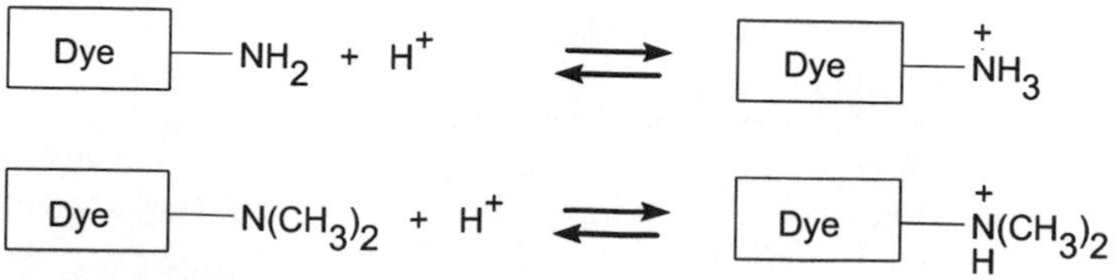

$$\boxed{\text{Dye}} - NH_2 \ + \ H^+ \ \rightleftharpoons \ \boxed{\text{Dye}} - \overset{+}{N}H_3$$

$$\boxed{\text{Dye}} - N(CH_3)_2 \ + \ H^+ \ \rightleftharpoons \ \boxed{\text{Dye}} - \overset{+}{N}(CH_3)_2 \\ \qquad\qquad\qquad\qquad\qquad\qquad\qquad\quad H$$

and of amino groups of proteins:

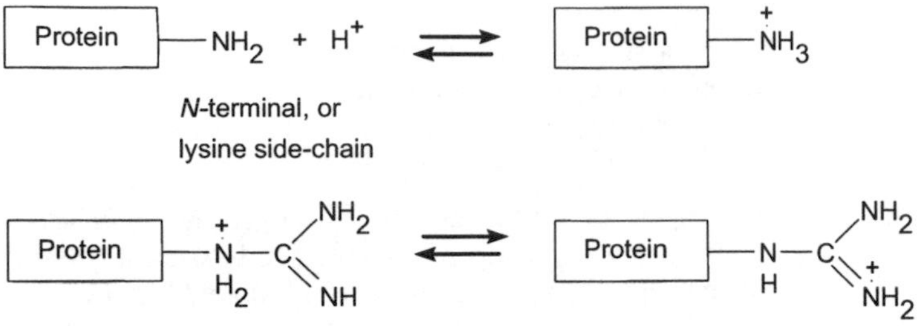

N-terminal, or
lysine side-chain

Guanidino group (arginine side-chain) is always ionized

The ionization of carboxyl groups is suppressed in acid media:

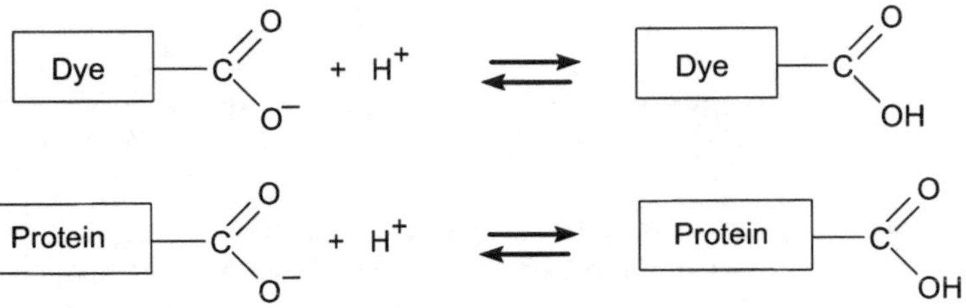

and so is that of the phosphoric acids of DNA and RNA:

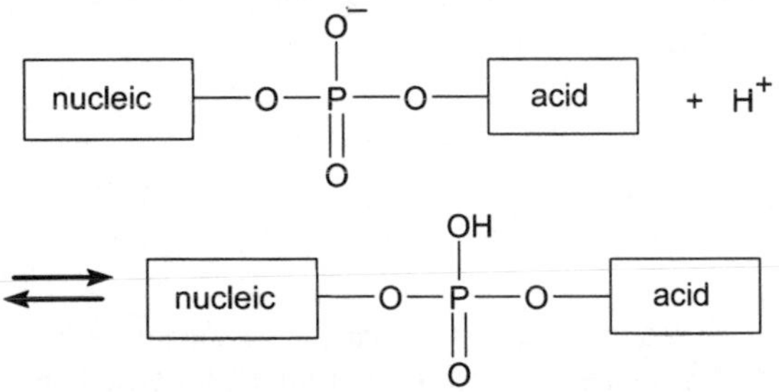

though in this case a higher $[H^+]$ is needed, because phosphoric acid is stronger than carboxylic acids.

These effects of acidification are simple applications of the law of mass action to the reversible chemical reactions of protonation of bases and dissociation of weak acids. Sulphonic acids are strong, so sulphonated dyes exist as anions even at very low pH. The half-sulphate ester groups of proteoglycans (Chapter 11) are also strong acids, as are any sulphate or sulphonate radicals introduced into tissues by treatment with histochemical reagents (Chapter 10).

The order of acidic strength of the acid (potentially anionic) groups normally present in tissues is sulphate > phosphate > carboxylate > phenol. Cationic dyes are ordinarily used at a pH sufficiently low to suppress the ionization of phenolic and carboxyl groups but high enough to allow the esters of phosphoric and sulphuric acids (i.e. nucleic acids and proteoglycans respectively) to exist as anions, and therefore to be stained. The uses of cationic dyes will be discussed further in Chapters 6, 9, and 11.

Electrostatic attractions operate over longer distances than the other forces involved in dye binding. They are probably important in pulling dye molecules towards oppositely charged parts of tissues. Ideally, an insoluble ion-pair or 'salt' should be formed if the dyeing is to be permanent, but this does not usually happen in histological staining. Ionic bonds may be the only forces holding dye to substrate when staining is by a dilute solution of a cationic or anionic dye with small molecules. Other types of binding are also involved when dyes with larger molecules are used, as will be seen below.

5.5.3.
Hydrogen bonding

Hydrogen bonds form between hydrogen atoms (which must be bonded covalently to oxygen, nitrogen, fluorine) and bicovalent oxygen, tricovalent nitrogen or fluorine. The bond is represented by a dotted line thus:

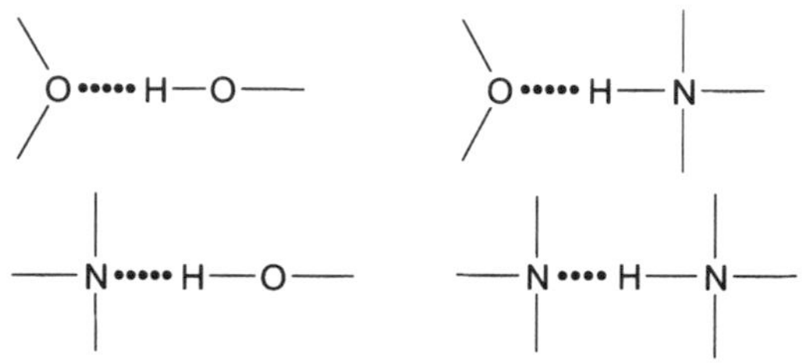

The bond is due to attraction between the lone pair of electrons (i.e. the pair not used in the covalent bond) on the oxygen or nitrogen atom, and the nucleus of the hydrogen atom. This nucleus is partly exposed because the electron orbital around it is drawn towards the strongly electronegative oxygen, nitrogen or fluorine atom to which the hydrogen is covalently bonded. Another type of hydrogen bond can join the delocalized π-electrons of an olefinic double bond or of an aromatic ring to the hydroxyl group of an alcohol or phenol:

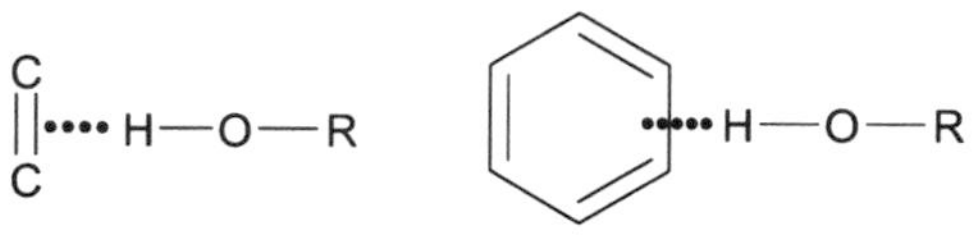

Each of the electrical charges resulting in the hydrogen bond is of lower magnitude than the full charge of an electron or proton. The bond is weaker than a covalent bond but stronger than a van der Waals attraction.

The hydrogen atoms of water are hydrogen-bonded to the oxygen atoms of other water molecules. Many dyes and components of tissues have hydrogen, oxygen, and nitrogen atoms capable of forming hydrogen bonds with water. It is therefore unlikely that bonds of this kind contribute significantly to the attachment of dyes to substrates when staining is carried out in aqueous media. The molecules of water, being much more numerous than those of the dye, would successfully compete for the available hydrogen bonding sites of the substrate. Horobin (1982) suggests that hydrogen bonding occurs when dyes are applied from non-aqueous solvents for staining glycogen, which has numerous –OH groups. There is evidence also for hydrogen bonding of some dyes to collagen (Prento, 2001; see also Chapter 8).

5.5.4.
Charge-transfer bonding

This is another type of rather weak bonding that results in the formation of non-covalent 'addition compounds'. On one side of the charge-transfer bond is a molecule with electrons available for donation. These are commonly the delocalized π-electrons of systems of double bonds or of aromatic rings, though they may be lone-pair electrons of amine nitrogen atoms. On the other side of the bond is an organic molecule capable of acting as an electron-acceptor, though the exact mechanism of acceptance is not fully understood (see Smith and March, 2007, for more information). Picric acid, which is used as both a fixative and a dye, is well known for its ability to form charge-transfer complexes with aromatic hydrocarbons, olefins, and amines. Some other aromatic nitro compounds share this property.

It is conceivable that charge-transfer bonding could be involved in the binding of picric acid and other nitro dyes to stained tissues, but this possibility has not been investigated.

5.5.5.
van der Waals forces

The van der Waals forces are the electrostatic attractions that always exist between the electrons of one atom and the nucleus of another. They are weak forces, and can act only between molecules that are already very close together. Three types of force are recognized. The strongest are **Polarization (Keesom) forces**, which are between dipoles. A dipole is a molecule in which the electrons are unsymmetrically distributed, so that one end carries a fractional electric charge relative to the other end. Water is a dipole, and so are most organic compounds that are not hydrocarbons. The strength of a polarization force varies inversely with the sixth power of the distance separating the dipoles. A symmetrical molecule with many delocalized electrons, such as a dye, is induced to become a dipole when close to an ion or a permanent dipole. **Debye forces** are the weak attractions between dipoles and induced dipoles. **Dispersion (London) forces**, which exist between symmetrical molecules that are both induced dipoles, are most effective between large molecules, and can cause long dye molecules to become aligned on long molecules of a fibre (Giles, 1975).

The van der Waals forces may be important in the 'direct' dyeing of cellulose, discussed later in this chapter, in the staining of elastin (Chapter 8), and in the attachment of some dye–metal complexes (Section 5.5.8) to their substrates, including cell nuclei.

5.5.6.
Hydrophobic interaction

When immersed or suspended in water, non-polar molecules or parts of molecules adhere to one another. This mutual affinity of hydrophobic substances is due to van der Waals forces between the hydrophobic groups, and to hydrogen bonding among nearby water molecules. Water exists as hydrogen-bonded clusters, probably mostly of 4 or 5 molecules (Starzak and Mathlouthi, 2003), but some containing as many as 280 molecules (Chaplin, 1999; Muller et al., 2003). The clusters change constantly with the making and breaking of hydrogen-bonds. In pure water the clusters fill all the space occupied by the liquid. An added non-polar substance, such as an oil, cannot form hydrogen bonds and is concentrated in the narrow spaces between water clusters. With increasing cohesion, due to van der Waals forces, the oil forms discrete droplets, which eventually coalesce to form a separate non-aqueous phase. Polar parts of otherwise hydrophobic molecules, such as phospholipids (Chapter 12), are hydrogen-bonded to clumps of water molecules, so the non-polar regions are the only parts that can approach one another closely enough to be held together by van der Waals forces. Hydrophobic interaction is important when a non-polar substrate such as cellulose acetate or polyester is dyed from an aqueous solution. The dye molecules can enter pores that are inaccessible to water clusters, and stay there.

In histology, hydrophobic interactions are responsible for the penetration of oil-soluble dyes into lipids and for their retention at hydrophobic sites in the tissue. Dyes of this type (solvent dyes; see Section 5.7) are applied as solutions in moderately polar organic solvents (e.g. 70% alcohol), and the stained preparations must be mounted in aqueous media. For staining to occur it is necessary for the dye to have a lower affinity for its solvent than for the hydrophobic substrate. The solvent should therefore be as polar as possible and saturated with the dye. Coloured, non-polar compounds are often formed as end-products in histochemical methods for enzymes (Chapter 14). Such products may become attached by hydrophobic interaction to lipids, and thus lead to faulty localization of the enzymes. The uses of solvent dyes in lipid histochemistry are discussed in Chapter 12.

5.5.7. Covalent combination

Covalent bonds are not formed as the result of reactions between ordinary anionic or cationic dyes with substrates. Many histochemical reactions, however, certainly produce covalent bonds between chromogens and reactive groups in the tissue. Covalently bound coloured material cannot be washed out of a section by simple solvents or salt solutions, but resistance to extraction does not prove the existence of covalent binding; the coloured product may simply be insoluble.

Reactive dyes (Section 5.3) are not used as ordinary histological stains because they are not selective enough in their reactions. Auxochromes like the dichlorotriazinyl group combine with free hydroxyl, amino and other groups, so dyes containing them would stain everything in the tissue, with no selectivity.

5.5.8. Coordinate bonds, chelation and mordants

A **mordant** is a substance that serves to bind a dye to a substrate. Thus, cotton can be impregnated with tannic acid, with which cationic dyes form insoluble salts. The tannic acid serves as a mordant for the dye, which would not adhere to the uncharged cellulose molecules of the cotton. In histological parlance, however, the term is restricted to metal ions that are able to bind covalently to suitable dye molecules, forming **complexes** (also known as coordination compounds or dye–metal complexes). An ion or molecule that combines with a metal ion is called a **ligand**. A ligand must contain at least one atom, the **donor**, with an unshared pair of electrons in its outermost shell. These electrons become shared by the metal ion and the donor to produce the covalent bond between the two atoms.

A bond of this type resembles an ordinary covalent bond, in which each atom contributes one of the electrons of the shared pair, in that it may be very strong and resistant to harsh physical and chemical treatments, or it may be weaker, having some ionic character. Bonds with two electrons donated by the same atom are often called **coordinate, dative,** or **semi-polar** bonds, and several conventional representations are used in structural formulae. These include such symbols as:

$Cu-NH_3$ (indistinguishable from any other covalent bond)

$\overset{\ominus}{Cu}-\overset{\oplus}{NH_3}$ (indicating acquisition of the electron by the copper atom, which then has a higher density of negative charge surrounding its nucleus than does the nitrogen)

$Cu \longleftarrow NH_3$ (showing clearly that the nitrogen atom was the donor; relative electronegativity at the head of the arrow)

$Cu \cdots NH_3$ (in which the covalent or ionic character of the bond is deliberately made vague).

None of these notations are entirely satisfactory. The first one shown (representation as a simple covalency) is used in this book, following the example of Pauling (1970).

The total number of atoms bonded to a metal atom or ion is the **coordination number** of the latter. The charge remaining on an atom stripped of all its ligands is its **oxidation number**. For the rules governing the assigning of oxidation numbers to elements, the reader should consult a textbook of general and inorganic chemistry. It is important to remember that the oxygen atom of the water molecule has an unshared pair of electrons and therefore serves as a donor. Thus, the copper(II) or cupric ions in an aqueous solution of $CuSO_4$ exist as $[Cu(H_2O)_4]^{2+}$, or tetraaquocopper(II) ions. The water molecules of this complex ion can be displaced by other ligands, such as ammonia in the copper(II) tetrammine ('cuprammonium') complex $[Cu(NH_3)_4]^{2+}$. In these complexes the coordination number of the copper atom is 4 and the oxidation number, represented by the Roman numeral, is +2.

When a ligand has two or more atoms suitably positioned to form coordinate bonds with the same metal ion, the latter will be incorporated into a ring. This arrangement commonly confers stability upon the complex, which is then known as a **chelate**. Thus, cupric ions combine with sulphosalicylate ions:

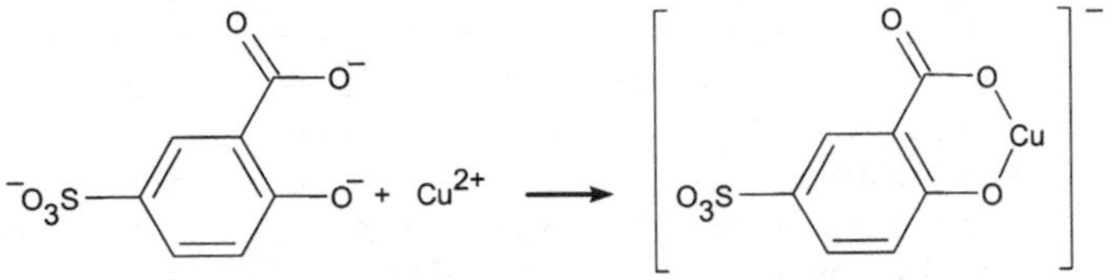

1:1 complex anion

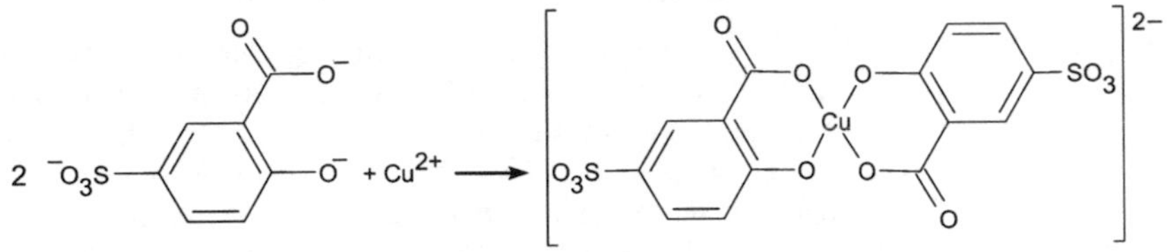

1:2 complex anion

Complexes of the chelate type are involved in the interactions of metal ions with dyes. The cations most often encountered in conjunction with histological stains are those of aluminium, iron, and chromium. Chelation of other metals is important in a wide variety of histochemical techniques.

The most important donor atoms of dyes are oxygen (of phenolic hydroxyl, carboxyl groups or quinones) and nitrogen (of azo, amine, and nitroso groups). These donor atoms must, of course, be suitably positioned on the dye molecule for the latter to be able to serve as a chelating ligand. Substituents *ortho* to one another on a benzenoid ring or at the 1 and 8 positions of naphthalene, or at sterically equivalent positions on other fused aromatic rings, are usually present in dyes that form complexes with metals. For a more thorough account of the chemistry of dye–metal complexes, with special reference to those of azo dyes, the reader is referred to Zollinger (1994).

When a metal ion acts as a mordant, coordinate bonds are formed with both the dye molecule and the substrate. The donor atoms in tissues stained by mordant dyes cannot be identified with certainty. It may reasonably be presumed, however, that any suitably positioned oxygen or nitrogen atoms that are not already fully coordinated with parts of other molecules in the tissue will be potentially available for binding a mordant metal ion. Dye–mordant–substrate complexes may have such forms as:

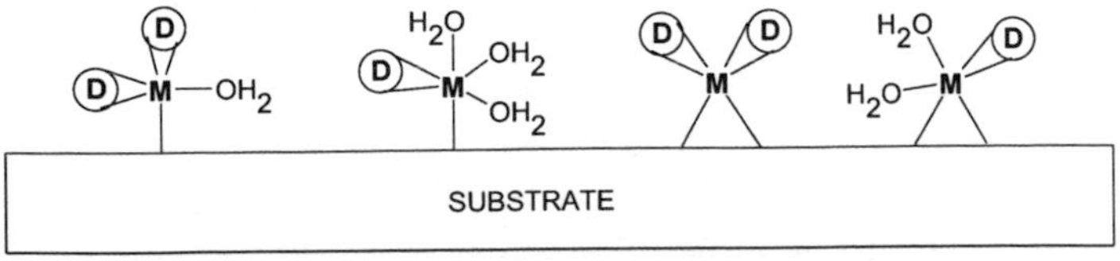

D = dye molecule; **M** = metal ion that can form six covalent bonds.
H_2O, OH_2 = coordinately bound water molecules.

A mordant is sometimes applied before a dye, but is usually mixed with it. Occasionally a metal salt is applied after the dye. In a mixture of dye and mordant there will be competition among the various potential ligands (dye, water and substrate) for the metal ions. Such a mixture also contains fully coordinated dye–metal (often 2:1) complex molecules, and these have their own characteristic staining properties, different from those of the dye alone. In most practical staining mixtures there is a large excess of mordant ions over dye molecules.

True mordant dyeing may occur in the staining of nuclei with iron– or aluminium–haematein (Chapter 6). It is known that nucleic acids are not the only substances involved in the binding of these dyes, and experimental evidence supports the contention that metal ions are interposed between the molecules of the dye and those of the tissue. For example, nuclear staining can be obtained by applying the aluminium salt before the dye, and stained preparations can be differentiated by treating with aqueous solutions of the salts and used as mordants. Nuclear staining by mordant dyes can also be differentiated by treatment with acids, which work, at least in some cases, by cleaving the bonds between metal atoms and tissue (see Baker, 1962).

Other dye–metal complexes, including chromium–gallocyanine, are simply large coloured cations (Berube *et al.*, 1966; Marshall and Horobin, 1972a), and there is no evidence for the interposition of a 'mordant' metal atom between the tissue and the chromogen (see Lillie, 1977). It has been suggested (Marshall and Horobin, 1973) that preformed dye–metal complexes may be held to their substrates by van der Waals forces more than by ionic attraction or covalent bonds. For such a mechanism to be effective it is necessary that the molecules of the complex be large and able to conform to their macromolecular substrate. This condition is likely to be met in complexes with two dye molecules bound to each metal ion.

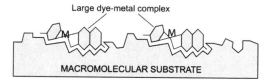

It is generally characteristic of histological staining by mordant dyes that the colours imparted to the tissues are not easily extracted by water, alcohols, or weakly acidic solutions used in the counterstaining and later processing of the preparations. Stronger acids decolorize the stained sections and are used for differentiation. Solutions of the mordant salt alone may also be employed for this purpose.

5.6. Nomenclature and availability of dyes

5.6.1.
Names and numbers

The formal chemical names of most dyes are too long for ordinary writing and conversation, so trivial names are used instead. Some of these have been in use long enough to be considered 'traditional' (e.g. haematoxylin, methylene blue, acid fuchsine). Others are trade names of manufacturers (e.g. alcian blue 8GX, procion brilliant red M2B). Letters or numbers following names are called 'shade designations' and form integral parts of the names. Thus, eosin Y and eosin B are different, though related, compounds. Unfortunately, the trivial names of dyes give no clues to their chemical natures or their uses.

In the *Colour Index* (3rd edn, 1971, and later supplements), published by the Society of Dyers and Colourists, dyes and other useful coloured compounds are given numbers (the '**C.I. numbers**'), based on chemical constitution, and also names that indicate their modes of industrial application and their colours. For example, methyl blue is C.I. 42780, Acid blue 93. Eriochrome cyanine R is C.I. 43820, Mordant blue 3. Natural dyes are named as a separate class, so that haematoxylin is C.I. 75290, Natural black 1, despite the fact that it is a mordant dye. The C.I. numbers are used in other works as well as the *Colour Index* itself and they should always be specified when ordering dyes from suppliers. Some of the dyes and related compounds used in biological work are not included in the *Colour Index*, but are described and discussed in *Conn's Biological Stains* (9th edn, Lillie, 1977; 10th edn, Horobin and Kiernan, 2002). The preferred names given in the 10th edn of *Conn's* are used in this book, and C.I. numbers and commonly encountered synonyms are also given.

> Authors have been inconsistent in their spelling of the names of dyes and in the use of initial capital letters. In this book and in the 10th edn of *Conn's Biological Stains*, initial capitals are used in the preferred names only for words that are also proper names of people or places. Other words, including trade names, are printed entirely in lower case letters, but shade designations are capitalized (e.g. Victoria blue 4R; methylene violet, Bernthsen; alcian blue 8G). The C.I. applicational names are treated as a botanist or zoologist would treat the generic and specific names of a species, with an initial capital for the class and lower case for the colour (e.g. Basic violet 10; Mordant black 37). Many words in traditional preferred names end in -in or -ine. The ending -ine is used when the dye is an amine or a derivative of an amine (e.g. fuchsine, **not** fuchsin; safranine, **not** safranin). For a dye that is not an amine, there is no terminal e (e.g. eosin, **not** eosine; haematein, **not** haemateine). This convention is used by dye chemists (e.g. Hunger, 2003; Zollinger, 2003) and was used by Baker (1958). For many years biologists, even Lillie (1977) have been inconsistent and often incorrect in their spellings of names of dyes. Some variations are not incorrect, such as diphthongal ae (e.g. haematoxylin rather than hematoxylin), and that of ph rather than f in such words as 'sulphur' and 'sulphonic'. These minor discrepancies merely reflect differences between English and American spellings.

Dyes for use as stains and histochemical reagents can be purchased from many suppliers of laboratory chemicals. Some firms specialize in biological stains. A few dyes (e.g. aldehyde–fuchsine; Chapter 8) are easy to synthesize in the laboratory. Dyes are not usually manufactured by the firms that sell them. They are made for the primary purpose of supplying the textile and other industries. Some stains, however, are obsolete as industrial dyes and are now produced solely for laboratory use.

Because of the different requirements of the dyer and the histologist, **most dyes are not marketed as pure compounds**. The dye is nearly always mixed with a substantial proportion of inactive filler (often sodium chloride or dextrin) and several different coloured substances are often present in a sample sold as a single dyestuff. Fillers are added to standardize the potency of different batches of dye so that they will behave similarly towards textiles. Some salt is often inevitably present as a result of the salting-out process used to recover the dye in solid form from the solution in which it was synthesized. The chemical reactions by which dyes are generated are usually accompanied by side reactions. These often lead to the production of other dyes, which end up as contaminants in the final products. Changes occur after dissolving some dyes, and this process may lead to deterioration of a staining solution (as with gallocyanine) or to improvement in its properties (as with haematoxylin and methylene blue). Occasionally a dye with a single name is a deliberate mixture of two quite different substances (e.g. alcian green). Nearly every histological stain tested by paper or thin layer chromatography has been shown to contain several coloured components. Often one of these predominates and this usually corresponds to the name on the bottle, but some commonly used dyes have been shown to be mixtures of two or three major components with 10 or more minor contaminants. It is hardly surprising that the properties of a biological stain vary from one batch to another of what is supposed to be the same single dyestuff.

5.6.2.
Certification and standardization

It is necessary for the histologist to have dyes that can be relied upon to give satisfactory and repeatable results. Such constancy of performance has assumed even greater importance in recent decades than in the past with the advent of automated screening devices for the examination of blood and exfoliated cells in pathology laboratories.

In the early days of staining, microscopists depended on a few suppliers, notably Dr Georg Grübler and Co. of Berlin, who tested the products of various manufacturers and then bought up and packaged batches that proved satisfactory as stains. In 1914 Grübler's dyes were no longer available outside Germany, and most biologists had to rely on the dye industries of other countries. Difficulty in obtaining usable stains led to the founding of the **Biological Stain Commission** (BSC) in the United States in 1920. This independent body tests batches of dyes submitted by manufacturers and suppliers and certifies those suitable for their intended uses. For the history of the BSC, see Conn (1980,1981).

A bottle containing a certified stain shows the percentage by weight of dye in the solid material. (The BSC tests only powders, not solutions.) For most dyes this is an inclusive assay of substances decolorized by titration with $TiCl_3$, which include the named dye and any coloured contaminants. Spectrophotometry and other analytical tests check the identity and purity of the dye, and each sample is evaluated for its performance in prescribed staining procedures. A certified dye's label also shows the C.I. number, and a batch number. Newly certified batches of dyes are reported bimonthly in the Commission's journal, *Biotechnic and Histochemistry*, and the Commission's laboratory in Rochester, NY, USA answers questions and receives comments about difficulties with obtaining or using the dyes.

Certification serves all biologists, but vendors submit mainly the dyes used in pathology and bacteriology, which account for most of the market. Many dyes used in other biological sciences are not tested. All uncertified samples of dyes should be viewed with suspicion and carefully tested by the user before applying them to valuable specimens. The history of the availability and standardization of biological stains is recounted by Lillie (1977), who also provides practical instructions for assaying and testing many dyes. Satisfactory assay methods are not available for a few dyes. These are tested empirically in appropriate staining procedures. The BSC's assay and testing procedures are all published (Penney *et al.*, 2002).

Certified dyes are sold worldwide, but outside North America there is no organization like the BSC that carries out simple assays and practical tests. The European Union has adopted principles of standardization based on the precept that a dyestuff ideally should be a single compound with no contaminants or inert filler (Schulte,1994; Lyon *et al.*, 1994; Lyon, 2002). Ready-made solutions of dyes, notably alum–haematoxylins, eosin and blood stains (Chapters 6 and 7) have been articles of commerce for nearly a century, for the convenience of those users who cannot spare the few minutes needed for weighing and measuring. Many suppliers sell pre-made solutions, but there is no independent assessment of their worth.

When a weight or concentration of any dye is specified in the instructions for a method, in this or any other text, it refers to the material constituting an acceptable sample of the dye, not to the pure dyestuff. For commonly used stains the acceptable percentages of active substances present in the commercial products are given with the descriptions of dyes in Section 5.9 of this chapter. Most of the data are from Lillie (1977) and Horobin and Kiernan (2002). If dye content stated on the label of a bottle differs by more than a few percent from the recommended acceptable value, appropriate correction must be made in preparing a working solution. With uncertified samples the dye content is seldom stated on the label, and must be guessed. Most dyes can be stored as dry powders for many years without deterioration (Emmel and Stotz, 1986; Titford, 2001, 2002).

5.7. Classification of dyes by methods of application

Dyes and other colorants may be arranged in 16 groups according to the ways they are applied to textile fibres and other substances. These techniques are not all used in histological practice but they are briefly set out below to give the reader some idea of the variety of colouring methods employed in industry. For more information, see Allen (1971), Bird and Boston (1975), Waring and Hallas (1990), Christie *et al.* (2000), Shore (2002b), Hunger (2003) and Zollinger (2003).

Basic dyes. These are coloured cations, which attach by electrostatic forces to anionic groups in the substrate. They are used on proteinaceous fibres, cellulosic fibres that have been pretreated with tannic acid, and polyacrylonitrile fibres. Cationic dyes form an important group of histological stains and histochemical reagents.

Acid dyes. These are coloured anions, with sulphonic or carboxylic acid auxochromes. Many dyes in this group are amphoteric, having amine as well as acid groups. An excess of anionic substituents confers a net negative charge on the molecule. The sulphonic acids are the most important industrial dyes in this group because they are strong acids, fully ionized even at low pH. They are applied from acidic dyebaths, mainly to proteinaceous fibres such as wool and silk with free amino and guanidino groups. As will be seen later, ionic interactions are not the only forces involved in the binding of acid dyes to their substrates. Anionic dyes are important as stains for cytoplasm and extracellular structures.

Direct dyes. These are anionic dyes with large molecules. Nearly all are azo dyes. They bind to cellulosic fibres directly (i.e. without the need for a mordant). Some are used as histological stains. The mode of dyeing by direct dyes is discussed in Section 5.9.3.8.

Mordant dyes. Mordants and their functions have already been discussed (Section 5.5.8). By convention (*Colour Index*), the mordant dyes are defined as those used in conjunction with metal salts. The mordant may be applied **before** the dye, together **with** the dye as a soluble dye–metal complex (the 'metachrome' process) or **after** the dye (the 'afterchrome' process). In some instances a mordant dye is also an anionic or, rarely, a cationic dye in its own right. Mordant dyes have many uses in histology and histochemistry.

Reactive dyes. These combine covalently with their substrates. The most important are those whose auxochromes unite with the hydroxyl groups of cellulose. A reactive dye bound to an insoluble hydrophilic polymer can be used for purification of enzymes by affinity chromatography. The active sites that bind coenzymes are the only parts of the apoenzyme molecules flat enough to have strong non-ionic affinity for the bound dye. The enzyme is eluted with a solution of the coenzyme (see Clonis *et al.*, 1987).

Solvent dyes. The simple solvent dyes are coloured substances that dissolve in hydrophobic materials but not in water. Solvent dyes are used in wood stains, lacquers, polishes, printing inks, inks for ball-point pens, and in the mass colouring of wax, some plastics, and soap. Other solvent dyes are salts formed by the interaction of anionic chromogens with hydrophobic cations. The latter are released during dyeing, leaving the coloured anions behind in the substrate. Biologists sometimes use the term **lysochromes** for solvent dyes, which are used to stain lipids (Chapter 12).

Vat dyes. These are important in the textile industry but are not used by biologists. A vat dye is applied to cloth as its leuco compound (which is not usually colourless in practice). This is then oxidized, commonly by treatment with air and steam, to the fully coloured form of the dye, which is insoluble. Vat dyes are used mainly on cotton. The oldest vat dye is indigo, derivatives of which are produced in the indigogenic techniques of enzyme histochemistry (Chapter 15).

Sulphur dyes. These are mixtures of uncertain composition made by heating a variety of organic compounds with sulphur or with alkali metal polysulphides. A sulphur dye is applied (mainly to cellulosic fabrics) mixed with aqueous sodium sulphide, which causes reduction to the leuco compound. The insoluble coloured dye is regenerated by exposure of the dyed material to air. The process is similar in principle to vat dyeing. Sulphur dyes are not used in histology.

Ingrain dyes. Originally this term included all dyes generated within the substrate, but it is now used specifically for temporarily solubilized dyes change into insoluble pigments after application to their substrates. The phthalocyanines are discussed later in this chapter. Alcian blue, used in carbohydrate histochemistry, is the most important biological stain in this class.

Polycondensation dyes (condense dyes). This category includes dyes with a variety of chromophoric systems and two or more *S*-alkyl thiosulphate side-groups such as –CH$_2$SSO$_3$⁻. On treatment of the dyed fabric with sodium sulphide, the dye molecules react with one another to form insoluble polymers in which the dye molecules are joined by –SS– linkages (Schimmelschmidt *et al.*, 1963). Such dyes are not used as biological stains.

Azoic dyes. These are formed within the substrate by reaction of diazonium salts (**azoic diazo components**) with suitable phenols or aromatic amines (**azoic coupling components**). They are important to the histochemist and are discussed later in this chapter and in Chapters 14 and 15.

Oxidation bases. Certain colourless bifunctional amines and aminophenols are used as dyes, especially for fur and hair. Oxidation, usually by hydrogen peroxide, produces insoluble brown or black polymers containing the quinonoid chromophore. The colour that develops may be modified by adding metal salts or phenolic compounds to the oxidation base. Similar chemical reactions are encountered in several histochemical techniques for peroxidases and oxidases (Chapter 16).

Disperse dyes. These are insoluble coloured compounds used as aqueous suspensions (particle size 1–10 μm) for dyeing cellulose acetates and polyesters. The colouring process is enhanced by the presence in the dyebath of suitable oily agents (**carriers**), which are believed to promote the entry of the dye particles into the interstices of the hydrophobic fibres, where water cannot penetrate. Disperse dyes are not used in histology.

Pigments. These are finely divided white, black, or coloured materials, insoluble in water and organic solvents. They are used as suspensions or emulsions in liquid media, as paints, and for the mass coloration of plastics, rubber and synthetic fibres. There are many inorganic and organic pigments. They are often formed as the visible end-products of histochemical reactions.

Fluorescent brighteners. These compounds (see reviews by Gold, 1971 amd Shore, 2002b) serve to increase the amount of visible light reflected from white or coloured objects. Invisible ultraviolet radiation absorbed by the brightening agent is emitted at a higher, visible wavelength. Most fluorescent brighteners contain the stilbene configuration. Some are used in microscopy as fluorochromes. Their staining properties resemble those of the direct cotton dyes.

Food colours. This group includes dyes of various kinds whose principal industrial applications are in the manufacture of foodstuffs. Fast green FCF, an anionic triphenylmethane dye, is the only one commonly used as a histological stain.

5.8. Traditional classification of stains by microscopists

Biological stains have traditionally been designated by their users as basic, acid, or mordant dyes or as 'fat stains', the last-named being the lysochromes or solvent dyes. These four groups reflect in a rough and ready way the purposes for which the dyes are used. Thus, **basic (cationic) dyes** are used to stain nuclei and the major anionic compounds of cytoplasm and extracellular structures. **Acid (anionic) dyes** demonstrate cytoplasmic and extracellular proteinaceous material. **Mordant dyes** are used mainly as nuclear stains, and **solvent dyes** (lysochromes) are for fats and other lipids.

This classification has the advantages of simplicity and widespread usage, but it is not adequate for the student trying to understand the reasons why different dyes are used, alone or in combination, for the demonstration of structural and chemical features of tissues. The uses of the dyes are determined by their physical and chemical properties. Any dye used as a stain should be thought of in terms of its colour, its molecular size and shape, its solubility, and its potential chemical reactivity. All these properties affect the method of use and the results obtained.

5.9. Classification of dyes by chromophoric systems

We now consider the major groups of dyes following a chemical scheme of classification based on the structures of the major chromophoric systems, following Gregory (1990) and Zollinger (2003). This is the scheme followed in the 10th edn of *Conn's Biological Stains*. In contrast to the *Colour Index* and the 9th edn of *Conn's*, dyes of natural origin are placed in their chemical categories, rather than in a heterogeneous group of 'natural dyes'. The more important members of each group, including all the dyes mentioned in later parts of this book, will be described. Some groups of dyes have little or no importance as biological stains, so for these only single representative examples are given. The number of dyes used in histology and histochemistry is likely to increase in the future, so the potential user should be aware of the variety available. For more information about individual dyes, see Venkataraman (1952–1978), Lillie (1977) and Horobin and Kiernan (2002). For a brief introduction to the literature of dye chemistry and usage, see Horobin (1983).

**5.9.1.
Inorganic
colouring agents**

Iodine, silver and gold salts (Chapter 18) and osmium tetroxide (Chapters 12 and 18) have a wide range of uses in microtechnique. Insoluble coloured or black inorganic compounds such as Prussian blue, copper ferrocyanide and cobalt and lead sulphides are formed as the end products of several histochemical reactions.

**5.9.2.
Nitroso dyes**

Nitrous acid reacts with phenols to give nitrosophenols in which the radical $-N{=}O$ replaces hydrogen *ortho* or *para* to the phenolic hydroxyl group. There is tautomerism between the nitroso compounds and the corresponding quinone oximes. Thus, for *p*-nitrosophenol:

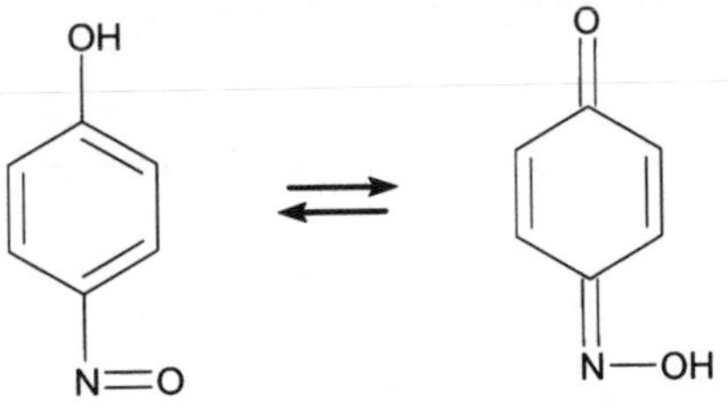

p-nitrosophenol

p-benzoquinone oxime
(can also be made from hydroxylamine
and *p*-benzoquinone)

The *o*-nitroso compounds can form coloured chelates with metal ions and so function as mordant dyes. Nitroso dyes have found hardly any uses in histology, though they have properties that might well be exploited.

Examples
NAPHTHOL GREEN Y (C.I. 10005; Mordant green 4; MW 173)

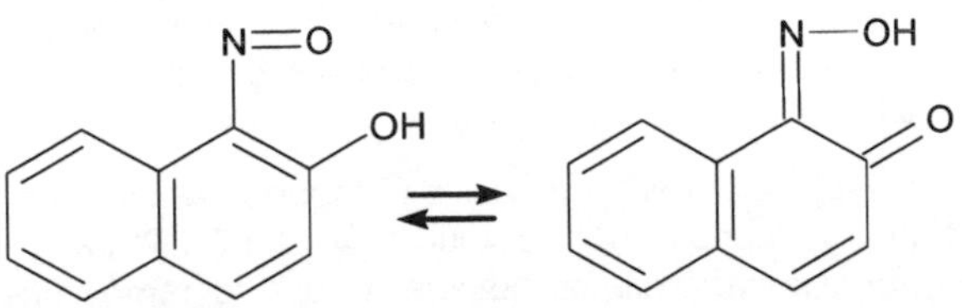

With ferrous ions and NaOH, this forms an important pigment, **pigment green B** (C.I. 10006; Pigment green 8), with the formula $Na^+[(Dye)_3Fe]^-$.

NAPHTHOL GREEN B (C.I. 10020; Acid green 1; MW 901)

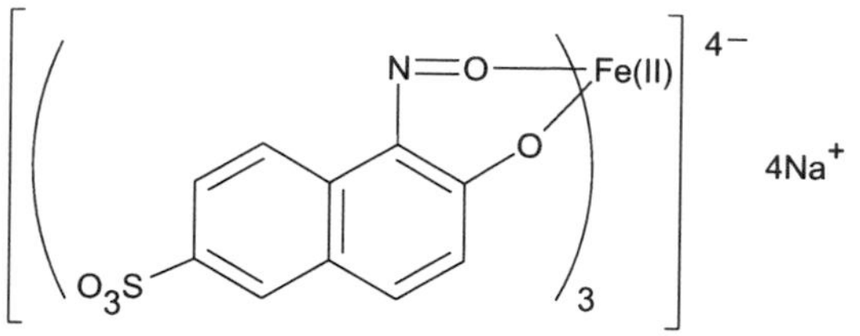

This stable dye–metal complex is used as the stain for collagen in some mixtures of anionic dyes.

5.9.3.
Nitro dyes

The nitro group may be present as a substituent in dyes with other chromophoric systems, but there are some in which it is the only chromophore. Hydroxyl or amino groups are also present in such dyes, and aromatic and quinonoid tautomers exist as is shown below for picric acid. The nitro group, formally represented as $-NO_2$, is a resonance hybrid of the two structures, with the two bonds between nitrogen and oxygen being equivalent to one another.

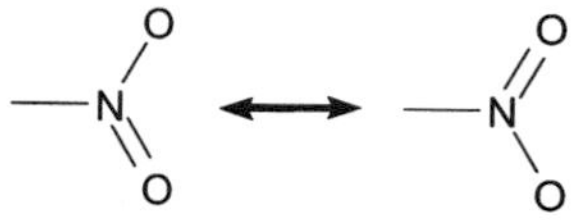

The single N—O bond can alternatively be represented as N$\longrightarrow$O or $\overset{+}{N}$—$\overset{-}{O}$, the symbols having the same meanings as when used in formulae of metal complexes.

Examples
PICRIC ACID (2,4,6-trinitrophenol; C.I. 10305; MW 299)

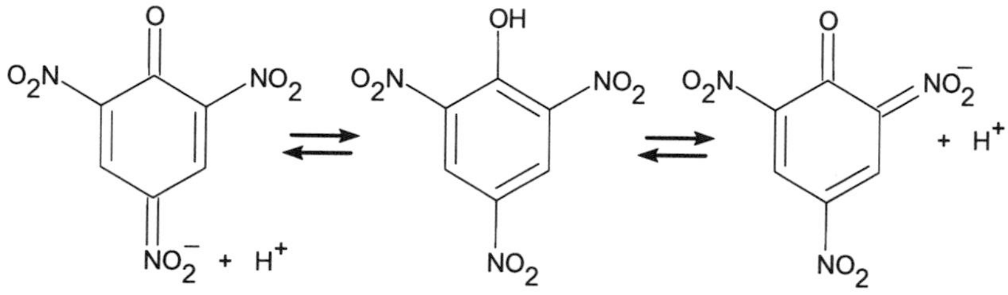

(*p*-quinonoid)   (aromatic)   (*o*-quinonoid)

The phenolic hydroxyl group is ionized because of the electron-withdrawing effect of the three nitro groups. Picric acid is a yellow anionic dye of low molecular weight. It can also form 'addition compounds', which are charge-transfer complexes, with a variety of substances. In these, the bonding is neither ionic nor covalent (see Smith and March, 2007, for discussion).

Picric acid is also used as a fixative (Chapter 2, where precautions attendant on its use are also mentioned). It is soluble in water (1.3%) and more soluble in alcohol and aromatic hydrocarbons, but xylene does not remove the dye from stained sections.

MARTIUS YELLOW (C.I. 10315; Acid yellow 24; naphthol yellow; 2,4-dinitro-1-naphthol; MW 256 (sodium salt), 251 (ammonium salt), 273 (calcium salt), 234 (the unionized phenol))

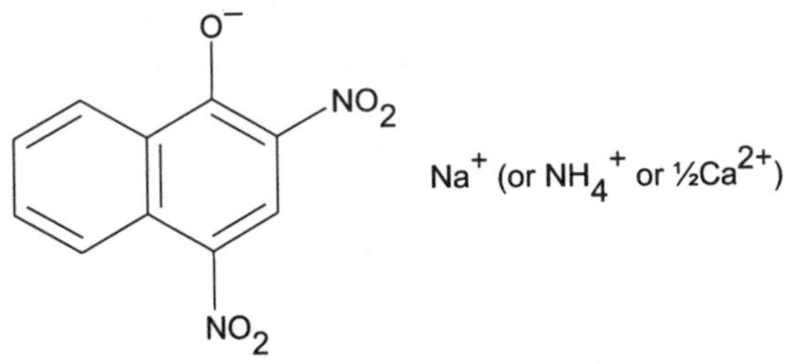

Na^+ (or NH_4^+ or $\frac{1}{2}Ca^{2+}$)

This dye is more deeply coloured (approaching orange) than picric acid, and is somewhat more soluble in water and less soluble in alcohol. The calcium salt is less soluble in water than the ammonium and sodium salts. Like picric acid, martius yellow is used as a cytoplasmic stain in conjunction with other anionic dyes.

A related compound, 2,4-dinitro-naphthol-7-sulphonic acid, is **flavianic acid,** well known to biochemists as a precipitant for the amino acid arginine. The sodium salt of flavianic acid is **naphthol yellow S** (C.I. 10316), an anionic dye more soluble than martius yellow.

5.9.4.
Azo dyes

This very large group of dyes is of great importance in industry and to the biologist. It will be described in some detail because many points of theoretical and practical interest are conveniently illustrated by members of the azo series. The chromophore is the azo group (–N=N–), which connects two aromatic ring systems. Dyes may contain one (monoazo), two (bisazo), three (trisazo), four (tetrakisazo) or more (polyazo) azo groups. The aromatic rings are usually benzene or naphthalene, and they may bear a variety of substituents.

5.9.4.1. Synthesis
Azo dyes are made by coupling diazonium salts with phenols or aromatic amines. The diazonium salts are made by reacting primary aromatic amines with nitrous acid, in acid solution, at temperatures at little above freezing:

$$Ar\text{---}NH_2 + HNO_2 + H^+ \longrightarrow Ar\text{---}\overset{+}{N}\equiv N + 2H_2O$$

Most diazonium salts are unstable and cannot be isolated in pure form as solids, but some are available as stable complexes. Usually the solution containing a diazonium salt is used immediately. Excess nitrous acid can be decomposed by adding a little urea:

$$2HNO_2 + (NH_2)_2CO \longrightarrow 3H_2O + 2N_2(g) + CO_2(g)$$

Coupling with phenols and amines occurs preferentially at the *para* position, but at the *ortho* position if another substituent is present *para* to the hydroxyl or amino group. With naphthols and naphthylamines, coupling is usually *ortho* to the hydroxyl or amine group. For example:

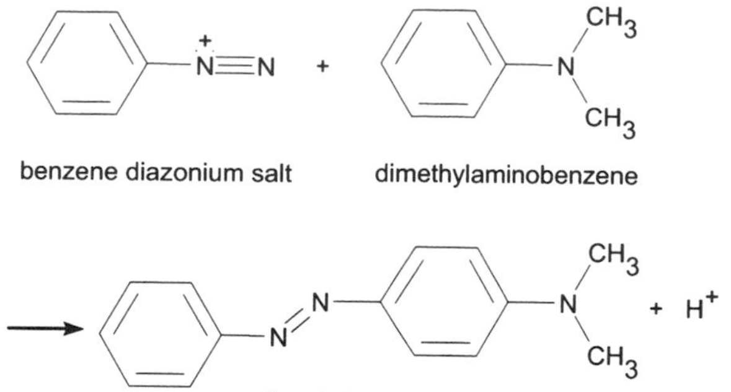

benzene diazonium salt   dimethylaminobenzene

p-dimethylaminoazobenzene
(oil yellow II; C.I. 11020; Solvent yellow 2)

The product of this reaction is the well-known carcinogen 'butter yellow' (which is neither a constituent of, nor an additive to, butter). It is insoluble in water and is not used in histology, but it is a dye on account of the auxochromic tertiary amine group. Solubility in water can be conferred by introducing a hydrophilic substituent. The sulphonic acid group is the one most often chosen and the sodium salt of the para-sulphonic acid derivative of butter yellow (formed from diazotized sulphanilic acid and p-dimethylaminobenzene) is a water-soluble dye.

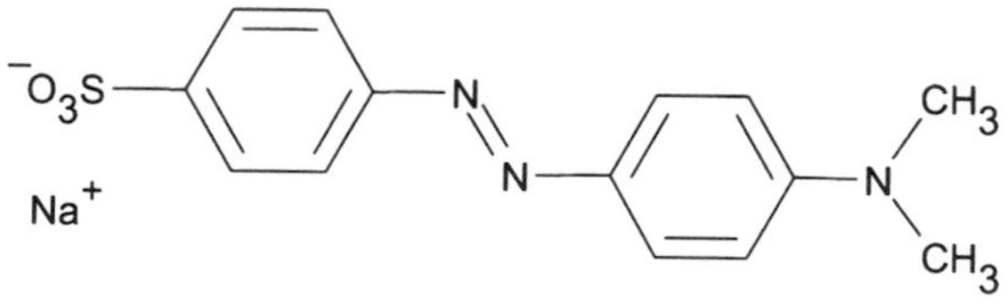

It is seldom used as a stain, but is familiar as an acid–base indicator, **methyl orange** (C.I. 13025; Acid orange 52).

In coupling with diazonium salts, phenols react as their anions whereas amines react as the unprotonated bases. Both these species exist in alkaline solutions. A diazonium ion, however, is changed in the presence of excess alkali into a diazotate anion, $Ar-N=N-O^-$, which does not participate in coupling reactions. Consequently, there is an optimum pH for every reaction between a diazonium salt and a phenol or amine. Usually a more strongly alkaline medium is required for coupling with phenols than with amines.

Azo dyes can also be produced by reactions of quinones with aryl hydrazines, but they are always manufactured by the coupling reactions of diazonium salts. For more complete accounts of chemistry of azo compounds, the reader should consult a textbook of organic chemistry (such as Smith and March, 2007) or the monograph of Zollinger (1994).

5.9.4.2. Structure

The azo group can exist in two isomeric forms:

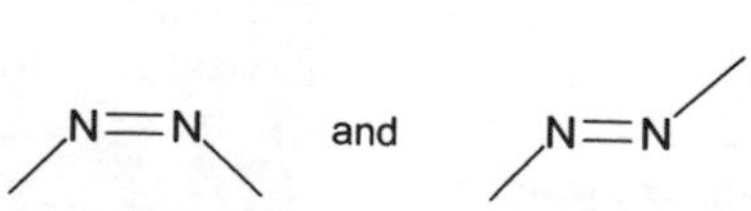

(cis form)   (trans form)

In dyes, the *trans* configuration is usually present because of intramolecular hydrogen bonding between one of the azo nitrogen atoms and a substituent in the *ortho* position on at least one of the aromatic rings:

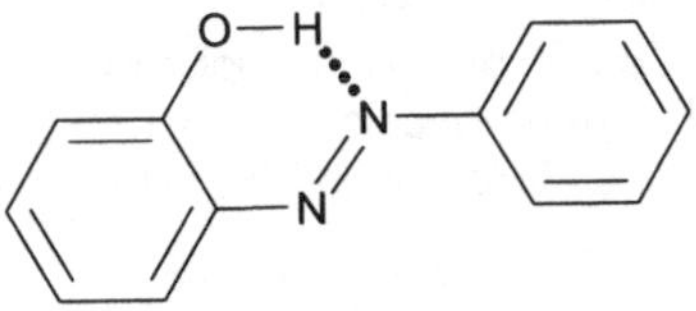

In some dyes, this arrangement provides a molecular shape conducive to the chelation of metal ions.

Phenolic azo dyes exist in tautomeric equilibrium with quinonoid forms:

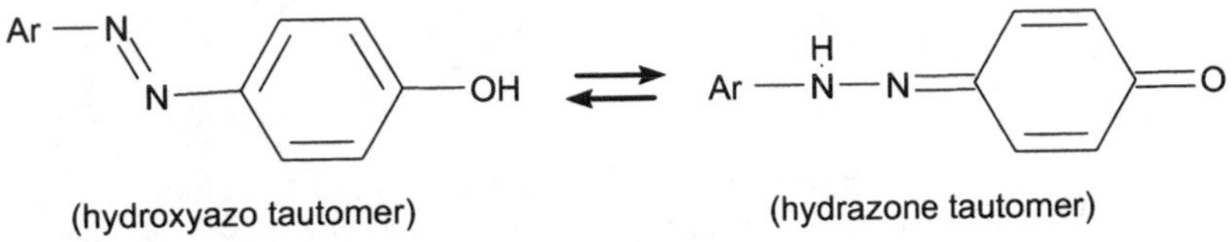

(hydroxyazo tautomer)   (hydrazone tautomer)

The dyes that are amines, however, usually occur only in the aminoazo form because of intramolecular hydrogen bonding.

5.9.4.3. Anionic azo dyes

The simpler anionic azo dyes are the 'leveling' dyes. They are mostly monoazo compounds with sulphonic acid and phenolic substituents. An example much used in histology is orange G.

Examples

ORANGE G (C.I. 16230; Acid orange 10; MW 452)

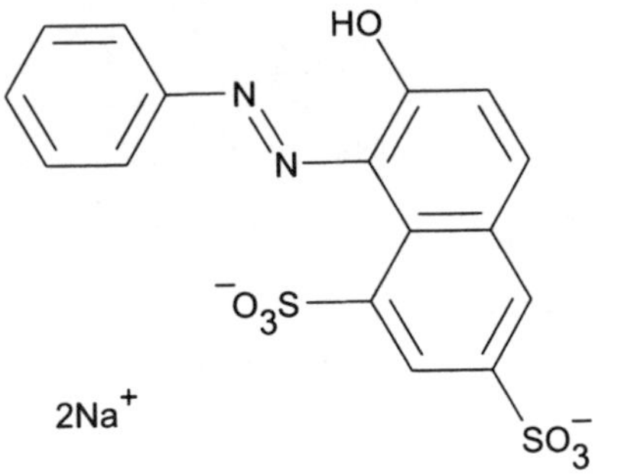

This dye is used as a cytoplasmic stain, usually in conjunction with other anionic dyes. It is very soluble in water but much less soluble in alcohol. Samples should contain at least 80% by weight of the anhydrous dye.

METANIL YELLOW (C.I. 13065; Acid yellow 36; MW 375)

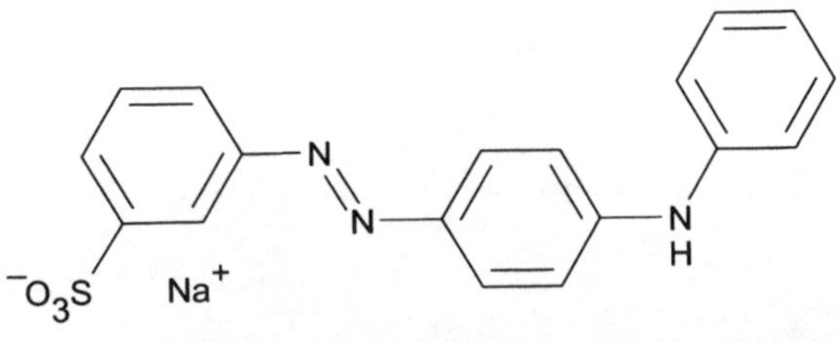

This dye, which is freely soluble in water and somewhat less so in alcohol, is used as a cytoplasmic stain in contrast to more deeply coloured dyes.

The 'milling' dyes have larger molecules. They are bis- and trisazo compounds. They are used as anionic stains of moderate to large molecular size in methods for connective tissue (Chapter 8). Some anionic triphenylmethane dyes are used for the same purposes. Another group of anionic dyes with large molecules is that of the direct dyes, to be described below. Biebrich scarlet is a milling dye.

BIEBRICH SCARLET (C.I. 26905; Acid red 66; MW 557)

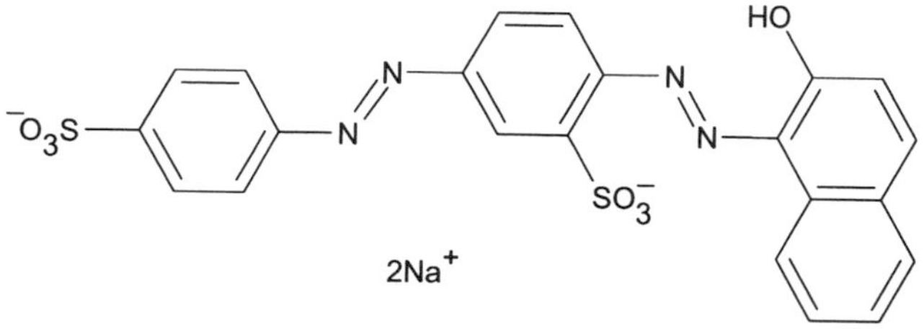

This dye is soluble in water but only slightly soluble in alcohol. It is used in several staining methods, as a counterstain for collagen. Biebrich scarlet does not change colour over a wide pH range. Alkaline solutions of it can be used for selective staining of strongly basic proteins (Spicer and Lillie, 1961).

AMARANTH (C.I. 16185; Acid red 27; MW 604; also called azorubin S)

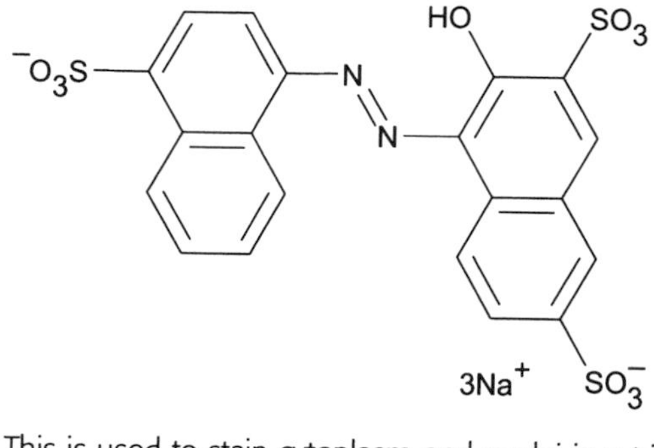

This is used to stain cytoplasm and nuclei in a trichrome method (Chapter 8).

5.9.4.4. Metal complexing azo dyes
These have functional groups capable of chelating chromium or similar metals. The commonest arrangements are:

(a)   Hydroxyl groups *ortho* to both azo nitrogens:

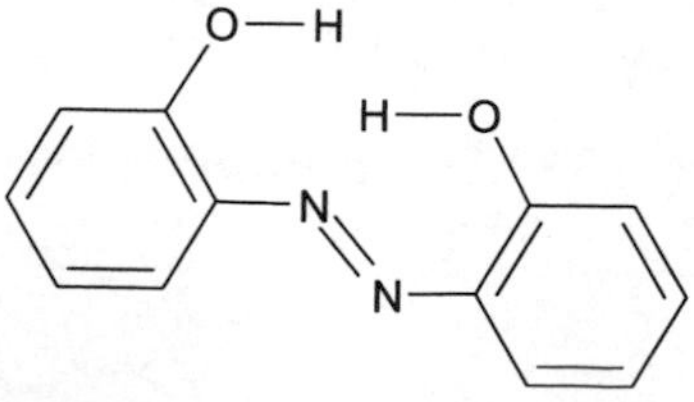

The chelate formed with an ion of a metal M has the structure:

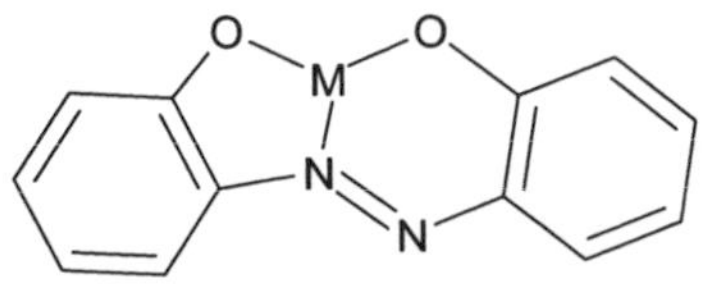

It is possible for only one of the azo nitrogen atoms to be linked with one metal ion, the other being too far away as a consequence of the *trans* configuration of the azo group. However, it can be seen from the structural formula above that a metal with a coordination number higher than 3 could combine with another molecule of dye. In this way large aggregate molecules of the dye–mordant complex may be formed.

(b)   Hydroxyl and amino groups *ortho* to both azo nitrogens:

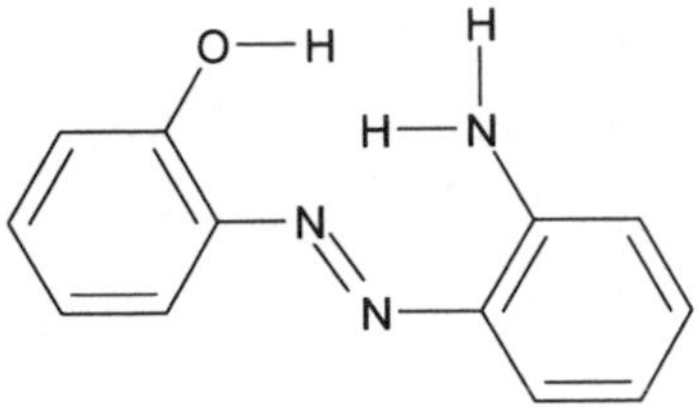

Chelates have structures analogous to that shown for (a) above.

(c)   The salicylic acid arrangement on one of the aromatic rings:

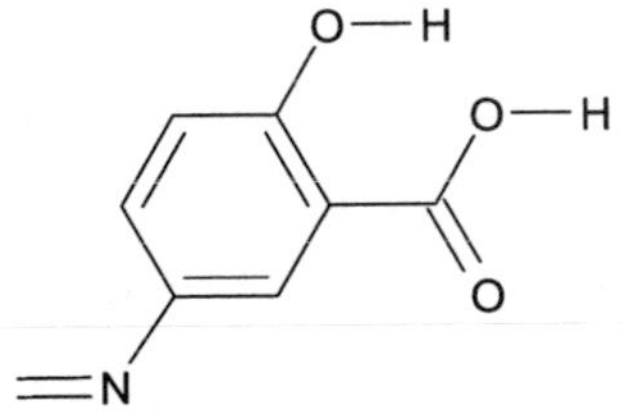

The formation of chelates by the salicylate ion was described in Section 5.5.8.

Examples

MAGNESON (4-(4-nitrophenylazo)resorcinol; diazo violet; (no C.I. number); MW 259)

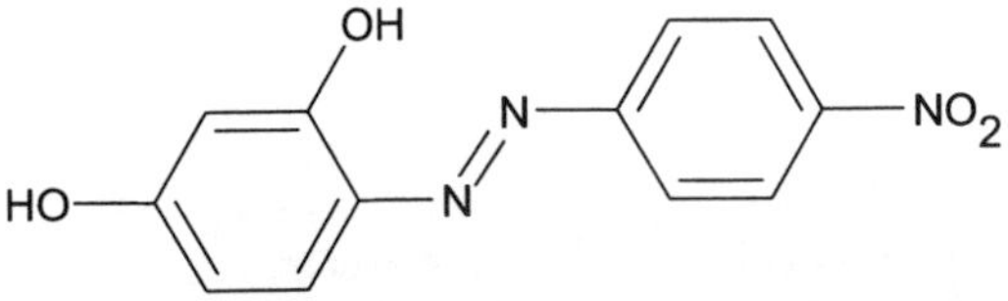

This is slightly soluble in water and alcohols; more soluble in dilute aqueous sodium hydroxide. It has been used as an analytical and a histochemical reagent for magnesium, with which a bright blue complex is formed.

ACID ALIZARIN VIOLET N (C.I. 15670; Mordant violet 5; MW 366.3)
Soluble in water; slightly soluble in acetone and ethanol. The chromium complex is violet; the copper complex is red. The fluorescent aluminium complex has been used as a fluorochrome for nuclei.

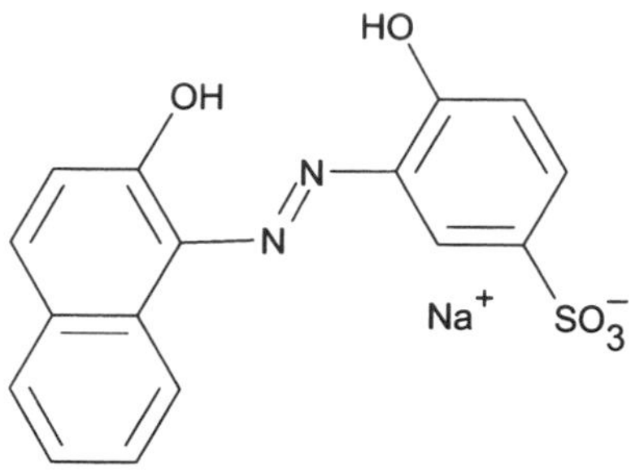

SALICIN BLACK EAG (solochrome black A; C.I. 15710; Mordant black 1; MW 461)

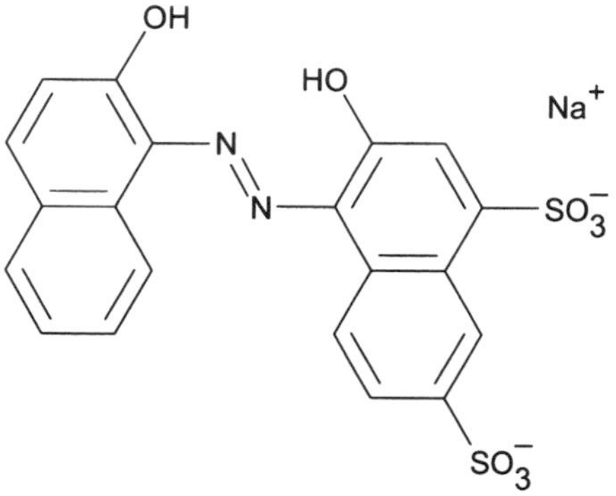

Soluble in water; slightly soluble in alcohol and acetone. The aluminium complex is fluorescent (orange emission) and is sometimes used as a fluorochrome.

5.9.4.5. Cationic azo dyes

Bismarck brown Y, which was the first commercially produced azo dye, is still used for colouring leather.

BISMARCK BROWN Y (Bismarck brown G; vesuvin; leather brown; C.I. 21000; Basic brown 1; MW 419)

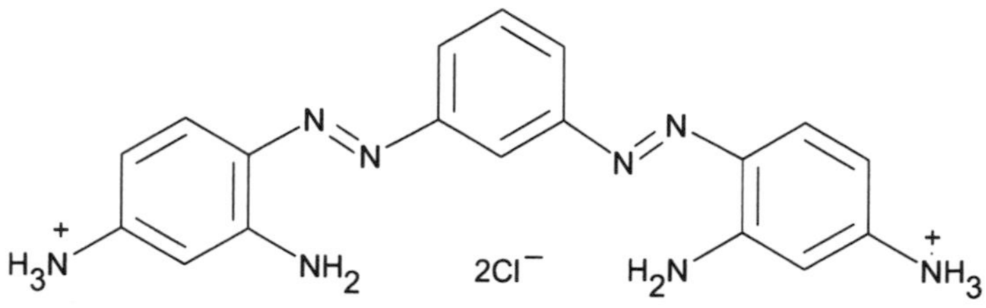

This dye is used in a variety of techniques for staining sections and smears. It is soluble in water and alcohol but insoluble in acetone and most other organic solvents. Samples should contain at least 45% of the anhydrous dyestuff. Solutions should not be heated because the dye is changed by raising the temperature.

CHRYSOIDINE (chrysoidine Y; C.I. 11270; Basic orange 2; MW 249)

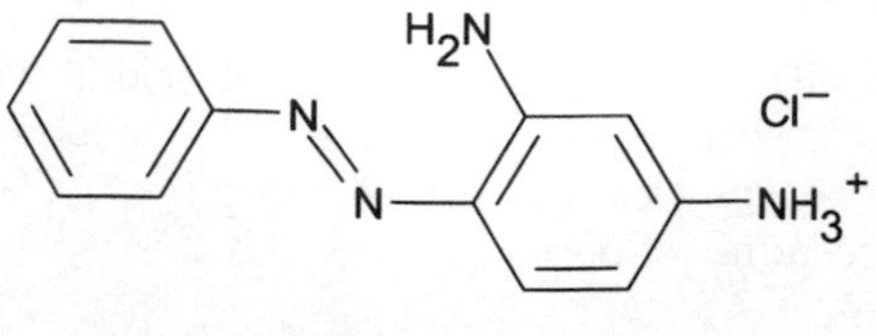

This dye can be used in the same way as Bismarck brown Y and is similarly unstable if heated.

JANUS GREEN B (diazene green; C.I. 11050; MW 511)

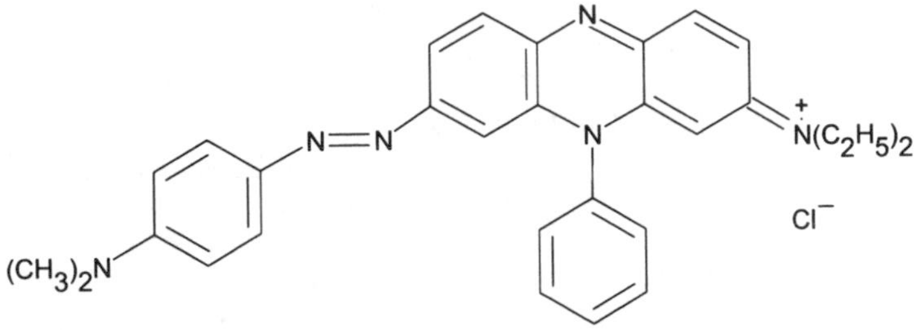

This dye contains both the azo and the azine chromophores. It is occasionally used as a simple cationic stain, especially for bacteria, but its principal application is for vital staining of mitochondria (Chapter 6).

ALCIAN YELLOW (C.I.12840; Ingrain yellow 1; MW 838)

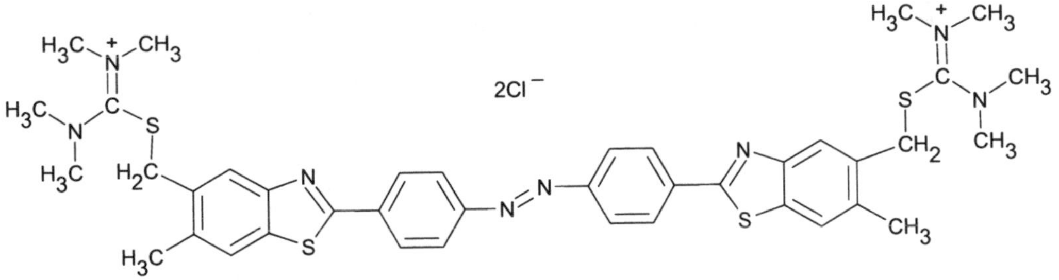

This dye contains both the azo and the thiazole chromophores and is fluorescent (blue emission when excited by near-UV). It is more soluble in ethanol (1%) than in water (0.2%). The cationic isothiouronium groups are split off when the dye binds to a negatively charged substrate, leaving behind an insoluble pigment. Alcian yellow has been used in the same way as alcian blue; it is currently used in a staining method for detecting bacteria (*Helicobacter*) in sections of gastric biopsies (Leung *et al.*, 1996; see also Section 10.10.5.1).

5.9.4.6. Reactive azo dyes

Reactive dyes form covalent bonds with the dyed substrate and are used mainly on cotton, where the attachment is to the hydroxyl groups of cellulose. The commonest reactive auxochromes are the dichlorotriazinyl and monochlorotriazinyl groups. The following is a dichlorotriazinyl azo dye.

PROCION BRILLIANT RED M2B (C.I. 18158; Reactive red 1; MW 717)

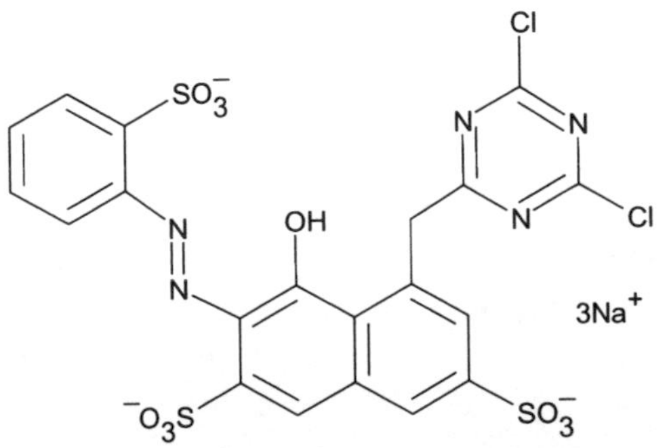

Reactive dyes are not used as stains for sections. An application of this dye in vital staining of bones and teeth is cited by Lillie (1977), and Burnell (1988) used it in a study of intercellular exchange through plasmodesmata between adjacent plant cells. The dye is an irreversible inhibitor of ribulose-5-phosphate kinase, whereas the hydrolysed dye, being unable to bind covalently, is a reversible inhibitor of that enzyme (Ashton, 1984).

5.9.4.7. Solvent azo dyes

These dyes have largely non-polar molecules with few or no atoms that can form hydrogen bonds. Groups such as $-SO_3^-$ and $-NH_3^+$ that confer water solubility are absent. Phenolic hydroxyl groups are usually present, but may be esterified without affecting the staining properties. Solvent dyes move from somewhat polar solvents into less polar (more hydrophobic) domains of the substrate. A traditional statement with almost the same meaning (Baker, 1958) is that a solvent dye is more soluble in lipids than in the solvent from which it is applied. Sudan black B and oil red O are the most frequently used stains for lipids (Chapter 12).

Examples

SUDAN IV (C.I. 26105; Solvent red 24; MW 380)

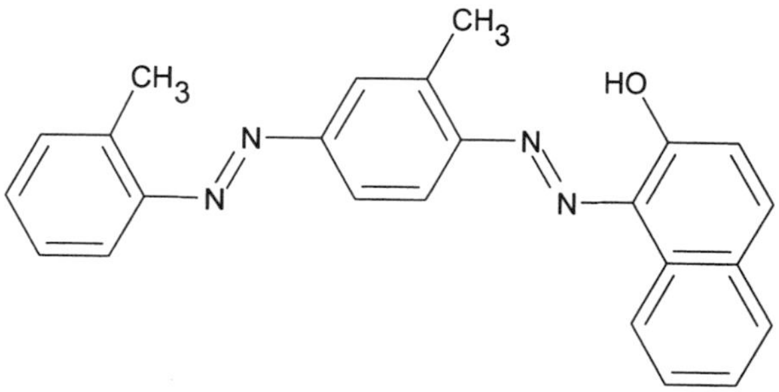

Sudan IV is suitable only for staining conspicuous accumulations of lipids, as in adipose tissue. The dye content should be at least 80% by weight. **Sudan III** (C.I. 26100; Solvent red 23; MW 352), which is less deeply coloured, lacks the two methyl groups of Sudan IV.

OIL RED O (C.I. 26125; Solvent red 27; MW 409)

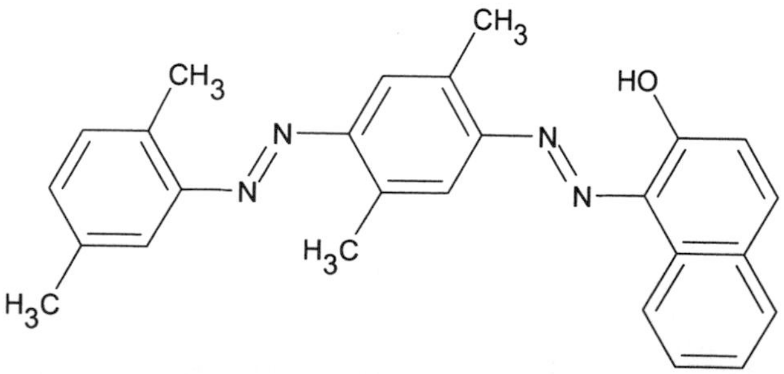

This dye is more intensely coloured than Sudan IV and therefore allows the resolution of smaller lipid-containing structures, such as intracellular droplets. Oil red O is often present as a contaminant in Sudan III and Sudan IV. All three dyes are mixtures of up to eight coloured components (Marshall, 1977).

SUDAN BLACK B (C.I. 26150; Solvent black 3; MW 457)
The dyestuff contains two major components (Pfüller et al., 1977), with these structures:

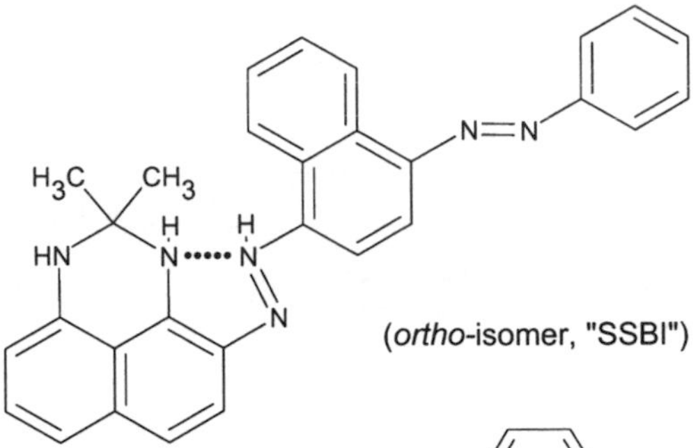

(*ortho*-isomer, "SSBI")

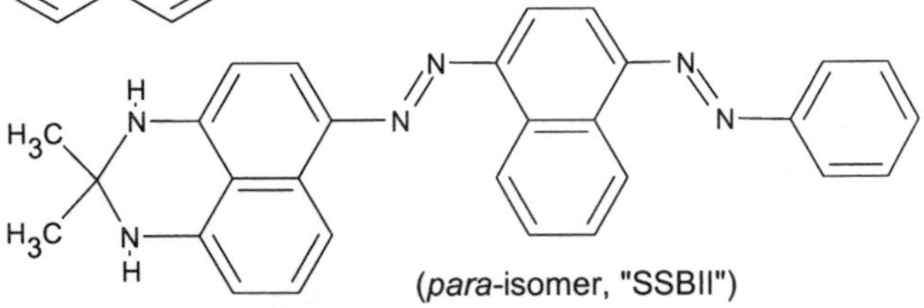

(*para*-isomer, "SSBII")

The second formula (SSBII) corresponds to the Sudan black B (C.I. 26150; Solvent black 3; MW 457) of *Conn's Biological Stains* (Lillie, 1977). There is no satisfactory assay method for Sudan black B. Batches of the dye are evaluated by the Biological Stain Commission on the basis of their absorption spectra and their performance in methods for staining lipids.

Sudan black B can dissolve in hydrophobic lipids but, by virtue of its two potentially protonatable nitrogen atoms, it may also behave like a cationic dye and bind to the hydrophilic phosphate–ester groups of phospholipids, in which it is more soluble than the other Sudan dyes. The *para* isomer (SSBII) is more strongly basic than the *ortho* (SSBI) isomer because in the latter an internal hydrogen bond between one of the secondary amine nitrogens and an azo nitrogen tends to inhibit protonation. A *bis-N*-acetylated derivative of Sudan black B can be prepared in the laboratory and some workers prefer this reagent to the commercially supplied dyestuff. Acetylated Sudan black B should not be able to form cations, but Marshall (1977) was unable to find in it any chromatographically distinct components that were not present in the parent dye.

5.9.4.8. Direct azo dyes

These, which are also called cellulose-substantive dyes, can colour cellulosic fibres (cotton and linen) without the help of metal salts or special reactive auxochromic groups. Ionic auxochromes cannot be attracted by unionized –OH, which is the only functional group present in cellulose. The dyes are all anionic. Most are dis- or trisazo dyes and all have long molecules with usually at least five aromatic rings (naphthalene counting as two). The rings must not be sterically hindered from assuming a coplanar configuration. In aqueous solution, direct dyes form molecular aggregates at room temperature but not at 90–100°C, the temperature at which they are applied to textiles.

The entry of direct dyes into porous cotton or linen fibres is facilitated by interfacial effects (Section 5.5.1). When the dye molecules are in the pores, they are probably close enough to the cellulose to be attracted by weak intermolecular forces. Hydrogen bonds are believed to form between the hydroxy hydrogen atoms of the substrate and the extensive delocalized π-electron system of the dye (see also Section 5.5.4, and Gordon and Gregory, 1983). Additional dye molecules may be retained in the pores as a result of aggregation due to van der Waals forces between the hydrophobic parts of dye molecules (see Allen, 1971).

Some of the direct azo dyes are used in histological work, especially in techniques for the demonstration of fibrin, collagen, elastin and amyloid. The various possible modes of dyeing of cotton may or may not be involved in these procedures, which are carried out at room temperature. The dyes can, of course, behave as ordinary anionic dyes towards cationic components of a tissue. In this respect the direct dyes resemble anionic azo dyes of the 'milling' class described earlier.

Some direct azo dyes have been shown to be carcinogenic in rats and mice (National Toxicology Program, 1978).

Examples
CONGO RED (C.I. 22120: Direct red 28; MW 697)

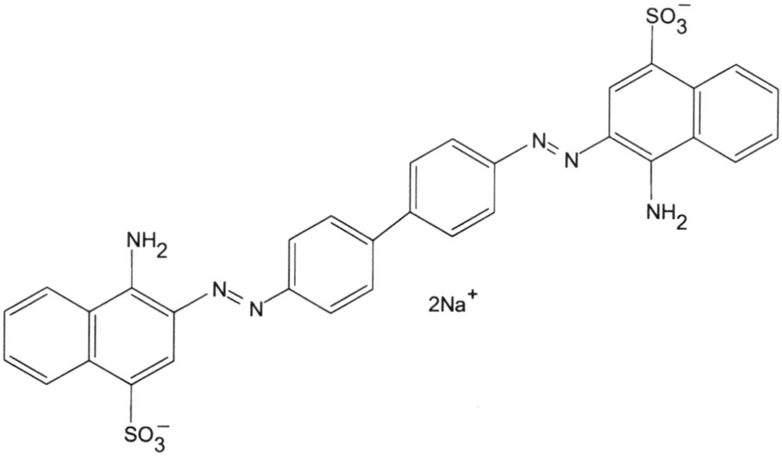

This dye is much more soluble in water than in alcohol. It is an indicator, changing from red to blue when the pH is less than about 3.0. It has several uses in histology, the best known being as a stain for amyloid (Chapter 11). Samples should contain at least 75% by weight of the anhydrous dye.

BENZO BLUE BB (direct blue 2B; C.I. 22610; Direct blue 6; MW 713)

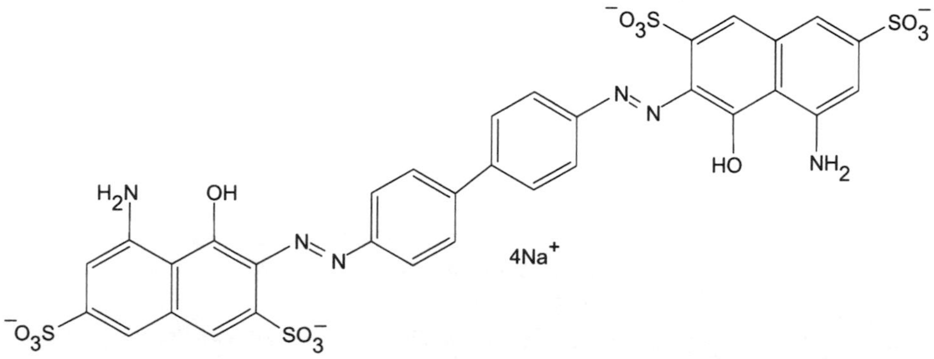

This is used in a method that enhances the birefringence of collagen fibres (Chapter 8). The additional sulphonate and amino groups make the dye more hydrophilic than Congo red. A closely related dye, **Chicago blue 6B**, has been used to suppress autofluorescence (Chapter 1, Section 1.1).

CHLORAZOL BLACK E (C.I. 30235; Direct black 38; MW 782)

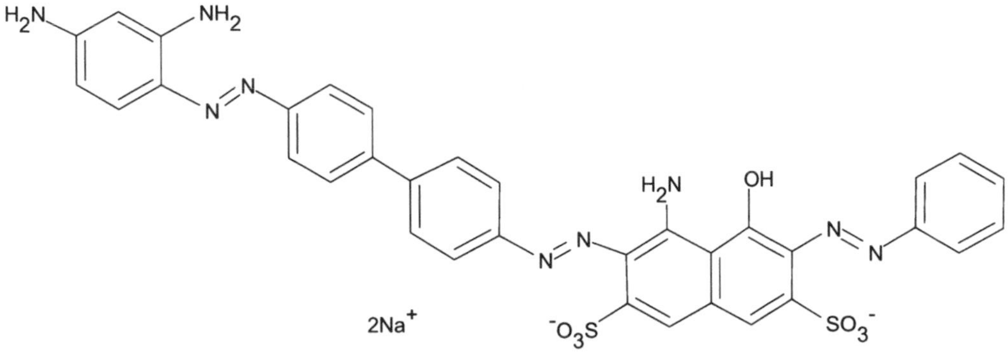

This dye is soluble in water and alcohol but not in most other organic solvents. It is used alone as a stain for sections, especially of plant tissues. The dye is amphoteric; in strongly acid solutions the molecule will bear a net positive charge. Samples of this dye contain small amounts of green, red and yellow dyes in additional to the main black component (Rosenthal *et al.*, 1965). Chlorazol black E is a general purpose stain for tissue sections, microorganisms and fungi.

SIRIUS RED F3B (C.I. 35780; Direct red 80; MW 1372)

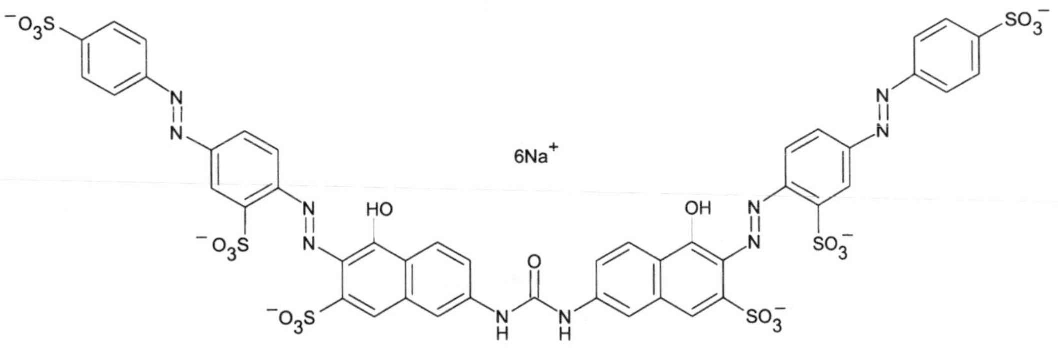

The long molecules of this tetrakisazo dye can align themselves along the fibrillary molecules of collagen, staining it red and also greatly increasing its natural birefringence when examined by polarizing microscopy (Chapter 8). The dye is more soluble in water than in alcohol and other organic solvents. It is used extensively but mainly by research workers, who often know it only as 'sirius red'. The name 'sirius' has no chemical significance. There are other 'sirius red' dyes, and sirius red F3B has many other names that do not include 'sirius' (see Lillie, 1977 and the *Colour Index*: Society of Dyers and Colourists, 1971–1996).

5.9.4.9. Azoic dyes

Azoic dyes are insoluble azo compounds synthesized within or upon substrates by the combination of diazonium salts with suitable aromatic amines or phenols (known as **azoic coupling components**). In histological sections, attachment to protein, or uptake into lipids may occur as the dye is being formed. The importance of azoic dyes in microtechnique is due to their formation as the end-products of many histochemical methods. Some of these will be discussed in Chapters 14–16. Diazonium salts and azoic coupling components are commonly used reagents in histochemistry. The diazonium salts are occasionally prepared immediately before use but more often they are bought ready-made as **stabilized diazonium and tetrazonium salts**. These are commonly zinc chloride double salts of the form:

$$(Ar - \overset{+}{N} \equiv N)_2 \ [ZnCl_4]^{2-}$$

Others are salts of sulphonic acids, such as the naphthalene-1,5-disulphonates:

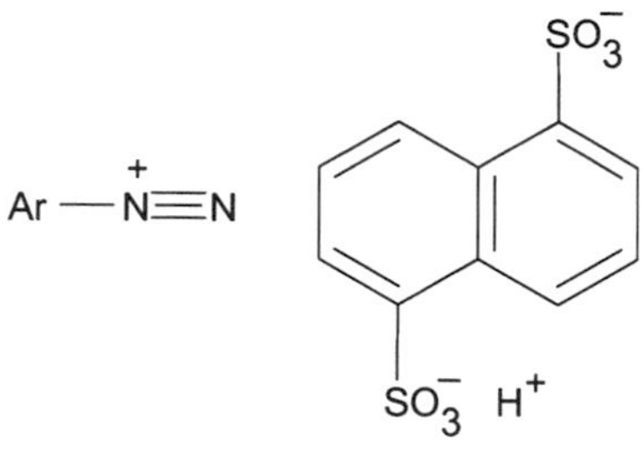

and yet others are borofluorides:

A few are simple chlorides, $R-N_2^+ \ Cl^-$ or bisulphates, $R-N_2^+ \ HSO_4^-$. The diazonium salt is mixed with an inert diluent such as sodium sulphate, and other substances may also be present as stabilizers. The original amine usually accounts for less than half the weight of the commercially obtained powder. Stabilized diazonium salts are also called **azoic diazo components**. They should *not* be referred to as 'stable diazotates'; diazotate ions have the structure $R-N=N-O^-$ and are formed when strong alkalis react with diazonium ions. The terms 'tetrazonium' and 'hexazonium' are used for salts with two and three diazotized amino groups per molecule.

Examples of azoic diazo components
FAST RED B SALT (diazotized 5-nitroanisidine acid 1-5-naphthalene disulphonate; C.I. 37125; Azoic diazo 5; MW 467)

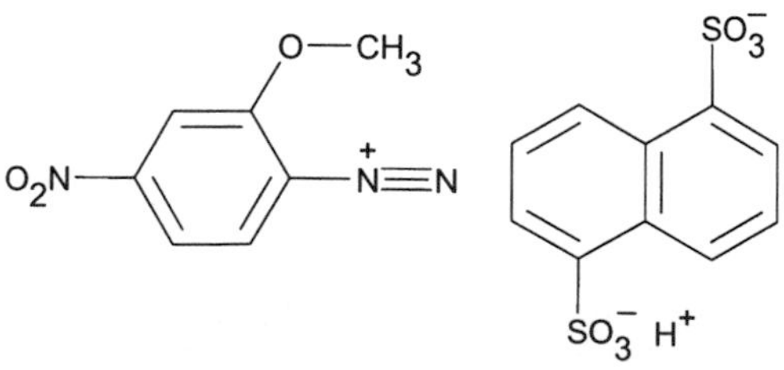

The primary amine represents 20% by weight of the commercial product (theoretical: 36% of formula weight). This diazonium salt is the one most often used for staining argentaffin cells (Chapter 17). It does not give satisfactory results in histochemical methods for hydrolytic enzymes.

FAST BLUE RR SALT (C.I. 37155; Azoic diazo 24; MW 776 including two molecules of diazo)

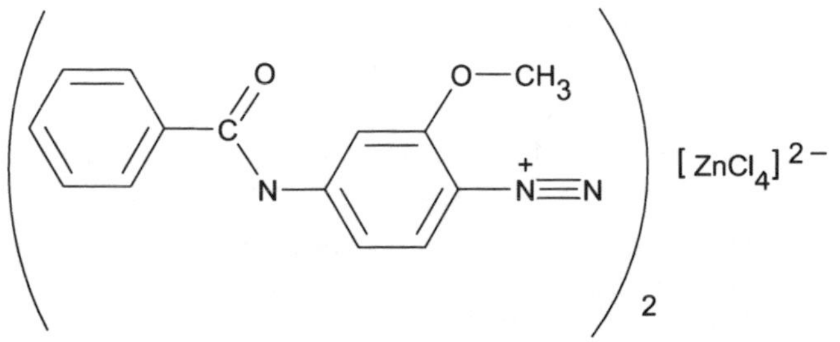

The primary amine accounts for 36% of the weight of the commercial product (theoretical: 71%). This diazonium salt is used in many methods for hydrolytic enzymes (Chapter 15).

FAST BLUE B SALT (Tetraazotized *o*-dianisidine zinc chloride double salt; C.I. 37235; Azoic diazo 48; MW 476)

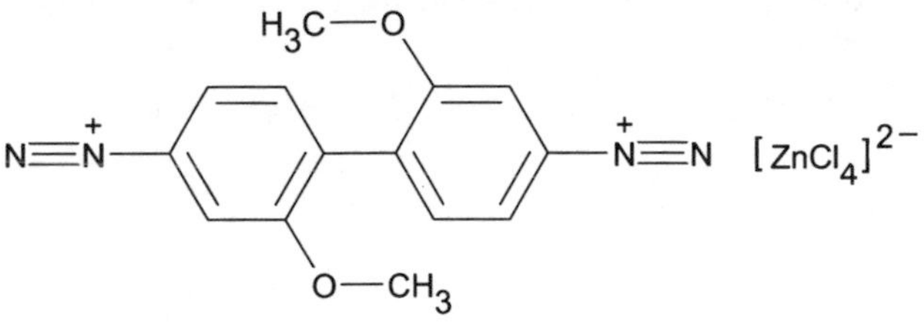

The theoretical content of the bifunctional primary amine (*o*-dianisidine) is 51% by weight but the commercial product contains about 20%. This is a 'tetrazonium' salt with a diazotized amine group at each end of the molecule. It is used in the coupled tetrazonium reaction for proteins (Chapter 10) and in some methods for enzymes (e.g. Chapter 7, Section 7.4.1).

FAST GARNET GBC SALT (C.I. 37210; Azoic diazo 4; MW 334)

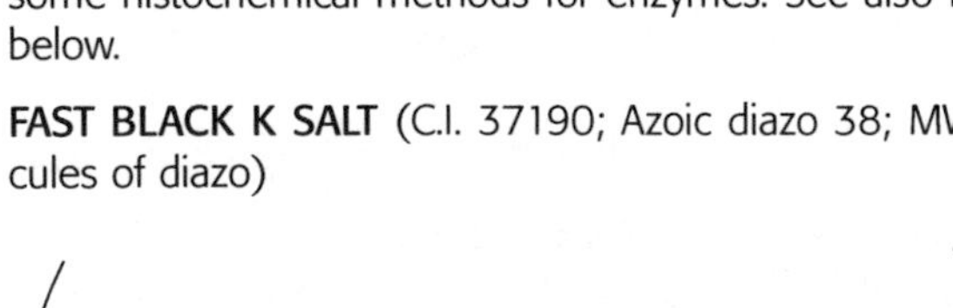

Contains 15–20% by weight of primary amine (theoretical: 67%). It is used in some histochemical methods for enzymes. See also note under fast black K salt, below.

FAST BLACK K SALT (C.I. 37190; Azoic diazo 38; MW 836; including two molecules of diazo)

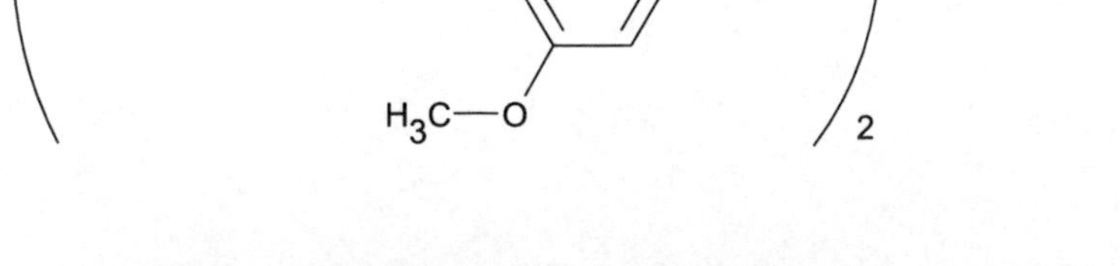

Lillie (1962) assumed that the primary amine represented 20% by weight of the commercial product (theoretical, from formula above, is 72%).

In fast garnet GBC salt and fast black K salt, azo linkages are already present in the diazonium ions. These salts are therefore coloured. Coupling with a phenol or amine produces a disazo dye, which has a darker colour.

Many dyes that are primary amines can be diazotized with nitrous acid to give coloured diazonium salts. Subsequent coupling with suitable aromatic molecules in sections of tissues results in the formation of new azo compounds with colours different from and often darker than those of the parent dyes. Pararosaniline and safranine O (Lillie et al., 1968a) are two dyes from which histochemically useful diazonium salts are easily prepared in the laboratory. An enzyme histochemical technique using hexazonium pararosaniline is described in Chapter 7 (Section 7.4.2).

Azoic coupling components

Most of the coupling components used in industry are derivatives of naphthalene, with hydroxyl, amine, and sulphonic acid groups substituted in various positions. An example is:

H-ACID (8-amino-1-naphthol-3,6-disulphonic acid; MW 319)

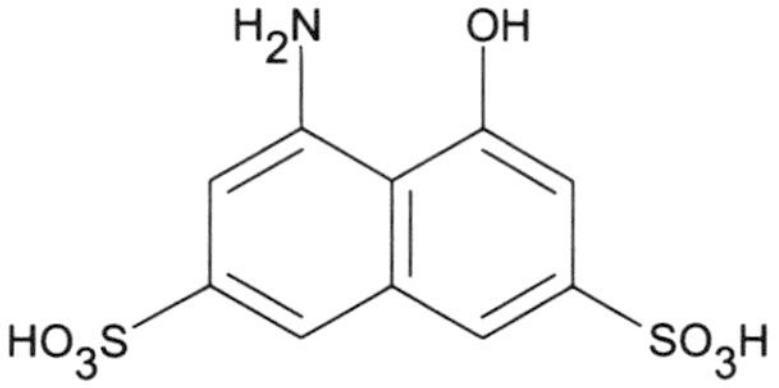

This is also available as a sodium salt (MW 341). Coupling occurs in alkaline solution, principally at position 2 (*ortho* to the hydroxyl group). This reagent is used in the coupled tetrazonium reaction (Chapter 10) for the histochemical detection of proteins.

In enzyme histochemistry, azoic coupling components are released by enzymatic hydrolysis of certain of their derivatives, notably esters and amides. Such methods are discussed in Chapter 15. The coupling components most often liberated in histochemical methods for enzymes are **naphthols:**

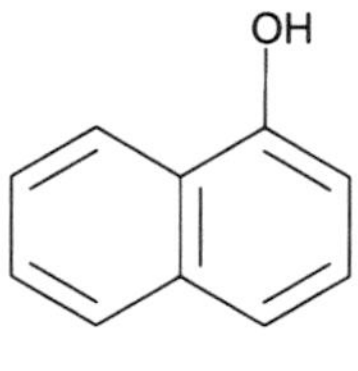

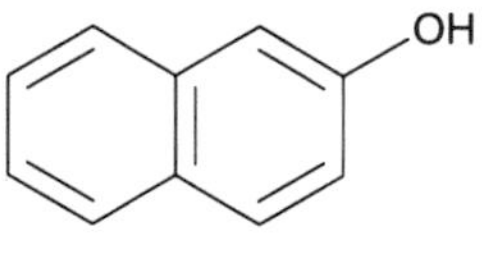

α-naphthol   β-naphthol

More intensely coloured azo dyes are formed from β-naphthol, but these are more soluble and form larger particles than the coupling products of α-naphthol. The advantages of both the simple naphthols are found in **naphthol-AS** (also known as **benzosalicylanilide**):

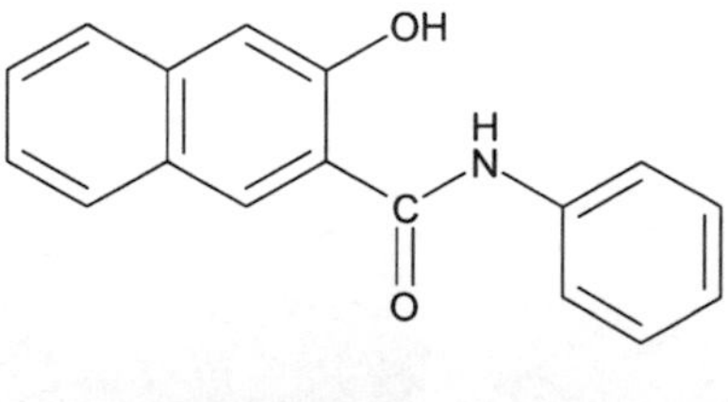

This compound couples with diazonium salts to give finely granular, brightly coloured insoluble products, but the rate of coupling is slower than with α- and β-naphthols.

5.9.5.
Arylmethane
dyes

These are compounds have the general formula:

$$R-\underset{\underset{R''}{|}}{C}=R'=X \qquad (X = N \text{ or } O)$$

in which two or three of the hydrogen atoms of methane are replaced by benzene or naphthalene rings (R, R', R''; in diarylmethanes one of these is H). The aromatic rings resonate between quinonoid and truly aromatic configurations. The chromophoric chain of conjugated bonds extends through all parts of the molecule, so that a large number of equivalent structures can be drawn for each dye. There are two major groups of triarylmethane dyes: aminotriarylmethanes (X=N) and hydroxytriarylmethanes (X=O).

5.9.5.1. Diarylmethane dyes

The only member of this group used as a microscopical stain is auramine O.

AURAMINE O (C.I. 41000; Basic yellow 2; Anhydrous MW 304; the commercial product has one molecule of water of crystallization; MW 322)

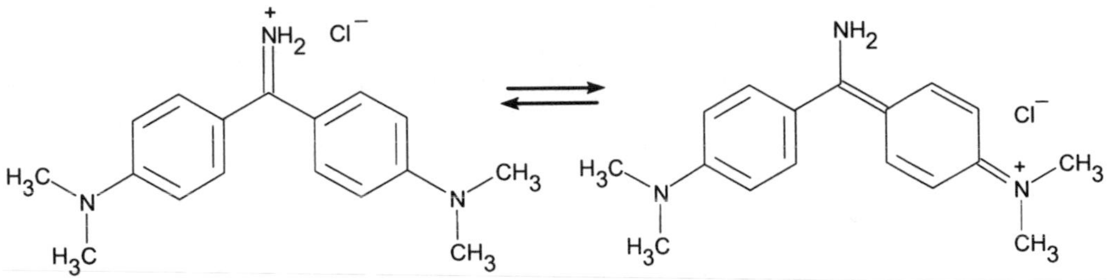

These formulae depict two of the possible resonance structures: an imine (left) and a quinonoid form. This yellow cationic dye is used mainly as a fluorochrome to detect tubercle bacilli in smears or sections (see Clark, 1981 for methods).

5.9.5.2 Aminotriarylmethane dyes

The simplest members of this class are the triphenylmethanes. Of these, pararosaniline, a red cationic dye, has the most easily understood structure. This dye, which has many uses in histology, histochemistry and bacteriology, is described at some length. Other important triarylmethane dyes are more briefly treated.

Examples
PARAROSANILINE (C.I. 42500; Basic red 9; MW 324)

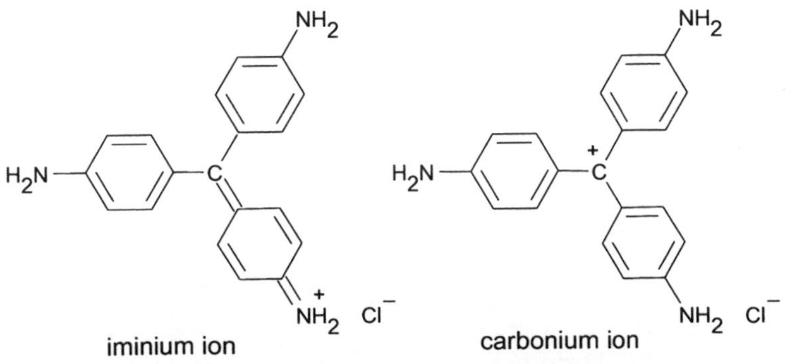

iminium ion   carbonium ion

Two of the possible resonance structures are shown. Any one of the three rings may transiently assume the aromatic or the quinonoid configuration. The positive charge may be assigned to any of the nitrogen atoms or to the central carbon. Similar resonance occurs in all triarylmethane dyes. By convention, iminium ion forms are usually shown in structural formulae. Acetate replaces chloride as the balancing ion in some samples of pararosaniline. For notes on purity, see under basic fuchsine (the next entry).

When pararosaniline is treated with strong alkali (pH > 12), one proton is removed and an imine, called a **colour base**, is instantly formed:

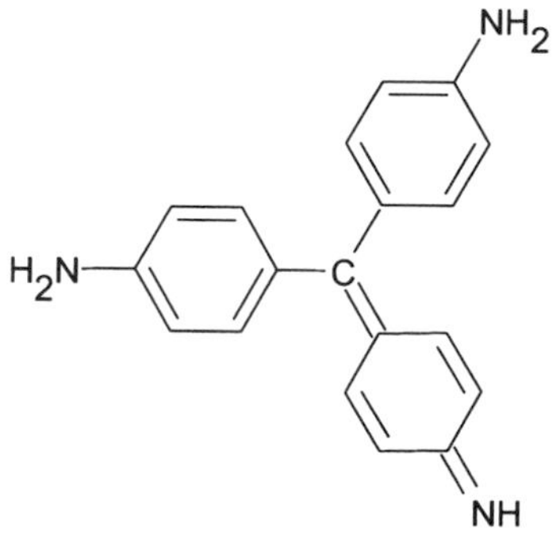

This imine is coloured (p-quinonoid arrangement in the above structure) and it is less hydrophilic than the cation. The pararosaniline cation also reacts more slowly with hydroxide ions, adding a hydroxy group to the central carbon to form a stable, colourless **carbinol base**, also called a **pseudobase**:

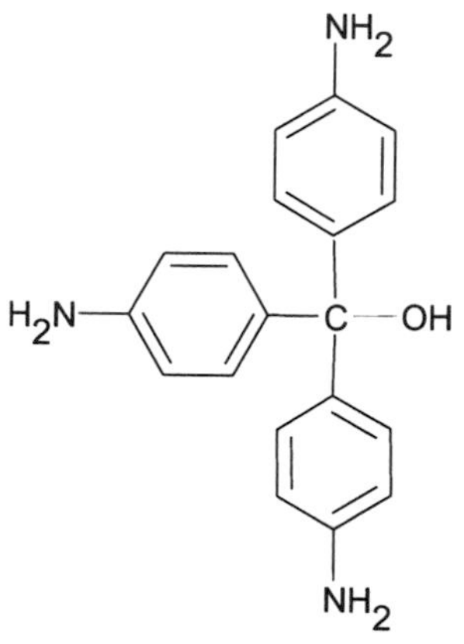

The carbinol base is a tertiary alcohol. It is named as a derivative of methanol (carbinol; H_3COH). It is a stable compound. Acidification converts it to the original dye.

Colourless derivatives of two other kinds are easily prepared from pararosaniline and related dyes. Reduction destroys the chromophoric structure and gives a **leucobase**:

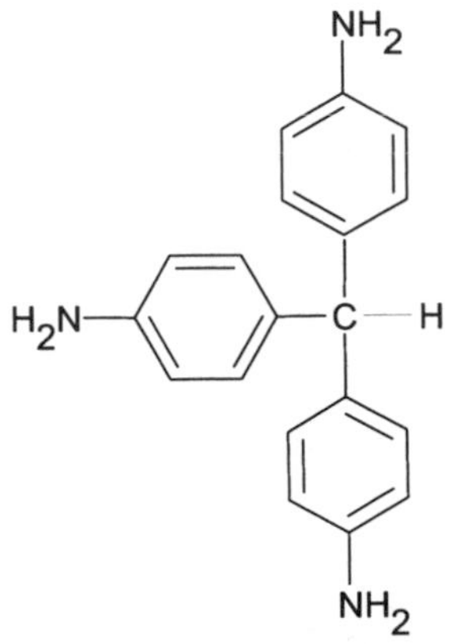

The third way of decolorizing pararosaniline involves treatment with sulphurous acid, to give **Schiff s reagent**, the chemistry and uses of which are described in other chapters.

Some derivatives of pararosaniline are prepared in the laboratory for use in some special staining methods. These include **hexazonium pararosaniline** (used in enzyme histochemistry, see Section 7.4.2) and **aldehyde–fuchsine** (Chapter 8, Section 8.4.3).

BASIC FUCHSINE
This is a mixture of triphenylmethane dyes. Modern samples of basic fuchsine consist almost entirely of either **pararosaniline** or **new fuchsine**. Older samples usually contained both dyes, together with rosaniline and magenta II. The balancing anion is sometimes acetate rather than the chloride shown in the formulae below.

ROSANILINE (C.I. 42510; Basic violet 14; Anhydrous: MW 338)

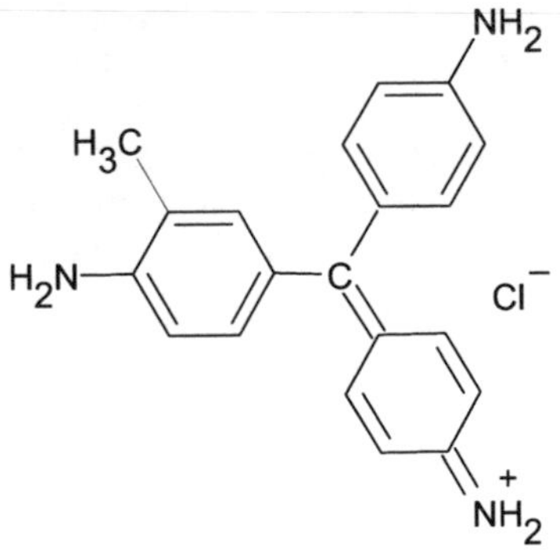

This dye is closely similar to pararosaniline and can replace it for all purposes except the preparation of aldehyde–fuchsine (Chapter 8). It is not commercially available as a pure compound.

NEW FUCHSINE (Magenta III) (C.I. 42520; Basic violet 2; MW 366)
This dye is frequently used in the same way as pararosaniline, to prepare a hexazonium salt for use in enzyme histochemistry. It is commercially available as a pure compound, but is not certified by the Biological Stain Commission.

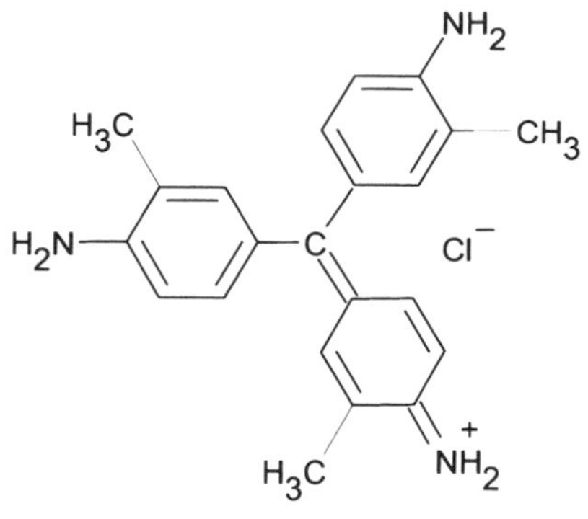

MAGENTA II (No C.I. number; MW 352)

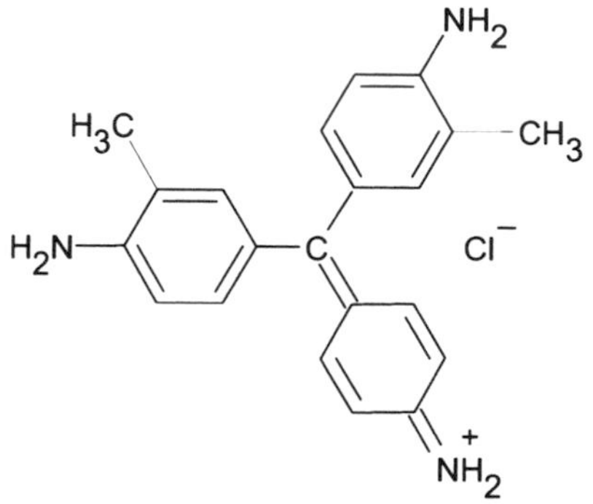

Magenta II is a component of basic fuchsine but it is not commercially available as a single dye.

All the components of basic fuchsine are soluble in water and more soluble in alcohol. For critical work it is desirable to use pure pararosaniline. To be certified by the Biological Stain Commission, samples of basic fuchsine must contain at least 88% anhydrous dye (estimated as pararosaniline or rosaniline) and must perform adequately in a variety of staining procedures, including those that use Schiff's reagent. Pararosaniline must also serve as a starting material for an aldehyde–fuchsine stain.

CRYSTAL VIOLET (C.I. 42555; Basic violet 3; MW 408)

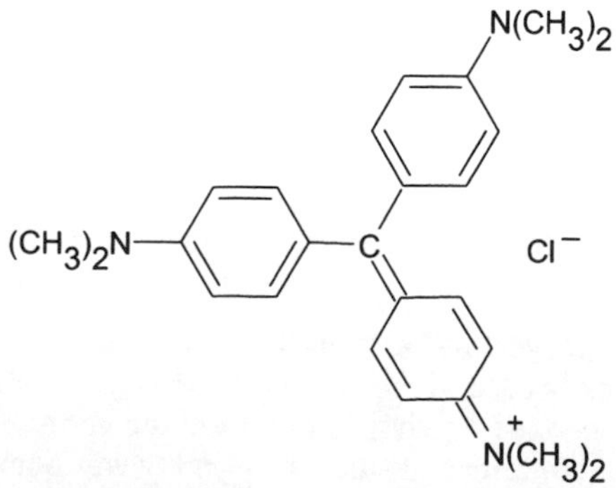

The *N*-hexamethylated derivative of pararosaniline is used in bacteriological techniques, notably the Gram stain (Chapter 6) more than in histology. Samples should contain at least 88% by weight of the anhydrous dye.

METHYL GREEN (C.I. 42585; Basic blue 20; MW of the dichloride: 458) This dye was supplied as a zinc chloride double salt, $[C_{26}H_{33}N_3]^{2+}$ $[ZnCl_4]^{2-}$, MW 595 (Lillie, 1977)

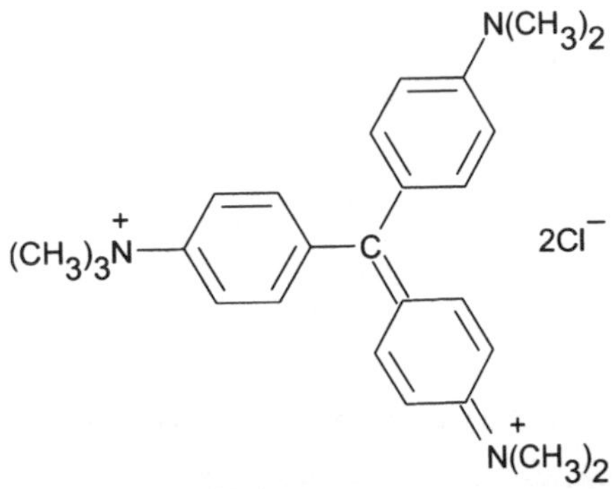

One of the alkyl groups on the quaternary nitrogen (left-hand side of formula above) detaches easily. Consequently, samples of methyl green were always contaminated with crystal violet, which had to be removed by repeated extractions into chloroform. Ethyl green, which is more stable and altogether preferable, is commonly sold as methyl green. Methyl green has not been manufactured for about 40 years, but the name is still seen on bottles of the next dye.

ETHYL GREEN (C.I. 42590; $C_{27}H_{35}Cl_4N_3Zn$ MW 609)
One of the quaternary methyl groups of methyl green is replaced by ethyl, and bromide may replace one of the four chloride ions of the zinc double salt (MW 653).

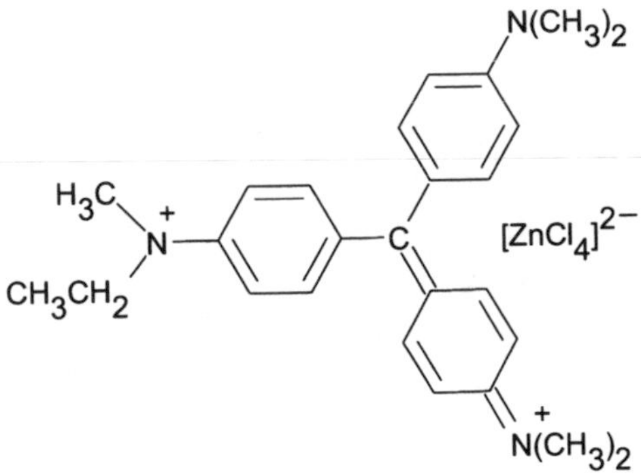

According to Lillie (1977), Lyon *et al.* (1987) and Green (1990), dyes sold as 'methyl green' are always ethyl green. This bluish-green dye is used in several techniques, including the ethyl green–pyronine method for nucleic acids (Chapter 9). The Biological Stain Commission requires that ethyl green ('methyl green') should contain at least 65% of anhydrous, zinc-free dye (MW 458.5). Ethyl green is used as a nuclear counterstain (Chapter 6) and in staining methods that colour RNA red and DNA bluish-green (Chapter 9).

ACID FUCHSINE (C.I. 42685; Acid violet 19)
This is a sodium, calcium or ammonium salt of a trisulphonic acid derivative of basic fuchsine. The acid fuchsine derived from rosaniline ($C_{20}H_{17}N_3Na_2O_9S_3$, MW 586) is:

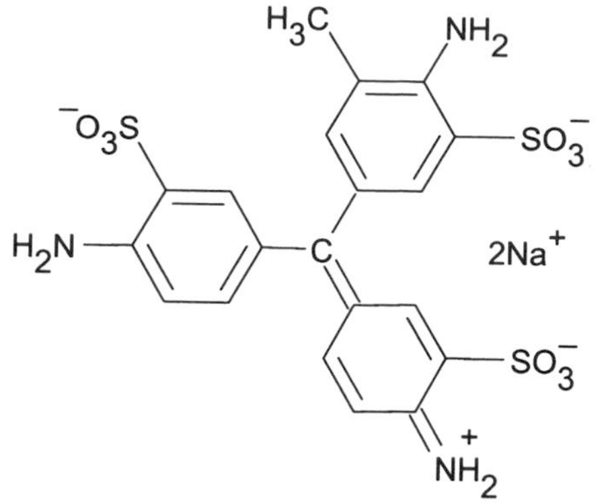

The one related to pararosaniline lacks the methyl group.

This red anionic dye has many uses, especially in conjunction with other anionic dyes (Chapter 8). It is very soluble in water but only sparingly so in alcohol.

For analytical purposes acid fuchsine is assumed to consist of equal parts of the anhydrous disodium salts of trisulphonated pararosaniline and rosaniline (average MW 578.5). Samples should contain at least 55% by weight of this hypothetical dyestuff.

FAST GREEN FCF (C.I. 42053; Food green 3; MW 809)

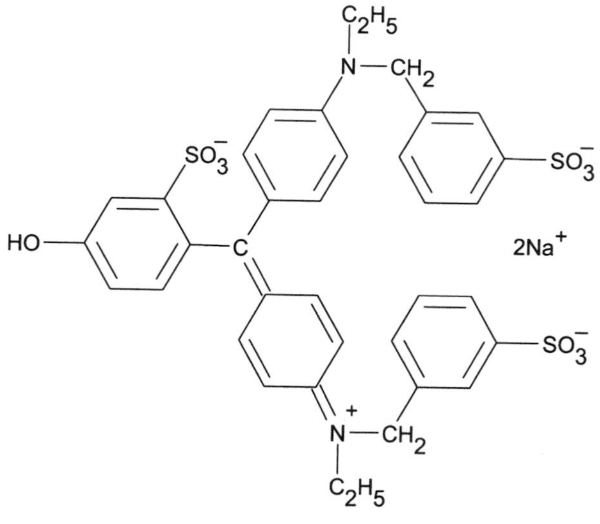

This bluish-green anionic triphenylmethane dye is used in methods for connective tissue and as a counterstain to methods that produce strong blues, purples, and reds. It is very soluble in water and considerably less so in alcohol.

A closely related dye is **light green SF** (light green SF yellowish; C.I. 42095; Acid green 5; MW 793), which lacks the phenolic hydroxyl group of fast green FCF. The two dyes are almost exactly the same colour and can be used for the same purposes, but C.I. 42053 is preferred because it is less prone to fading. Samples of fast green FCF should contain at least 85% by weight of the anhydrous dye. Light green SF should be at least 65% dye. There was a shortage of light green SF in the mid-1990s, and some suppliers substituted other, unsuitable dyes (Penney and Powers, 1995).

PATENT BLUE VF (C.I. 42045; Acid blue 1; MW 567)

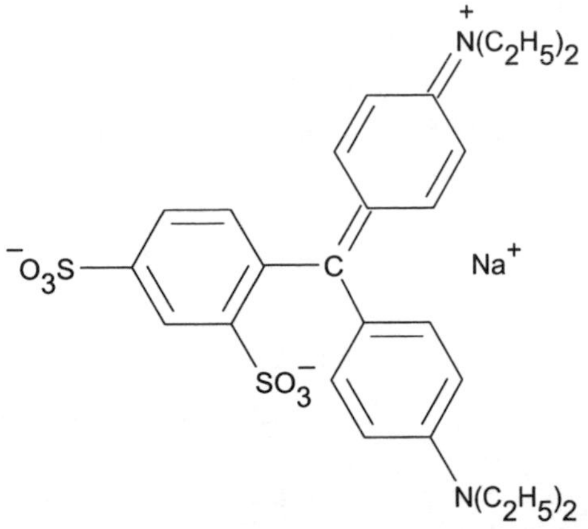

This blue anionic dye changes colour to orange when strongly acidified. It can easily be reduced to a colourless leuco compound, which is used in a histochemical method for the peroxidase-like activity of haemoglobin (Chapter 16). The dye is more soluble in water than in alcohol. Patent blue V (C.I. 42051, Acid blue 3) has a hydroxy group at position 5 on the sulphonated ring; it is used in the same way as patent blue VF.

ANILINE BLUE (methyl blue; C.I. 42780; Acid blue 93; MW 800)

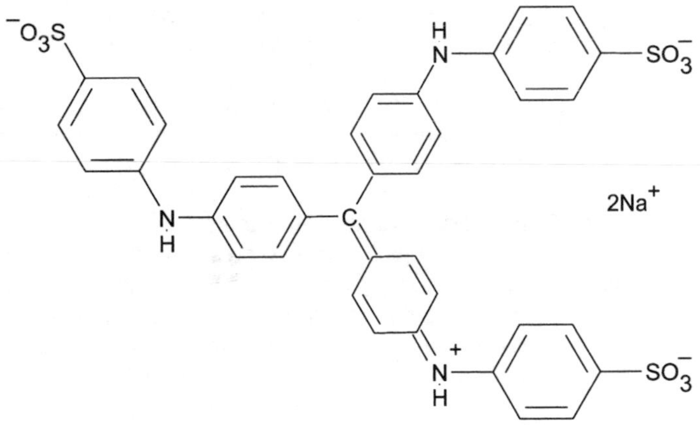

Methyl blue can be manufactured in fairly pure form, and some samples of aniline blue consist largely of this dye. It is also available as the diammonium salt (MW 787). Aniline blue is, however, commonly a mixture of methyl blue with several related dyes, including methyl blue and **water blue** (C.I. 42755, Acid blue 22), which cannot be produced as a pure compound. Methyl blue and its mixtures with related dyes have been known in the past as **water blue, soluble blue, aniline blue (water-soluble)** and **aniline blue WS**. They are very soluble in water, insoluble in alcohol, and have identical staining properties. The colour changes to red with strong alkalis. They are used as anionic dyes of large molecular size, especially in methods for connective tissue (Chapter 8). These dyes cannot be assayed very precisely. The criteria for certification by the Biological Stain Commission are given by Penney *et al.* (2002).

In addition to blue triphenylmethane dyes, aniline blue contains an impurity known as **sirofluor**, which is a useful fluorescent histochemical reagent for staining certain carbohydrates of plants (Chapter 11).

Spirit blue (C.I. 42775; Solvent blue 3) also known as **aniline blue, alcohol-soluble**, is a mixture of diphenyl and triphenyl pararosanilines (i.e. aniline blue without the sulphonic acid groups). Spirit blue is a cationic dye but is insoluble in water. Its alcoholic solutions are occasionally used in histology.

COOMASSIE BRILLIANT BLUE R250 (brilliant blue R; brilliant indocyanine 6G; C.I. 42660; Acid blue 83; MW 826)

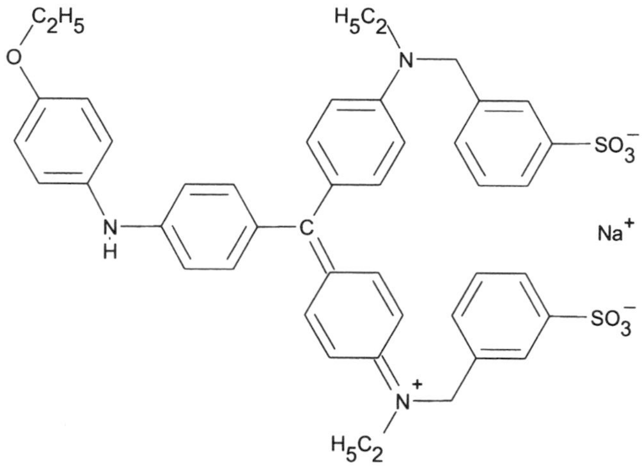

This anionic dye is only slightly soluble in water because of its hydrophobic side-chains; it is even less soluble in alcohol. When coomassie brilliant blue R250 binds to protein the absorption maximum is shifted, and this forms the basis of a sensitive spectrophotometric assay. The dye is also in widespread use for staining protein in polyacrylamide electrophoresis gels. A method for staining protein in sections is described in Chapter 10 (Section 10.9.1.1).

5.9.5.3. Hydroxytriarylmethane dyes
There are three subgroups in this class. **Simple hydroxytriphenylmethanes** are compounds in which all three nitrogen atoms of pararosaniline or rosaniline (Section 5.9.5.2) are replaced by oxygen, giving **pararosolic acid** or **rosolic acid** respectively. A mixture of the two, with various impurities is called **aurin** (C.I. 53800) and is used as an indicator (yellow below pH 6.8, red above pH 8.2).

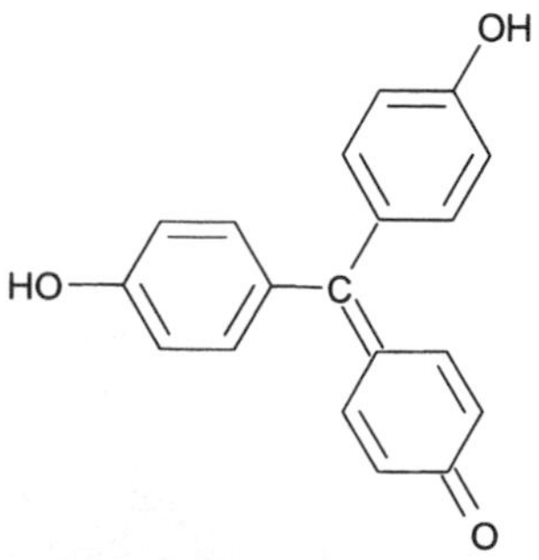

pararosolic acid, M.W. 290 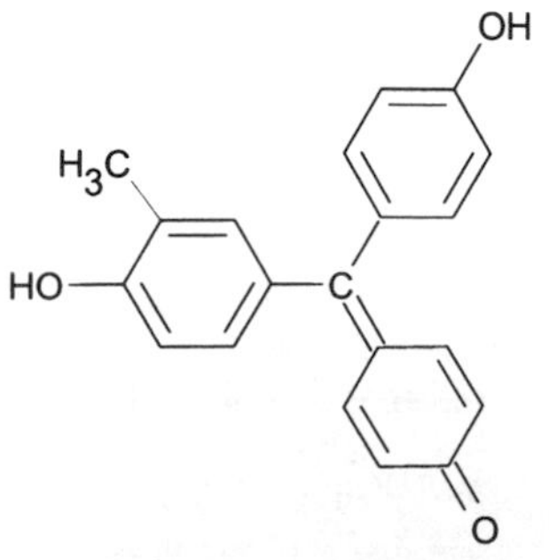   rosolic acid, M. W. 304

In the **phthaleins** (also called phenolphthaleins), only two of the rings carry oxygen atoms *para* to the central carbon. The third ring has a carboxyl group *ortho* to the central carbon. Many phthaleins are sold as white or palely coloured lactones, in which the carboxyl group forms a cyclic internal ester (a **lactone**) with the central carbon. An example is the well known indicator and purgative phenolphthalein, which becomes red as the pH changes from 8.2–9.4.

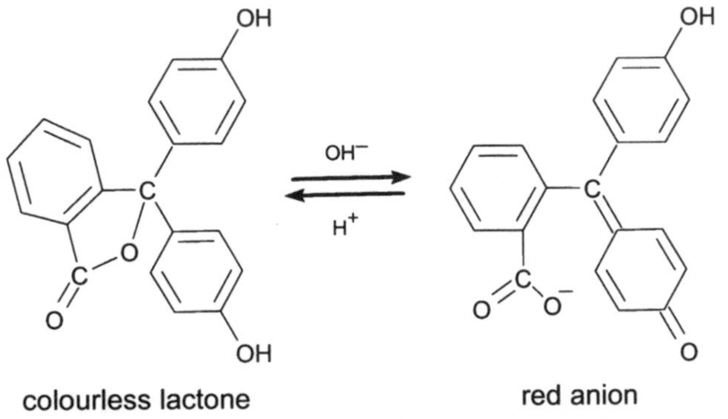

colourless lactone   red anion

Sulphonphthaleins differ from phthaleins in having a sulphonic acid group *ortho* to the central carbon. If a cyclic internal ester is formed with the central carbon, the resulting compound is called a **sultone**. (It is *not* a sulphone, which is an organic compound with two carbon atoms joined to a sulphur atom that also has double bonds to two oxygen atoms: $RR'SO_2$. There is confusion in the scientific literature and in vendors' catalogues!) The phthaleins and sulphonphthaleins include many valuable pH indicators, and a few have been used as stains for proteins. Only a few hydroxytriarylmethane dyes are used as biological stains.

Examples
AURIN TRICARBOXYLIC ACID (ATA, MW 422) The triammonium salt is aluminon, MW 473, and the trisodium salt is chrome violet CG, C.I. 43810, Mordant violet 39. MW 488

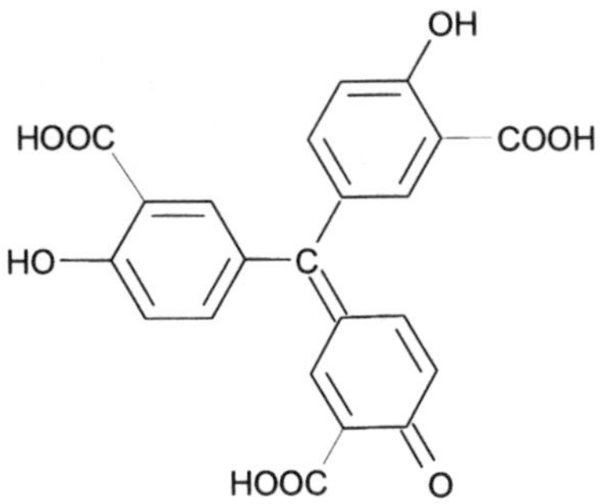

This dye has been used for histochemical detection of aluminium and other metals in tissues, and is also of great pharmacological interest as an inhibitor of angiogenesis, apoptosis and thrombosis; it inhibits nucleases and other enzymes (Bina-Stein and Tritton, 1976). The cationic chromium complex was used as a nuclear stain by Berube and Clark (1964).

ERIOCHROME CYANINE R (chromoxane cyanine R; solochrome cyanine R; C.I. 43820; Mordant blue 3; MW 448)
This useful sulphonphthalein dye is an acid–base indicator (red with acid, blue with alkali) and it can be used as either a red anionic dye or a dye–metal complex. It has been used as a substitute for haematoxylin (Lillie et al., 1968b). The metal is ferric iron in histological practice, though coloured complexes are also formed with aluminium (red) and chromium (blue).

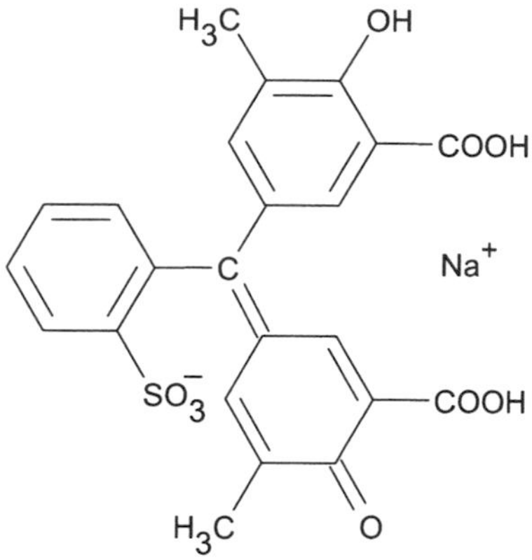

Red and blue iron complexes are involved in staining (Kiernan, 1984a,b). The dye is used as a general purpose blue and red single stain and in selective methods for nuclei and for myelin (Chapter 6). Eriochrome cyanine R is sold as a powder containing about 50% by weight of the dye, usually as its monosodium salt (shown above) rather than the trisodium salt indicated in most catalogues and works of reference.

5.9.6.
Xanthene dyes

The chromophoric system is:

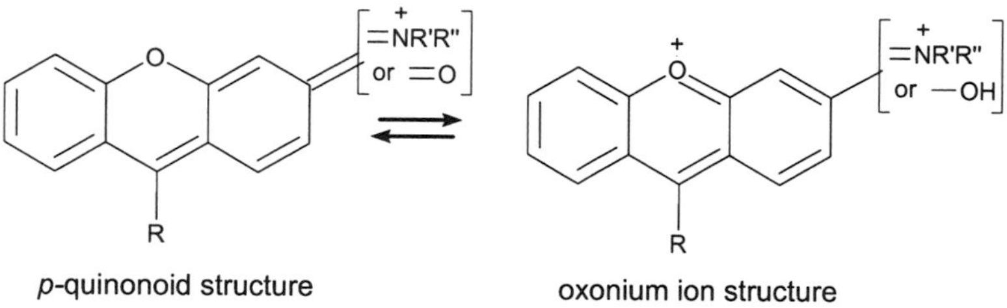

p-quinonoid structure   oxonium ion structure

R, R', and R'' may be hydrogen or any of a variety of alkyl or aryl radicals. Other substituents may also be present. If R is a phenyl group, the dye is also a triphenylmethane derivative in which two of the benzene rings are joined by an ether linkage. Many xanthene dyes are fluorescent and some are used primarily as fluorochromes. The *p*-quinonoid structure is adopted in the structural formulae for the examples of xanthene dyes given below. The dyes are classified by ionic charge rather than as hydroxy- and amino-xanthenes.

5.9.6.1. Anionic xanthene dyes

Examples
FLUORESCEIN SODIUM (uranin; C.I. 45350; Acid yellow 73; MW 376)

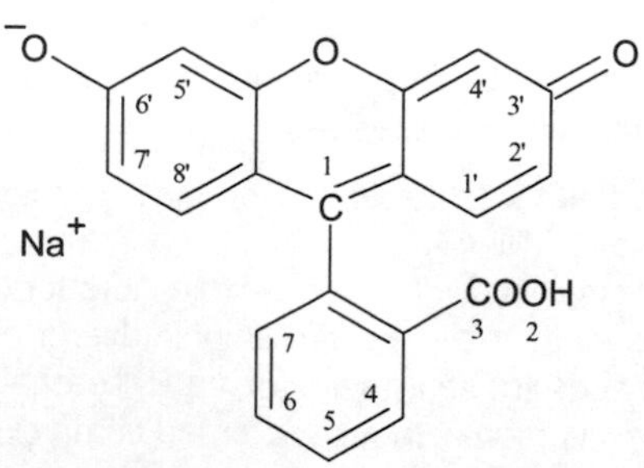

The numbering is as given by Lillie (1977).

This yellow anionic dye is used only as a fluorochrome. An isothiocyanate can be prepared, and this is used as a fluorescent label for proteins (Chapter 19). Optimal excitation is by blue-violet or ultraviolet light and the fluorescent emission is green. Fluorescein is the parent compound of several red xanthene dyes, of which eosin is the most important.

EOSIN AND ITS CONGENERS

These halogenated derivatives of fluorescein are also fluorescent but they are used principally as red dyes. The substitutions in the fluorescein molecule are set out in *Table 5.1*. All the dyes in the table are red, in various shades. All are freely soluble in water, rather less soluble in alcohol, and are precipitated (as the colour acids) by mineral acids. All can be used for similar purposes, though certain dyes are traditionally associated with particular techniques. For certification by the Biological Stain Commission, the percentage by weight of anhydrous dyes in a sample must not be less than 80% (eosin Y), 85% (eosin B), 80% (phloxin B), or 80% (rose Bengal).

Table 5.1. Eosin and related dyes

| Name and molecular weight | C.I. number | Substituent on fluorescein skeleton at carbon number | | | | | | | | | |
		1'	2'	4'	5'	7'	8'	4	5	6	7
Eosin (eosin Y; eosin yellowish) C.I. Acid red 87 MW 692	45380	H	Br	Br	Br	Br	H	H	H	H	H
Eosin B (bluish) C.I. Acid red 91 MW 624	45400	H	NO_2	Br	Br	NO_2	H	H	H	H	H
Phloxin C.I. Acid red 98 MW 761	45405	H	Br	Br	Br	Br	H	Cl	H	H	Cl
Phloxin B C.I. Acid red 92 MW 830	45410	H	Br	Br	Br	Br	H	Cl	Cl	Cl	Cl
Erythrosin (erythrosin Y) C.I. Acid red 95 MW 628	45425	H	H	I	I	H	H	H	H	H	H
Erythrosin B C.I. Acid red 51 MW 880	45430	H	I	I	I	I	H	H	H	H	H
Rose Bengal C.I. Acid red 94 MW 1018	45440	H	I	I	I	I	H	Cl	Cl	Cl	Cl

ETHYL EOSIN (eosin, alcohol soluble; C.I. 45386; Solvent red 45; MW 714)
This, the ethyl ester of eosin, is only slightly soluble in cold water but dissolves freely in alcohol. It is occasionally used when staining with eosin is to be done from an alcoholic solution. Unlike the water-soluble red derivatives of fluorescein, ethyl eosin must be differentiated by alcohol rather than by water. Samples of ethyl eosin should contain at least 78% by weight of the anhydrous dye.

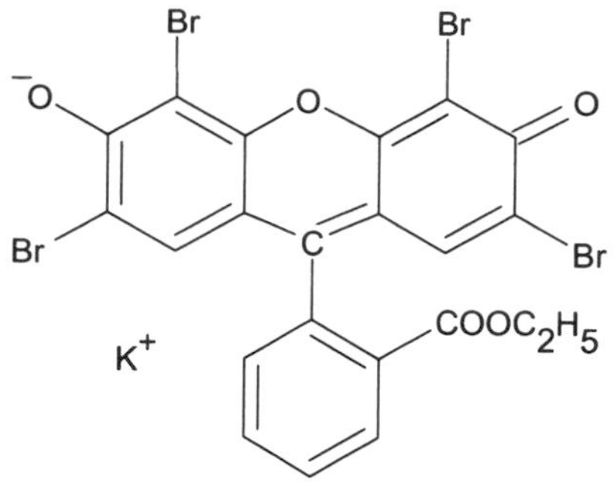

5.9.6.2. Cationic xanthene dyes

PYRONINE Y (pyronine G) (C.I. 45005; MW 303)

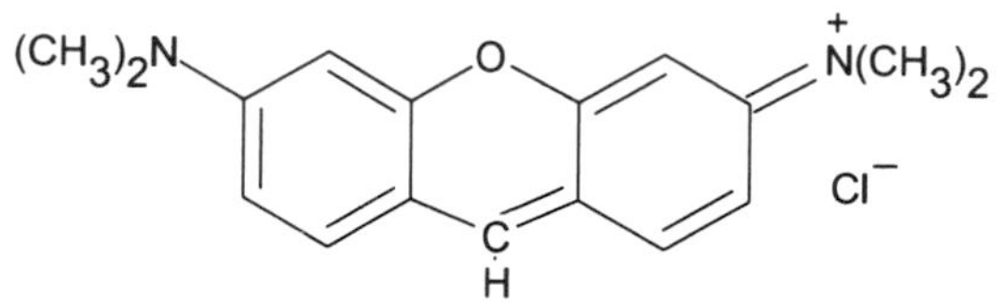

This red dye is used, together with ethyl green, in a method for nucleic acids (Chapter 9). The dye is very soluble in water and alcohol. Samples should contain at least 45% by weight of anhydrous dye. In the 1980s pyronine Y became available with much higher purity than in the past (Lyon *et al.*, 1987), leading to an increase in the popularity of the ethyl green–pyronine method.

Pyronine B (C.I. 45010) differs only in having ethyl instead of methyl groups on the nitrogen atoms, but it cannot be substituted for pyronine Y. Pyronine B is used in some bacteriological staining methods.

RHODAMINE B (C.I. 45170; Basic violet 10; MW 479)

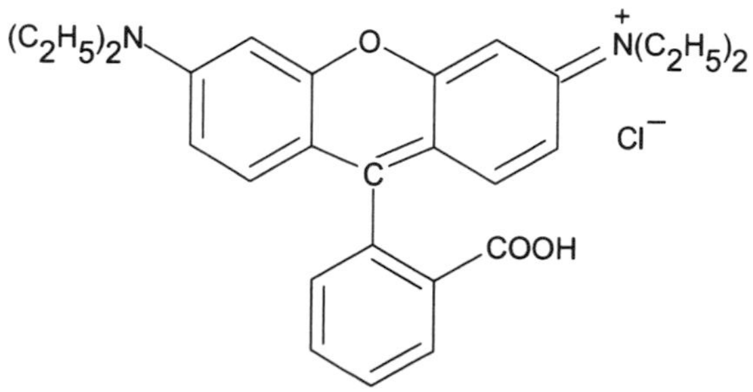

This red-violet dye emits a strong orange fluorescence when excited by either ultra-violet or green light. An isothiocyanate radical (S=C=N–) can be substituted in the carboxyphenyl group to give **rhodamine B isothiocyanate**, a reactive dye capable of conjugating with proteins to yield fluorescently labelled derivatives (Chapter 19).

OREGON GREEN 488 (no C.I. number or name)
This is fluorescein with fluorine replacing hydrogen at positions 2' and 7'. It is used as a fluorescent label for macromolecules (maximum absorption/emission: 494/517 nm).

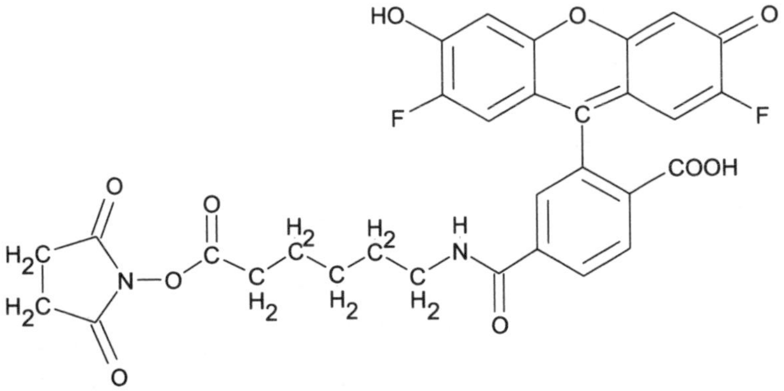

The reactive derivative shown is Oregon green 488-X succinimidyl ester, with a 7-atom aminohexanoyl spacer ('X') separating the protein-reactive group from the chromophore. Several other reactive Oregon green reagents are available (Haugland, 2002).

5.9.7. Acridine dyes

These dyes are similar to the xanthenes, but with a nitrogen rather than an oxygen atom linking the benzene rings. As with the xanthenes, the chromophoric system resonates between *o*- and *p*-quinonoid forms:

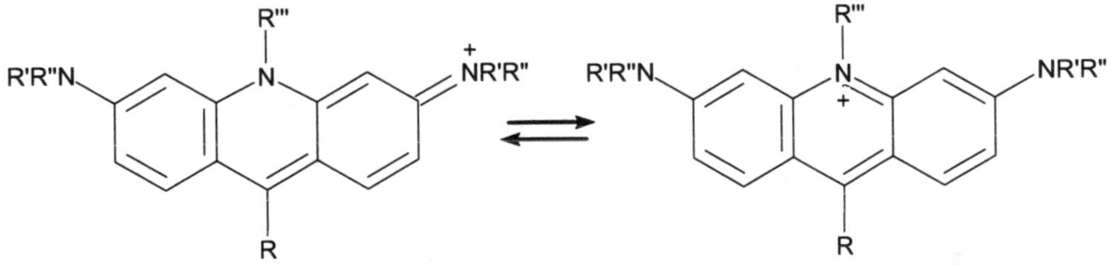

R, R', R'' and R''' may be hydrogen atoms or alkyl or aryl radicals. If R is a phenyl group the dye will also be a triphenylmethane derivative with two of its benzene rings linked by a nitrogen atom. The acridine dyes used in histology are all strongly fluorescent. The related **phenanthridine** fluorochromes are discussed in Chapter 9.

Examples
ACRIFLAVINE (trypaflavine) (C.I. 46000; MW 260)

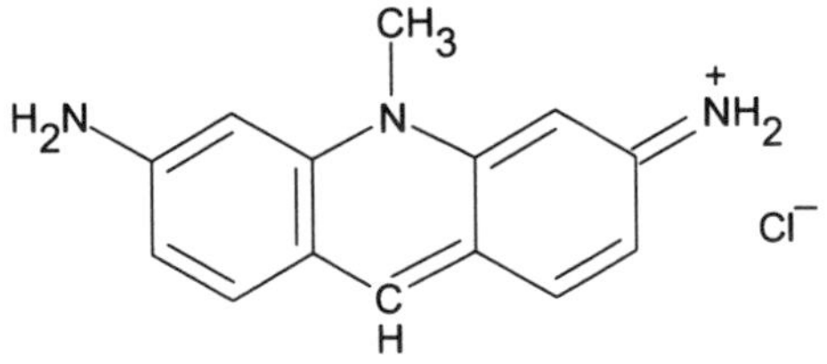

This may be used on the rare occasions when a yellow cationic dye is needed in ordinary light microscopy, and also as a fluorochrome. It is soluble in water and in alcohol. Acriflavine is better known as an antiseptic than as biological stain. The dye binds to plasma proteins, and, more strongly, to DNA. Small doses injected intra-venously into animals can be used to distinguish permeable from impermeable blood vessels in fluorescence microscopy (Rodriguez, 1955; Allen, 1992; Kiernan, 1996c).

ACRIDINE ORANGE (C.I. 46005; Basic orange 14; MW 302; Lillie (1977) states that this dye is usually supplied as a zinc chloride double salt: $[C_{17}H_{20}N_3]^{2+}$ $[ZnCl_4]^{2-}$, MW 740))

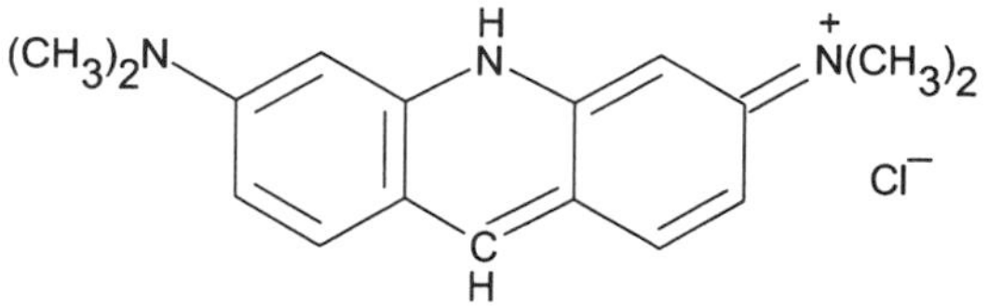

Used only as a fluorochrome, this dye is well known for its ability to impart fluorescent emissions of different colours to DNA and RNA (Bertalanffy and Bickis, 1956). The possible mechanism of this fluorescent metachromasia has been discussed by Horobin (1982). Acridine orange has also been used in carbohydrate histochemistry and as a vital stain.

5.9.8.
Azine dyes

In these dyes, the chromophore is a pyrazine ring:

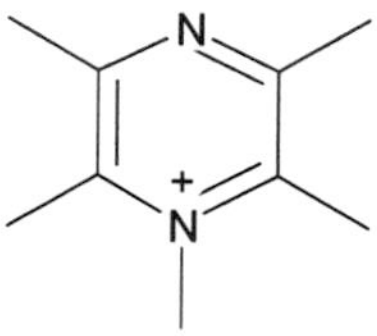

sandwiched between two aromatic systems, with o- and p-quinonoid configurations contributing to the resonance. These two structures are shown below for neutral red. For the other examples only one form is shown.

Examples
NEUTRAL RED (C.I. 50040; Basic red 5; MW 289)
Two forms are shown; in another the positive charge is on the primary amine nitrogen atom.

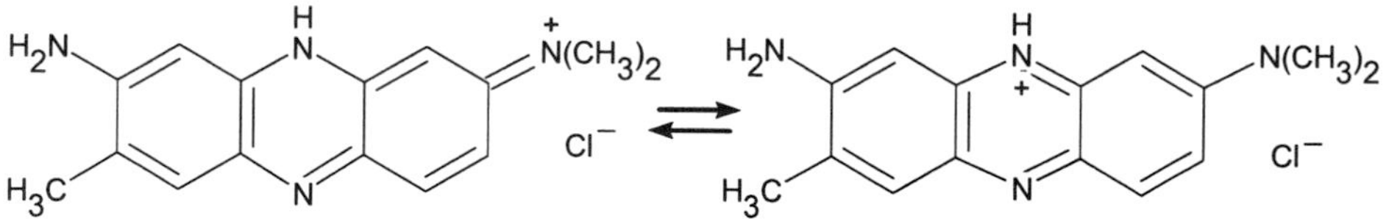

p-quinonoid form   o-quinonoid form

Neutral red is a cationic dye, freely soluble in water and alcohol. Aqueous solutions turn yellow on addition of alkali, the change occurring over the range pH 6.8–7.0. Strongly acidic solutions are blue-green, and a brown precipitate is formed with an excess of alkali. An acceptable sample of neutral red contains at least 50% by weight of the anhydrous dye.

Neutral red is valuable as a simple red cationic dye (Chapter 6). Dilute solutions of neutral red have been used as a fluorescent stain for cell nuclei (Allen and Kiernan, 1994) and for hydrophobic material (suberin) in plant tissues (Lulai and Morgan, 1992). This dye is also used to stain living cells; it enters vacuoles and lysosomes, and its red colour indicates the relatively low pH in these organelles (Rashid et al., 1991). It is used to test for viability in cultured animal cells (Ciapetti et al., 1996) and protozoa (Vdovenko and Williams, 2000). Neutral red in living cells is fluorescent, and this property has been exploited to distinguish malignant from normal cells (Paramanatham et al., 1997) and in functional imaging of the surface of the brain (Chen et al., 1998).

SAFRANINE O (safranine, safranine T; C.I. 50240; Basic red 2; MW 351)

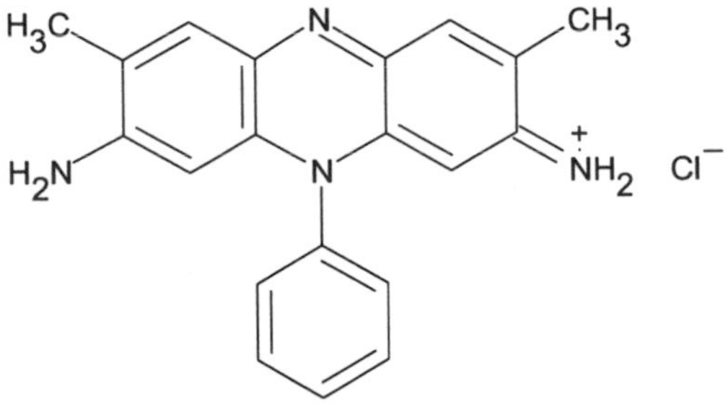

This is always a mixture of the compound formulated above with dyes that have differently positioned methyl groups. It dissolves in water and alcohol. An acceptable mixture absorbs maximally at 530 nm. Samples should contain at least 80% by weight of the anhydrous dye. Safranine O is valuable as a red cationic dye, and is much used in plant anatomy to colour lignin and nuclei, and to stain Gram-negative bacteria (Chapter 6).

AZOCARMINE G and **AZOCARMINE B** (C.I. 50085, Acid red 101 and C.I. 50090, Acid red 103)

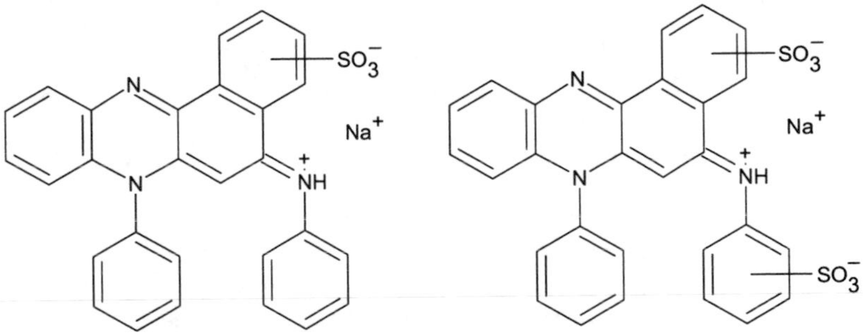

azocarmine G   azocarmine B

These two acid dyes are used for staining nuclei and cytoplasm in the AZAN procedure (Chapter 8) and some related methods. Azocarmine B, with its second sulphonate group, is more soluble in water but some authors claim that azocarmine G imparts a brighter red colour. These compounds are unfortunately named because they are not azo dyes and have no similarity to carmine.

5.9.9.
Oxazine dyes

The oxazine chromophore:

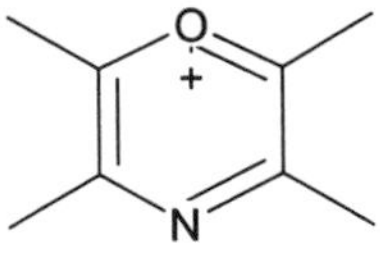

has obvious similarity to those of the azine and thiazine dyes and exists in o-quinonoid form (with positive charge attributed to the oxygen) and p-quinonoid form (as shown for the dyes described below). The natural dyes **orcein, litmus,** and **azolitmin** belong to the oxazine series. Orcein is used as a biological stain, litmus and azolitmin as pH indicators (see Lillie, 1977, for chemistry and properties).

Examples

CRESYL VIOLET (cresyl violet acetate; no C.I. number; MW 321)

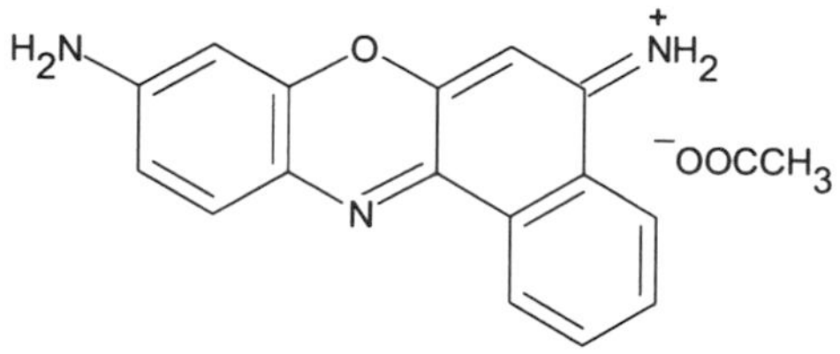

The structure shown is the major component of modern dyes sold as cresyl violet. The name was formerly applied to a methylated derivative of this compound, which was sometimes mixed with pyronine Y (Green, 1990). Cresyl violet is a cationic dye, soluble in water and alcohol. Its principal application is in Nissl stains (for nervous tissue; see Section 6.4.5.) An oxazone (see also under Nile blue) is present as an impurity, and solutions of the dye do not keep well.

GALLOCYANINE (C.I. 51030; Mordant blue 10; MW 337)

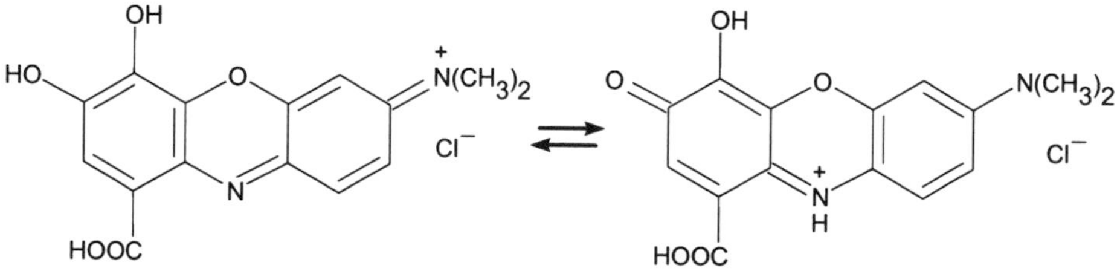

Two of several tautomers are shown. Gallocyanine is not used alone, but as a pre-formed chromium complex, which is formed when the staining solution is made up in the laboratory. Infrared spectroscopy and other chemical studies (Marshall and Horobin, 1972a) indicate that the formulation shown on the right is the one that combines with chromium(III), in a 2:1 dye–metal complex with the structure:

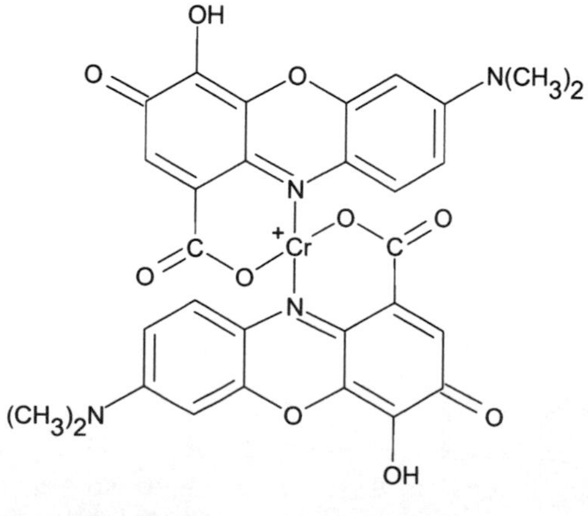

This complex is cationic, and is used principally to stain nucleic acids. The blue-grey colour is more resistant to extraction by water and alcohols than are simple cationic dyes. Chromium-gallocyanine staining solutions are stable for only about one week. Berube et al. (1966) precipitated and dried the dye–metal complex, to make a stable powder that could be dissolved in water when needed. My attempts to repeat this procedure were disappointing; staining by the redissolved material was paler than that achieved with solutions recently made from the dye and chrome alum.

NILE BLUE (Nile blue A, Nile blue sulphate; C.I. 51180; Basic blue 12; MW 354)

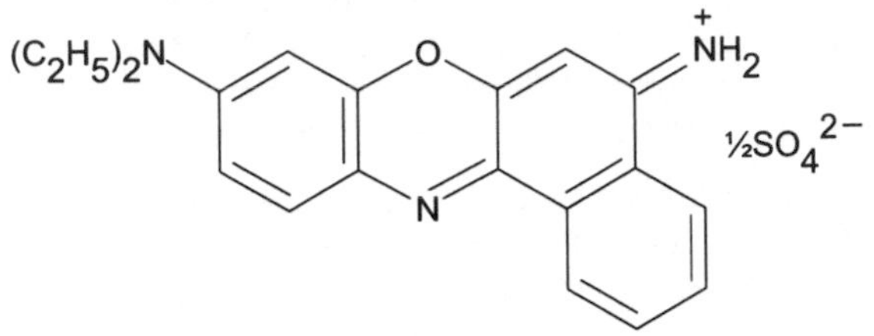

Nile blue is soluble in water, and can be used as an ordinary basic dye, which imparts blue and green colours to paraffin sections of fixed tissue. It has also been used in experimental embryology as a vital stain for transplanted tissues. For use in histochemistry, this dye is partly oxidized by boiling in dilute sulphuric acid. This generates an **oxazone**, known as **Nile red:**

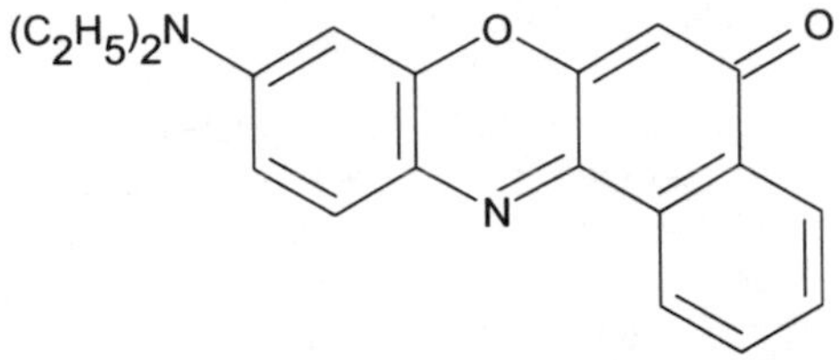

The oxazone, though insoluble in water, dissolves in aqueous solutions of Nile blue sulphate. The mixture can be used to stain lipids, in which the red compound dissolves. Furthermore, Nile red becomes fluorescent in a hydrophobic environment, so the oxidized Nile blue is also useful as a fluorochrome for lipids (Chapter 12). A sample of Nile blue sulphate should be at least 70% dye for certification by the Biological Stain Commission.

ORCEIN (C.I. Natural red 28; no C.I. number)
Orcein is made by oxidation of orcinol (3,5-dihydroxytoluene) in the presence of ammonia. Orcinol, an compound formerly made by alkaline hydrolysis of compounds present in certain lichens, is now made synthetically. Orcein is a mixture of 14 oxazine dyes, of which two are shown below. For more information, see Beecken *et al.* (2003).

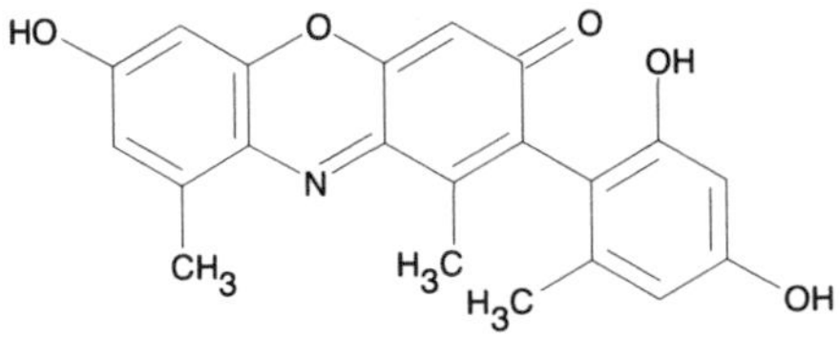

α-hydroxyorcein (MW 363)

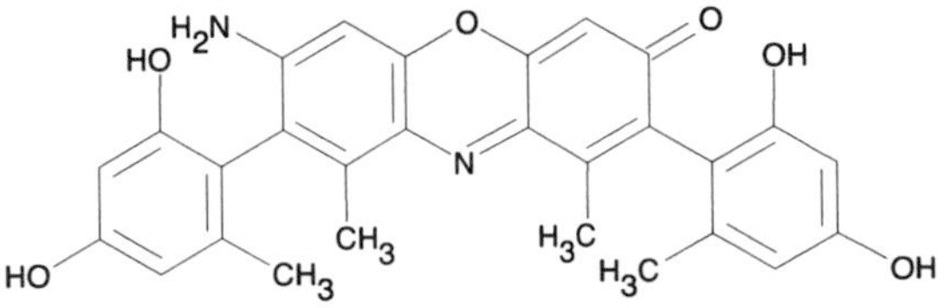

γ-aminoorcein (MW 485)

Orcein is used for staining elastin (Chapter 8) and also in methods for chromosomes and to detect a hepatitis B antigen in sections of infected livers (Panicker *et al.,* 1996). Batches of the dye vary, and solutions change with age, giving optimum staining after storage at room temperature for 3 weeks to 6 months. See Henwood (2003) for coloured micrographs of variations in orcein staining and a review of techniques.

5.9.10. **Thiazine dyes**	The chromophore of the thiazines is like that of the oxazines, with sulphur replacing oxygen. The thiazine dyes used in histology are all cationic and all except methylene green are blue or violet. All except methylene violet Bernthsen are soluble in water. In addition to their general usefulness as blue cationic dyes, some of the thiazines, especially the demethylation products of methylene blue, are used as eosinates in haematological staining. This will be discussed in Chapter 7. Most of the thiazine dyes can be used for metachromatic staining (Chapter 11).

The following examples include most of the thiazine dyes that are used as biological stains. Structures are shown in the p-quinonoid configurations, with positive charges formally attributed to the most strongly basic nitrogen atoms.

THIONINE (C.I. 52000; Lauth's violet; MW 264 [chloride]; 287 [acetate])

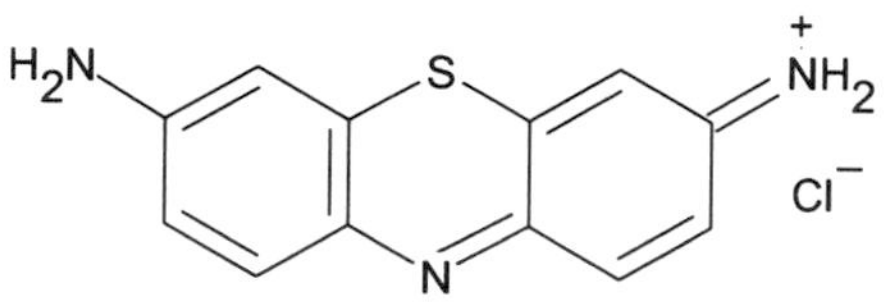

The simplest of the thiazines is a blue dye, soluble in water and in alcohol, but less so than most other members of the series. An acceptable sample should contain at least 85% anhydrous dye. Thionine must not be confused with **thionine blue** (C.I. 52025, Basic blue 25), which has different staining properties (Taylor, 1961). Unsatisfactory or mislabelled batches of thionine are often encountered. Allison (1995) compared dye samples from several sources in a method for staining bone, and obtained consistent success only with thionine that had been certified by the Biological Stain Commission.

A 'thionine–Schiff' reagent can be made in the laboratory. It is comparable to Schiff's reagent made from basic fuchsine (Chapter 9) and is used in carbohydrate histochemistry (Chapter 11).

AZURES A, B and C

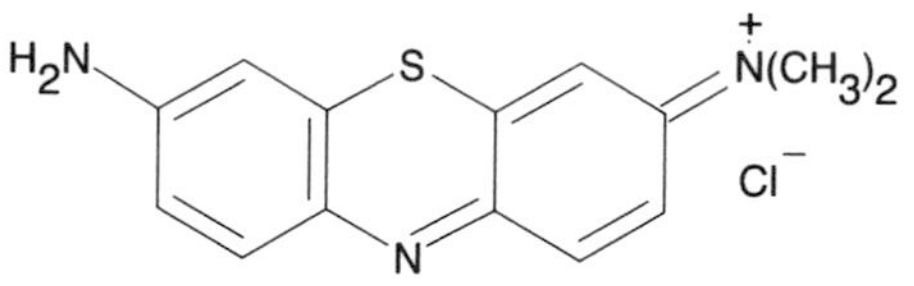

azure A (C.I. 52005; MW 292) 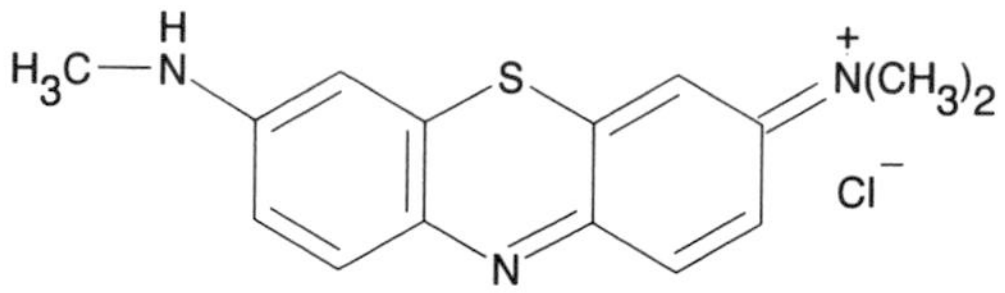   azure B (C.I. 52010; MW 306)

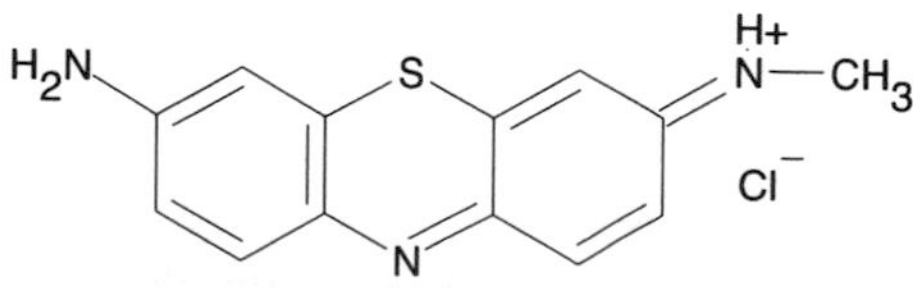

azure C (C.I. 52002; MW 278)

These blue, water-soluble cationic dyes are products of demethylation of methylene blue. Azure B (which has also been called azure I and methylene azure) is the one responsible for the special properties of the Romanowsky–Giemsa stains for blood (Chapter 7) Pure azure B (prepared by direct synthesis rather than from methylene blue) is available, and is the desired material for preparing a standardized stain for blood. The other azures are included in older formulations such as those of Giemsa and Wright (Chapter 7).

Azure A is used in Lillie's original azure–eosin method (Chapter 6). Azure C has been used for staining cleared whole-mounts of botanical specimens (Hodnett *et al.*, 1997). Toluidine blue (see below) is closely similar to azure A.

METHYLENE BLUE (C.I. 52015; Basic blue 9; MW anhydrous chloride 320, chloride trihydrate 374, zinc chloride double salt with 0.5 $ZnCl_2$, 406)

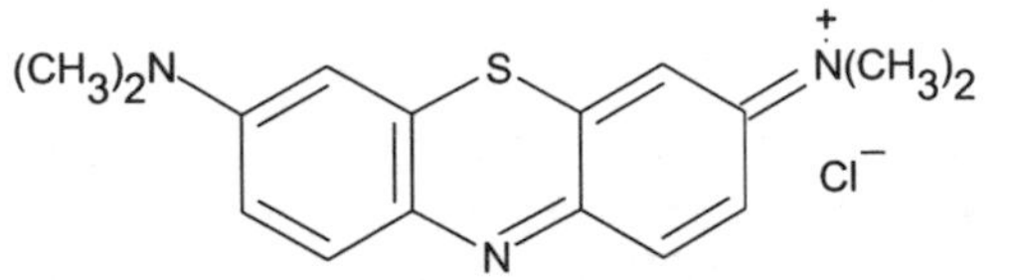

Many samples of methylene blue contain zinc chloride, which reduces the solubility in water and may render the dye too toxic for use as a vital stain (though this is disputed; see Richardson, 1969). If possible, a pharmacopoeial grade certified as zinc-free should be used. The dye is freely soluble in water and in alcohol. With time or heating and exposure to air and alkali, a methylene blue solution is variably demethylated to yield azure B, azure A, and other thiazine dyes, a change known as polychroming. For use in bacteriology and haematology the dye is hydrolysed and oxidized in this way to give the mixture of dyes known as **polychrome methylene blue**.

For certification by the Biological Stain Commission, a sample must contain at least 82% by weight of anhydrous methylene blue chloride and must be satisfactory as a nuclear and bacterial stain.

METHYLENE GREEN (C.I. 52020; Basic green 5; MW 365)

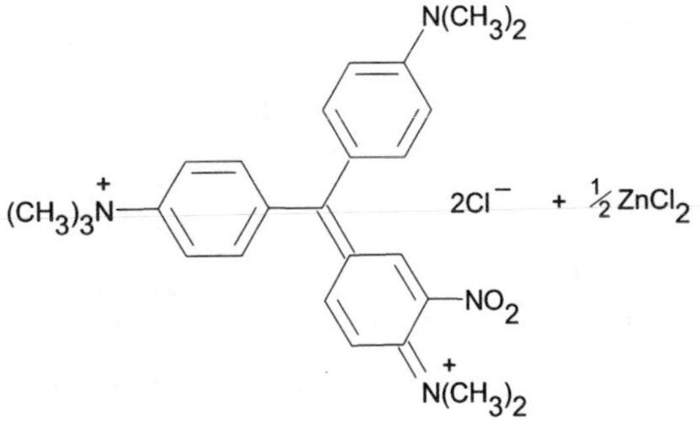

The exact position of the nitro group is uncertain. The bluish green colour is presumably due to mixed light absorption of the thiazine and nitro chromophores. The dye is soluble in water and slightly soluble in alcohol. It has been used as a counterstain for nuclei, following a histochemical method that imparts a dark purple colour to mucus (McNulty *et al.*, 2004; see also Chapter 6). Ethyl green (Section 5.9.5.2) is more frequently used for such purposes.

NEW METHYLENE BLUE (new methylene blue N; C.I. 52030; Basic blue 24; MW 348)

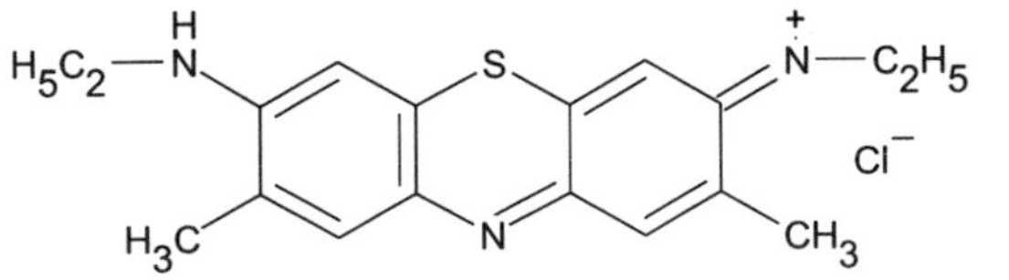

This dye provides strong metachromatic staining but it cannot replace methylene blue in vital staining methods. Its principal use is in Brecher's stain for reticulocytes (see Clark, 1981). New methylene blue is also used to trace the distribution of injected liquids (Lee *et al.*, 2004).

TOLUIDINE BLUE (toluidine blue O; C.I. 52040; Basic blue 17; MW 306)

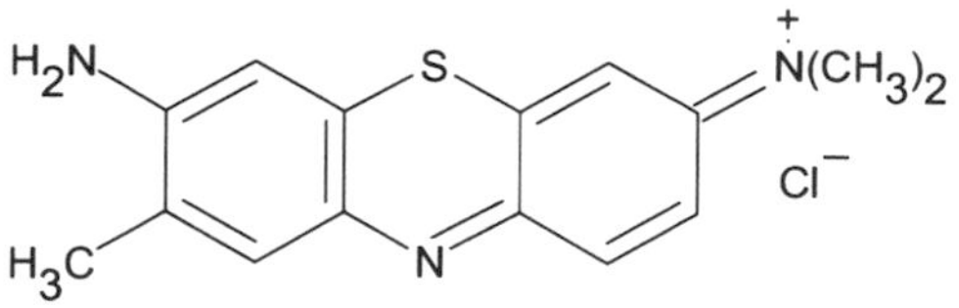

This is perhaps the most useful of all the blue cationic dyes, being similar to but cheaper than azure A. Metachromatic effects are easily obtained. Lillie (1977) points out that older samples of this dye are of the zinc chloride double salt (dye content about 60%) but that toluidine blue O is now sold in the zinc-free state (over 90% dye). An acceptable sample must contain at least 50% by weight of the anhydrous dye (MW 306). The variable dye content must be taken into account when making solutions, and the quantities of dye called for in older recipes should be reduced. Toluidine blue O is freely soluble in water and slightly soluble in alcohol.

METHYLENE VIOLET BERNTHSEN (C.I. 52041; MW 256)

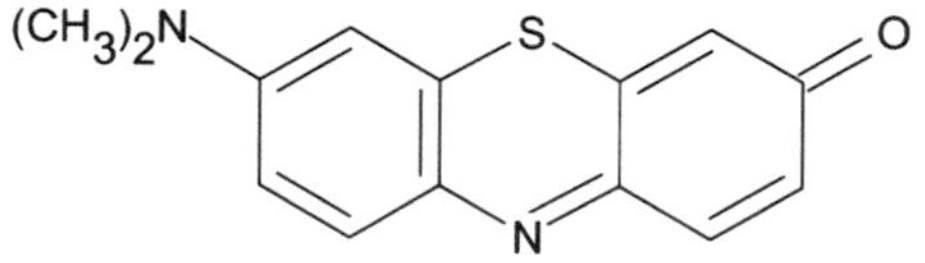

This dye is formed by oxidation of methylene blue. It is a component of traditional staining mixtures for blood, and was formerly thought to account for the staining of leukocyte and protozoan nuclei. The pure dye is insoluble in water but dissolves in the presence of other thiazine dyes. It is more soluble in chloroform. **Methyl thionoline** (with $-NHCH_3$ replacing $-N(CH_3)_2$ in formula above) and **thionoline** (with $-NH_2$ replacing $-N(CH_3)_2$ of methylene violet, Bernthsen) are related dyes also formed in the polychroming of methylene blue (Marshall, 1978).

Methylene violet Bernthsen should not be confused with **methylene violet RR** (C.I. 50205; Basic violet 5), which is an azine dye related to safranine O.

5.9.11.
Polyene dyes

In these compounds the chromophore is a chain of methine (−CH=) groups. The two major groups of polyene dyes are **carotenoids**, which are coloured substances in plants with long aliphatic methine chains, and the synthetic **stilbene dyes**.

Examples
SAFFRON (safran du Gatinais; C.I. 75100, Natural yellow 6)
Saffron is an expensive spice and food colorant. It consists of the dried thread-like reddish stigmas of *Crocus sativus*, a plant cultivated in Spain, Iran and elsewhere. The principal colorant is **crocin 1**, which is an ester formed from two molecules of gentobiose (6-β-D-glucosyl-D-glucose) and one of the dicarboxylic acid crocetin.

In crocin 2, one gentobiosyl group is replaced by glucosyl; Crocins 3 and 4 are monocarboxylic acids, with one end of the crocetin molecule not esterified and respectively, gentobiose or glucose at the other end. These compounds all susceptible to degradation, especially in solution; light and heat can cause *trans* to *cis* isomerization of the crocetin moiety, and acidity and alkalinity bring about hydrolysis of the glycoside linkages (Tarantilis *et al.*, 1994). Other compounds in saffron account for the dye's flavour, odour and possible medicinal properties. Adulteration with other naturally coloured or dyed plant fragments was discussed in detail by Maisch (1885).

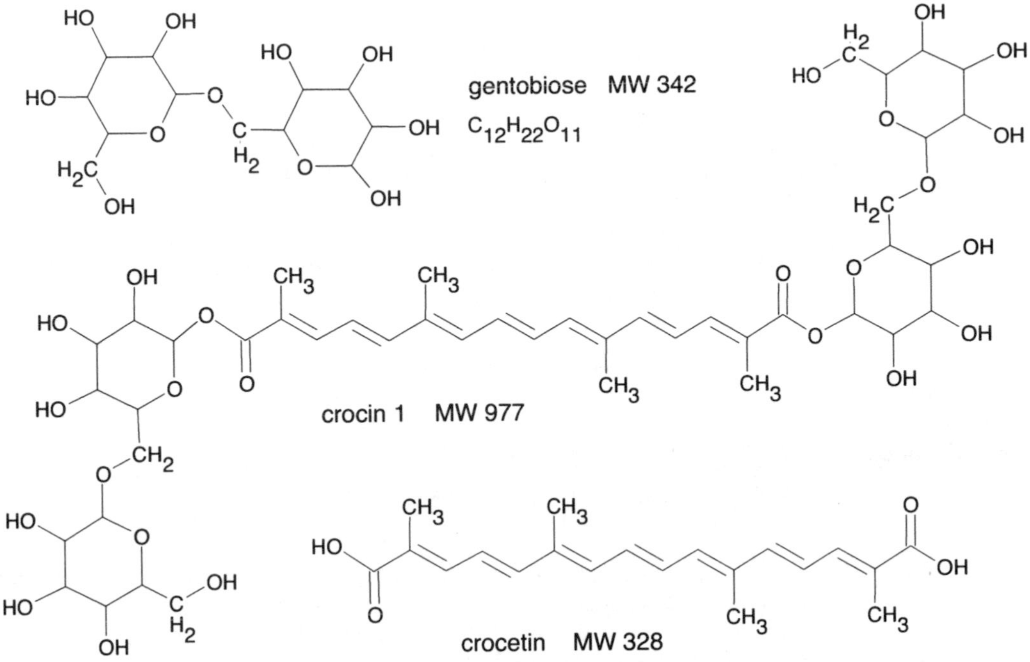

gentobiose MW 342 $C_{12}H_{22}O_{11}$

crocin 1   MW 977

crocetin   MW 328

Saffron was probably the first microscopical stain, used in 1714 by van Leuwenhoek to demonstrate muscle fibres (Conn, 1933; Kiernan, 2006). Its modern use dates from Masson (1911) and Movat (1955), as a yellow collagen stain in trichrome (Chapter 8) techniques, but the thinnest collagen fibres are not shown by these methods (Pickering et al., 1996). A solution containing saffron and phloxin B was recommended by Garvey (1991) as an alternative to eosin Y following nuclear staining with haemalum. The green fluorescence of saffron was exploited by Trigoso and Stockert (1995) in a stain for eosinophil leukocytes. When staining with saffron takes place from an alkaline solution or following treatment of sections with a strong acid, the active dye may be crocin 3 or 4 or crocetin, formed by hydrolysis of crocin 1.

CALCOFLUOR WHITE M2R (C.I. 40622; Fluorescent brightening agent 28; MW 897)

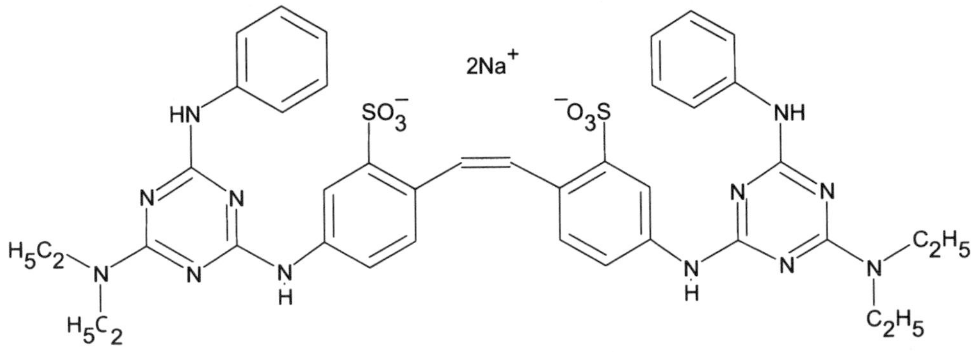

This belongs to a subgroup of polyenes known as stilbene dyes, many of which are derivatives of 4,4'-diaminostilbene-2,2'-disulphonic acid, $HO_3S(NH_2)C_6H_3CH=CHC_6H_3(NH_2)SO_3H$. Fluorescent brighteners absorb ultraviolet radiation and emit blue or green light. A fabric containing one of these compounds appears more vividly white than it otherwise would. Thus, fluorescent brighteners can offset the tendency of white materials to turn yellow with age.

Fluorescent brighteners are used in microscopy as fluorochromes, especially for plant tissues. The extended molecule of Calcofluor white M2R binds to cellulose, perhaps in the same way as a direct cotton dye, but does not enter living cells (Fischer et al., 1985; Mori and Bellani, 1996). A method for differential fluorescent staining of cellulose and lignin is described in Chapter 6. In addition to their occasional use in histology, various fluorescent brighteners have been used for staining pathogenic fungi (Fraire et al., 1996) and for automated counting of bacteria and spores in liquids (Davey and Kell, 1997).

5.9.12. Polymethine dyes and fluorochromes

The chromophore has the general structure:

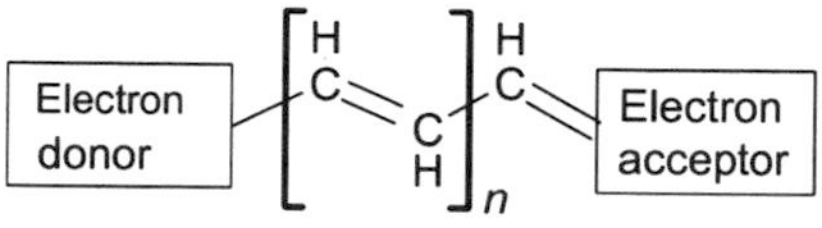

The value of n in the general formula may be zero, in which case only one methine (=CH–) group separates the donor from the acceptor. The hydrogen of a methine group may be replaced by an alkyl group or a bond to another part of the dye molecule. The =CH– may also be replaced by an azamethine (indamine, =N–) group. The polymethine class includes about 10 groups of dyes, some having structures that do not strictly conform to the general polymethine formula. The nomenclature and definition of the groups, and of the individual compounds, is confusing and inconsistent (Kiernan and Horobin, 2002; Zollinger 2003). Examples from three of the groups in the polymethine family of dyes follow.

Many fluorescent polymethines are used in research as vital stains or probes that enter living cells and localize to organelles such as nuclei, mitochondria, the Golgi apparatus and the endoplasmic reticulum (see Haugland, 2002 and the associated web site for more information and extensive bibliography). The entry of these compounds into cells and their affinities for different organelles can generally be predicted from systematic (quantitative) interpretation of their structural formulas in terms of molecular size, charge and hydrophilic or hydrophobic character (Horobin, 2001).

5.9.12.1. Cyanines

In these dyes the donor and acceptor of the general polymethine formula are aromatic rings with at least one being heterocyclic with a positively charged nitrogen atom. Most cyanines are cationic dyes. The relation of colour to chemical structure has been thoroughly studied in the cyanines (see Brooker, 1966), which are used as sensitizing agents in photographic emulsions. Many modern fluorochromes belong to this group of dyes (see Haugland, 2002). Many cyanines fade on exposure to light, so only a few are used in microscopy or for textiles.

Examples
PINACYANOL (Not in recent editions of C.I.; MW 389; also known as quinaldine blue)

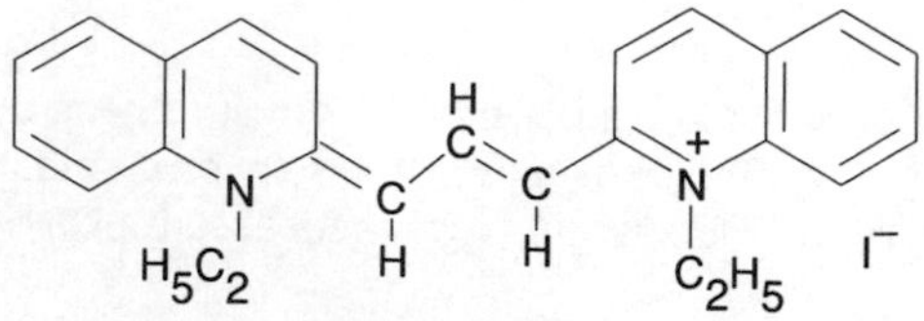

This blue cationic dye provides metachromatic (red) staining of mast cells (Bensley, 1952; see also Cook, 1974; Bancroft and Cook, 1984).

STAINS-ALL (no C.I. number; MW 560)

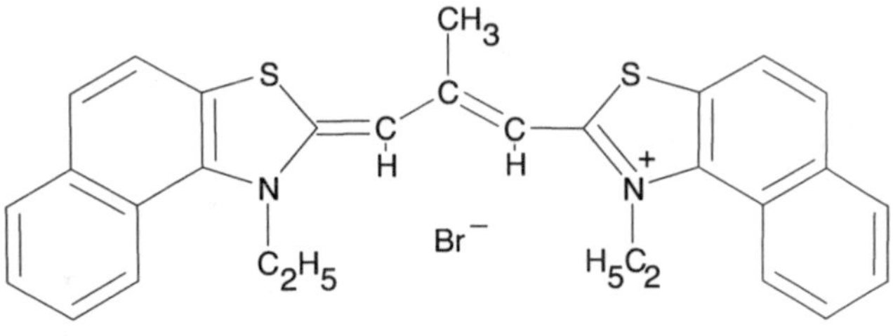

This dye, also known as **carbocyanine DBTC**, is used alone to stain sections in various shades of blue, purple, and red (Green and Pastewka, 1974a,b, 1979), but its usefulness is unfortunately rather limited because the stained sections fade rapidly on exposure to light. Stains-all is used for staining electrophoresis gels; most proteins are coloured pink but calcium-binding proteins become dark blue (Campbell et al., 1983; Hruba et al., 2005).

DiI (No C.I. number; MW 934)

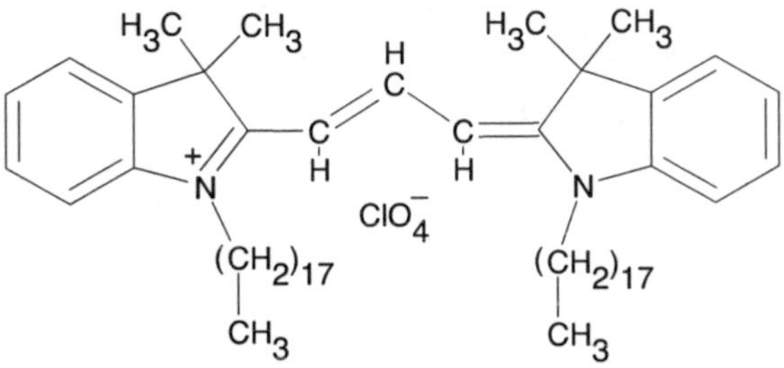

The name DiI is used for strongly fluorescent cyanines with long lipophilic side chains (see Haugland, 2002). The one illustrated is more correctly designated DiI-C_{18}(3) perchlorate or 1,1'-dioctadecyl-3,3,3',3'-tetramethylindocarbocyanine perchlorate. These dyes were first used in biochemical studies of cell membranes (Klausner and Wolf, 1980) and were later found to enter and remain in the membranes of living cells (Honig and Hume, 1986; Purves et al., 1987). The compounds can also enter the cytoplasm by endocytosis. They are used for tracing neuronal connections in living and fixed tissue and for examining the migration of cells in developing animals (e.g. Serbedzija et al., 1991; Henkel et al., 1996).

5.9.12.2. Thiazole dyes
The benzothiazole ring:

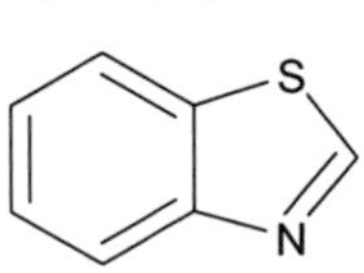

is the chromogen in dyes of this group, considered by Zollinger (2003) to be closely related to cyanines, but lacking a methine bridge between the two ring systems. Dyes with other chromophoric systems (especially azo dyes) sometimes also contain benzothiazole rings.

Examples
PRIMULINE (C.I. 49000; Direct yellow 59)
This greenish–yellow dye (amphoteric: here shown as anionic) is a mixture, the principal component of which is:

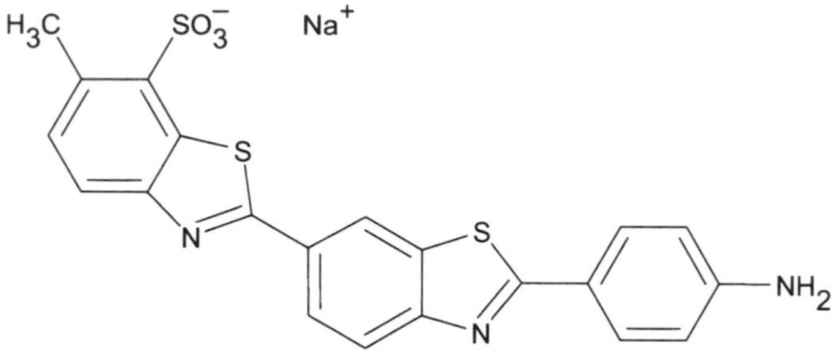

It has been used as a vital stain and fluorochrome, with UV excitation and blue emission (e.g. Kuypers *et al.*, 1977). With textiles, primuline can function as a direct dye for cellulosic fibres. It can be diazotized on the fibre and then coupled with suitable phenols or amines to give more intense, faster colours.

Methylation and sulphonation of primuline yields **thioflavine S** (C.I. 49010; Direct yellow 7), an anionic dye of uncertain composition that is is used as a fluorescent stain for amyloid (Guntern *et al.*, 1992; Sun *et al.*, 2002).

THIOFLAVINE T (Thioflavine TCN) (C.I. 49005; Basic yellow 1; MW 319)

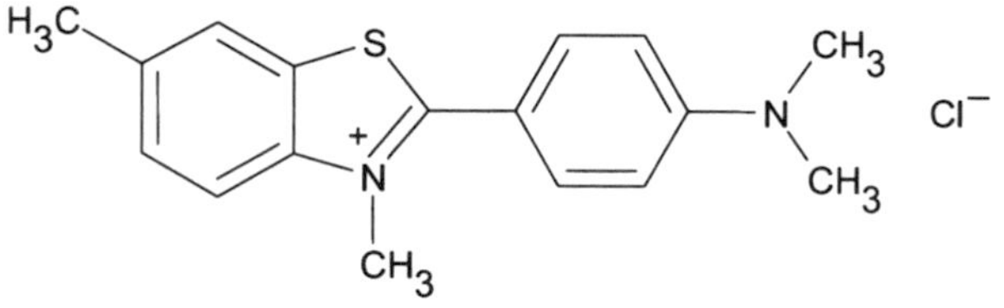

This yellow cationic dye is used principally as a fluorochrome. An insoluble yellow pigment is formed with phosphotungstomolybdic acid. Its principal use in microtechnique is for staining amyloid (see Culling, 1974), though not with complete specificity (McKinney and Grubb, 1965; Burns and Whitehead, 1966).

5.9.12.3. Flavonoids
In these dyes, included in the 'hydroxyketone' group by Allen (1971) and Lillie (1977), the chromogen is the flavone structure:

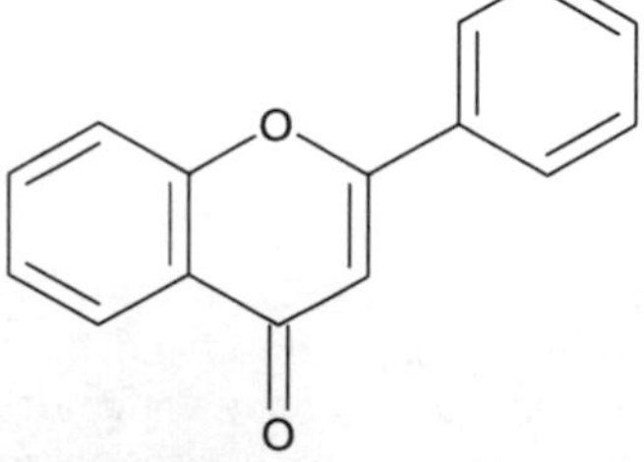

The group includes naturally occurring and synthetic dyes, of which only the former are important in histology. Haematein and brazilein are formed by oxidation of the naturally occurring flavone compounds haematoxylin and brazilin.

HAEMATOXYLIN and HAEMATEIN (C.I. 75290; Natural black 1)

Haematoxylin is extracted from the heart-wood of *Haematoxylon campechianum*, the logwood tree of South and Central America. Haematoxylin is soluble in both water and ethanol but dissolves more rapidly in the latter. Haematein is less soluble than haematoxylin in water, but more soluble in ethanol, ethylene glycol and glycerol, which are also solvents for haematoxylin. Haematoxylin is not a dye. Its solutions are colourless when pure and protected from contact with air (Bettinger and Zimmermann, 1991a). Partial oxidation changes haematoxylin into **haematein**, which is the active ingredient of the many 'haematoxylin' stains used in histology. Haematein solutions are red at pH <1, yellow at pH 1–5, and violet at pH > 6.

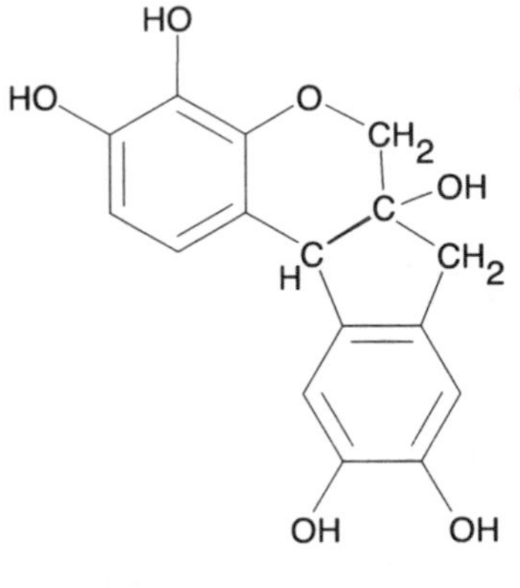

haematoxylin

(anhydrous: MW 302; yellow powder.
trihydrate: MW 356; clear brownish
crystals). Colourless when pure.

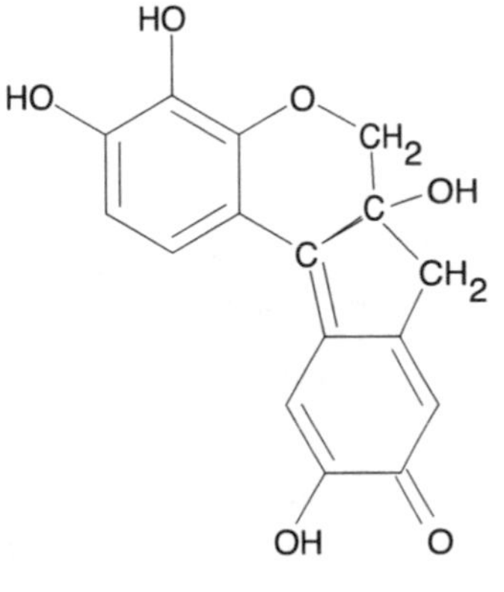

haematein

(MW 300)
Colour varies with pH.

The oxidation of haematoxylin to haematein may be brought about slowly (weeks) by exposure to air or rapidly (minutes) by adding an oxidizing agent such as sodium iodate. One gram of anhydrous haematoxylin (a pale brown powder) is fully oxidized to haematein by 218 mg of $NaIO_3$. Haematoxylin was formerly sold as transparent brown crystals of its trihydrate, which needed 185mg of $NaIO_3$ per gram of dye precursor. Smaller amounts of oxidizing agents are commonly used because haematein itself is slowly oxidized by atmospheric oxygen to give useless products. A reservoir of initially unoxidized haematoxylin in a staining solution allows for the continued production of haematein by slow atmospheric oxidation, thereby prolonging the useful life of the reagent.

The real value of haematein resides, however, with its metal complexes, which are more strongly coloured and can bind selectively to many components of cells and tissues. Solutions containing aluminium ions and haematein are used for staining cell nuclei blue. Such solutions are called **haemalum** or (very commonly but incorrectly) 'haematoxylin'.

If a haemalum is made from haematoxylin without any added oxidizing agent, the solution must, before using, be stored in contact with air for a few weeks to build up an adequate concentration of haematein. This slow oxidation is called ripening.

Ferric salts also oxidize haematoxylin to haematein. Iron–haematoxylin mixtures, which stain nuclei black, can be used immediately, with no requirement for ripening. The concentration of ferric ions in such stains is usually greatly in excess of that needed to oxidize the haematoxylin and form the metal–haematein complex.

Consequently, these solutions deteriorate from over-oxidation. This can be in a few days or a few weeks, depending on the formulation of the mixture.

The main product of over-oxidation of haematein is an orange-yellow substance known as **oxyhaematein**. It is formed more quickly by oxidation with hydrogen peroxide, potassium permanganate, or sodium iodate than by exposure to oxygen. Marshall and Horobin (1972b) have provided strong (though not conclusive) evidence that oxyhaematein has the structure:

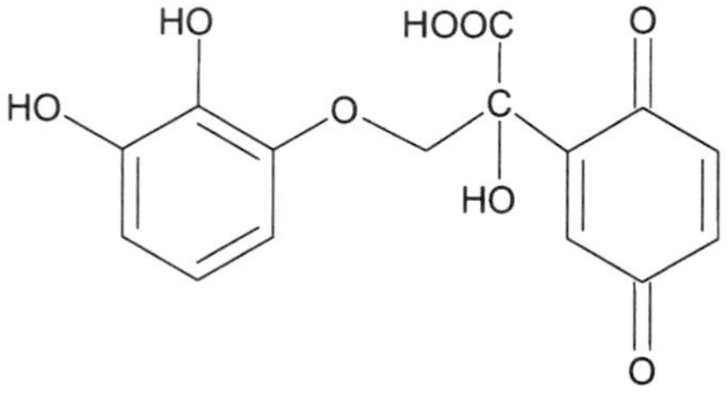

and have shown that it can behave as an ordinary anionic dye whose properties are unaffected by mixing with aluminium salts.

Staining with haematein is carried out in conjunction with a metal salt, most often aluminium (for staining nuclei blue) or iron (for staining nuclei, myelin or other elements blue-black, according to technique). Preformed dye–metal complexes are used for most purposes, though in the classical method of Heidenhain a ferric salt and the dye are applied sequentially to the sections. Many other metals are used for special purposes. Several recipes for mixtures containing haematoxylin are given by Bancroft and Stevens (1996), and lists of metals and structures demonstrated are given by Culling (1974) and Culling et al. (1985). Staining methods using metal–haematein complexes are described in Chapter 6 of this book. A histochemical method in which the dye is used for the localization of certain lipids is given in Chapter 12.

Spectrophotometric studies have shown that commercial samples of haematoxylin are usually quite pure, containing 90–95% of the anhydrous compound, which is a pale brown powder. The trihydrate (crystals with a reddish hue) is offered by some vendors. Materials sold as 'haematein' are variable, with dye contents ranging from 1% to 75% (Marshall and Horobin, 1974). When haematein is required, it should always be made by oxidizing haematoxylin in the laboratory (Llewellyn 2005).

BRAZILIN and BRAZILEIN (C.I. 75280; Natural red 24)

Brazilin is extracted from brazil wood (*Caesalpina sappan* from Indonesia and *C. brasiliensis* from Central and South America). The country of Brazil was named after the discovery there of trees yielding the dyestuff, which had previously been imported into Europe from oriental sources. Brazilin differs from haematoxylin only in lacking one hydroxyl group. Upon oxidation, a red dye, **brazilein**, is produced.

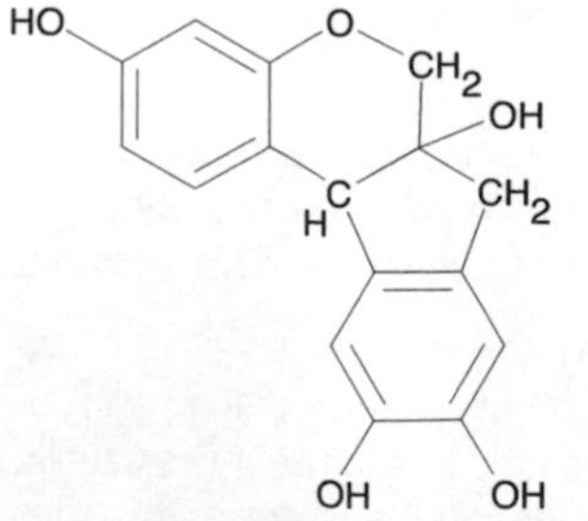

brazilin (MW 286) 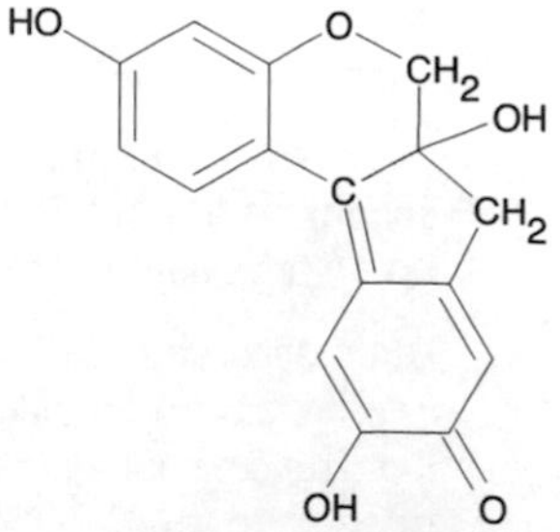   brazilein (MW 284)

Like haematein, brazilein is used as a complex with a metal. The aluminium complex is a useful red nuclear stain (Chapter 6; see also Anatech Ltd, 2002).

5.9.13.
Carbonyl dyes

Several groups of dyes that are quinones or other ketones are included in the family of carbonyl dyes recognized by Zollinger (2003). The general structure is:

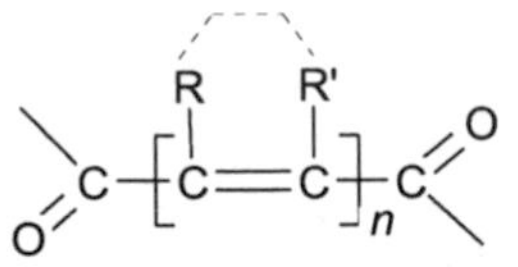

$$n = 1 - 4$$

in which the conjugated system includes at least two C=O groups. R and R' in the general formula may or may not be identical and may be separate (as in indigoid dyes) or joined (as in the anthraquinones). Two of the groups of carbonyl dyes are significant in histology and histochemistry.

5.9.13.1. Indigoid dyes and pigments

Natural **indigo** is the classical examples of a vat dye (Section 5.7): a soluble precursor, in this case a colourless leuco compound, is applied to a fabric and then oxidized to an insoluble coloured substance. Indigo is manufactured by oxidizing indoxyl, which is now a synthetic product.

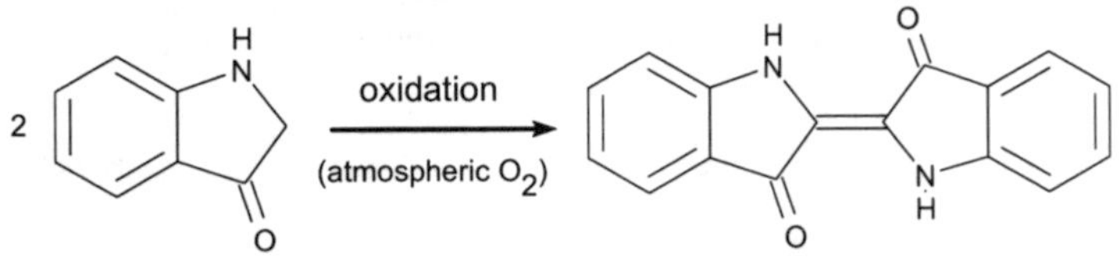

indoxyl

(traditionally made by hydrolysis
of **indican**, a glycoside from
Indigofera species)

indigo blue (indigotin)

(C.I. 73000; Vat blue 1)

For use in dyeing, the indigo blue is reduced, usually by sodium dithionite ($Na_2S_2O_4$), to its soluble leuco compound, **indigo white** (C.I. 73001):

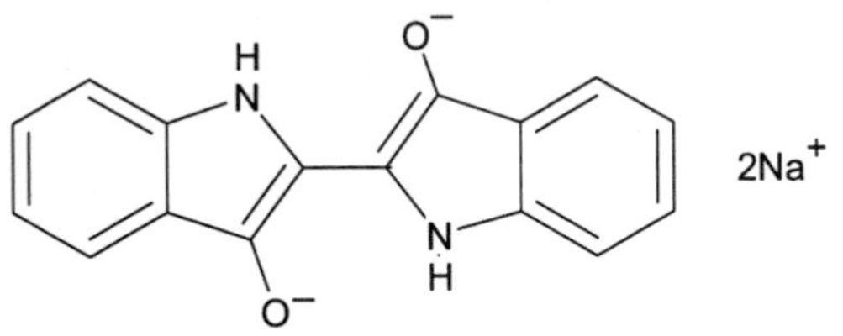

$2Na^+$

This, after application to the textile, is reoxidized by air to the insoluble indigo blue.

The chromophoric system of the indigoid dyes is the conjugated chain:

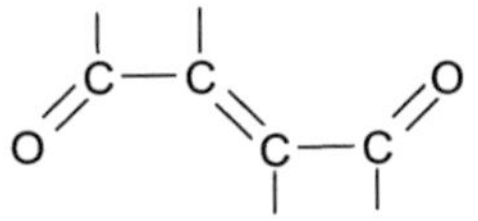

The colour is due to resonance among structures such as these:

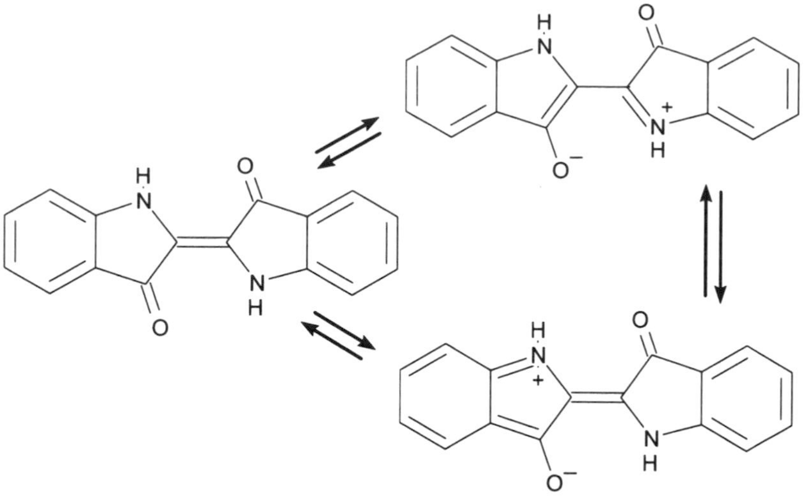

Insoluble indigoid compounds are produced as the coloured end-products of some histochemical reactions (Chapter 15 and Kiernan, 2007a). In addition, one soluble indigoid dye is used in histology.

INDIGOCARMINE (C.I. 73015; Acid blue 74; MW 466)

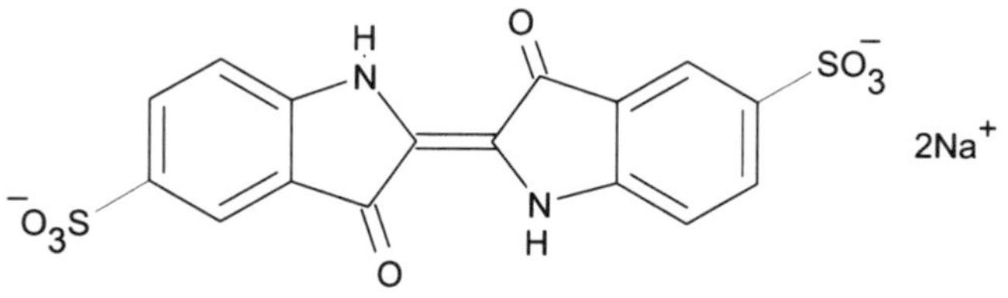

This blue anionic dye is soluble in water but almost insoluble in alcohol. It is used in a variety of procedures, the best known being a combination with picric acid (picroindigocarmine) used for staining connective tissue. Samples should contain at least 80% by weight of the anhydrous dye.

5.9.13.2. Anthraquinone dyes
Anthraquinone:

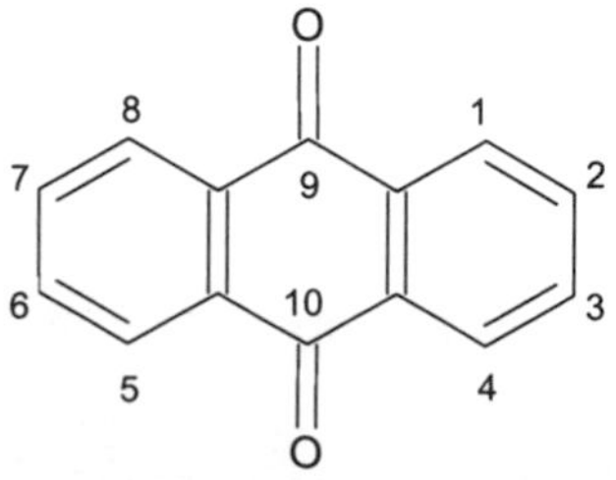

with its p-quinonoid configuration, is the chromophore of all the members of this large class of dyes. Anthraquinones of industrial importance, include vat dyes, disperse dyes, and pigments (Gregory, 1990; Zollinger, 2003), but only the metal-complexing members of the group are in regular use as biological stains.

Examples

ALIZARIN RED S (alizarin red, water soluble; sodium alizarin sulphonate; C.I. 58005; Mordant red 3; MW 342)

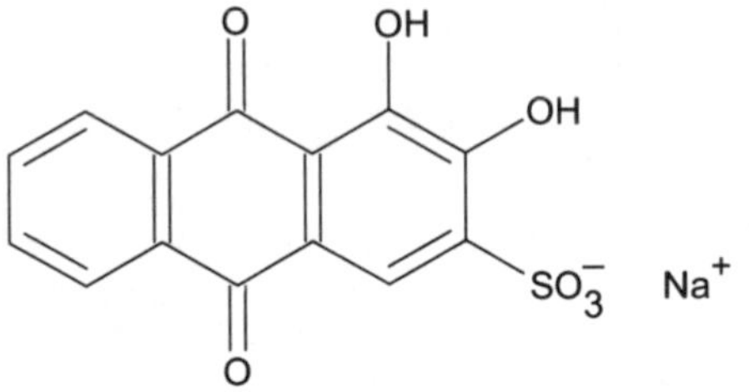

As an anionic dye this will stain tissues red. Its principal use, however, is as a histochemical reagent for calcium, with which an orange chelate is formed under appropriate conditions of use (Chapter 13). The Biological Stain Commission tests alizarin red S as a stain for bone in whole-mounts of small animals. Samples unsatisfactory for histochemical purposes are quite frequently encountered.

Alizarin (C.I. 58000; Mordant red 11) lacks the sulphonic acid group. It was extracted from the roots of madder (*Rubia tinctoria*), but is now a synthetic product. Alizarin has been used only rarely as a biological stain (Lillie, 1977).

NUCLEAR FAST RED (Kernechtrot; calcium red; C.I. 60760; MW 357)

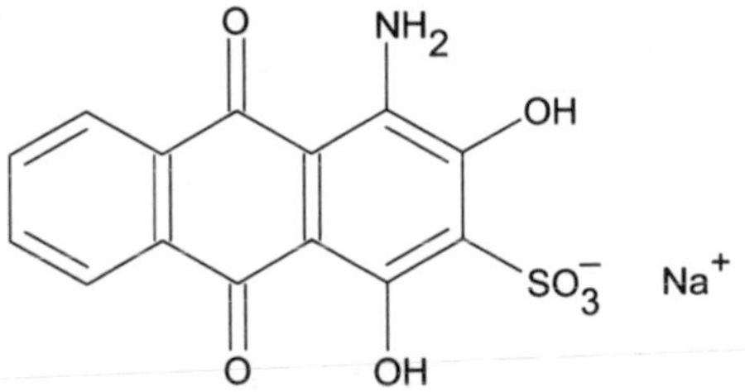

Like alizarin red S, this dye is sometimes used as a histochemical reagent for calcium. The aluminium complex is commonly used as a stain for nuclei. For the latter purpose nuclear fast red is similar to carminic acid and brazilein. Unsatisfactory dyes labelled with the name of this dye are quite frequently encountered, and the name nuclear fast red is sometimes applied to neutral red, C.I. 50040, a cationic dye with completely different staining properties (Frank *et al.*, 2007).

CARMINIC ACID (C.I. 75470; Natural red 4; MW 492)

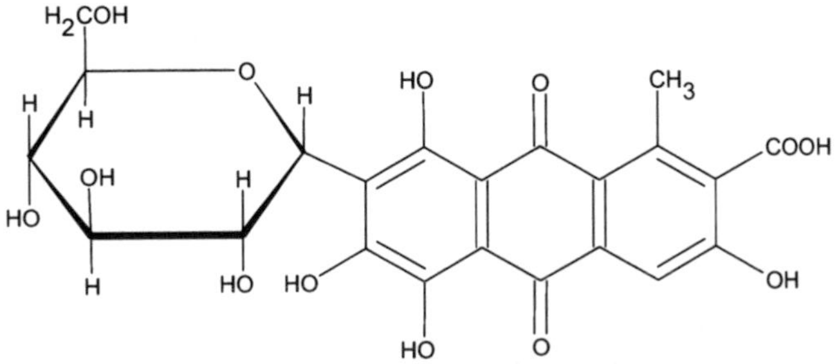

This red glycoside-like substance is the principal colouring matter of **cochineal**. Cochineal is made by grinding the dried bodies of female *Coccus* insects (from Central America). The cyclic side chain shown on the left side of the structural formula is derived from D-glucose, which is joined by a C-glycosyl linkage (without intervening oxygen) to the polyhydroxyanthraquinone carboxylic acid. Carminic acid is slightly soluble in water and alcohol, but in the presence of an aluminium salt it dissolves in larger amounts, with the formation of the complex. This dye–mordant complex is used as a red nuclear stain for sections and whole-mounts. Carminic acid decomposes if heated above 100°C (Lancaster and Lawrence, 1996). Solutions of the aluminium-carminic acid complex deteriorate after a few weeks of storage at room temperature.

Carmine, which is also made from cochineal, is used as a nuclear stain in general histology and in staining methods for glycogen and mucus. It contains 20–25% of protein (some from the insects and some added during manufacture), together with calcium ions and an anionic dye–metal complex of carminic acid and aluminium. The structure of carmine is uncertain and probably varies according to the method of manufacture. Calcium may not always be present. A suggested formula is shown in *Fig. 5.1*. Because carmine is a material of uncertain composition it should not be used as a histological stain without preliminary testing, and supposedly histochemical methods involving its use must be viewed with suspicion. The name carmine is applied to at least three substances used in food colouring; analytical procedures have been developed to distinguish these (Dapson, 2005b), and to characterise samples of carmine that are suitable for microscopical staining (Dapson *et al.*, 2007).

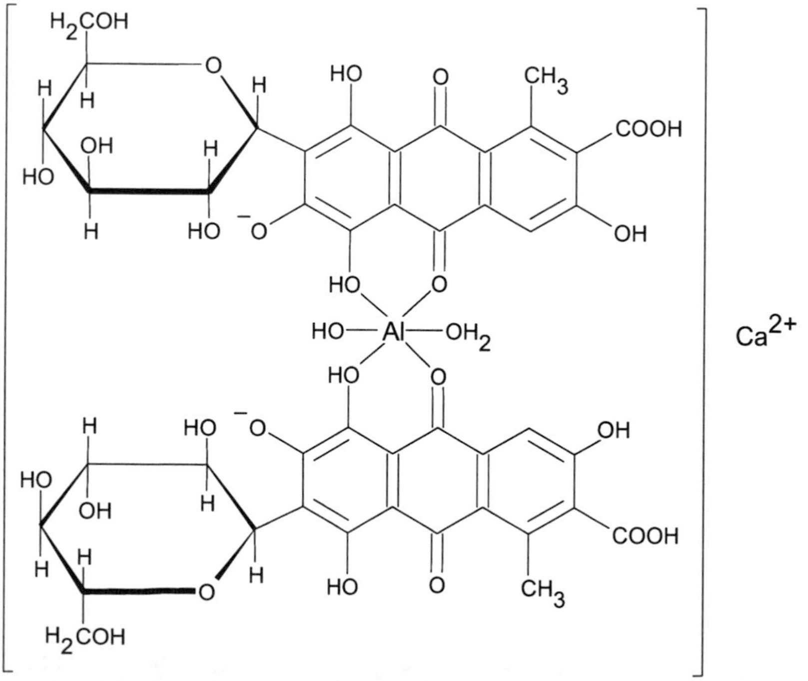

Figure 5.1. Structure of carmine as suggested by Meloan *et al.* (1971). Their formula has been slightly modified to conform with the conventions used in this book. Ionization of the phenolic hydroxyl groups *ortho* to the sugar substituents is said to be necessary for chelation of Al^{3+} with the nearby oxygen atoms. Presumably the carboxyl groups are also at least partly ionized in solution, but it is not known whether carmine contains enough Ca^{2+} to balance these. Al^{3+} could also form complexes with the free quinonoid and phenolic oxygens shown on the sides of the carminic acid molecules facing away from the Al atom. This would give the dye–metal complex a net positive charge and might occur when Al^{3+} is present in excess, as in mixtures used for nuclear staining. The mode of attachment of the dye–metal complex to tissues has not been determined.

5.9.14.
Phthalocyanine dyes

Most of these are derivatives of **copper phthalocyanine**, a blue pigment of high physical and chemical stability (C.I. 74160; Pigment blue 16; MW 576):

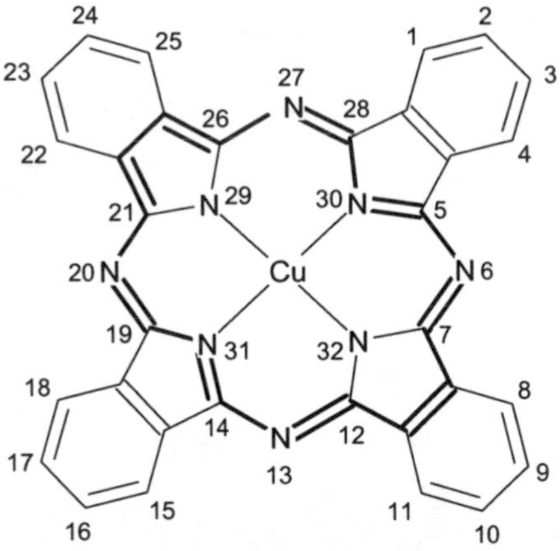

(Numbering of the phthalocyanine
ring follows Patterson *et al.*, 1960.)

The carbon and nitrogen atoms form a fully conjugated aromatic system, stabilized by resonance so that the *o*-quinonoid benzene ring (here shown at the upper left-hand corner) has no fixed location in the molecule. Colour is due to the extensive conjugation. The dark lines in the formula above show the **aza[18]annulene** chromophore, which occurs also in many naturally occurring coloured compounds including porphyrins, chlorophyll and haem. The bonds to the metal atom in copper phthalocyanine are shown as simple covalencies, though other representations are permissible (Section 5.5.8). In dyes, solubilizing groups are introduced as substituents on the phthalocyanine ring. Copper may be replaced by cobalt or other metals.

An intravenously injected suspension of copper phthalocyanine, often called **monastral blue** for this purpose, is used in laboratory animals for identifying permeable blood vessel walls at sites of inflammation or injury (Dux and Jancso, 1994; Baluk *et al.*, 1997).

Examples

SIRIUS LIGHT TURQUOISE BLUE GL (C.I. 74180; Direct blue 86; MW 760)
Two sulphonic acid groups (as their sodium salts) are present on benzenoid rings at opposite corners of the copper phthalocyanine molecule. This is the simplest phthalocyanine dye. It has been tried in histology but is not used in any important staining methods (see Lillie, 1977). The tetrasodium salt of copper phthalocyanine tetrasulfonic acid (MW 984) has been used as a surface stain for grey matter in slices of human brain (Wu and Kiernan, 2001).

ALCIAN BLUE 8G ((alcian blue 8GS, 8GX); C.I. 74240: Ingrain blue 1)
The exact chemical compositions of these dyes were not revealed by Imperial Chemical Industries Ltd., the manufacturers, but Scott (1972a) determined that alcian blue 8GX contained four tetramethylisothiouronium groups:

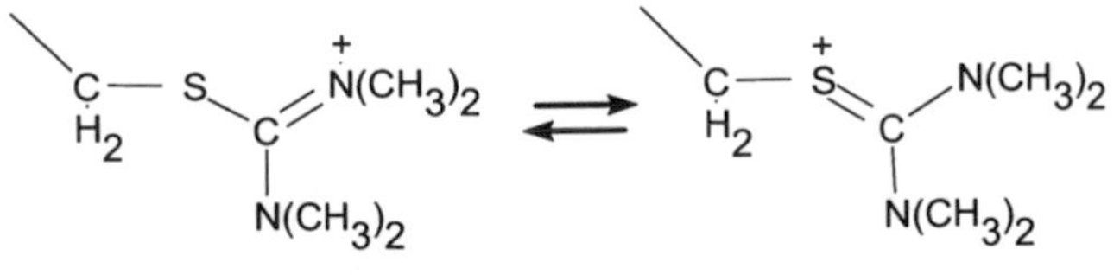

one on each of the benzenoid rings of the copper phthalocyanine structure, at positions 2 or 3, 9 or 10, 16 or 17, and 23 or 24. The dye is a mixture of the four possible geometrical isomers. The other alcian blues are believed to bear either two or three thiouronium substituents. All these dyes are supplied mixed with boric acid, sodium sulphate, and dextrin. The solubilizing side-chains of alcian blue can be easily removed by base-catalyzed hydrolysis, leaving insoluble copper phthalocyanine in the textile or tissue.

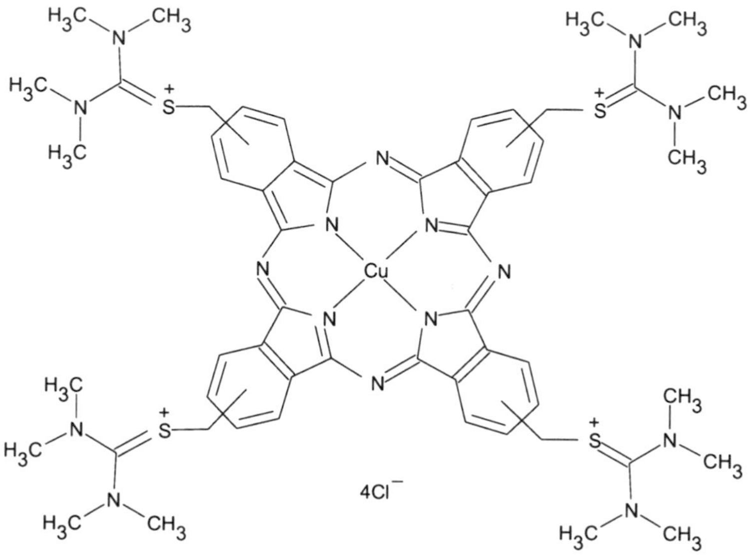

The most important applications of alcian blue are in carbohydrate histochemistry (Chapter 11). Two other 'alcian' dyes, mentioned below, have been used for similar purposes. Unsatisfactory samples of alcian blue are often encountered, so it is necessary to test every new batch before applying the dye to important material. It seems that the dye powder can deteriorate with storage: it becomes insoluble, perhaps from loss of its solubilizing tetramethylisothiouronium side chains. Variants of alcian blue with more stable solubilizing groups are available and can be substituted for alcian blue 8G in some commonly used staining techniques (Churukian et al., 2000; Henwood, 2002). Acidic solutions of alcian blue 8G sometimes give good service for more than 5 years.

The dye **alcian yellow** is not a phthalocyanine but a monoazo dye which also contains the benzothiazole chromophore and a thiouronium auxochrome. **Alcian green** is a mixture of alcian blue with alcian yellow.

CUPROLINIC BLUE (quinolinic phthalocyanine; no C.I. number)

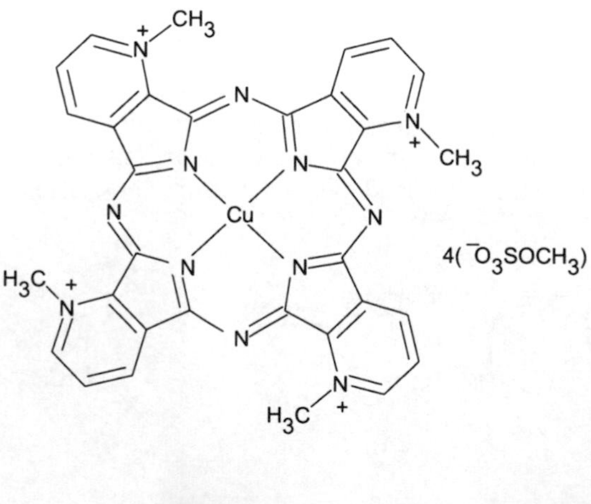

This basic dye has a modified phthalocyanine chromophore with quaternary nitrogen atoms replacing four of the carbons. This arrangement provides a positively charged planar molecule without the bulky side-chains of alcian blue. The dye cations can enter the intramolecular crevices of nucleic acids, which are not accessible to alcian blue. The use of cuprolinic blue for staining RNA is discussed in Chapter 9.

LUXOL FAST BLUE MBS (C.I. 74180; Solvent blue 38)

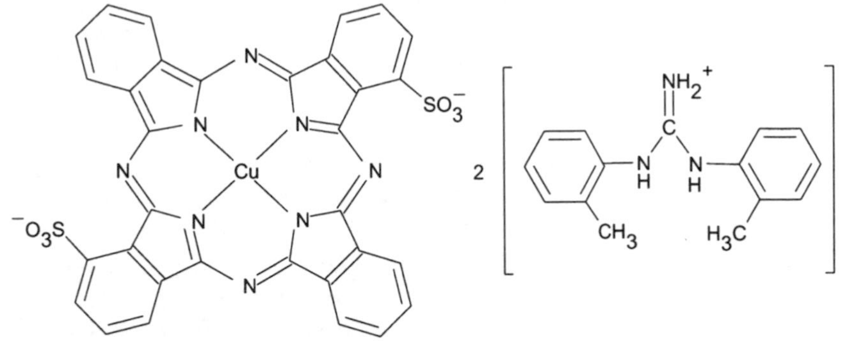

This is the ditolylguanidinium salt of a copper phthalocyanine disulphonic acid. It is soluble in alcohols but almost insoluble in water.

The 'luxol' dyes are anionic chromogens that are balanced not by H^+ or Na^+ but by **arylguanidinium** cations such as those of diphenylguanidine or ditolylguanidine. These dyes are insoluble in water but soluble in alcohols. Luxol fast blue MBS has a copper phthalocyanine chromogen, whereas **luxol fast blue G** and **luxol fast blue ARN** (C.I. Solvent blue 37) are azo dyes (Salthouse, 1962, 1963; Horobin and Kiernan, 2002). Dyes with similar properties but of known chemical constitution can be produced in the laboratory from suitable direct cotton dyes and diphenylguanidine (Clasen *et al.*, 1973), but have not become popular.

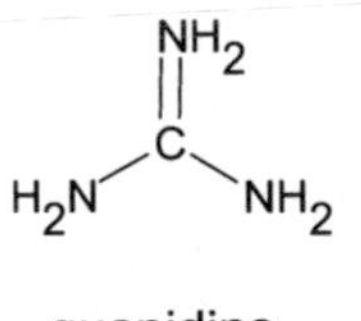

guanidine
(imino-urea)

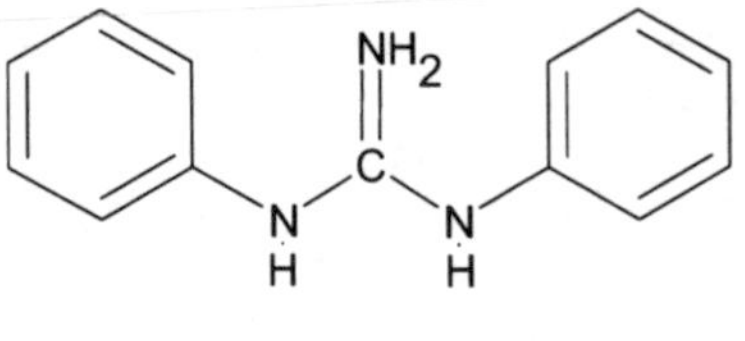

diphenylguanidine

The luxol dyes are used for staining myelin (Chapter 6).

Several **anionic metal phthalocyanine dyes** (with Co, Cu, Ni and Zn) were tested by Achar *et al.* (1993) and found to be suitable green and blue counterstains for plant tissues in which lignin had been stained red by safranine O.

5.10 Structure–staining correlations

The objects or substances to which a dye will bind can be predicted, to some extent, from an examination of its structural formula. The estimation of physical, chemical and pharmacological properties of organic compounds, a field of great importance to many industries, is reviewed by Lyman *et al.* (1982) and Hansch and Leo (1995). To evaluate a dye, one looks at the formula for information concerning electric charge, ability to form chelates or covalent bonds, the shape and size of the dye ion or molecule, and features favourable to non-ionic bonding (see also Section 5.5).

Quantitative structure–activity relations (QSAR) are determined on the basis of quantities calculated from a structural formula. Horobin (1980, 2002, 2004) has discussed the subject from the viewpoint of biological staining, and Dapson (2005a) has derived numerical parameters from the structures of 436 dyes that have been or might be used as biological stains. These data can be used to predict whether a compound will stain, for example, nucleic acids, lipids, basic proteins or mucus in sections of fixed tissue. QSAR calculations can predict whether a fluorescent compound that enters living cells will be concentrated in the nucleus, endoplasmic reticulum, Golgi apparatus, lysosomes or mitochondria (Rashid and Horobin, 1991; Rashid et al., 1991; Horobin, 2001; Horobin et al., 2006).

5.10.1
Type of dye

The **overall charge** of the coloured ion is easily seen, and usually determines whether the staining will be principally of nuclei and acid carbohydrates (cationic dyes) or principally of cytoplasm and collagen (anionic dyes). Uncharged dyes may be reactive dyes (which stain everything), solvents (which stain lipids) or mordant dyes (which are used most frequently for nuclei or myelin).

5.10.2
Size

The size of a dye ion or molecule affects its **penetration** of different components of the tissue, and its **substantivity** (Section 5.9.3.8). The molecular or ionic weight is a reasonable estimator of size. It should be remembered that many dyes consist of aggregated molecules in aqueous solution, but large molecules join to one another more readily than small ones, and form correspondingly larger particles. Another easily obtained value is the size (in number of bonds or atoms) of the **longest conjugated chain** in the molecule. This increases with the size of the chromophoric system, and high values are associated with strong non-ionic binding.

When a tissue is stained by two or more dyes with a charge of the same sign, the larger coloured ions enter the more porous parts of the tissue. For example, when eosin (MW 692; anion 646) and methyl blue (MW 800; anion 753) are used together, as in Mann's method (Chapter 6), collagen and chromatin become blue, and erythrocytes and cytoplasm are red. Porosity is not the only factor in differential staining; some others are discussed in Chapters 6 and 8.

Except when covalent bonds are formed, the strength of the bonding between a tissue and any coloured substance depends largely on non-ionic forces of attraction. As explained in Sections 5.5.4–5.5.7, these forces are weak, and require intimate contact between dye and substrate. A large molecule that can be planar, such as a disazo dye or a phthalocyanine will stick to a tissue more strongly than a small planar dye. There are some dyes that can never assume planar configurations because of steric hindrance. The triphenylmethanes, for example, have their rings arrayed like the blades of a propeller. Among such dyes, those with the largest molecules are the most difficult to remove from stained sections.

5.10.3
Hydrophobic–hydrophilic balance

The hydrophobic or hydrophilic nature of a dye is indicated by **log P**, which is the logarithm of its **partition coefficient** (P) between a moderately hydrophobic solvent (such as octanol) and water. Log P can be measured in a laboratory or estimated from the formula by attributing scores (see Horobin, 1980, 1982) to the different parts of the structure and summing the scores. The result is informative when it is compared with the values for dyes with known staining properties. Instead of log P, Dapson and Dapson (2005) provides for each dye a hydrophobic index (**HI**), which is the reciprocal of the mean of the charges associated with all the atoms in the structure. This index is high (8–9.5) for dyes used as fat stains, which are strongly hydrophobic, and low (1.3–5) for most anionic dyes. Most cationic dyes are somewhat hydrophobic, with HI in the range 5–8. Generally, the more hydrophobic dyes exhibit stronger binding in an aqueous environment. The most hydrophobic dyes are, of course, insoluble in water. Hydrophilic dyes are used in non-aqueous solution, for staining hydrophilic substrates. Hydrogen bonding probably contributes to the substantivity in these cases (Section 5.5.4).

6 Histological staining in one or two colours

For the study of microscopic anatomy and of pathological material it is usual to stain sections of tissue in such a way as to impart a dark colour to the nuclei of cells and a lighter, contrasting colour to the cytoplasm and extracellular structures. With simple methods of this type, of which the most widely practised is alum–haematoxylin (haemalum) and eosin ('H and E'), it is not possible to make deductions concerning the chemical natures of any of the components of the tissue. Identification of the different types of cells and of the fibres and matrices of the intervening connective tissue must be based solely on morphological criteria. The H and E method is perhaps the least revealing of the two-colour techniques because in most cell-types the alum–haematein component colours only the nuclei. Nevertheless, this procedure is used more than any other in the teaching of normal histology and by pathologists. Other simple staining methods provide more informative preparations than does H and E, but familiarity with the latter has not yet led to contempt.

Nuclear stains and simple counterstaining procedures are considered in this chapter. A few methods for staining in various shades of one colour are also described. The rationales of the techniques are discussed, but methods of higher chemical specificity (e.g. for nucleic acids, carbohydrates, and functional groups of proteins) are not covered. The special methods for blood and for connective tissue are likewise described elsewhere (Chapters 7 and 8).

6.1. Nuclear stains

The nucleus of a eukaryotic cell contains the two **nucleic acids**: DNA in the chromosomes, and RNA in the nucleolus. Both are associated with strongly basic **nucleoproteins**: these are **histones** in diploid cells or **protamines** in haploid cells such as spermatozoa. Nucleoproteins are rich in the amino acids arginine and lysine. The cations of these amino acids are neutralized by phosphoric acid residues of the nucleic acids (see also Chapter 9). The DNA and nucleoprotein of the chromosomes together constitute the material known as **chromatin**, named for its prominence in most stained preparations. In interphase cells the chromosomes are extended and cannot be seen individually. The chromatin seen in stained preparations of interphase nuclei may be evenly distributed through the nucleoplasm or aggregated in a pattern characteristic of the cell type. The dyes used as nuclear stains impart colour to the chromatin by binding to the nucleic acids, the nucleoprotein or both these substances.

6.1.1.
Cationic dyes

The modes of binding of cationic dyes to substrates were discussed in Chapter 5, where descriptions of several dyes of this type can be found. The dyes are applied from acidified solutions in order to ensure the ionization of their primary, secondary, or tertiary amine groups. Three types of anions capable of binding cationic dyes occur in tissues. These are the phosphates of nucleic acids, sulphate esters of certain macromolecular carbohydrates (Chapter 11), and carboxylate ions of carbohydrates and proteins. As explained in Chapter 5, the ionization of carboxyl groups is suppressed if the concentration of hydrogen ions in the staining solution is too high (in practice, pH <3–4), while sulphate groups remain ionized even in strongly acidic media. Phosphoric acid is of intermediate strength. A basic protein, such as haemoglobin, contains an excess of free amino over carboxyl groups, so that the latter can be made available for binding cationic dyes only from alkaline solutions (e.g. at pH 8). The staining properties of cationic dyes are profoundly influenced by the pH of their solutions. *If they are too acid, only the structures rich in sulphated carbohydrates will be coloured; if they are neutral or alkaline, everything will be stained.*

The interpretation of the results obtained with cationic dyes at various pH levels has been studied in some depth (see Gabe, 1976; Lillie and Fullmer, 1976; Prento, 2001 for reviews and discussion). It is convenient to think of staining by cationic dyes as a process of ion-exchange, in which small cations such as H^+ are competitively displaced from the tissue by the larger cations of the dye (see Horobin, 1982). When the tissue and the dye solution are together for a long enough time, there is an equilibrium:

$$Tissue^- \cdots H^+ + Dye^+ \rightleftharpoons Tissue^- \cdots Dye^+ + H^+$$

Binding of dye by non-ionic forces (Chapter 5) favours staining (pulling the above reaction from left to right), whereas a high concentration of H^+ or Na^+ in the solution opposes staining (pushing the reaction from right to left). This simple explanation applies only to dilute solutions of dyes with small molecules. In most real staining techniques non-ionic forces cause aggregation of dye, so that more than one coloured molecule is bound at each anionic site in the tissue.

The following list will serve as a rough guide to the use of dilute (e.g. 0.01–0.2%) solutions of cationic dyes. It applies especially to those of the thiazine series.

pH 1.0   Only sulphated carbohydrate components are stained. Sulphonic acid groups or sulphuric acid esters can be artificially produced in the tissue (Chapters 10 and 11) and these, too, will bind cationic dyes from strongly acid solutions.

pH 2.5–3.0   Staining of the above, and also phosphate of nucleic acids (DNA and RNA), and of phospholipids (in frozen sections).

pH 4.0–5.0   Staining of the above, and also carboxyl groups of carbohydrates and of the more acid proteins. Carboxyl groups of free fatty acids may be stained in frozen sections.

pH > 5.0   Staining of the above with increasing staining of neutral and basic proteins with increasing pH.

With higher concentrations of dye, the rules set out above are not followed, and staining is generally less specific. The duration of exposure to the dye has only minor effects on the results, though longer times are needed to achieve the greatest possible depth of staining (equilibrium) if very dilute solutions are used. The end result is also affected by treatments after staining.

Most cationic dyes are rather readily extracted from sections by 70% alcohol. Absolute ethanol, *n*-butanol, and acetone are usually less active in this respect. In any critical work with cationic dyes the conditions of rinsing and dehydration must be carefully standardized. *The water used for rinsing the sections after staining should be buffered to the same pH as the dye solution.* Fixatives generally do not directly affect sulphate, phosphate, and carboxylate groups, but combination with or removal of amine groups has the effect of lowering the pH at which proteins are stained. Thus, fixation by osmium tetroxide, which causes oxidative deamination (Chapter 2) renders almost all components of tissues stainable by cationic dyes at pH 4 or higher.

For general purpose staining of nuclei, cationic dyes are used in dilute solution (0.1–0.5%) at pH 3–4.5. The aqueous solution of the dye is usually acidified by addition of acetic acid or a suitable buffer. Objects that are coloured by cationic (basic) dyes are said to be **basophilic** (Baker, 1958, argued in favour of 'basiphil'). When nuclei are stained by cationic dyes, basophilia will also be evident at sites of accumulation of cytoplasmic RNA such as the Nissl substance of neurons, and in structures containing sulphated carbohydrates such as mast cell granules, cartilage matrix, and many secretory products. In this propensity cationic dyes differ importantly from some of the metal complexing (mordant) dyes used as nuclear stains. As explained above, cationic dyes will not stain nuclei specifically. The following solutions are suitable for use either alone or as counterstains to other methods.

6.1.1.1. Toluidine blue (C.I. 52040)
A 0.5% aqueous solution, acidified by adding approximately 1.0 ml of glacial acetic acid to each 100 ml of dye solution. Alternatively, make up in 0.1 M acetate buffer, pH 4.0. The optimum pH may vary between 3.0 and 5.5 according to the fixative and the tissue to be stained. Stain in this solution for 3 min, rinse in water, dehydrate in 95% followed by two changes of absolute alcohol, clear in xylene, and mount in a resinous medium.

If too much colour is lost during washing or alcoholic dehydration, move the slides directly onto filter paper and blot firmly with two or three layers of filter paper. Transfer to a clean, dry staining rack or coplin jar and dehydrate in two changes (each 4–5 min) of *n*-butanol. Clear and mount as above. If detachment of the sections seems imminent, the clearing in xylene may be omitted, but the resinous medium will then take longer to become fully transparent.

The dye may also be immobilized in stained structures by converting it to an insoluble molybdate. After staining, wash in water and immerse for 5 min in 5% aqueous ammonium molybdate (ammonium paramolybdate, $(NH_4)_6Mo_7O_{24}.4H_2O$) solution (which may be used repeatedly until it becomes cloudy; usually stable for 1 or 2 weeks). Wash in running tap water for 2–3 min. The molybdate of toluidine blue is not extracted by water or alcohols and even resists counterstaining by acidic mixtures of dyes, such as that of van Gieson (Chapter 8).

Nuclei and acid carbohydrate components are stained blue. Some carbohydrate-containing structures are metachromatically stained (red) as explained in Chapter

11. Cytoplasmic RNA (e.g. Nissl bodies of neurons) is also blue. Other thiazine dyes (e.g. Borrel's methylene blue, azure A) may be substituted for toluidine blue.

6.1.1.2. Neutral red (C.I. 50040)

Use a 0.5% aqueous solution for 1–5 min. Acidification with acetic acid (Section 6.1.1.1) is usually desirable. Wash, dehydrate, and clear as described for toluidine blue.

Nuclei and other basophilic structures are stained red. Safranine O (C.I. 50240) gives a similar result, but longer staining times (often 30 min) are usually required.

Neutral red can also be used as a fluorochrome. Stain hydrated paraffin sections for 5 min in 0.002% aqueous neutral red, then dehydrate, clear and cover in the usual way. With excitation by near UV or blue light (325–500 nm) nuclei and cytoplasmic RNA emit yellow-orange fluorescence (Allen and Kiernan, 1994).

6.1.1.3. Ethyl green (C.I. 42590) and methylene green (C.I. 52020)

These unrelated dyes are useful counterstains when objects of greater interest than nuclei have been coloured red, purple or brown. Ethyl green is still sold as 'methyl green', a dye that has been obsolete for more than 30 years (Section 5.9.5.2).

For staining with ethyl green, immerse slides for 15 min in a 0.2% solution of the dye at pH 4.0–4.5. An acetate buffer (Chapter 20) is a suitable solvent. Rinse quickly in water, blot the slides dry, and dehydrate in two changes of acetone or of n-butanol (as described above for toluidine blue). Clear in xylene and cover, using a resinous mounting medium. Nuclei and other basophilic structures are stained bluish green.

A methylene green counterstain for nuclei (McNulty et al., 2004) is a 0.5% (w/v) solution of the dye in 2.4% aqueous boric acid. After 5 min in this solution, the slides are washed in two 2–min changes of water followed by three 3–min changes of 100% ethanol, clearing in xylene and application of a resinous mounting medium.

6.1.1.4. Polychrome methylene blue

The staining solution is a mixture of thiazine dyes produced by oxidation and demethylation (polychroming) of methylene blue. The polychroming (Chapters 5 and 7) may be accomplished in various ways. The following method, in which silver oxide is used as an oxidizing agent, is recommended for its simplicity and speed.

Borrel's methylene blue

Add 25 ml of 4% aqueous sodium hydroxide (NaOH) to 100 ml of 1% silver nitrate (AgNO$_3$). Allow the precipitate of silver oxide (Ag$_2$O) to settle, decant off the supernatant, and wash the precipitate by shaking and decantation, with two changes of 100 ml of water. Dissolve 1.0 g of methylene blue (C.I. 52015) in 100 ml of water, boil, and add to the washed Ag$_2$O. Boil for 5 min, leave to cool, then filter. This stock solution is diluted to five times its volume with water to give the working solution. Both the stock and the diluted solutions are stable for at least 10 years.

Method

(1) Stain frozen sections or hydrated paraffin sections for 2 min in the diluted solution of Borrel's methylene blue.
(2) Rinse rapidly in running tap water, blot slides dry, and dehydrate in two changes (each 30 s, with agitation) of absolute ethanol.
(3) Clear in xylene and cover, using a resinous mounting medium.

Result

All components of the tissue are stained in various shades of blue. Strongly acid carbohydrates stain metachromatically (red), especially if some differentiation is allowed to occur in the water wash. With deliberate overstaining, as described, the objects that are normally metachromatic will be dark blue or purple.

6.1.2.
Anionic dyes

For reasons given in Chapter 5, anionic dyes are applied from acidic solutions. Used alone, an anionic dye will colour almost all the components of a tissue, but differential staining effects can sometimes be obtained when two or more dyes are applied simultaneously or in sequence. A method of this type is Mann's eosin–methyl blue. Nuclei, cartilage, and collagen acquire the blue colour, and cytoplasms are stained pink or red by eosin. The reasons for these results are not fully known, but it is widely held that the large molecules of methyl blue are excluded by the smaller ones of eosin from the supposedly 'dense' network of cytoplasmic protein molecules. Collagen and chromatin, with their presumed 'looser' textures, would admit molecules of both dyes, but the eosin would diffuse out more rapidly than the methyl blue when the sections are washed following immersion in the mixture. The influence of molecular size on the staining properties of dyes will be discussed in more detail in Chapter 8. Nuclear staining by methyl blue was studied by McKay (1962) who found that the presence of nucleic acids was necessary. He was unable to obtain evidence for binding of the dye by ionic attraction and suggested that the staining of nuclei was analogous to the direct dyeing of cotton (Chapter 5). McKay compared methyl blue with chlorazol black E, a direct azo dye. Chlorazol black E was found to behave like most other anionic dyes, including eosin, and was, therefore, thought to be bound to tissue principally by electrovalent forces. Useful staining of nuclei and cytoplasm can be obtained with chlorazol black E. This dye also stains elastin, but probably by a non-ionic mechanism (Goldstein. 1962).

6.1.2.1. Mann's eosin–methyl blue

The procedure given below is the 'short method' of Mann (1902). The 'long method' (Mann, 1902; Cook, 1974; also discussed at length by Gabe, 1976) is more controllable and is used for demonstrating intracellular objects such as secretory granules and viral inclusion bodies. Fixation is not critical, but superior contrast is obtained if mixtures containing mercuric chloride, potassium dichromate, or picric acid have been used.

Preparation of stain

Mix:

1% aqueous eosin (C.I. 45380):	45 ml
1% aqueous methyl blue (C.I. 42780):	35 ml
Water:	100 ml

The stock solutions and the mixture can be kept for two years. Precipitates may form in the mixture; they should be removed by filtration. Any water-soluble 'aniline blue' (C.I. 42755; see Chapter 5) may be used in place of methyl blue.

Procedure

(1) De-wax and hydrate paraffin sections.
(2) Stain in eosin–methyl blue for 10 min.
(3) Wash in running tap water for a few seconds to remove excess dyes from slides.
(4) Dehydrate in 95% and two changes of absolute alcohol.
(5) Clear in xylene and cover, using a resinous mounting medium.

Result

Nuclei and collagen blue; erythrocytes, cytoplasm, and nucleoli red. With this 'short' method the colours obtained are rather variable. Like Borrel's methylene blue, this is a 'quick look' stain for determining which of a series of sections or specimens are worthy of more critical examination.

6.1.2.2. Chlorazol black E

Staining solution

Chlorazol black E (C.I. 30235):	3.0 g
70% aqueous ethanol:	300 ml

Dissolve the dye (magnetic stirrer; 30 min at room temperature), then filter the solution. It keeps for about 9 months, gradually losing strength as a black precipitate forms on the bottom and sides of the bottle.

Procedure

(1) De-wax paraffin sections and take to 70% alcohol.
(2) Stain in the chlorazol black E solution for about 10 min. The time is not critical.
(3) Rinse in 95% ethanol, two changes, 1 min in each. (See *Note 2* below.)
(4) Complete the dehydration in two changes of absolute alcohol.
(5) Clear in xylene and cover, using a resinous mounting medium.

Result

Nuclei black. Elastin black. Other components of tissue in various shades of grey. Cytoplasm often has a greenish tinge and cartilage matrix is usually pinkish grey. Collagen is rather lightly stained. Cytoplasmic organelles such as mitochondria and secretory granules are well displayed in suitably fixed material. The colour does not fade. (See also *Note 3* below.)

Notes

(1) The method will work after any fixation but, as with most other dye staining methods, greater contrast is obtained after fixation in a mixture containing picric acid, mercuric chloride or potassium dichromate than after fixation in formaldehyde alone.
(2) Over-staining seldom occurs if the time at Stage 2 is less than 20 min. Differentiation occurs slowly and controllably in 95% ethanol. Cannon (1937), the originator of the method, recommended terpineol as a differentiator. He also commented on the similarity of the end result to that obtained with Heidenhain's iron–haematoxylin, a traditional but time-consuming technique involving a critical differentiation (Section 6.1.3.1).
(3) The most informative preparations are thin sections (5 µm or less) examined at high magnification. Other methods of staining with chlorazol black E are given by Clark (1981).

6.1.3.
Metal complexing dyes

For nuclear staining, mixtures of mordant dyes with appropriate metal salts are applied to sections of tissue. The modes of action of metal ions in binding dye molecules to their substrates have already been discussed in Chapter 5. There it was pointed out that some dye–metal complexes, such as that of chromium with gallocyanine, behave as if they were simple cationic dyes. For others, including haematein, brazilin and eriochrome cyanine R, the interactions of dye, metal and substrate are more complicated than the attraction of oppositely charged ions. These latter dyes are used to obtain selective staining of chromatin.

Haematein (the principal product of oxidation of **haematoxylin**) is used in solutions containing ferric, aluminium or, more rarely, chromium ions. In other mixtures, used only for specialized purposes, the metal ion may be lead, copper or zirconyl, or phosphotungstic or phosphomolybdic acid. For nuclear staining, the solution must contain a considerably greater proportion of ferric or aluminium ions than of haematein and it must be acidified. The word 'haematoxylin' is commonly used in the names of staining methods and mixtures, even though 'haematein' would be more correct.

Solutions containing oxidized haematoxylin (haematein) and Al^{3+} are the 'H' (haemalum) of H and E, and are used everywhere to stain the nuclei of cells. The reactions of aluminium ions with haematein have been studied by Bettinger and Zimmermann (1991a,b), who found that a cationic dye–metal complex was present in acid solutions. The complex was bound by DNA in sections of tissue, even though the pH was lower than that at which nucleic acids can be stained by ordinary cationic dyes. The haemalum mixtures in common use contain a large excess of Al^{3+} ions over haematein molecules. Aluminium ions have considerable affinity for DNA, and can prevent its subsequent staining by cationic dyes. Acids used to increase the selectivity of nuclear staining probably disrupt the bonding between Al^{3+} and parts of the tissue other than chromatin, rather than between Al^{3+} and the dye (Baker, 1960, 1962).

Unfortunately, affinity of Al^{3+} or the Al–haematein complex for DNA does not account for the selectivity of nuclear staining by the commonly used haemalum solutions. This is inhibited only slightly by prior extraction of DNA from the tissue, but it is considerably reduced after chemical blocking of lysine and arginine residues (Lillie *et al.*, 1976). Furthermore, measurements of the colour intensity in haemalum-stained nuclei do not vary in proportion to the content of DNA (Schulte and Fink, 1995). These observations suggest that the dye–metal complex attaches mainly to a component of the nucleus other than DNA. The non-DNA component of chromatin is the basic nucleoprotein, which would be expected to bind an anionic rather than a cationic dye–metal complex. However, alum–haematein does not stain other tissue components that have affinity for anionic dyes, so there must be a high affinity for chromatin that is unrelated to DNA or the basic amino acids of its associated nucleoprotein.

Horobin (1988) suggests that dye–metal complexes are bound to chromatin by both ionic and non-ionic forces. The latter are likely to be enhanced by the other substances present in alum–haematein staining solution. Most formulations contain a highly polar substance such as glycerol, ethylene glycol or chloral hydrate, which would be expected to associate by hydrogen bonding with hydrophilic components of the tissue and to interfere with short-range forces (van der Waals, hydrophobic etc; see Chapter 5) that would hold the dye–metal complex to some potential substrates. A shape of the dye–metal complex ion that favourably conforms with the nucleoprotein and nucleic acid molecules would be bound closely enough to resist disruption by hydrogen bonding substances. Any colorant intimately adherent to DNA or the histone molecules of chromatin would not easily be removed by aqueous or other hydrogen-bonding rinses.

Alum–haematein staining may be **progressive** or **regressive**. The former is usually preferred, but if overstaining has to be corrected the sections are differentiated in 70% or 95% alcohol containing a little hydrochloric acid. Aqueous acid may also be used, but the differentiating action is then slower. Addition to the staining bath of more acid or more of the aluminium salt also suppresses the tendency to overstain, thereby making the mixture more selective as a progressive nuclear stain. The acid-lability of nuclei stained by alum–haematoxylin precludes counterstaining with solutions that are more than slightly acidic. Eosin is suitable but the van Gieson mixture (Chapter 8) is not. The aluminium–haematein complex changes colour from reddish brown to blue at about pH 6. The latter colour is the one desired, so stained sections are washed in tap water, to which a trace of alkali may have to be added. This process is called **blueing**. An eosin counterstain imparts pink and red colours to all components of the tissue, including nuclei previously made blue by alum–haematein. Consequently, the nuclei in a typical H and E preparation are purple, from mixing of the colours.

The **iron–haematein complex** has a deep blue-black colour and can be removed from stained sections only by strongly acid differentiating solutions. If the iron salt and the haematein are applied sequentially to the section, as in **Heidenhain's method**, a great variety of structural details can be revealed by careful differentiation. The progressive mode is the method of choice for pure nuclear staining, so the dye solutions are then made with large excesses of ferric salt and acid (usually hydrochloric). **Weigert's haematoxylin** is a typical mixture of this type. The ferric ions eventually over-oxidize the haematein, so the stain deteriorates gradually (over several days), until it is no longer usable. Some iron–haematoxylins have better keeping properties than Weigert's. The more stable iron–haematoxylin mixtures contain both ferric and ferrous ions. The reducing action of the latter is assumed to restrain the oxidation of the dye (see Lillie and Fullmer, 1976). Little is known of the mechanisms of nuclear staining by iron–haematein. Extraction of DNA has no effect, and chemical blocking of lysine and arginine residues causes only partial inhibition of staining (Lillie *et al.*, 1976).

Sections containing nuclei stained by iron–haematoxylin do not lose their colour when treated with strongly acidic reagents, including the mixtures of anionic dyes used for differential coloration of cytoplasm and collagen (Chapter 8).

It is also possible to stain nuclei with synthetic metal complexing dyes that are cheaper than haematoxylin. A suitable substitute is **eriochrome cyanine R**, used with a ferric salt. This behaves like alum–haematein when used as a nuclear stain. Several other alternatives to haematoxylin have been described by Lillie *et al.* (1976).

Often red is preferred to the blue and black imparted to nuclei by the metal–haematein stains. This may be achieved by using an aluminium salt with **carminic acid** ('carmalum'), **brazilein** ('brazalum'), or **nuclear fast red**. Red nuclear stains are most often employed as counterstains to histochemical or other specialized methods that impart other colours to the objects in which the microscopist is primarily interested.

6.1.3.1. Heidenhain's iron–haematoxylin

This simple classical technique is used principally to resolve structural details within cells, so the tissue should be fixed in a mixture that preserves cytoplasmic organelles. Helly's or Altmann's fixative meet this requirement (Chapter 2). Paraffin sections should be no more than 5 μm thick. The sections are soaked in a solution containing ferric ions and then immersed in a haematein solution, which forms a black complex with the bound iron, everywhere in the tissue. The haematein serves only to demonstrate iron (Wigglesworth, 1952), which is bound principally to carboxyl groups of proteins. The iron alum solution is then used again, to differentiate the preparation until the desired staining is obtained.

The differentiating solution acts partly because it is acidic and partly because its ferric ions form soluble complexes with haematein, thereby extracting the dye from the stained section. Differentiation by acid alone leaves the nuclear chromatin as the last material to be destained. A neutral or alkaline solution of a compound containing iron(III), such as potassium ferricyanide, extracts colour first from the nuclei and last from membranous structures such as myelin and mitochondria. Iron alum is between these extremes, and allows the staining of nuclei, secretory granules, cilia, brush-borders, centrosomes, mitochondria, the various transverse bands of striated muscle fibres, and bundles of cytoskeletal filaments. Even structures that can be properly resolved only by electron microscopy, such as the endoplasmic reticulum (ergastoplasm) and some of the organelles of protozoa, were described originally in preparations stained by Heidenhain's haematoxylin technique. Complete extraction of nucleic acids from sections has no effect on nuclear or cytoplasmic staining by this method; the binding of iron is principally to carboxyl groups of proteins (Puchtler, 1958).

Solutions required
5% iron alum

Ferric ammonium sulphate FeNH$_4$(SO$_4$)$_2$.12H$_2$O:	10 g
Water:	200 ml

Iron alum is also called ammonium ferric sulphate. It should consist of violet crystals that dissolve completely in water to make a light orange-brown solution. If the crystals are large, it may be necessary to leave the mixture overnight on a magnetic stirrer. There are many bad batches of this compound, which contain insoluble white or light brown material. Even with clean iron alum, a precipitate forms after several months, and the solution should then be discarded.

Matured 10% alcoholic haematoxylin

Haematoxylin:	20 g
95% alcohol:	200 ml

Atmospheric oxidation slowly generates haematein in this stock solution, which should be ready to use in about 2 months. To accelerate the oxidation, add 50 mg of potassium or sodium iodate for each gram of haematoxylin. This will oxidize about one-quarter of the dye precursor to haematein and allow the stock solution to be used immediately. The atmosphere works slowly on the remaining haematoxylin.

This valuable stock solution should be kept in a screw-capped bottle in a dark or dimly lit place. It will serve you well for 20 years if you inspect it from time to time and make up any loss of volume due to evaporation of the solvent.

Working solution of matured haematoxylin

Matured 10% alcoholic haematoxylin:	5 ml
Water:	95 ml

This solution can be kept (in a dark place) and used repeatedly for about one year.

Procedure
(1) De-wax and hydrate paraffin sections. Remove mercury deposits if necessary. (See also *Note 1* below.)
(2) Put the slides in 5% iron alum solution: overnight or for 24 h. (See also *Note 2* below.)
(3) Rinse in 3 changes of water, each for 1 min.
(4) Put the slides in the working solution of matured haematoxylin: overnight or for 24 h. (See also *Note 2* below.)
(5) Wash in running tap water for 5 min.
(6) Shake and wipe off excess water from one of the slides. Put a few drops of the 5% iron alum solution on the sections. Put the slide on the stage of a microscope, and watch the destaining process through a ×10 objective.
(7) When the desired appearance has been achieved, put the slide into running tap water, and leave it there for at least 30 min. (See also *Note 3* below.)
(8) Dehydrate through graded alcohols.
(9) Clear in xylene and cover, using a resinous mounting medium.

Result
Nuclei, cytoplasmic structures and erythrocytes black, blue-black or grey, depending on the degree of differentiation.

Notes
(1) If the sections are stained with eosin or a similar red anionic dye before Step 2, there will be less staining of collagen by the iron–haematoxylin (Gabe, 1976).

(2) It is a common practice to pre-heat the iron alum and the working solution of matured haematoxylin to about 55°C. Steps 2 and 4 can then be shortened to 1 h, but the black colour will not be as strong as with the traditional long method.

(3) A counterstain is not usually necessary or desirable, but may be applied after Step 7. Cook (1974) recommends eosin or light green.

6.1.3.2. Alum haematoxylin: haemalum and eosin
The method described here is typical of the many H and E procedures. The traditional recipe for Mayer's haemalum has been modified by reducing the amount of sodium iodate for the reasons given in Chapter 5. Alternative alum–haemateins of equal value are described in *Note 5*. Do not expect a satisfactory result by following the numbered steps of this method uncritically: careful attention to the appended notes is essential.

Solutions required
A. Mayer's haemalum
This is the 1901 variant of Langeron, which is ready to use immediately; Mayer's original mixture, published in 1891, did not include an oxidizing agent and it was necessary to wait several months for sufficient atmospheric oxidation of haematoxylin to haematein (see Llewellyn, 2005).

Dissolve the following, in the order given, in 750ml of water. A magnetic stirrer will hasten dissolving of the alum, haematoxylin and haematein formed by iodate oxidation.

Aluminium potassium sulphate ($KAl(SO_4)_2.12H_2O$):	50 g
Haematoxylin (C.I. 75290):	1.0 g
Sodium iodate ($NaIO_3$):	0.1 g
Citric acid (monohydrate):	1.0 g
Chloral hydrate:	50 g
Water:	to make 1000 ml

To prolong the working lifetime of the stain, this solution is made with only half the quantity of sodium iodate stipulated in Langeron's formulation. Mayer's haemalum often keeps for a year but some batches lose their potency after only a few months. The solution may be reused many times. Some authorities recommend boiling the solution and filtering when it has cooled, but boiling does not seem to be necessary. The function of the chloral hydrate is questionable; some workers simply omit it, and some make up to 1 l with 250–300 ml of glycerol or ethylene glycol.

See *Note 5* below for some alternative alum–haematein solutions.

B. Eosin

Eosin Y (C.I. 45380):	2.5 g
Water:	495 ml
Glacial acetic acid:	0.5 ml

This solution keeps for several months, and may be used repeatedly. Moulds often grow in it and need to be removed by filtration. Addition of a crystal of thymol to the solution helps to retard the growth of moulds.

C. Acid–alcohol

| 95% alcohol: | 500 ml |
| Concentrated hydrochloric acid: | 5 ml |

Keeps for several weeks in a bottle or staining vessel. Discard when it becomes strongly coloured by extracted dye.

Procedure

(1) De-wax and hydrate paraffin sections. Frozen sections should be dried onto slides.

(2) Stain in Mayer's haemalum (Solution A) for 1–15 min (usually 2–5 min, but this should be tested before staining a large batch of slides). Overstained sections can easily be differentiated by agitating for a few seconds in acid–alcohol (Solution C), then washing thoroughly in tap water.

(3) Wash in running tap water for 2 or 3 min or until the sections turn blue. If the tap water is not sufficiently alkaline to blue the sections, add a few drops *either* of ammonium hydroxide (SG 0.9) *or* of saturated aqueous lithium carbonate, *or* a small pinch of calcium hydroxide to about 500 ml of water and leave the washed sections in this for 30–60 s, then rinse in tap water again. Examine the wet slide under a microscope to check that selective nuclear staining has been achieved. Any blue coloration of cytoplasm and connective tissue should be extremely faint. (See also *Note 3* below.)

(4) Immerse the slides in eosin (Solution B) for 30 s with agitation. (See also *Note 4* below.)

(5) Wash (and differentiate) in running tap water for about 30 s. (See *Note 1* below.)

(6) Dehydrate in 70%, 95%, and two changes of absolute ethanol (with agitation, about 30 s in each change; without agitation, 2–3 min in each change). (See also *Note 2* below.)

(7) Clear in xylene and cover, using a resinous medium.

Result

Nuclear chromatin blue to purple; cytoplasm, collagen, keratin, erythrocytes pink.

Notes

(1) The ideal balance between the two components of the H and E stain is a matter of personal taste and is determined by the intensity of coloration due to the eosin. For a weaker counterstain, use 0.2% eosin or prolong the differentiation (stage 5). Differentiation also occurs in the 70% alcohol used for dehydration and, to a lesser extent, in the higher alcohols. A yellow to orange cast can be discerned in some objects stained by eosin Y. This is most easily seen in erythrocytes. Staining by eosin should never be so strong that the nuclei are obscured.

   Many workers use a mixture of two xanthene dyes (such as eosin Y and phloxin) to increase the variety of shades of the background colour. Garvey (1991) favours a combination of phloxin with saffron, a yellow dye that can be bought as a food colouring agent.

(2) For nitrocellulose sections, avoid absolute alcohol and complete the dehydration in two changes (each 10 min) of *n*-butanol. Frozen sections usually require shorter times in the dyes and longer times for differentiation, washing, dehydration, and clearing.

(3) Poor nuclear staining may be due to prior excessive exposure of the tissue to acidic reagents (e.g. unneutralized formalin or decalcifying fluids). To restore the chromophilia, Luna (1968) recommends treatment of the hydrated sections with *either* 5% aqueous sodium bicarbonate ($NaHCO_3$) *or* 5% aqueous periodic acid, overnight, followed by a 5-min wash in water before staining.

(4) A satisfactory alternative to eosin is **fast green FCF** (0.5% aqueous), which is differentiated by water more readily than by alcohol. This dye stains acidophilic elements a bluish-green colour. It is valuable if some components of the section have already been stained pink or red with, for example, the periodic acid–Schiff method (Chapter 11).

(5) There are several alternatives to Mayer's haemalum. Baker's 'haematal-16', which contains 16 ions of Al^{3+} for every one molecule of haematein, is a slow, progressive nuclear stain and should be applied to the sections for 10–30 min. Another popular solution is Gill's haematoxylin, which has higher concentrations of ingredients and a 1:8 dye:Al^{3+} ratio (approximately). It usually gives adequate staining in less than 10 min. Ehrlich's haematoxylin, one of the oldest of these mixtures, also has a low dye:Al^{3+} ratio.

Ehrlich's haematoxylin (Ehrlich, 1886)

Water:	100 ml
Alcohol (100%):	100 ml
Glycerol:	100 ml
Glacial acetic acid:	10 ml
Haematoxylin:	2 g
Aluminium potassium sulphate (alum; $AlK(SO_4)_2.12H_2O$):	to excess

The 'excess' of alum means enough to make a saturated solution, with undissolved material in the bottom of the bottle. This is Ehrlich's original formulation. It is often misquoted, with a smaller amount (10 g) of alum. The solution is ready to use in about a month, when it is dark red. Nuclei are stained progressively. The solution can be used repeatedly for several years.

Haematal-16 (Baker, 1962)

Dissolve 0.5 g of haematoxylin in a mixture of water (125 ml) and ethylene glycol (125 ml). Bubble air through the solution for about 4 weeks. Every few days make up again to 250 ml with water to compensate for evaporation. Add to the above solution 250 ml of ethylene glycol followed by 500 ml of an aqueous solution of aluminium sulphate ($Al_2(SO_4)_3.18H_2O$ 8 g; water to 500 ml). The final volume is 1000 ml. When the haematein is made by atmospheric oxidation, as described here, the haematal-16 solution is stable for approximately 2 years.

Gill's haematoxylin (Gill, Frost and Miller, 1974)

Dissolve 2.0 g of haematoxylin in a mixture of ethylene glycol (250 ml) and water (750 ml). With continuous stirring (magnetic stirrer) add 2.0 g of haematoxylin, 200 mg of sodium iodate ($NaIO_3$), 17.6 g of aluminium sulphate ($Al_2(SO_4)_3.18H_2O$) and 20 ml of glacial acetic acid.

6.1.3.3. Weigert's iron–haematoxylin

Stock solutions

These stable solutions can be kept for at least 5 years.

Solution A

Haematoxylin (C.I. 75290):	5 g
95% ethanol:	500 ml

Solution B

Ferric chloride (FeCl$_3$.6H$_2$O):	5.8 g
Water:	495 ml
Concentrated hydrochloric acid:	5 ml

Working solution

Mix equal volumes of A and B. Put A in the staining jar first for more rapid mixing. The mixture should be made just before using, but can be kept for a few days on the bench or for about 2 weeks at 4°C. (See also under van Gieson's method in Chapter 8.)

Procedure

(1) De-wax and hydrate paraffin sections.
(2) Stain in the working solution of Weigert's haematoxylin for 5 min (10 min if the solution is more than a few days old).
(3) Wash in running tap water. Check with a microscope (See *Note* below).
(4) (Optional) Apply other staining procedures, as desired.
(5) Dehydrate, clear and cover, using a resinous mounting medium.

Result

Nuclei black or blue-black (may be dark brown if the working solution has been stored for more than a few days).

Note

This should give selective nuclear staining without the need of differentiating. If overstaining occurs, the sections can be destained by immersion in acid–alcohol (1% v/v concentrated hydrochloric acid in 95% alcohol, as for alum–haematein; see previous method, Section 6.1.3.2), though the process is slow. Overstaining can be prevented on future occasions by using a higher proportion by volume of Solution B in the working mixture. Conversely, if staining is too slow or too weak, even with a freshly mixed working solution, the proportion of Solution A should be increased. Slight grey coloration of the cytoplasm does not usually matter; it disappears when a counterstain is applied.

6.1.3.4. Lillie's modification of Weigert's iron–haematoxylin

This stable solution is prepared as follows:

(1) Make 1% alcoholic haematoxylin by dissolving 1.0 g of haematoxylin in 100 ml of 95% ethanol.
(2) Make the following solution:

Ferric chloride (FeCl$_3$.6H$_2$O):	2.5 g
Ferrous sulphate (FeSO$_4$.7H$_2$O):	4.5 g
Water:	298 ml
Concentrated hydrochloric acid:	2.0 ml

Stir until dissolved. (Filter if necessary, to remove undissolved impurities.)

(3) Add the solution containing the iron salts to the alcoholic haematoxylin solution. The mixture goes black. It can be used immediately, in the same way as the original Weigert's iron–haematoxylin. Lillie's solution is stable for 2–3 months at room temperature.

6.1.3.5. Brazilin

This dye (Chapter 5) is closely related to haematoxylin. Its oxidation product (brazilein) forms with aluminium ions a complex that stains nuclei red. The colour (like that imparted by alum–haematein) is extracted by acids, so alum–brazilein is best applied as a counterstain to follow a method that imparts green or blue colours to other components of the tissue.

A suitable mixture is **Mayer's brazalum**. This is made in exactly the same way as Mayer's haemalum, but substituting brazilin (C.I. 75280) for haematoxylin. It is more stable than Mayer's haemalum, perhaps because brazilin has only one pair of hydroxyl groups in the easily oxidized catechol configuration. The staining time is usually about 5 min, followed by differentiation, if necessary, in acid–alcohol. Nuclei are stained red. Brazalum is an excellent nuclear counterstain to follow alcian blue (Chapter 11) or Perls' Prussian blue method for iron deposits (Chapter 13).

6.1.3.6. Mayer's carmalum

Staining mixture (after Gatenby and Beams, 1950)

Carminic acid (C.I. 75470; not to be confused with carmine):	1.0 g
Aluminium potassium sulphate, $KAl(SO_4)_2.12H_2O$:	10 g
Water:	200 ml

Heat until it boils, then allow to cool to room temperature. Filter. Add 1.0 ml formalin (37–40% HCHO) as an antibacterial preservative. The solution loses most of its potency after 2–3 weeks.

Procedure
(1) Stain hydrated sections for 10–30 min. Overstaining does not occur. See also *Note* below.
(2) Wash in running tap water for about 1 min.
(3) Dehydrate, clear, and cover.

Result
Nuclei crimson. Like alum–brazilein, carmalum is valuable as a counterstain. It gives pleasing appearances following alcian blue (Chapter 11), indigogenic methods for esterases (Chapter 15) or silver methods for nervous tissue (Chapter 18).

Note
Mayer's carmalum is often used for whole specimens such as embryos and small invertebrates. For these, dilute the staining mixture 20 times in 0.5% (v/v) acetic acid, and stain for 24–48 h. See Chapter 4 for information about dehydrating, clearing and covering whole-mounts.

6.1.3.7. Alum–nuclear fast red

Staining solution (after Luna, 1968; Humason, 1979; Presnell and Schreibman, 1997)

Nuclear fast red (Kernechtrot; C.I. 60760):	0.2 g
Aluminium sulphate ($Al_2(SO_4)_3.18H_2O$):	10 g
Water:	200 ml

Heat with stirring until it is nearly boiling, then leave overnight to cool. There is a substantial residue of insoluble material, which must be removed by decanting and filtering. Keeps for about a year; may need to be filtered before each use.

Procedure
(1) Stain hydrated sections for 5–10 min.
(2) Wash in running tap water, about 1 min.
(3) Dehydrate, clear and cover.

Result
Nuclei crimson. Usually there is also pale pink staining of cytoplasm and collagen. If staining is unsatisfactory, the cause may be a mislabelled or otherwise unsatisfactory batch of the dye (see Frank *et al.*, 2007).

6.1.3.8. Iron-eriochrome cyanine R for nuclei or myelin

This method (Kiernan, 1984b) is derived from the methods of Page (1965), Llewellyn (1974,1978), Hogg and Simpson (1975) and Clark (1979a). It has two variants, and can be used *either* for selective nuclear staining (similar to that seen with aluminium–haematein) *or* for staining myelin sheaths of nerve fibres. A related method that stains in two colours is described later in this chapter (Section 6.3.1). The dye is also sold under the names solochrome cyanine R, chromoxane cyanine R, and Mordant blue 3. The iron–dye complex stains everything. Differentiation in acid–alcohol removes colour from everything except nuclear chromatin, and the blue colour develops when the sections are washed in water. Differentiation in alkali or a ferric salt removes colour from everything except myelin and erythrocytes.

Solutions required

A. Staining solution

0.21 M aqueous ferric chloride (5.6% w/v $FeCl_3.6H_2O$):	20.0 ml
Eriochrome cyanine R (C.I. 43820):	1.0 g
Concentrated (95–98% w/w) sulphuric acid:	2.5 ml
Water:	to make 500 ml

The ingredients take 2–5 min to dissolve, with stirring. Filtration should not be necessary. The solution can be kept and used repeatedly for at least 8 years.

B(1). Differentiating solution for nuclei

Ethanol:	500 ml
Water:	500 ml
Concentrated (12 M) hydrochloric acid:	5 ml

Keeps for several months, but use it only once.

B(2). Differentiating solutions for myelin

Any one of the following aqueous solutions may be used. See also *Note* below.

Ferric ammonium sulphate (iron alum, $NH_4Fe(SO_4)_2.12H_2O$):	10% w/v
Ferric chloride ($FeCl_3.6H_2O$):	5.6% w/v
Ferric nitrate ($Fe(NO_3)_3.6H_2O$):	7.3% w/v

The differentiating solution keeps for a few years, but may be used only once. Discard if it is cloudy or if there is a thick layer of pale insoluble material in the bottom of the bottle.

C. Counterstain

After a nuclear stain, use a red anionic dye such as eosin. Van Gieson's picro-fuchsine (Chapter 8) may also be used. After a myelin stain, use a red basic dye (0.5% aqueous neutral red or safranine is suitable) to stain nuclei and Nissl substance.

Procedure

(1)   Stain hydrated sections in Solution A. For nuclear staining 5 min is sufficient. For myelin staining 15–20 min are needed. (For either method the slides may remain in the dye solution for 30 min without harm.)

(2)   Wash in running tap water, 30 s, or in 3 changes of distilled water. This is to remove unbound dye.

(3a)   **Differentiation for nuclear staining.** Immerse in Solution B(1) with continuous agitation for 10 s, wash in running tap water for about 30 s and examine with a microscope to check that only the nuclei are stained. If other structures are also stained, put the slides back into Solution B(1) for another

10 s, and check again. (Differentiation usually takes 10–30 s.) If too much colour is extracted, go back to Step 1 and use a shorter differentiation next time.

(3b) **Differentiation for myelin staining.** Immerse in Solution B(2) until only the myelin (white matter of CNS) retains the stain. This usually takes 5–10 min. It is sometimes impossible to decolorize the nuclei completely without losing some intensity in myelin.

(4) Wash in tap water (running, or three or four changes) for about 5 min.

(5) Apply a counterstain, as desired.

(6) Dehydrate, clear, and cover using a resinous mounting medium.

Results

Nuclear stain: Nuclei blue. The colour is more resistant to aqueous acids than that of alum–haematein, allowing the use of a greater variety of counterstains.

Myelin stain: Myelin blue. Erythrocytes are also blue.

Note

Clark (1979b) recommended an alkaline differentiating solution for myelin staining: a freshly prepared 1% (v/v) dilution of ammonium hydroxide. This acts in a few seconds, and it is easy to remove too much of the blue dye–metal complex. The mechanisms of differentiation by Fe(III) or alkali have been discussed by Kiernan (1984b, 2007b).

6.1.3.9. Gallocyanine chrome alum

Gallocyanine chrome alum is a blue cationic complex of chromium(III) with an oxazine dye (Chapter 5). It is a useful stain for nucleic acids that resists extraction by alcohols or acidic counterstains to a greater extent than simpler cationic dyes. Specimens may be fixed in any mixture that preserves DNA and RNA. The method is used mainly on paraffin sections, but frozen sections of formalin-fixed material may also be used.

Preparation of staining solution

Gallocyanine (C.I. 51030):	300 mg
Chrome alum (chromium potassium sulphate):	10 g
Water:	200 ml

Boil in a conical flask for 20 min and leave until cool. Filter, and then make up the volume of the filtrate to 200 ml by pouring water through the precipitate in the filter paper. The staining properties of this solution begin to weaken after a week.

Procedure

(1) De-wax and hydrate paraffin sections.

(2) Stain either for 2 h at 50–60°C (coplin jar in oven), or for 24 h at room temperature.

(3) Wash in tap water, and counterstain (e.g. with eosin) if desired.

(4) Dehydrate, clear, and mount in a resinous medium.

Result

Nissl substance of neurons and nuclear chromatin (including nucleoli) blue. Deposits of ribosomal RNA in the cytoplasm of cells other than neurons are also blue. Proteoglycans (mast cells, cartilage matrix) and some types of mucus containing acidic carbohydrates, such as intestinal goblet cells, are also stained.

6.2. Anionic counterstains

In most of the general 'oversight' methods used in histology a blue, purple, or black nuclear stain is followed by a paler, usually pink, counterstain, which colours all the other components of the tissue. **Eosin Y** is suitable for this purpose. It is an anionic dye, so it is bound principally by ionized cationic groups of protein molecules. The most numerous of these are the β-amino group of the side-chain of lysine and the guanidino group of arginine. Nearly all proteins contain these two amino acids, so eosin and other anionic dyes are bound by almost all the structures present in any tissue. A few objects are, however, missed by anionic counterstains. Thus, the extra-cellular matrix surrounding the collagen fibres of connective tissue is composed largely of proteoglycans (Chapter 11), which have negatively charged molecules and therefore cannot bind anionic dyes. The same is true of many glycoprotein secretory products and of the matrix of cartilage. Glycogen, a neutral polysaccha-ride, is unable to bind anionic or cationic dyes. The granules of mast cells contain a basic protein, but this is already neutralized by heparin, a strongly acid proteogly-can also present in the granules. These are therefore stained by cationic dyes but not by dye–metal combinations such as haemalum or by the usual anionic coun-terstains. Usually it is not possible to see very fine fibres (e.g. reticulin, nerve fibres) or cytoplasmic organelles in sections coloured by a single anionic counterstain. Although these delicate structures bind the dye, the degree of contrast is insuffi-cient to permit their resolution in sections more than 0.5–1.0 µm thick.

Anionic dyes other than eosin may also be used as counterstains, but those with strong tinctorial power (e.g. methyl blue, acid fuchsine) are usually avoided because they might obscure the primary staining of the nuclei. When a red nuclear stain has been used, **metanil yellow** (Quintero-Hunter *et al.*, 1991) or **fast green FCF** is suitable.

The composition of a solution of an anionic counterstain is not critical. The follow-ing usually work well if applied for about 1 min. The lowest indicated concentration is sufficient for most specimens, but stronger solutions may be needed for very thin sections, for osmicated material, or for specimens that have spent months in formaldehyde.

Eosin Y (C.I. 45380):
0.1–0.5% in 0.05–0.1% acetic acid. (Stable for several months.)

Fast green FCF (C.I. 42053):
0.1–0.2% in 0.5–1.0% acetic acid. (Stable for at least 5 years.)

Metanil yellow (C.I. 13065):
0.25–0.5% in 0.25–0.5% acetic acid. (Darkens, with deterioration of staining power, after 3 weeks.)

For a longer list of suitable counterstains, see Presnell and Schreibman (1997).

If the maximum amount of anionic dye is to be retained in the tissue, the wash after staining should be in 0.5% acetic acid, not water. There is usually some loss of dye into 70% ethanol. This may be desirable, but for maximum retention of colour, blot the slides after washing, and take directly to the first of 3 changes of absolute alcohol.

6.3. Single solution methods

It has already been pointed out that a cationic dye applied from a solution whose pH is higher than about 5 will stain nearly all the components of a tissue. Neutral or alkaline solutions of cationic dyes can therefore be used as single reagents for general purpose oversight staining. The contrast is less than when two dyes are used, but the speed and simplicity of a one-step method are sometimes advanta-geous. Although most anionic dyes are of no value when used alone, **chlorazol**

black E is exceptional, for reasons that are obscure. The blackness of this dye and its content of coloured impurities (Chapter 5) may be more important than its physical and chemical properties in producing optical contrast in stained sections.

A moderate amount of detail can be seen, in addition to the nuclei, in a section slightly overstained by alum–haematein, alum–brazilein, or alum–carminic acid, but these dye–metal complexes are hardly ever used alone in this way. **Heidenhain's iron–haematoxylin** (Section 6.1.3.1) requires critical differentiation but is capable of revealing considerable cytoplasmic detail.

Eriochrome cyanine R used with an excess of a ferric salt has already been mentioned as a blue nuclear stain. If the ratio of iron to dye in the solution is low, nuclei are stained blue and cytoplasm and collagen are red (see below). Both colours are attributed to dye-iron complexes, because the metal-free dye imparts a different shade of red and its colour, unlike that from the mixture, is easily washed out of the sections by alkali. Experimental evidence indicates that the iron complexes of eriochrome cyanine R are bound to tissues by the dye moiety, without the interposition of iron atoms (Kiernan, 1984b).

Mann's eosin–methyl blue is a mixture of anionic dyes used as a one-step oversight stain. Its possible mechanism of action has already been described. Mann's mixture is also used in pathology for the detection of viral inclusion bodies in diseased cells.

The **azure–eosin** technique is a valuable one-step staining method in which an anionic and cationic dye are applied simultaneously from a single solution at a carefully controlled pH. Results are similar to those obtained using the same dyes in sequence, but a greater variety of shades of colour is seen when the single solution is employed. This technique was developed from those used for staining blood. The properties of mixtures containing eosin and cationic thiazine dyes will be discussed in Chapter 7. The only disadvantage of the azure–eosin technique is the instability of the staining mixture. Brief instructions are given here, and a full account of the method and the results obtained with it is given by Lillie and Fullmer (1976).

6.3.1.
Two colours with eriochrome cyanine R

This technique (Kiernan, 1984b) is a modification of the original method of Hyman and Poulding (1961) and of Chapman's (1977) variant.

Staining solution

0.21 M aqueous ferric chloride (5.6% w/v $FeCl_3.6H_2O$):	2.5 ml
Eriochrome cyanine R (C.I. 43820):	1.0 g
Concentrated (95–98% w/w) sulphuric acid:	2.5 ml
Water:	to make 500 ml

The ingredients take 2–5 min to dissolve, with stirring. Filtration should not be necessary. *The pH must be 1.5*, or the correct colours will not be obtained. The solution can be kept and used repeatedly for at least 6 years, but the pH may change with storage, especially in the first few weeks after making the solution. It should be checked from time to time, and adjusted as necessary by adding a few drops of 1.0 M hydrochloric or sulphuric acid, or 1.0 M sodium hydroxide.

Procedure
(1) Slides bearing hydrated sections are stained for 3 min in the above solution.
(2) The stained slides are washed in 3 changes of water (must be distilled), each 20s, with agitation.
(3) Dehydrate in 95% and 2 changes of absolute alcohol.
(4) Clear in xylene or toluene, and cover, using a resinous medium.

Result

Nuclei blue-purple; cytoplasm pink to red; collagen mostly pink, but some fine fibres in loose connective tissue purple; myelin sheaths of nerve fibres blue-purple; red blood cells orange-red.

6.3.2.
Azure–eosin
method (Lillie's
technique)

Staining solution

This is made from stock solutions, which all keep for several months.

Azure A (C.I. 52005) (0.1% aqueous stock solution):	16 ml
Eosin B (C.I. 45400) (0.1% aqueous stock solution):	16 ml
0.2 M acetic acid:	6.8 ml
0.2 M sodium acetate:	1.2 ml
Acetone:	20 ml
Water:	100 ml

This working solution should be mixed immediately before using. The quantity above suffices for one batch of 10 slides in a 100ml or 125ml staining vessel. Its pH is 4.0, which is usually optimum for formaldehyde-fixed tissues. (See also *Note 2*, below.)

Procedure

(1) De-wax and hydrate paraffin sections.
(2) Stain in the working solution for 1 h.
(3) Pour off the staining solution and replace it with acetone, three changes, each 45–60s, with agitation. (See also *Note 1*, below.)
(4) Clear in two changes of xylene.
(5) Apply coverslips, using a synthetic resinous mounting medium.

Result

Nuclei and cytoplasmic RNA blue. Cartilage matrix and other metachromatic materials red to purple. Muscle cells pink. Cytoplasm of other cells pale blue to pink according to type. Collagen and erythrocytes pink. (See *Notes 2* and *3* below.)

Notes

(1) As an alternative to dehydration in acetone, the sections may be blotted dry and passed through two changes of *n*-butanol, each 3–5 min with occasional agitation.
(2) If satisfactory results are not obtained, the pH of the staining solution should be changed. The acetic acid and sodium acetate may be replaced by 8 ml of 0.2 M acetate buffer (Chapter 20) of any pH from 3.5–5.5. Phosphate and other buffers may be used outside this range. Before applying this method to large numbers of slides, test it from pH 3.5–5.5 at intervals of 0.5 pH unit. Staining solutions buffered beyond this range are unlikely to be needed. Solutions of pH > 4.0 are often needed after fixation in agents other than formaldehyde.
(3) A full account of this technique, with descriptions of the tinctorial effects in normal and pathological tissues, is given by Lillie and Fullmer (1976).
(4) Similar results can be obtained with Giemsa's stain, which is described in Chapter 7.

6.4. Miscellaneous two-colour methods

This section contains methods in which two dyes are used for a variety of purposes.

6.4.1.
Safranine and
fast green FCF

Combinations of safranine (a red cationic dye) and light green (an anionic dye) are popular for staining plant tissues. The preparations will not fade with time if light green is replaced with the closely similar dye fast green FCF. The following method is taken from Berlyn and Miksche (1976). It is applicable to paraffin sections of specimens fixed in an alcohol–formaldehyde–acetic acid mixture or other general purpose fixative.

Solutions required
Aqueous safranine

Safranine O (C.I. 50240):	2 g
Water:	195 ml
Methanol:	5 ml

This solution is stable for at least 2 years, and may be reused many times. Filter if necessary before using. (The methanol is added to discourage growth of micro-organisms.)

Alcoholic fast green FCF

Fast green FCF (C.I. 42053):	1 g
95% ethanol:	200 ml

This solution is stable for at least 5 years and may be reused many times. Old solutions may need to be filtered.

Procedure
This technique includes a critical differentiation, so it is advisable to handle the slides individually through Steps 4–7.

(1) De-wax and hydrate paraffin sections.
(2) Immerse slides in aqueous safranine for 1 h (or longer if necessary or convenient). There should be considerable overstaining).
(3) Wash in running tap water until no more red dye comes out of the sections, then rinse in distilled water.
(4) Pass slide through 30%, 50%, 70% and 95% alcohol, about 30 s with agitation in each. Some safranine is extracted into these alcohols.
(5) Stain in alcoholic fast green FCF for 5–10 s.
(6) Rinse in 100% alcohol and check under a microscope. The red colour should be seen only in cuticle, lignified cell walls, nuclei and some plastids. If it is necessary to remove more safranine, repeat Step 5. The time in the fast green solution may need to be as long as 2 min. If too much safranine has been removed, wash the slide in running tap water until no more green remains in the sections, and return to Step 2.
(7) Dehydrate in three changes of 100% alcohol, 20–30 s, with agitation, in each.
(8) Clear in two changes of xylene and cover, using a resinous mounting medium.

Result
Lignified cell walls, cuticle and the nuclei of cells are red. Cellulose cell walls are green. Plastids (including chloroplasts) may be red or green. In animal tissues nuclei, cartilage matrix and some cytoplasms are red; collagen and the cytoplasm of most cells are green.

Note
Safranine and light green (or fast green FCF) are not often used together for animal tissues, but they can be valuable for revealing intracellular detail in specimens that have been fixed in mixtures containing osmium tetroxide. The reagents and procedure (Benda's method) are different from the technique described here (see Gabe, 1976 for discussion and technical details). Benda's method works on semi-thin (0.5–1.0 μm) sections of glutaraldehyde-fixed and postosmicated tissue that

has been embedded in epoxy resin. The colours are pale, however, and the preparations are less informative than sections that have been strongly stained with a single basic dye.

6.4.2.
Twort's method

Twort's stain was originally made by mixing saturated aqueous solutions of neutral red and light green, collecting the resulting precipitate, dissolving it in 80% alcohol to make a stock solution, and diluting this before use with an equal volume of water. A modification by Ollett (1951) is easier to make, and light green is replaced by fast green FCF, which is less prone to fading. The working solution contains red cations and green anions, which impart their colours simultaneously to different components of the tissue. Usually neutral red's contribution to the staining is too strong, so it is differentiated in acidified alcohol.

This method was originally devised as a counterstain for Gram-positive bacteria that had been selectively stained with crystal violet. The nucleic acids in Gram-negative bacteria and in nuclei of eukaryotic cells take up the neutral red cations, and most of the background of cytoplasm and collagen is green. (The Gram stain for bacteria is discussed in Section 6.4.4.)

Solutions required
Ollett's modified Twort stain
Stock solution

Neutral red (C.I. 50040):	0.36 g
Dissolve in 180 ml of 95% alcohol.	
Fast green FCF (C.I. 42053):	0.04 g
Dissolve in 20 ml of 95% alcohol.	

Mix these two solutions and store in a screw-capped bottle. It is stable for at least a year.

Working solution
To one volume of stock solution, add three volumes of either distilled water or 0.2 M acetate buffer, pH 4.9. This mixture is used only on the day it is made.

2% acetic acid–alcohol

Absolute ethanol:	200 ml
Glacial acetic acid:	4 ml

Usually this is made up as needed, but it can be stored for several weeks without deterioration. It is used only once.

Procedure.
(1) De-wax and hydrate paraffin sections. Remove mercury deposits if necessary.
(2) Immerse in the working solution of Twort's stain for 5–10 min.
(3) Wash quickly in distilled water.
(4) Immerse slides in 2% acetic acid–alcohol for about 15 s, with agitation.
(5) Complete the dehydration in two changes of 100% alcohol.
(6) Clear in two changes of xylene and examine. If there is too much red in the sections, repeat Step 4.
(7) Apply coverslips, using a resinous mounting medium.

Result
Nuclei, mast cell granules and sites of high RNA concentration are red. Cytoplasm and collagen are green. Purple colours are seen in some sites, such as the matrix of cartilage and bone, that take up both dyes. The staining is influenced by the fixative and the thickness of the sections. Do not expect too much of a procedure that allows little visual control of the staining achieved by simultaneously applied dye ions.

Note

In a variant of this method (Monroe and Frommer, 1967) the sections are placed in 1% phosphotungstic acid (PTA) for 2–3 min and rinsed in water before staining, and the acetic acid–alcohol at Step 4 is replaced by 2–3 min in 70% alcohol. The PTA treatment introduces large negatively charged ions into collagen and most cytoplasms, so that these, like nuclei, are stained in shades of red and pink, whereas striated muscle, erythrocytes and keratin are green. (Staining methods making use of PTA and anionic dyes are called trichrome methods; the commonly used ones are described in Chapter 8.)

6.4.3.
Lendrum's phloxin-tartrazine method

Phloxin is similar to eosin (Chapter 5), so it stains everything, but in a brighter shade of red than eosin Y. Lendrum (1947) showed that a yellow anionic dye, tartrazine, when applied from a solution in cellosolve, displaced phloxin in an orderly way, first from collagen, then from muscle, then from erythrocytes, and finally from elastin, Paneth cell and eosinophil granules, spermatozoa, and various pathological intracellular inclusions. Tartrazine itself is removed quickly by water but is almost insoluble in absolute alcohol, so it is possible to impart any desired intensity of yellow background to structures that do not contain phloxin (See also *Note 1* below). Although collagen can be selectively stained yellow, the purpose of this technique is to display cellular components of the tissue in the strong red colour of phloxin; it is widely used to demonstrate intracellular inclusions. Staining methods that display collagen fibres in brighter and darker colours are discussed in Chapter 8.

Tissues to be stained by the phloxin-tartrazine method may be fixed in acidified alcohol, formaldehyde, or (preferably) in a mixture containing mercuric chloride. The Lendrum method is valuable for emphatic staining of basic proteinaceous material in cells and connective tissue.

Solutions required
Aqueous phloxin

Phloxin B (C.I. 45410):	1 g
Calcium chloride ($CaCl_2$):	1 g
Water:	200 ml

Keeps for one year. Lendrum found that calcium chloride increased both the strength of staining and the shelf life.

Tartrazine in cellosolve

Tartrazine (C.I. 19140):	Approx. 4 g
Cellosolve (2-ethoxyethanol, or ethylene glycol monoethyl ether):	200 ml

This should be a saturated solution, with some undissolved dye in the bottom of the bottle. It is stable for several years, but becomes increasingly contaminated with phloxin when used repeatedly in the present technique.

Procedure
(1) De-wax and hydrate paraffin sections.
(2) (Optional) Stain the nuclei selectively with an alum–haematoxylin or a suitable iron–haematoxylin.
(3) Wash in running tap water for 5 min.
(4) Immerse in aqueous phloxin solution for 30 min.
(5) Rinse with water.
(6) Treat with tartrazine in cellosolve, either in a staining jar or with the slide on a horizontal rack. At 10 min intervals, wash in water and examine with a microscope. Continue the treatment with tartrazine in cellosolve until the desired appearance is obtained. The speed of differentiation varies with the

material. Typically it takes 20–30 min to decolorize the collagen, 30–40 min for muscle and 40–50 min for erythrocytes. The most resistant structures may remain red or pink for several hours.

(7) When the desired staining by phloxin remains in the section, immerse the slide in tartrazine again for about 10 s to stain the background yellow. (See *Note 2* below.)

(8) Rinse in 70% alcohol, which will slowly extract some tartrazine and make the yellow background paler.

(9) Complete the dehydration in 3 changes of 100% alcohol, clear in xylene and apply a coverslip, using a resinous mounting medium.

Result

Nuclei (if stained) blue or black. Phloxinophilic structures red and pink, according to the duration of Step 6. Collagen and other destained materials yellow.

Notes

(1) Clark (1979b) preferred a 1% aqueous solution of rose Bengal (C.I. 45440) to phloxin, and used a 0.05% solution of Bismarck brown Y (C.I. 21000) in cellosolve instead of tartrazine, because it was able to displace the red dye without staining the decolourized parts of the tissue. He suggested that the displacing dye formed hydrogen bonds with phloxin or rose Bengal, extracting the red dye preferentially from the sites to which it was most weakly bound. Non-ionic, non-covalent bonds are certainly involved in the attachment of dyes to one another and to substrates. Hydrogen bonding is unlikely, however, when the competition for dye binding occurs in an aqueous solution (Chapter 5).

(2) If a yellow background is not wanted, replace Step 7 with a thorough wash in water to remove all the residual tartrazine.

6.4.4.
The Gram stain for bacteria

A simple staining method provides the basis for classification of bacteria into two groups. The technique, which involves trapping of an insoluble derivative of a dye, was introduced in 1884 by Christian Gram. The procedure has three steps:

(1) Staining with crystal violet (Chapter 5) or a related cationic triphenylmethane dye. This imparts colour to everything.

(2) Treatment with an aqueous solution of iodine and potassium iodide. This reagent contains triiodide ions (I_3^-), which form a water-insoluble complex with the dye:

$$[\text{crystal violet}]^+ \; + \; I_3^- \; \longrightarrow \; [\text{crystal violet}]\!\!-\!\!I_3$$

Any dye that gives a precipitate with I_3^- may be used instead of crystal violet. Such dyes are all cationic triarylmethanes. Dye precipitants other than I_3^- may be used if they yield products that are insoluble in water and slowly soluble in organic solvents. For example, picric acid is suitable; potassium permanganate is not, because the crystal violet–permanganate complex is insoluble in alcohol.

(3) Extraction of the dye–iodine complex with an organic solvent such as ethanol, acetone or aniline. The solvent extracts dye from some types of bacteria (Gram-negative) but leaves other types (Gram-positive) fully stained unless the extraction is greatly prolonged. A second dye of contrasting colour is then applied, to stain the Gram-negative bacteria. Gram used Bismarck brown; nowadays safranine, a red cationic dye, is preferred.

Nucleic acids are stainable by cationic dyes, but the crystal violet of the Gram stain has no histochemical specificity for these substances and has been shown to bind also to phospholipids, lipoproteins, proteins and several carbohydrate-containing components of the bacterial cell (see Popescu and Doyle, 1996). In sections of animal tissue stained in the same way, nuclear chromatin, collagen fibres, various intracellular granules, keratin and fibrin are Gram-positive, but they are less resistant to destaining than are Gram-positive bacteria (see Pearse, 1972). It is generally agreed that some special property of the cell walls of Gram-positive bacteria retards extraction of the dye-triiodide complex by organic solvents (see Horobin, 1982; Murray *et al.*, 1994).

Using an electron-opaque organic platinum complex in place of Gram's iodine, Beveridge and Davies (1983) examined the deposition and extraction of precipitated crystal violet by electron microscopy. They determined that the outer (peptidoglycan) layer of the bacterial cell membrane retarded the extraction of the dye complex. In Gram-negative bacteria this layer is thinner than in Gram-positive bacteria, and it is also damaged by the solvent used in the third stage of the staining procedure. The damage increases the permeability of the outer part of the membrane, facilitating extraction of the dye complex. Fungal hyphae and spores, which are Gram-positive, also have thick peptidoglycan-containing outer membranes (see Popescu and Doyle, 1996). Some bacteria (*Archaea*, which are recognized as a distinct kingdom on the basis of DNA composition) have outer membranes so thick and dense that they prevent the entry of crystal violet. These organisms are Gram-negative because they contain no dye for the organic solvent to extract (Beveridge and Schultze-Lam, 1996).

Procedure
This is the procedure recommended by Bartholomew (1962; see also Clark, 1973 and Sanderson, 1994).

Solutions required
A. Hucker's crystal violet
Crystal violet (C.I. 42555):	4.0 g
95% ethanol:	40 ml
Ammonium oxalate [$(NH_4)_2C_2O_4.H_2O$]:	1.6 g
Water:	160 ml

Dissolve the dye in the alcohol and the ammonium oxalate in the water, then mix the two solutions. Stable for 2 years.

B. Gram's iodine
Water:	200 ml
Potassium iodide (KI):	4 g
Iodine:	2 g

The iodine takes several hours to dissolve; the process can be accelerated by grinding the I_2 and the KI together in a mortar before adding the water. This solution can be kept for many years, in a glass-stoppered bottle. It is also called Burke's iodine and often misnamed Lugol's iodine, which, according to Gray (1954) is 6% iodine in 4% aqueous potassium iodide.

C. Extracting solvent
Either 95% ethanol *or* 95% isopropanol (Add 5 ml water to 95 ml of isopropyl alcohol). Isopropanol acts somewhat more slowly than ethanol.

D. Counterstain
Either 0.25% **safranine O** (C.I. 50240) in 9.5% ethanol.(Dissolve the dye in 95% ethanol, then add 9 volumes of water.)
Or 1% **neutral red** (C.I. 50040) in water.

Both solutions can be kept for about 2 years. See also the *Notes* at the end of this method.

Procedure

Smears may be fixed by heating the slide over a flame or by immersion in alcohol. Sections are assumed to be dewaxed and hydrated sections of formaldehyde-fixed specimens. Staining is carried out by dropping the reagents onto horizontal slides, supported on a rack over a sink.

(1) Flood slide with Hucker's crystal violet (Solution A) for 1 min.
(2) Rinse briefly (2 or 3 s) in running tap water, to remove most of the excess dye.
(3) Flood slide with Gram's iodine (Solution B), pour it off immediately, replace with new Gram's iodine and wait for 1 min.
(4) Wash with water until all the iodine (brown) is removed. Shake off excess water.
(5) Pour the extracting solvent (C) slowly onto the slide, letting it run over the edges, for about 30 s, until the release of dye into the solvent has largely stopped. This step is critical and the time may need to be varied. Too much extraction removes crystal violet from the Gram-positive organisms; too little will fail to remove the dye from Gram-negative bacteria.
(6) Wash quickly in a large volume of tap water. (This stops the de-staining.)
(7) Flood with the counterstain (Solution D, or see *Note 1* below) for 1 min.
(8) Rinse the slides in tap water, blot with wet filter paper, and allow the smears or sections to dry by evaporation.
(9) Smears are usually examined without coverslips. An oil immersion objective is used.
(10) For sections (or for permanent preparations of smears) immerse the dry slides in xylene for about 3 min and then apply coverslips, using a resinous mounting medium.

Result

Gram-positive bacteria and fungi, dark blue-violet. Gram-negative bacteria, red. See also *Note 2* below. In sections, the result can be varied with the duration of exposure to 95% alcohol or isopropanol at Stage 5. Nuclei of cells should be red. If they are blue or purple, the extraction at Stage 5 was inadequate. In a correctly differentiated section some crystal violet is likely to be retained in keratin and fibrin, but their blue colour should be much lighter than that of Gram-positive organisms. Collagen fibres and cytoplasm are usually pink from over-staining by the counterstain (Stage 7). The counterstain can be weakened by a longer wash at Stage 8.

Notes

(1) For bacteria in sections of tissue, the counterstain at step 5 can be replaced with Ollett's variant of Twort's method (Section 6.4.2). Gram-negative bacteria and cell nuclei will then be red, and collagen and most cytoplasm green.
(2) A control slide bearing smears or sections containing known Gram-positive and Gram-negative organisms should be stained alongside the specimen under investigation.

6.4.5.
Luxol fast blue and cresyl violet

As explained in Chapter 5 (Section 5.9.14), the 'luxol' dyes are arylguanidinium salts of anionic chromogens. They are insoluble in water and are used as solutions in alcohol or other moderately polar organic liquids. Phospholipids are stained by these dyes, though probably not very specifically (Salthouse, 1963; Lycette *et al.*, 1970). Luxol dyes probably also enter hydrophobic domains of protein molecules (Clasen *et al.*, 1973; Kiernan, 2007b). It has been shown that the arylguanidinium cation is liberated into the solvent during the process of attachment of the dye to its substrate, leaving the coloured anion behind. The staining is then differentiated and made specific for myelin by treatment with dilute aqueous lithium carbonate, followed by 70% ethanol. The mechanism of differentiation is in need of investigation. A red or violet cationic dye subsequently applied as a counterstain binds not only to the nuclei and Nissl substance but also to the luxol fast blue anions present in the myelin sheaths, thereby increasing the intensity of coloration of the latter (Clasen *et al.*, 1973).

Luxol fast blues MBS, G, and ARN, and methasol fast blue 2G are some of the dyes that can be used to stain myelin in the manner described above. The first such technique was that of Kluver and Barrera (1953), which is still widely used. A somewhat simpler version is described below. Luxol fast blue is easy to use but slow in its action. It does not give such a strong colour to the myelin, especially in the peripheral nervous system, as iron-eriochrome cyanine R (Section 6.1.3.8). The latter is therefore preferred for the demonstration of myelinated axons of narrow calibre. Fixation is not critical; aqueous formaldehyde-containing mixtures are usually used, followed by preparation of paraffin sections. Somewhat stronger coloration is seen in frozen sections, especially with formal–calcium fixation, possibly because of greater retention of phospholipid.

Solutions required
A. Staining solution

Luxol fast blue MBS (C.I. 74180):	0.25 g
95% ethanol:	250 ml

Many workers add glacial acetic acid (2.5 ml) but this does not appear to confer any advantage. The solution keeps for at least 5 years and may be used repeatedly.

B. Differentiating solution (0.05% Li$_2$CO$_3$)

Lithium carbonate (Li$_2$CO$_3$):	0.25 g
Water:	500 ml

This keeps indefinitely and can be used repeatedly, but the solution should be discarded when it is more than faintly blue from extracted dye.

C. Counterstain

Cresyl violet acetate:	0.1 g
Water:	100 ml
Oxalic acid:	5 mg
(0.5 ml of 1% aqueous H$_2$C$_2$O$_4$.2H$_2$O)	

Dyes labelled 'cresyl fast violet' or 'cresyl echt violet' may be suitable, but cresyl violet acetate certified by the Biological Stain Commission should be used if possible. Filter the solution before using. The solution can be kept for a few months, but should be replaced if its colour has faded or if it contains a deposit of dark, insoluble material. See also *Note 2* below.

Procedure
(1) De-wax paraffin sections and take to absolute ethanol. Frozen sections should be dried onto slides (from water) and then equilibrated with absolute ethanol.
(2) Stain in Solution A in a screw-capped staining jar at 55–60°C (in an oven or water bath) for 16–24 h (overnight).
(3) Rinse in 70% ethanol and then in water.
(4) Immerse in the differentiating solution (B) until grey and white matter can be distinguished. This commonly takes 2–30 s for thin paraffin sections, but thick frozen sections may require up to 30 min. Move to Step 5 early rather than late, to avoid extracting too much blue dye.

(5) Transfer slides to 70% ethanol, two changes, each 1 min. More dye leaves the sections at this stage.

(6) Rinse in water. Check with a hand-lens or low power microscope. Grey matter should be largely unstained; white matter should be a greenish shade of blue. Carefully repeat Steps 4 and 5 if there is still blue colour in neuronal cell bodies in grey matter.

(7) Counterstain for 5 min in cresyl violet (Solution C).

(8) Wash in water and blot dry.

(9) If necessary, differentiate the counterstain in 70% ethanol until only the nuclei and Nissl substance are purple. There should be no 'background' colour in the neuropil between neuronal cell bodies in grey matter. The colour of the stained myelin is deepened by counterstaining.

(10) Blot dry and dehydrate in three changes of 100% ethanol (each 30 s with agitation) or n-butanol (each 3–5 min, without agitation). (Use n-butanol if you find that ethanol extracts too much cresyl violet.)

(11) Clear in xylene and cover, using a resinous medium.

Result

Myelin blue; nuclei and Nissl substance purple.

Notes

(1) Some batches of luxol fast blue do not work very well. For other techniques, see Cook (1974). Churukian (2000) describes a variant in which the staining is accelerated by heating in a microwave oven.

(2) Neutral red (Section 6.1.1.2) is an excellent counterstain for luxol fast blue. Another counterstain that is sometimes used is the PAS procedure (Chapter 11), which provides a pink background in the neuropil, without nuclear or other cellular staining.

6.5. Fluorescent staining

Fluorescence microscopy is commonly used for histochemical purposes, such as the localization of specific sequences of nucleotides in DNA or RNA (Chapter 9) and the detection of antigens by means of labelled antibodies (Chapter 19). A typical fluorescence microscope is equipped with filter blocks for the observation of the three types of fluorescent label that are in common use:

(a) Compounds optimally excited by the longer ultraviolet wavelengths (330–385 nm); most of these emit blue or yellow light.

(b) Fluorescein and other compounds optimally excited by blue light (350–460 nm); these emit green or yellow light.

(c) Rhodamine and other compounds optimally excited by green light (530–560 nm). These emit orange or red light.

Ultraviolet filter blocks have barrier (suppression) filters that appear transparent or pale grey to the eye, so the true colour of the emitted fluorescence can be seen. The observed colour of fluorescence evoked by blue or green excitation is modified by the barrier filters, which must subtract all radiation with wavelength near to and shorter than that of the visible exciting light.

The excitation component of a filter block may provide a wide band of the spectrum, as indicated by the wavelength ranges quoted above, or it may provide a narrow band, optimal for a particular fluorescent label within that range. Many fluorescent compounds emit adequately when excited by wavelengths well away from the maxima of their absorption spectra. Consequently there is usually some background autofluorescence (Chapter 1), which may helpfully display the background architecture of the tissue or may hinder the observation of important fluorescent objects. Some of the guesswork can be removed, and the autofluorescence overcome, by counterstaining with a second fluorochrome that emits a colour that contrasts sharply with histochemically significant fluorescent objects in a tissue.

Fluorochromes are used in much the same way as ordinary dyes, but usually from much more dilute solutions. Cationic fluorochromes impart fluorescence to nuclei and other basophilic structures, and anionic fluorochromes bind to nuclei, cytoplasm and collagen. Many dyes that are used as ordinary stains are fluorescent. There are other dyes that suppress (quench) any fluorescence previously present in the stained components of tissues. For example, fluorescence microscopy of an H and E-stained section reveals a green background in which the nuclei stand out as black objects. This is due to eosin being an anionic fluorochrome, whereas alum–haematein quenches fluorescence.

Table 6.1. Properties of some fluorochromes

Name	Wavelength (nm) for excitation) (wide-band excitation filter)	Wavelength (nm) of emission (observed colour varies with barrier filter used)
Cationic fluorochromes		
Acridine orange	460 & 500 (blue)	526 & 650 (green & red)[a]
Acriflavine	480 (UV or blue)	550-600 (yellow, orange)
Auramine O	460 (UV or blue)	550 (yellow)
Berberine sulphate	430 (UV or blue)	550 (yellow)
Chlortetracycline	395 (UV or blue)	520 (green)
Ethidium bromide[a]	520 (UV, blue, green)	605-620 (orange, red)
Hoechst dyes[a]	350-365 (UV)	460-480 (blue)
Neutral red	540 (green or blue)	(orange, yellow)
Propidium iodide[a]	520-535 (UV, blue, green)	610-620 (orange, red)
Basic fuchsine (pararosaniline)[b]	560-570 (blue or green)	625 (brown, red)
Quinacrine	440 (UV or blue)	530 (blue, green)
Rhodamine B	540 (UV, blue or green)	625 (orange, red)
Tetracycline	390 (UV or blue)	560 (green, yellow)
Anionic fluorochromes		
Acid fuchsine	530-540 (blue or green)	630 (brown, red)
Eosin	524 (UV, blue or green)	544 (green)
Erythrosin	530 (UV, blue or green)	555 (green, yellow)
Fluorescein	494 (UV or blue)	518 (green)
Primuline	410 (UV or blue)	550 (yellow)
Thioflavine S	430 (blue)	550 (green, yellow)
Fluorochromes covalently bound to protein[c]		
Cascade blue labels	396-400 (UV)	410-420 (violet, blue)
Coumarin labels	340-390 (UV)	405-455 (blue)
Dansyl labels	340-380 (UV)	475-520 (blue)
Fluorescein labels	490-495 (UV or blue)	515-520 (green, yellow)
Oregon green labels	495-510 (UV or blue)	520-530 (green, yellow)
Rhodamine labels	540-560 (green)	580-600 (orange, red)
Texas red labels	583-595 (green)	603-615 (red)

Data are taken from various sources, notably Pearse (1980), Lillie and Fullmer (1976), Haugland (2002) and trade literature from the Zeiss and Leica/Leitz microscope companies.
[a]These reagents are used in the histochemical study of nucleic acids (see Chapter 9).
[b]The coloured product of the reaction of aldehydes with Schiff's reagent has similar fluorescent properties.
[c]The labelling of antibodies and other proteins is discussed in Chapter 19.

**6.5.1.
Cationic and
anionic
fluorochromes**

Table 6.1 shows the properties of some cationic dyes and other compounds (used for fluorescent staining of nucleic acids, cartilage matrix and other basophilic components of tissues) and also of anionic fluorochromes, which will impart general background fluorescence to any tissue. Instructions for using neutral red as a fluorochrome are given in Section 6.1.1.2.

**6.5.2.
Simple
procedure for
fluorescent
counterstaining**

The method of application of a single fluorochrome is as follows. It is assumed that the sections have first been stained by an immunofluorescent or other histochemical method, and then rinsed in unbuffered saline (0.9% NaCl in water).

(1) A dilute solution of the fluorochrome is prepared, by diluting a stronger (e.g. 0.1% or 1%) stock solution with either distilled water or unbuffered saline. (Saline is generally preferable after immunofluorescent staining.) The amount of dilution varies with the particular fluorochrome and the desired strength of counterstaining. Typically the stock solution will need to be diluted to 100–1000 times the original volume and its colour will be almost imperceptible. The diluted solution is discarded after using.

(2) The preparation is rinsed in two changes of water or unbuffered saline. For immunofluorescence preparations the pH must be above about 4.5, because acidic solutions break the non-ionic attractions that keep antigens and their antibodies together (Chapter 19).

Either

(3a) (*Optimum fluorescence, but not permanent*) A coverslip is applied, using a slightly alkaline aqueous mounting medium such as buffered glycerol. Instructions for making and using some aqueous media suitable for fluorescence microscopy are described in Chapter 4 (Section 4.3.2). Media of this kind provide optimal fluorescence of labelled antibodies; they retain bound cationic fluorochromes but they are not compatible with anionic fluorochromes, which are extracted. The slides are examined and photographed as soon as possible. Slides may be stored in horizontal cardboard trays for several weeks in darkness at 4°C, but eventually the fluorescence will fade. Mounting in a slightly alkaline liquid aqueous medium dates from the early years of immunohistochemistry (Nairn, 1976). With modern antigen retrieval and signal amplification methods (Chapter 19 and **3c** below) it is possible to make permanent preparations.

Or

(3b) (*Good preservation of fluorescence, but no protection for the specimen*) The slides are air-dried and stored in boxes at 4°C. They are examined dry, without coverslips. This method is useful for fluorochromes that are easily extracted by water or other solvents.

Or

(3c) (*Permanent preparation*) Dehydrate in three changes of 100% alcohol (which coagulates antibodies and other proteins), clear in xylene and mount in a non-fluorescent resinous medium such as DPX (Chapter 4, Section 4.3.1.). Use new alcohol, because even slight traces of dyes can alter the fluorescent properties of the sections. Some diminution of fluorescence may occur when permanent preparations are made, but if the original immunofluorescent or other histochemical labelling was bright, the fluorescence remains unchanged for years (Espada *et al.*, 2005).

6.5.3.
Alum–tetracycline: a fluorochrome for nuclei

Tetracycline is a yellow antibiotic that could be classified as a cationic carbonyl dye:

It is strongly fluorescent and is able to form chelates with many metals. The simple procedure described below (Kiernan, 1981) is an alternative, for fluorescence microscopy, to alum–haematein. Similar staining cannot be obtained with tetracycline alone, but the action of aluminium ions in this method has not been studied.

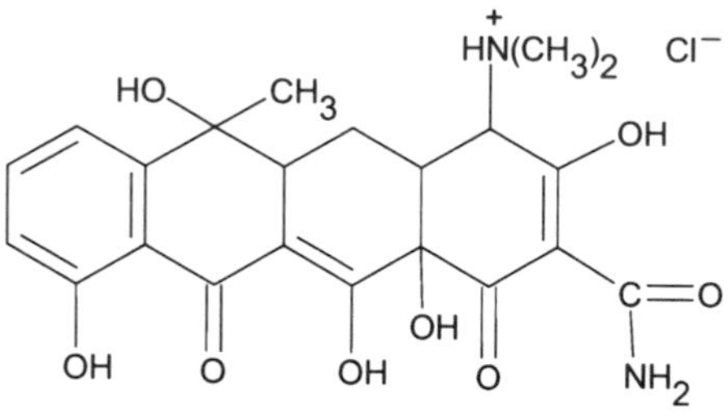

The alum–tetracycline staining solution is acidic and therefore potentially able to break antigen–antibody bonds, so it is not a suitable counterstain for immunofluorescent preparations unless the bound labelled antibody has been permanently insolubilized by treatment with a fixative such as formaldehyde or alcohol.

Fluorescent nuclear staining can also be achieved with an acidified solution of alum and acid alizarin violet N; for this latter combination the staining is due largely to nucleic acids (Grosman and Vardaxis, 1997).

Staining solution

Tetracycline hydrochloride:	0.5 g
Water:	100 ml
Aluminium potassium sulphate ($AlK(SO_4)_2.12.H_2O$):	5.0 g

The solution is stable for about one month, becoming decreasingly efficacious as its colour changes from yellow to orange-brown.

Procedure
(1) Stain hydrated sections for 5 min.
(2) Wash in 3 changes of water.
(3) Dehydrate through graded alcohols, clear in xylene, and mount in a non-fluorescent resinous medium.
(4) Examine by fluorescence microscopy, with excitation by ultraviolet or blue light.

Result
Nuclei emit a yellow to orange fluorescence.

6.5.4.
Fluorescent method for plant cell walls

This procedure (Mori and Bellani, 1996) is partly histochemical. Lignified cell walls contain free aldehyde groups and can therefore be stained with Schiff's reagent (Chapter 10). In addition to being magenta in colour, the product of the Schiff reaction emits brownish red fluorescence when excited by ultraviolet light. The non-lignified cell walls, composed mainly of cellulose, bind (by non-ionic, non-covalent forces) a fluorescent brightening agent (Chapter 5). This emits pale blue to white light. The method was devised for leaves or stems that had been fixed in 50% ethanol, dehydrated and embedded in plastic. Sections, 2 µm thick, are dried down onto glass slides.

Solutions required
A. Schiff's reagent.
This is described in connection with the Feulgen technique in Chapter 9 (Section 9.3.2). Read the instructions and precautions relating to Schiff's reagent before using it for the first time in this technique.

B. Calcofluor white M2R solution.

Calcofluor white M2R (C.I. 40622):	10 mg
Water:	100 ml

Procedure

(1) Immerse slides in Schiff's reagent (Solution A) for 2 h.
(2) Wash in running tap water for 5 min, then rinse in distilled water.
(3) Immerse in Calcofluor white M2R (Solution B) for 2 min.
(4) Rinse in 3 changes of distilled water and air-dry.
(5) Rinse briefly in xylene and apply coverslips, using a non-fluorescent mounting medium.

Result

The preparations are examined with broad-band utraviolet excitation (350–410 nm) and a barrier filter that stops light of wavelength shorter than 460 nm. Lignified cell walls (e.g. xylem) emit brownish red fluorescence. Non-lignified cell walls (e.g. in parenchyma) emit bright pale blue to white fluorescence, and partly lignified walls (e.g. sclerenchyma) emit various shades of pink and purple.

6.5.5.
DAB-induced fluorescence of lipids in frozen sections

3,3'-diaminobenzidine (DAB) is a versatile histochemical reagent, used principally in methods for the localization of oxidases and peroxidases (Chapter 16). Enzyme-catalyzed oxidation converts DAB into an insoluble brown product. Peroxidase is used to label large molecules, including lectins (Chapter 11) and antibodies (Chapter 19). The oxidized product of DAB oxidation contrasts well with blue or green dyes. Counterstaining may not be needed for frozen sections that have been exposed to DAB because this compound reacts with tissue-bound aldehydes formed by atmospheric oxidation of lipids. The product is fluorescent (von Bohlen und Halbach and Kiernan, 1999; see also Chapter 12) and it is prominent in lipid-rich tissues such as white matter in the nervous system. If a fluorescence microscope is available, a display of anatomical features can be seen in any frozen section that has been immersed in a solution containing DAB.

6.6. Vital staining

There are several techniques in which a dye or fluorochrome is administered to a whole living organism or applied to freshly removed tissue or to a culture or suspension of living cells. The word 'vital' implies that the cells remain alive and healthy while stained, but this is not necessarily so (see Baker, 1958; Barbosa and Peters, 1971). Toxic consequences of vital staining do not necessarily detract from the usefulness of a method, but it must be remembered that the intracellular distribution of colour may be caused by a pharmacological or toxic action of the dye. Vital staining may be watched as it proceeds, and with some methods, the preparations can be fixed and made permanent.

Accounts follow of two traditional applications: the demonstration of mitochondria and of nerve fibres.

6.6.1.
Mitochondria with janus green B

Janus green B is a cationic dye that contains both the azo and the azine chromophores (Chapter 5). A neutral solution binds to carbohydrates, nucleic acids and proteins, as would be expected (Section 6.1.1). Within poorly oxygenated tissues or cells, the dye is reduced (Chapter 16) to a colourless leuco compound. Reduction occurs more slowly in mitochondria than in other parts of the cell, because the cytochrome oxidase/cytochrome c system acts as an oxidizing agent, using the residual dissolved oxygen. The mitochondria therefore remain visible for longer than other cytoplasmic domains. Mitochondrial staining is prevented by inhibition of cytochrome oxidase (Lazarow and Cooperstein, 1953). Mitochondria can be stained in blood cells and protozoa (Chapters 5 and 13 in Clark, 1973), and in the presynaptic and postsynaptic parts of neuromuscular junctions (Couteaux and Bourne, 1973; Zacks, 1973). Costello and Henley (1971) recommended highly diluted janus green B for increasing the visibility of the jelly surrounding marine eggs and embryos. Yack (1993) used the dye to assist the dissection and photography of insect nerves and chordotonal organs, and suggested that in this application the staining might not be due to mitochondria.

The technique is simple, and applicable to small fragments of fungi, plants, invertebrates or vertebrate animals, or to any culture or suspension of living cells.

Staining solution

Janus green B (C.I. 11050):	20 mg
Saline or balanced salt solution:	100 ml

Use a sample of dye certified by the Biological Stain Commission; others are likely to be unduly toxic (Lillie, 1977). The saline is one appropriate for the cells or organisms to be examined. Several such solutions are described in Chapter 20. Water (or sea water) is appropriate for whole aquatic organisms. The dye solution can be stored for several months at 4°C. For protozoa, the staining solution may need to be diluted as much as 1000 times.

Procedure

(1a) *Suspended cells.* Mix equal-sized small drops of staining solution or cell suspension on a slide. Apply a coverslip and seal its edges with petroleum jelly (white petrolatum, Vaseline).

(1b) *Cells cultured on a flat surface.* Drain off the culture medium. Put a drop of staining solution on the layer of cultured cells, apply a coverslip, and seal the edges.

(1c) *Tissue fragments.* Tease or spread out the freshly dissected material to make a thin layer on a slide. Add a drop of staining solution, apply a coverslip, and seal the edges as described in 1a, above.

(2) Observe under a microscope. The mitochondria become visible in 10–20 min (2–5 min if a heated stage, 37°C, is available).

Result

Mitochondria appear as green or blue-green dots or threads. An oil- or water-immersion objective is needed to see them clearly. They may remain visible for as long as an hour. When a cell dies, the colour diffuses into the cytoplasm and then enters the nucleus.

6.6.2.
Nerve fibres with methylene blue

Methylene blue is a cationic dye (Chapter 5), but its value in neurohistology depends on properties other than basicity. When living or freshly removed tissue is treated with methylene blue under suitable conditions, axons and their terminal branches are selectively stained. The biochemical mechanisms underlying this coloration are poorly understood despite several studies of the phenomenon (see Schabadasch, 1930; Richardson, 1969; Kiernan, 1974; Muller, 1992). The ability to stain nerve fibres is shared by some other *N*-methylated derivatives of thionine, but methylene blue itself is generally considered to be the best dye for the purpose.

For staining peripheral innervation, the most satisfactory results are obtained by immersing freshly removed tissue in a dilute oxygenated solution of methylene blue buffered to pH 5.0–7.0, for about 30 min at 30°C. It is also possible to inject the dye locally or systemically into the living animal. The deposits of dye are soluble in water and in alcohol, so the stained tissues are fixed in ammonium molybdate, which forms an insoluble salt with methylene blue. The methylene blue-molybdate complex has been shown by electron microscopy to be associated with microtubules and to occur also as free crystals in the axoplasm of vitally stained nerve fibres (Chapman, 1982). Thin specimens are examined as whole mounts, but it is also possible to prepare frozen or paraffin sections of the vitally stained specimens. Ideally, the axons stand out as blue lines on a colourless background, but commonly there is also some staining of non-neuronal elements. Both somatic and autonomic fibres take up vital methylene blue, the former at pH 5.5–7.0, the latter at pH 5.0–5.5. Above pH 7.0, only the coarser, myelinated sensory axons are stained (FitzGerald and Fitter, 1971).

The following method (from Richardson, 1969 and Kiernan, 1974) is for the demonstration of peripheral innervation in freshly removed tissue.

Solutions required
A. Buffered diluent

Sodium succinate (CH2COONa)2.6H2O:	7.0 g
Sodium chloride (NaCl):	3.0 g
Glucose (dextrose):	1.5 g
Water:	800 ml
Concentrated hydrochloric acid:	add carefully until the pH
Water:	is 5.5 to make 1000 ml

Store at 4°C. It keeps for several weeks.

B. Methylene blue stock

Methylene blue (C.I. 52015):	100 mg
Water:	100 ml

It is advisable to use a zinc-free grade of dye designated for vital staining, but the presence of zinc does not prevent axonal staining (Richardson, 1969). This stock solution can be kept at room temperature for at least 5 years.

C. Staining solution

Solution A:	100 ml
Solution B:	1.5 ml

This is usually mixed just before use, but it can be kept for a few weeks at 4°C. Allow it to warm to 37°C before using.

D. Ammonium molybdate fixative
This keeps for only one day. It is made by dissolving ammonium molybdate in a stable buffer.

Buffer, pH 5.5:

Sodium phosphate, dibasic (Na_2HPO_4):	2.0 g
Citric acid ($C_6H_8O_4.H_2O$):	1.2 g
Water:	500 ml

This can be kept for a few weeks at 4°C.

Working fixative solution:

Buffer (above):	50 ml
Ammonium molybdate, $(NH_4)_6Mo_7O_{24}.4H_2O$:	3 g

It takes about 15 min for the ammonium molybdate to dissolve (magnetic stirrer). Make up the fixative while the specimens are incubating in the stain. Cool it to 0–4°C for use.

Procedure
(1) Remove fresh pieces of tissue, no more than 1.0 mm thick. The method can also be used for muscle biopsies. Collect into saline (0.9% NaCl) but do not leave them in it for more than 5 min.

(2) Put the pieces in the warm staining solution with continuous aeration at about 30°C. (These conditions are obtained by bubbling air through the solution and specimens while they are in a flask or beaker standing in a 37°C water bath. The air cools the staining solution to about 30°C). Leave for 30–40 min.

(3) Remove specimens from the staining solution, rinse quickly (5–10 s) in water and place in the working fixative solution (D) for 12–18 h at 0–4°C. (See also *Note 3* below.)

(4) Wash in water (0–4°C) for 10 min.

(5) Transfer to absolute methanol at 4°C for 30 min.

(6) Complete the dehydration in *n*-butanol at 4°C for 30 min.

(7) Clear in benzene, toluene or xylene, 15 min (at room temperature). 8. Prepare as whole mounts in a resinous medium (See also *Notes 2* and *3* below).

Result

Axons blue. The background should be largely unstained. Erythrocytes are sometimes blue.

Notes

(1) If the method fails, try varying the pH between 5 and 7.5. In general, thicker axons are stained at higher pH.

(2) Müller (1989) recommends post-fixation in a buffered formaldehyde-glutaraldehyde mixture after Step 3, followed by dehydration in *t*-butanol and paraffin embedding. The second fixation improves structural preservation.

(3) As an alternative to whole mounts, the specimens may be *either* **(a)** sectioned on a freezing microtome and collected into ice-cold water after Stage 4, and then mounted onto slides, dehydrated in **cold** absolute methanol (2 quick changes), cleared, and covered, *or* **(b)** embedded in wax after Stage 7 and the paraffin sections mounted onto slides, cleared, and covered. Sections should be thick: 50–100 µm.

7 | Staining blood and other cell suspensions

It is frequently desirable to stain cells that have been smeared or otherwise deposited onto a glass slide. The cells may be naturally suspended in liquid, as in the case of blood or an inflammatory exudate, or they may have been artificially suspended by disaggregating a piece of tissue or a colony of cultured cells. Cells may be washed or scraped from an epithelial surface, as they are in the clinical diagnostic practice known as **exfoliative cytology**, or they may be obtained as 'impression smears', by simply pressing the slide against a freshly cut surface of an organ or tumour. The present chapter is concerned with methods whereby whole cells are stained on the slide. Techniques in which cells are stained, sorted and counted while still suspended are outside the scope of this book. Other exduded topics include blood grouping, methods for the immunological study of subpopulations of lymphocytes, and special methods for chromosomes.

Special methods of preparation and staining are used for identifying the types of cells in smears of blood and haemopoietic tissues. The same techniques can reveal abnormal cells and the presence of pathogenic protozoa such as malaria parasites. These methods are also valuable for the examination of cells derived from other fluids (e.g. urine, pleural exudates, cerebrospinal fluid), and in smears of exfoliated cells.

7.1. Preparation of films, smears and sediments

7.1.1.
Preparation of blood films

Films are usually made with freshly drawn whole blood. Coagulation can be prevented by putting the blood in a specimen tube that contains an anticoagulant (e.g. sodium citrate: 25 mg of $Na_3C_6H_5O_7.2H2O$; or EDTA: 0.5 mg of $Na_2EDTA.2H_2O$ for each 1 ml of blood). If no anticoagulant is used, the film must be prepared immediately (*Fig. 7.1*). The glass slides must be clean and have been degreased in alcohol or acetone. A small drop of blood is spread over the slide as shown. The film is then allowed to dry. For a preparation enriched in leukocytes, the **'buffy coat'** is used. In blood that has been centrifuged, this is the greyish layer seen on the upper surface of the deposit of packed erythrocytes. A suspension enriched in leukocytes can also be obtained by density gradient centrifugation of blood in a solution of a suitable inert polymer.

If it cannot be stained within a few hours, the film should be fixed (by immersing the slide in 95% alcohol for 5 min), rinsed in water, air-dried, and stored in a dust-free box. With the Romanowsky–Giemsa staining techniques (e.g. Leishman's, Wright's), the alcoholic solvent of the mixture of dyes serves as a fixative. **No fixative other than alcohol is permissible for blood films that are to be treated with neutral stains**. Formaldehyde (even traces of the gas in the air, according to Boon and Drijver, 1986) and chromium compounds prevent the Romanowsky–Giemsa effect, presumably by combining with basic groups of proteins in nuclei, and altering the affinity for charged dye particles (Wittekind, 1983).

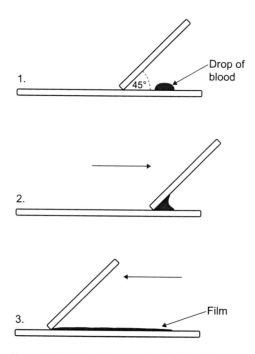

Figure 7.1. Technique for preparation of a blood film.

7.1.2.
Preparation and fixation of smears

A smear of exfoliated cells may be prepared directly by spreading the material scraped from a surface over a glass slide, to make a thin layer. Alternatively, the material may be mixed with an excess of a physiological saline solution (Chapter 20) and then spun for 5–10 min in a centrifuge (approximately 500 g). The supernatant is discarded. The pellet is taken up in a small volume of serum or of 1% bovine albumin in saline, and then smeared onto a slide. The presence of protein in the suspending medium protects the cells from breakage during smearing.

Many methods are available for the disaggregation of lumps and for getting rid of mucus and other unwanted substances (see Mayall and Gledhill, 1977; Bancroft and Cook, 1984; Koss and Melamed, 2006).

Unfixed cells will adhere to clean glass. The slide should then be fixed in ethanol or an acetic–ethanol mixture (Chapter 2) before the deposited cells have dried out. This is known as **wet fixation**, and it prevents much of the flattening and enlargement that occur in cells that have been allowed to dry. Even less distortion is seen if the cells are fixed by adding a fixative agent to the suspension, but some flattening is often advantageous, because the nuclear and cytoplasmic features are enlarged (see Boon and Drijver, 1986). For cells that have been fixed in the suspension, it is necessary to coat the slide with an adhesive. Chrome–gelatin or APES

(Chapter 4) is recommended. Blood is the only fluid that may be allowed to air-dry onto slides; the cells evidently are protected by the plasma.

**7.1.3.
Sedimentation
methods**

Cells suspended in saline or any other liquid less viscous than plasma will sink. Having sunk, they will adhere to a glass slide that forms the bottom of the container. An even layer can thus be obtained of cells that have not been squashed, torn, or otherwise distorted by smearing. A simple sedimentation method is illustrated in *Fig. 7.2*. This type of technique was originally introduced for use with cerebrospinal fluid (Sayk, 1954). The cells settle gently onto the slide as the liquid medium is slowly absorbed into the filter paper. Slides bearing sedimented cells should be wet-fixed and can be stored in 70% alcohol prior to staining.

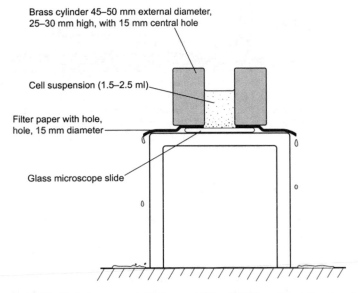

Brass cylinder 45–50 mm external diameter,
25–30 mm high, with 15 mm central hole

Cell suspension (1.5–2.5 ml)

Filter paper with hole,
hole, 15 mm diameter

Glass microscope slide

Figure 7.2. Method recommended by Boon and Drijver (1986) for sedimentation of a cell suspension. The weight of the metal chamber (about 300 g) presses on the filter paper, slowing down the drainage of the suspending solution, thus allowing enough time for the cells to settle onto the slide.

Sayk's method is slow; the absorption of 2 ml of fluid into the filter paper may take 2 h. A Cytospin centrifuge (Shandon Elliott) or a Cytospin assembly usable with a conventional centrifuge deposits cells in the same way as gravity-powered sedimentation (*Fig. 7.3*). There is more flattening of the cells, but preparations can be made in 5 min from samples much smaller than those needed for making smears.

Erythrocytes are more fragile than leukocytes and other types of cell. **Haemolysis** is the destruction of erythrocytes by brief exposure to a hypotonic solution or a low concentration of a detergent such as saponin. The haemoglobin is released into the surrounding medium, and all that remains of the erythrocyte is a **ghost** consisting of damaged membranes and some cytoskeletal proteins. Dilution of haemolysed blood with isotonic saline provides a suspension of leukocytes, which can be concentrated by centrifugation. These procedures are useful when the presence of erythrocytes would be intrusive, as in the mechanical counting of leukocytes or the examination of thick blood films for protozoan parasites (Petithory *et al.*, 1997).

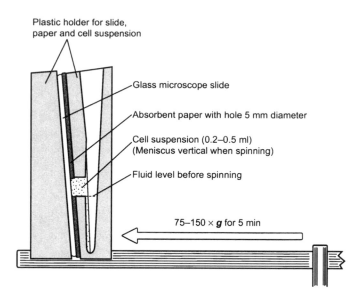

Plastic holder for slide,
paper and cell suspension

Glass microscope slide

Absorbent paper with hole 5 mm diameter

Cell suspension (0.2–0.5 ml)
(Meniscus vertical when spinning)

Fluid level before spinning

75–150 × **g** for 5 min

Figure 7.3. Principle of cell sedimentation by centrifugation. The absorbent paper has about the same thickness as the slide. The ideal concentration of the cell suspension is determined by trial. 1 to 5 × 10^3 cell/mm^3 (or a 10- to 50-fold dilution of whole blood) is satisfactory for most purposes.

7.2. Romanowsky–Giemsa stains

Useful staining reagents can be made by mixing aqueous solutions of suitable cationic and anionic dyes (e.g. methylene blue and eosin; neutral red and fast green FCF). The precipitate that forms contains ionic species of both dyes, and is almost insoluble in water but freely soluble in alcohol. It is also soluble in water containing an excess of either the anionic or the cationic dye. Mixed dyes of this type were often called '**neutral stains**', but this term has been dropped because neutral coloured molecules are not involved in their actions (Wittekind, 1983, 2002). When the anionic component is eosin, the mixture is called an 'eosinate'. The most important applications of these solutions are in haematology and exfoliative cytology, but they may also be used for general staining of any tissue. Lillie's azure–eosin method (Chapter 6) is an example.

7.2.1.
Theory of Romanowsky–Giemsa staining

The traditional stains for blood contain two or three thiazine dyes (methylene blue and its oxidation products) and eosin, dissolved usually in methanol and glycerol. The latter helps to stabilize the stock solution; it can be replaced by diethylamine hydrochloride, which does not increase the viscosity (Liao, Ponzo and Patel, 1981). These mixtures are known generically as 'Romanowsky–Giemsa stains', after the Russian and German haematologists who first described their properties in 1891. The commercially available ready-mixed preparations are more reliable than those made in the laboratory from the separate ingredients. However, extempore mixtures are quite satisfactory for non-haematological purposes (see Lillie and Fullmer, 1976). The alcoholic solution of an eosinate must be diluted with water (or a buffer) immediately before use, to liberate the colorant ions in an active form. The pH of the diluted stain and of the water for rinsing is a critical factor, especially when using these mixtures of dyes to stain blood cells in sections of fixed tissues.

Haematological staining solutions have been developed empirically. The main source of variation among different batches is the rather unpredictable assortment of dyes produced by the oxidation of methylene blue (Chapter 5). *It is now known that the properties of the Romanowsky–Giemsa stains are attributable only to azure B and eosin* (Marshall, 1978; Wittekind, 1983). Other thiazine dyes, notably methylene violet (Bernthsen), are always present in the mixtures, but at low concentrations they do not have adverse effects. Although eosin is usually impure, its contamination with other xanthene dyes is unimportant (see Lillie, 1977). It is now possible to make standardized staining solutions that conform to internationally agreed standards. Eosin and purified azure B are the only dyes in such mixtures. Abnormalities in blood and marrow smears are seen only from time to time, so it is essential for the pathologist that the stains give consistent results, even in the hands of inexperienced technicians.

The different cells in a blood film are identified by virtue of the colours imparted to the nuclei, cytoplasm and cytoplasmic granules of the cells. Erythrocytes are coloured by the eosin anions, with intensity proportional to their intracellular concentrations of haemoglobin. Immature mammalian red cells (reticulocytes) also contain material stained by the cationic dyes this representing the remnants of the nuclei of the cells. Leukocytes have purple (not blue) nuclei, and lilac-blue cytoplasm. Granules within the cytoplasm are red in eosinophils, blue in basophils and purple in neutrophils. Abnormal objects such as leukaemic white cells and malaria parasites also have characteristic tinctorial properties. The nuclei of protozoa should be coloured bright red by a satisfactory haematological staining solution.

The azure B in a diluted blood stain is present as dimers: two cations of dye are held together by van der Waals attractions between their planar phenothiazine rings (Chapter 5), giving a particle with a charge of +2. The purple coloration of leukocyte nuclei, known as the Romanowsky–Giemsa effect, is due to (a) the binding of cationic dimers to nuclear DNA, and (b) the binding of eosin anions to the already bound azure B cations. Ionic and non-ionic forces (Chapter 5) are involved in the binding of the dyes. The negatively charged phosphoric acid groups of DNA attract the azure B cations, and the attachment of the dye is reinforced by van der Waals and hydrophobic interaction between the aromatic rings of the dye and the purine and pyrimidine rings of the DNA (see also Chapter 9). Both types of force are also involved in the adherence of eosin to bound azure B (Horobin and Walter, 1987; Müller-Walz and Zimmermann, 1987; Friedrich *et al.*, 1990; Wittekind *et al.*, 1991).

7.2.2.
Leishman's and
Wright's stains

These are methods for blood films. The stock solutions can be bought ready-made or prepared by dissolving a powder, which is the precipitated and dried eosinate of a suitably polychromed methylene blue (see *Note 1* below).

A buffer solution, pH 6.8, is also required, but tap water, if not too alkaline, will often serve quite adequately in its place. Distilled water is usually rather too acid (pH around 5.5), owing to dissolved carbon dioxide derived from the atmosphere. A suitable solution for use with blood stains may be made by diluting a phosphate buffer (Chapter 20) with 5–10 times its volume of distilled water.

Procedure
(1) Place slide with film on a horizontal staining rack over a sink.
(2) Flood the slide with the stock solution of Leishman's or Wright's stain. Wait for 1 min. The solvent fixes the cells and plasma of the film. (See *Note 4* below.)
(3) Add buffer solution in sufficient quantity to dilute the stain two- or threefold. (The excess liquid will spill over into the sink.) Leave for 3 min.
(4) Wash off the stain with copious buffer solution (or tap water if satisfactory), making sure that the shiny skin of insoluble material on the surface of the stain does not deposit on the slide.

(5)   Stand the slide on end to drain and dry.

(6)   Clear and cover (see *Note 2* below) if a permanent mount is required.

Result

Erythrocytes pink; nuclei of leukocytes deep purple; cytoplasm of agranular leuko-cytes pale blue or lilac; basophil granules dark blue; neutrophil granules purple; eosinophil granules red to orange. Platelets blue to purple. Nuclei of protozoa, including malaria parasites bright red.

Notes

(1)   Both Leishman's and Wright's stains are made by dissolving in methanol the precipitated eosinates of polychromed methylene blue. They differ only in the methods of polychroming. If the stain is supplied as a powder, make a 0.15% solution in methanol. Shake well and leave to stand for 2 days or longer. Filter. The caps of the bottles in which the solution is kept should not have metal lin-ers; these have been shown to cause deterioration of the stains.

(2)   The preparations are commonly examined by placing immersion oil directly onto the dried films and examining with an oil immersion objective, which is necessary for resolution of the cytological detail. A permanent preparation is made by clearing in xylene for about 2 min (without prior exposure to alco-hols) and applying a resinous mounting medium and a coverslip.

(3)   Unsatisfactory staining can result from deterioration of the stain due to evap-oration of the solvent or from using water at the wrong pH. It is occasionally necessary to vary the pH of the buffer between 6.0 and 7.0 in order to secure optimum coloration of the film.

(4)   If blood films cannot be stained within about 2 h of preparation, they should be fixed by immersion for a few minutes in methanol. Stage 2 of the method described above is then unnecessary, and the films may be stained in freshly diluted Leishman's or Wright's solution.

7.2.3.
Giemsa's stain

Giemsa's stain is sometimes used for blood films, but is more suitable for sections, with which more consistent results are obtained than with Leishman's or Wright's staining mixtures. Giemsa powder is a mixture of 'Azure II' (21% w/w) with its eosinate (79% w/w). Azure II is believed to be a mixture of equal weights of methylene blue and azure B, originally marketed by the German firm of K. Hollborn, which bought Dr G. Grubler's business (Chapter 5, Section 5.6.2) in 1897 (Lillie, 1977). According to Lillie and Fullmer (1976), a Giemsa powder may be made by mixing methylene blue eosi-nate (4 g), azure B eosinate (5 g), azure A eosinate (1 g) and methylene blue (2 g if dye content is 85–88%, as the chloride). Giemsa powder obtained ready-made, from a reputable supply house and certified by the Biological Stain Commission, is recom-mended for all purposes. The glycerol added to the methanol used as solvent has the effect of increasing the stability of the diluted Giemsa stain, so that it is possible to expose sections to the aqueous working solution for several hours if necessary.

Helly's fixative is recommended for haemopoietic tissue, but zinc–formalin is cur-rently preferred because it does not contain mercury or chromium(VI). Decalcification may be necessary.

Preparation of stain

A. Giemsa stock solution

Giemsa powder:	2.0 g
Glycerol:	132 ml

Mix thoroughly in a 300 ml bottle with an air-tight screw cap. Put the bottle con-taining the mixture in an oven at 60°C for 2 h. Then add:

Absolute methanol:	132 ml

Mix gently. When cool, tighten the screw cap and shake. Stable for about 5 years. The eosin component is weakened after storage for 10–15 years.

B. Buffer solutions
Reagents should be available for the preparation of acetate or phosphate buffers from pH 4.0 to pH 7.0 (Chapter 20). **Buffered water** is made by diluting the buffer solutions 5–10 times with distilled water. See *Notes 1* and *4* below.

Procedure
(1) De-wax and hydrate paraffin sections.
(2) Immerse slides for 5 min in buffer solution at the optimum pH, as determined by experiment (see *Note 1* below). For Helly-fixed cancellous bone this is often pH 6.8. With formaldehyde- or Carnoy-fixed tissue, a pH as low as 4.0 is sometimes needed.
(3) Dilute the stock Giemsa solution (A) with 50 volumes of buffered water at the same pH as that used in Step 2. Immerse the slides in the diluted stain for 2 h
(4) Alternatively, preheat the diluted Giemsa solution in a closed coplin jar to 50–60°C (A microwave oven does this quickly.) Insert the slides and leave them for 15 min.
(5) Rinse the slides rapidly in buffered water and differentiate if necessary as described in *Note 2* below.
(6) Blot sections dry with filter paper.
(7) Dehydrate in two changes (each 3–5 min) of *n*-butanol. Alternatively, dehydrate rapidly in three changes of absolute ethanol
(8) Clear in xylene and cover.

Result
Nuclei blue to purple; erythrocytes, collagen, and keratin pink; leukocytes as described above for blood films except that basophil granules (and also mast cell granules) are deep purple rather than dark blue; cartilage matrix purple. Differentiation (see *Note 2*) accentuates the metachromasia (red purple colour) of cartilage and of mast cell and basophil granules. Bacteria are blue to purple.

Notes
(1) This and related methods are influenced greatly by the pH with which the section is equilibrated before staining, which should also be the pH of the staining solution itself. Distilled or tap water may or may not have the correct pH. Check the pH of buffered water with a meter *after* dilution. Adjustment is sometimes necessary, especially with acetate buffers.
(2) After rinsing with buffer, the section should be examined with a microscope. If the blue component of the stain is too strong, the slide should be differentiated by dipping it quickly into a 0.01% aqueous solution of glacial acetic acid and then returning it to the buffer. Several dips in the very weak acetic acid may be needed. If the pink component predominates, the pH of the stain is probably too low.
(3) Lillie and Fullmer (1976) strongly advocate this type of technique as a general oversight method, because more cytoplasmic details (granules, RNA, etc.) can be seen than with haematoxylin and eosin. The azure–eosin method (Chapter 6) is similar in principle, but does not provide the same differential coloration of leukocytes as the Giemsa stain.
(4) If blood-films are to be stained with Giemsa, fix them first in methanol. Dilute the stock Giemsa solution (A) with 40–50 volumes of distilled water and stain by immersing the slides for 15–40 min. The time will vary with different batches of Giemsa powder. Rinse in water, dry, and, if desired, clear and mount as described for Leishman's and Wright's stains (Section 7.2.2).

(5) Churukian (2000) recommends the addition of 1 ml of Triton X-100 (a cationic detergent) to every litre of the buffer used to dilute the Giemsa stock solution, to prevent formation of a precipitate in the working staining mixture.

7.2.4. Standardized Romanowsky–Giemsa method

This procedure, approved by the International Committee for Standardization in Haematology, makes use of pure dyes, which are commercially available but expensive. The procedure described below (Boon and Drijver, 1986) incorporates improvements recommended by Wittekind and Kretschmer (1987).

Stock solutions

1. Dye mixture
Combine the following two solutions:

Azure B thiocyanate:	1.0 g
Dissolve in dimethylsulphoxide (DMSO):	133 ml
Eosin Y disodium salt:	0.33 g

This is the usual form in which eosin Y (C.I. 45380) is supplied. Its dye content is about 85%. Eosin for use in this technique is sometimes supplied as the dye acid, which may be assumed to be 100% pure, so 0.27 g is equivalent to 0.33 g of the disodium salt.

Methanol:	200 ml

Store this stock solution in a brown glass bottle at room temperature. It keeps for about 6 months, and should not be used if it contains a precipitate. The life of the solution can be prolonged by adding a few drops of 1.0 M HCl until the apparent pH (the reading on a pH meter with its electrode in the non-aqueous solution) is 4.

2. Buffer
Ideally, use 0.03 M HEPES buffer, pH 6.5, but 0.033 M phosphate buffer, pH 6.8, is satisfactory. See Chapter 20 for instructions for making buffer solutions.

3. Staining solution

Solution 1 (Dyes):	2 ml
Solution 2 (Buffer):	30 ml

Mix when needed, use once and discard.

Procedure
(1) Make blood films or similar preparations and fix by immersion in either methanol or the stock dye solution (*Solution 1*, above).
(2) Immerse slides in the staining solution in a coplin jar or similar vessel: 25 min for blood films; 35 min for bone marrow smears.
(3) Wash in buffer (*Solution 2*), 1 min.
(4) Rinse briefly in water.
(5) Drain and allow to dry. A coverslip may be applied, but is neither necessary nor desirable (See *Note 2* following the instructions for Leishman's and Wright's methods).

Result
As for Leishman's or Wright's stain.

7.3. Other methods using dyes

Any method for staining sections should, in principle, to be applicable to fixed smears of whole cells. One of the main goals of clinical exfoliative cytoloy is the recognition of cells derived from malignant tumours. For this purpose, a staining method must show the shapes and sizes of the cells, provide crisp delineation of the nuclear chromatin, and demonstrate the presence in the cytoplasm of large amounts of ribonucleoprotein, or of deposits of keratin or mucus. The azure–eosin methods for blood cells (discussed earlier in this chapter) are often used for non-haematological purposes. Schulte and Wittekind (1989) recommend a standardized thionine-eosin method. Informative results can also be obtained with Mann's short eosin–methyl blue technique (Chapter 6) and with bacteriological staining procedures (such as the Gram stain; see Chapter 6, Section 6.4.4). The Papanicolaou method, however, is the one most used by clinical pathologists.

7.3.1.
Collection and preservation of cells

Preparative techniques vary with the materials being examined. For detailed accounts of techniques see Boon and Drijver (1986) and Koss and Melamed (2006). Cells from the vagina and cervix uteri are collected with a spatula and either smeared onto slides and fixed or immersed in Saccomanno's transport medium for smears to be made in the laboratory. Sputum usually contains viscous mucus, which must be dispersed before smears can be made, by incubating in two volumes of DTT–Carbowax. Cells from urine, cerebrospinal fluid or ascites fluid may be concentrated by centrifugation or by one of the methods described in Section 7.1.3. *Cells must not be allowed to air-dry after being smeared or otherwise deposited on slides*; drying artifacts include cracking and undue flattening and spreading of cells. The slide should be immersed immediately in a fixative. In some laboratories smears are preserved by spraying with a proprietary solution containing polyethylene glycol, or even with hair spray. Such mixtures of unknown composition should, however, be avoided in scientific work.

Saccomanno's transport medium

Carbowax 1540:	20 g
Melt (50°C) and add, with stirring, to:	
Water:	500 ml
Then add, with stirring:	
Ethanol:	to make 1000 ml

Carbowax 1540 is Union Carbide's trade-name for polyethylene glycol with molecular weight range 1300–1600. The generic name for the product is polyethylene glycol 1500 or PEG-1500.

Spatulas bearing cells may be immersed in this liquid. Sputum or deposits from centrifuged urine of other fluids may be mixed with 2 or 3 volumes of Saccomanno's medium.

DTT–Carbowax

Carbowax 1540:	30 g

Melt (50°C) and add, with stirring, to:

60% Ethanol:	1000 ml

This solution is stable, but Dithiothreitol (DTT) solutions can be kept for only a few days, so the working solution is made up as required:.

3% Carbowax 1540 in 60% ethanol:	50 ml
DTT:	1.0 g

DTT prevents the combination of –SH groups of cysteine to form –S–S– (cystine) bridges between polypeptide chains of proteins; DTT also reduces cystine to cysteine (Cleland, 1964). The resulting reduction of molecular size in the glycoproteins of mucus reduces the viscosity and facilitates the release of cells and formation of thin smears or films. Add two volumes of DTT–Carbowax to the sample.

Fixation

(See also Section 7.1.2 and Chapter 2, Section 2.5.1). The slide with a smear or other thin deposit of cells is immersed immediately in a suitable fixative: 100% methanol, 95% ethanol, methacarn or Carnoy's fluid. The last two of these cause lysis of erythrocytes, which is often desirable when the cells of interest are derived from an epithelium. Duration of fixation is 15–30 min.

7.3.2. Papanicolaou staining of smears

The name of G.N. Papanicolaou is associated with a family of techniques with which cytoplasms are coloured by eosin, mucus by light green, and keratin by orange G. Nuclear chromatin is stained blue with alum–haematein. After the nuclei have been stained, the small anions of orange G enter all the unstained components of the smear. This dye will bind to proteins only from a solution more acid than pH 3. The single ions and dimers of eosin and the large ions or aggregates of light green compete with one another for cytoplasmic binding sites, but they do not displace orange G from keratin. Single eosin ions enter erythrocytes, which become orange-pink (the colour of monomeric eosin, perhaps mixed with some residual orange G). Eosin dimers (red-pink) enter the cytoplasms of most cells, and are bound by proteins there. Light green is bound by mucus, which therefore acquires the bluish green colour of this dye. The optimum pH for competition between eosin and light green is 6.5. The pH of each dye solution is determined by the concentration of phosphotungstic acid (PTA) added to the solution. Hydrochloric acid may be substituted for PTA, but with some loss of distinctness in the selective staining. The large anions of PTA seem to assist in the exclusion of large dye particles (light green) from most cells.

These methods were probably derived empirically from procedures used for staining cells and connective tissue fibres in sections. The possible mechanisms of differential staining by mixtures of anionic dyes, with and without such additives as PTA, are discussed more critically in Chapter 8.

The following procedure (Boon and Drijver, 1986) is reliable because the pH of the dye mixtures is controlled, and all rinses and washings are clearly described.

Note that the term 'pH' is used incorrectly in the instructions below. The reading obtained when the glass electrode of a pH meter is in an aqueous-alcoholic solution is not the correct value of the logarithm of the reciprocal of the hydrogen ion concentration. A more accurate figure, known as the pH^*, can be calculated from the meter reading (see Perrin and Dempsey, 1974).

Solutions required

A. Mayer's haemalum

See Chapter 6. Any other alum–haematein that gives nuclear staining may be substituted.

B. Orange G with PTA

Orange G (C.I. 16230):	1.0 g
50% alcohol:	500 ml
Phosphotungstic acid:	approx. 75 mg

The pH, which must be between 2.0 and 2.8, is determined by the amount of phosphotungstic acid in the solution.

C. Eosin and light green with PTA

Eosin (C.I. 45380):	900 mg
Light green (C.I. 42095):	350 mg
Phosphotungstic acid:	1.5 g
50% alcohol:	500 ml

The pH should be 4.6. Add solid lithium carbonate, a little at a time, with continuous stirring, until the pH is 6.5. It is important to use light green that has been certified by the Biological Stain Commission, because some bad batches purporting to be this dye were sold in the early 1990s. Alternatively, fast green FCF may be used; the difference in colour is hardly discernable (Penney and Powers, 1995).

Solution A keeps for several months. Solutions B and C keep indefinitely. All may be used repeatedly.

Staining procedure
(1) Wash the slides with the fixed smears in 50% alcohol. (At least 1 h if the smears have been sprayed with a glutinous material such as polyethylene glycol to prevent drying; otherwise 1 min.)
(2) Rinse in tap water, 15 dips.
(3) Immerse in Solution A (haemalum) until nuclei are blue (2–10 min).
(4) Wash in tap water until no more colour comes away from the slides.
(5) Rinse in 50% alcohol, 15 dips.
(6) Immerse in orange G-PTA (Solution B) for 1 min.
(7) Two rinses, each 15 dips, in 50% alcohol.
(8) Immerse in Solution C (eosin-light green-PTA) for 2 min.
(9) Rinse in 50% alcohol, 15 dips.
(10) Dehydrate in two changes of absolute alcohol.
(11) Clear in *t*-butanol.
(12) Cover, using a resinous mounting medium.

Result
Nuclei, blue-purple, with blue or red nucleoli. Cytoplasm pink or blue-green, according to cell type. Keratinized cells orange. Erythrocytes pink to orange.

7.4. Enzyme methods for leukocytes

Some histochemical methods for enzymes are applied to blood and bone marrow smears, for the identification of normal and abnormal leukocytes, and for differential staining of B and T lymphocytes. The chemical principles of such techniques are explained in Chapters 14, 15 and 16. Practical instructions for two methods are given here. They differ in several practical details from comparable procedures used with sectioned tissues. For more information, and for other enzyme histochemical methods of haematological interest, see Elias (1982) and Hayhoe and Quaglino (1988).

7.4.1.
Alkaline phosphtase in granulocytes

This enzyme occurs in the cytoplasm of granulocytes (neutrophils and basophils, but not eosinophils) and their immediate precursors, but not in myeloblasts. In myelogenous leukaemia, the abnormal circulating leukocytes contain little or no alkaline phosphatase.

The enzyme catalyses the hydrolysis of naphthol-AS phosphate at high pH:

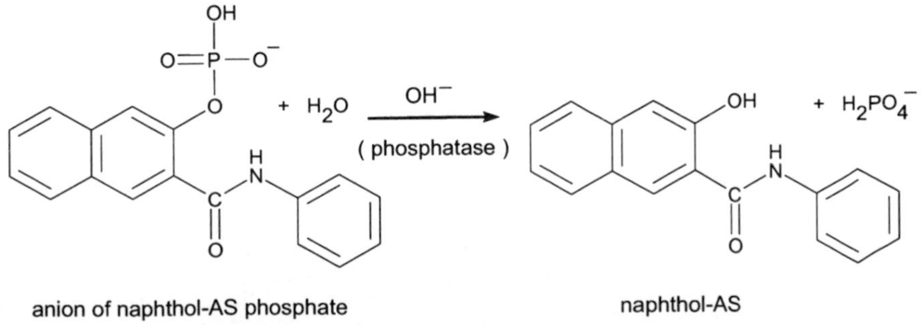

anion of naphthol-AS phosphate   naphthol-AS

The released naphthol AS molecules couple immediately with a diazonium salt that is included in the incubation medium, to form an insoluble azoic dye.

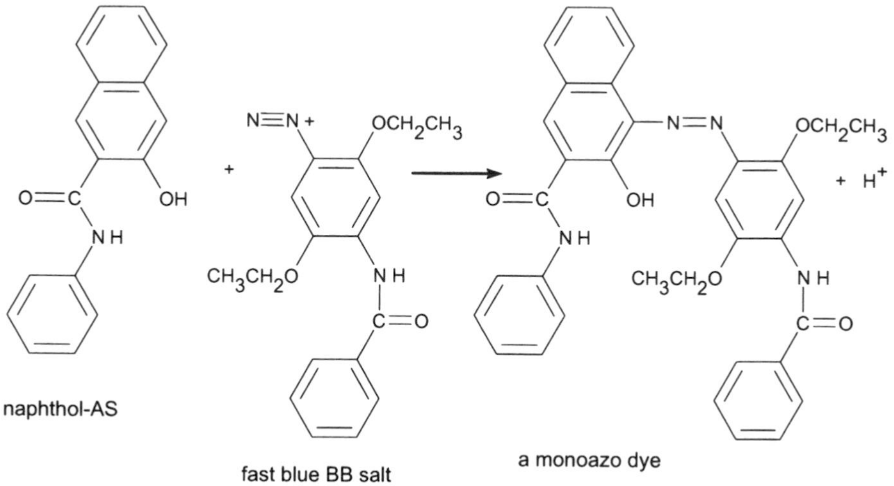

naphthol-AS

fast blue BB salt

a monoazo dye

(The azo coupling reaction is discussed in Chapter 5; alkaline phosphatase histochemistry is explained in Chapter 15). The following method (Rutenberg, Rosales and Bennett, 1965) is applied to air-dried films or smears.

Solutions required

Fixative

Methanol:	90 ml
Formalin (37–40% HCHO):	10 ml

Keeps indefinitely at 0–4°C.

Substrate stock solution

Naphthol-AS phosphate:	60 mg
N,N-dimethylformamide:	1.0 ml

Dissolve the ester in the solvent then add:

0.2 M TRIS buffer, pH 9.1:	200 ml

Keeps for several months at 4°C.

Working incubation medium

Substrate stock solution:	20 ml
Fast blue BB salt (C.I. 37175):	20 mg

Dissolve, then filter. Mix immediately before using, and use only once.

Neutral red (counterstain)

Neutral red (C.I. 50040):	0.2 g
Water:	200 ml

Keeps indefinitely. The pH may need to be adjusted (see Chapter 6).

Procedure

(1) Immerse slides with air-dried smears in the fixative, in a coplin jar, 30 s at 0°C to 4°C. For marrow smears, first extract fat with cold acetone (Chapter 12).

(2) Pour off fixative and replace with water (tap or distilled), 5 changes, then drain and leave until completely dry.

(3) Mix the working incubation medium. Pour it into the coplin jar containing the slides, and leave for 15 min.
(4) Wash gently in 5 changes of tap or distilled water, and air-dry.
(5) Counterstain nuclei with neutral red, for 3 min.
(6) Wash in running tap water for about 2 s, to remove unbound dye.
(7) Blot, and then allow to dry thoroughly in the air. A coverslip may be applied: immerse in xylene and use a resinous mounting medium. Alternatively, immersion oil may be placed directly onto the dry film or smear. (Aqueous mounting media and alcohol extract the product of the histochemical reaction.)

Results

Sites of enzymatic activity appear as blue granules in the cytoplasm. Nuclei are red-orange.

Notes

(1) The alkaline incubation medium loosens cells from the slides. Losses are reduced by careful handling and the air-drying in steps 2 and 4.
(2) Other substrates and diazonium salts can be used. Elias (1982) prefers naphthol-AS–MX phosphate, and states that fast blue RR salt (C.I. 37155) may used instead of fast blue BB salt. (One gram of fast blue RR salt is equivalent to three of fast blue BB salt, so only about 6 mg are needed in the method as described here.)

7.4.2
Esterases in monocytes and T cells

Various histochemically detectable esterases are present in the cytoplasm of monocytes and macrophages. These enymes are remarkable in that their activities can survive fixation and heat, though they are inhibited by alcohol. An esterase that catalyses the hydrolysis of α-naphthyl acetate is present in monocytes and also in type T lymphocytes (Ferrari et al., 1980).

The technique (Ranki et al., 1980, incorporating some modifications from Elias, 1982) is similar to the one for alkaline phosphatase (Section 7.4.1). α-Naphthol released by hydrolysis of the substrate couples with fully diazotized pararosaniline (known as 'hexazonium pararosaniline', because the parent compound has three diazotizable amino groups). The final product of the reaction is therefore a large insoluble dye molecule derived from one molecule of pararosaniline and three of α-naphthol:

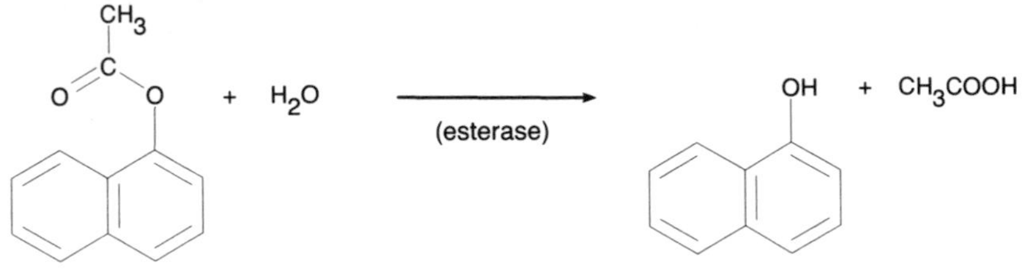

α-naphthyl acetate α-naphthol

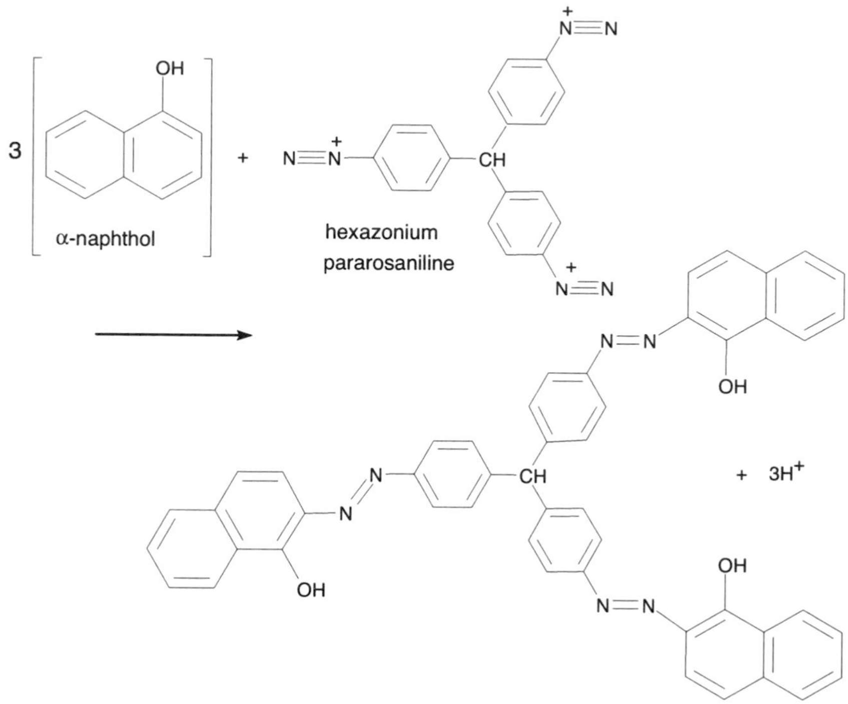

Solutions required

Formalin-acetone fixative

Dissolve 20 mg anhydrous disodium hydrogen phosphate (Na_2HPO_4) and 100 mg anhydrous potassium dihydrogen phosphate (KH_2PO_4) in 30 ml water. Add 25 ml of formalin (37% HCHO), and check that the pH is 6.6. Add 45 ml acetone.

Probably indefinitely stable in a tightly capped bottle. Use at 4°C.

Alternatively, use cold formal–calcium (Chapter 2), which keeps indefinitely and is useful for other purposes too.

Phosphate buffer, pH 5.0

See Chapter 20. Add 30 ml water to 70 ml of 0.1 M buffer, to make the 0.07 M buffer prescribed for this technique.

Some 0.1 M (0.4% w/v) sodium hydroxide will also be needed, for adjusting the final pH of the incubation medium.

Substrate stock solution

Dissolve 200 mg of α-naphthyl acetate in 10 ml of acetone. Keeps for several weeks in a tightly capped bottle.

Pararosaniline stock solution

Add 2.0 g pararosaniline (C.I. 42500) to 50 ml of 2.0 M hydrochloric acid (the concentrated acid diluted sixfold; see Chapter 20). Heat with stirring until it boils, leave to cool to room temperature, and filter. This stable solution is kept at 4°C.

Sodium nitrite solution

Dissolve 1.0 g sodium nitrite ($NaNO_2$) in 25 ml water. Keep at 4°C until needed. This solution should be made on the day it is to be used.

Hexazonium pararosaniline
This reagent is prepared immediately before using. Mix equal volumes (each about 2 ml) of the 4% aqueous sodium nitrite and the pararosaniline stock solution, stir and let stand for 1 min.

Incubation medium
Immediately before using, mix:

Substrate stock solution:	0.5 ml
0.07 M phosphate buffer, pH 5.0:	40 ml
Hexazonium pararosaniline:	2.4 ml

Add a few drops of 1.0 M NaOH to bring the pH to 5.8.

Counterstain
An alum–haematein such as Mayer's or Gill's haematoxylin, or any basic dye that will contrast with the red reaction product. Ethyl green is suitable. These stains are described in Chapter 6. A blue thiazine dye is not recommended, because it is likely to give red metachromatic staining of basophil and mast cell granules.

Procedure
(1) Air-dry the films or smears and fix by immersing the slides in fixative (formalin-acetone or formal–calcium) for 10 min at 4°C.
(2) Wash in 3 changes of water and air-dry for at least 30 min.
(3) Immerse for 60 min at room temperature in the freshly prepared incubation medium.
(4) Wash in water, 3 changes. (Optionally, the slides may now be post-fixed in neutral buffered formaldehyde (Chapter 2), which is said by Elias (1982) to improve the nuclear counterstain.)
(5) Counterstain nuclei with either an alum–haematein or methyl green (Chapter 6).
(6) Rinse in 3 changes of water and air-dry. When completely dry, rinse in xylene and cover, using a resinous mounting medium.

Result
Sites of α-naphthyl acetate esterase activity red. Cytoplasm of monocytes is strongly positive. The cytoplasm of the T lymphocyte contains one or more red dots. Neutrophils and B lymphocytes are negative. All nuclei are coloured blue or blue-green by the counterstain.

Notes
1. Sodium fluoride (0.1–0.2 M, in the incubation medium) inhibits the enzyme in monocytes and macrophages, but not in the granules of the T lymphocytes (Ranki *et al.*, 1980).
2. This method can be applied to paraffin sections of formaldehyde-fixed tissue. Acetone at 4°C (not alcohol) must be used for all dehydration and rehydration. Toluene or xylene may be used for clearing.

8 | Methods for connective tissue

A connective tissue stain is used to identify and study the various extracellular fibrous elements of animal tissues. Smooth and striated muscle fibres, erythrocytes, and the cytoplasms of other cell types are also clearly shown by the same techniques. Nuclei are commonly stained in the same section, to facilitate correlation of the multi-coloured histological picture with the more familiar appearance obtained with an oversight method such as haemalum and eosin. The amorphous ground substance of connective tissue, however, is most easily demonstrated by histochemical methods for proteoglycans (Chapter 11).

The histological techniques for connective tissues fall into three categories: those based on mixtures of anionic dyes that impart different colours to collagen and cytoplasm, the methods for reticulin (which are histochemical in nature), and a variety of methods for elastin.

8.1. Collagen, reticulin and elastin

The two principal types of fibre found in connective tissue are **collagen** and **elastin**. Apart from their morphological characteristics (for which consult a textbook of histology), these fibres have certain physical and chemical properties that enable them to be stained selectively.

8.1.1.
Collagen

Collagen is a family of basic glycoproteins containing high proportions of glycine, hydroxyproline and proline. Another amino acid, hydroxylysine, though present in smaller quantities, is found only in collagen. The conformation of the collagen molecule is maintained by hydrogen bonding between peptide groups (as in all proteins) and the peptide chains are joined to one another by various types of covalent linkage formed by condensation of hydroxylysine with lysine (see Bailey, 2003). This results in the formation of cables, each consisting of a triple helix of polypeptide strands. The carbohydrate components are mostly α-D-glucosyl and α-D-galactosyl residues, attached mainly to hydroxylysine. The triple helices are joined end to end and side to side by hydrogen bonds, electrostatic attractions, and covalent bridges to form structures visible in the electron microscope as collagen **fibrils** (see Kuhn, 1987, Kucharz, 1992). The collagen **fibres** seen with the light microscope are bundles of aligned fibrils.

A collagen fibre is birefringent, mainly because of the parallel alignment of its constituent protein molecules, and perhaps partly also because of the arrangement of carbohydrate macromolecules associated with the fibres (Kiraly *et al.*, 1997). It is therefore possible to see collagen fibres by examining unstained sections in a microscope with crossed polars. They appear as bright lines on a dark background. Certain staining methods, notably picro-sirius red, conspicuously enhance the birefringence of collagen fibres.

About 20 types of collagen, identified by Roman numerals, are recognized on the basis of amino acid sequences, physical and immunological properties, and fibrillary ultrastructure. The common collagens of mammalian tissues (Montes and Junqueira, 1991) are the following:

Type I   Thick fibrils assembled in parallel bundles. This is the principal collagen of bone, fascia and tendons.
Type II   Thin fibrils; in hyaline cartilage.
Type III Thin fibrils. Occurs in skin and muscle, and also in basement membranes.
Type IV The collagen molecules form a network rather than fibrils. Consequently, Type IV collagen is not birefringent. This is the principal collagen of all basement membranes, where it is intimately associated with another protein, laminin, and a glycosaminoglycan, heparan sulphate.

For information on other types of collagen, see Mayne and Burgeson (1987), Kornblihtt and Gutman (1988) and Ricard-Blum *et al.* (2000).

As a glycoprotein, collagen is stained, though not strongly, by the periodic acid–Schiff method (Chapter 11). By using reagents that are more sensitive than Schiff's it is possible to detect free aldehyde groups in collagen (Davis and Janis, 1966). These may arise from the oxidative deamination of the side-chains of lysine, as in immature elastin (see below).

The term **reticulin** includes the basement membranes of epithelia and blood capillaries and very fine (including immature) fibres that contain principally Type III collagen. Both types of reticulin contain more carbohydrate than does ordinary collagen. In the electron microscope, the reticular fibril shows the characteristic banding pattern of collagen. The staining methods for reticulin probably demonstrate a carbohydrate-containing matrix in which the collagenous fibrils are embedded, rather than the fibrils themselves (Puchtler and Waldrop, 1978).

8.1.2.
Elastin

About 90% of the volume of **elastic fibres** and **elastic laminae** consists of elastin, a protein different from collagen and reticulin. The remaining 10% is a glycoprotein that forms microfibrils within the largely amorphous elastin matrix (Franzblau and Faris, 1981; Chadwicke and Goode, 1995). **Oxytalan fibres**, present around the roots of teeth, are atypical elastin-containing structures in which the microfibrils predominate (Section 8.4.3).

Elastin is a hydrophobic protein, rich in glycine, alanine, and valine. It contains remarkably few amino acids with side-chains that can form ions. The peptide strands of elastin do not form fibrils but are united by **desmosine** and **isodesmosine** linkages to form a material with a predominantly amorphous appearance in the electron microscope. A desmosine bridge is formed from four lysine side-chains (see Bailey, 2003). Three of these are oxidatively deaminated to give aldehydes, which then unite, together with one unoxidized lysine side-chain, to form an aromatic ring similar to that of pyridine:

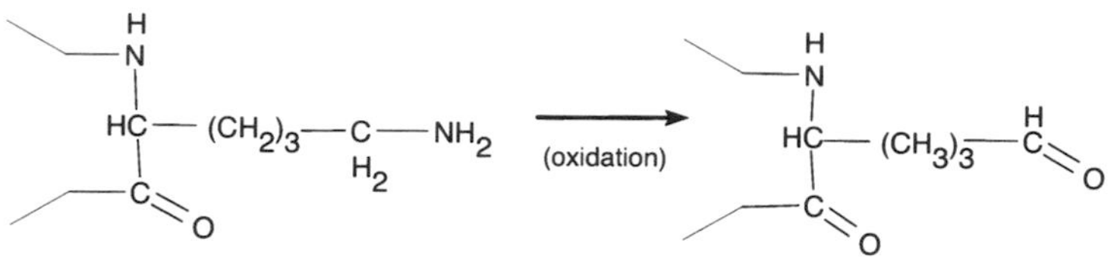

lysyl → (oxidation) → ε-lysylal

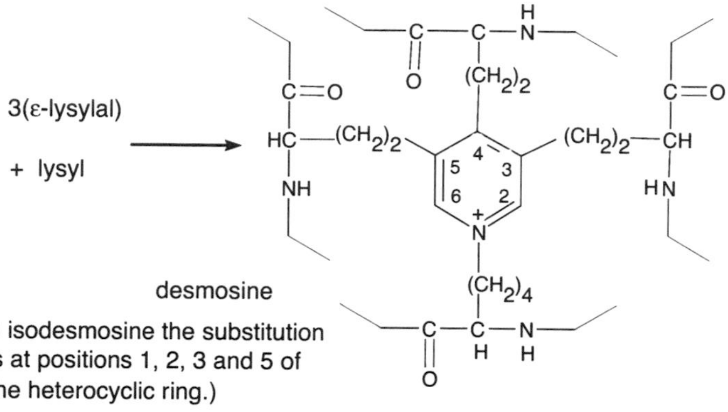

3(ε-lysylal) + lysyl → desmosine

(In isodesmosine the substitution is at positions 1, 2, 3 and 5 of the heterocyclic ring.)

In immature elastin, the formation of desmosine is incomplete, and free aldehydes can be detected histochemically (Nakao and Angrist, 1968; MacCallum, 1973). Elastin is resistant to digestion by most proteolytic enzymes. With ordinary staining methods it is acidophilic but contrasts poorly with other components of the tissue. Elastic fibres and laminae are autofluorescent (ultraviolet or blue excitation), and are commonly seen in sections examined by fluorescence microscopy for other purposes. They also contain magnesium ions, and can be stained with reagents that form coloured or fluorescent complexes with Mg^{2+} (Muller and Firsching, 1991), but this method is not in general use. The usual staining methods for elastin make use of dyes that are preferentially retained in the hydrophobic environment of the material.

8.2. Methods using anionic dyes

Numerous techniques are available for staining with mixtures of dyes, but most are variants of one of two main groups. In the first group, typified by van Gieson's method, a mixture of two anionic dyes imparts one colour to collagen and another to cytoplasm, including that of muscle fibres and erythrocytes. The second group embraces the 'trichrome' procedures in which two, three, or rarely four anionic dyes are used in conjunction with phosphotungstic or phosphomolybdic acid. Collagen, cytoplasm (of muscle and most other cells), and erythrocytes are all coloured differently, and other elements such as cartilage, fibrin, and secretory granules also acquire characteristic colours.

8.2.1.
van Gieson's method: principles

Following a black nuclear stain with an iron–haematoxylin, the sections are immersed in a solution of acid fuchsine in saturated or near-saturated aqueous picric acid. Collagen is stained red (acid fuchsine), and cytoplasm is yellow. In related techniques another anionic dye (most frequently aniline blue or sirius red F3B) is substituted for acid fuchsine and occasionally a third dye is used, either as an additional step or mixed with the other two. In all these methods, the mixture of anionic dyes is quite strongly acid, with a pH of 1.0–2.0 (see Lillie and Fullmer,

1976; Clark, 1981, for details). Other acid-resistant nuclear stains can replace iron–haematoxylin (Chapter 6). A picro-fuchsine mixture may also be applied as a counterstain after any other histological or histochemical methods that yield acid-resisting products with contrasting colours. For example, it works well after silver reduction methods (Chapter 18). It is easy to stain large numbers of sections by van Gieson's method and its modifications. These are excellent micro-anatomical stains, but they do not reveal many details within the palely stained cytoplasm.

Differential coloration of collagen and cytoplasm can be obtained with many other pairs of dyes; the collagen is always stained by the larger coloured particles while the smaller dye ions stain cytoplasm; the separation of ionic weight is greater than 200 in dye pairs that give selective staining of collagen and cytoplasm (Horobin and Flemming, 1988). Physical and chemical mechanisms contributing to the selectivity of these technically simple staining methods will now be discussed.

The differential dyeing cannot be simply explained. It is due partly to the physical properties of collagen and cytoplasm, partly to the different ways in which large and small dye ions attach to substrates, and partly to differences in the amino acid composition of collagen and cytoplasmic proteins. Different observations and experiments indicate that each of these three mechanisms is essential. It must be concluded that all are operative, even though they may not contribute equally to the resultant staining effect.

Baker (1958) reviewed earlier studies that explained differential staining of this type entirely on the basis of the different sizes of the anions of the dyes used. He suggested that when two anionic dyes were applied simultaneously to a section there would be competition between them for cationic binding sites on the protein molecules of the tissue. The dye with smaller, more rapidly diffusing ions would penetrate quickly into a tightly woven proteinaceous matrix. There it would occupy the binding sites (assumed to be protonated amino and guanidino groups of protein) and exclude the dye whose particles were larger. This latter dye would, however, enter the loosely textured and more easily permeated component of the tissue, collagen. It might not immediately attach to cationic groups in collagen, because these would already have been occupied by the anions of the first, more rapidly diffusing dye. The larger dye ions, however, have stronger affinity for their substrate, owing to their size (Horobin and Flemming, 1988) and their greater numbers of negatively charged sulphonic acid groups (Reid *et al.*, 1993), so they compete successfully against smaller dye ions. Moreover, when the section is washed in water or alcohol, the small dye ions are the first to leave the tissue, because of their smaller size and lower affinity, and can be expected to diffuse out of the more porous regions first. Consequently, only the larger dye ions remain attached to the vacated cationic binding sites. Early evidence in support of the permeability-and-diffusion hypothesis came from experiments in which gelatin gels were stained by mixtures of eosin Y (ionic weight 646) and methyl blue (ionic weight 754, with a tendency to form aggregates). Concentrated gels were coloured red by eosin and dilute ones blue by methyl blue (see Mann, 1902; Baker, 1958).

It is assumed in this hypothesis that fixed cytoplasm is in some way less porous to dye ions than fixed collagen, though there is no evidence other than that derived from the behaviour of dyes to support or refute such an assertion. In one variant of the van Gieson method (see Lillie and Fullmer, 1976) the sections are stained with fast green FCF, a dye with larger ions than either picric acid or acid fuchsine, prior to immersion in the van Gieson mixture. Collagen is coloured red, erythrocytes green, and the cytoplasm of muscle yellowish green. From Baker's hypothesis, one would have expected green collagen, yellow erythrocytes, and probably red muscle. (It might alternatively be argued, after knowing the result, that the van Gieson dyes displace fast green FCF from all parts of the tissue except stained erythrocytes, which have such a dense texture that they cannot be penetrated even by picrate ions.) Another paradoxical observation is even more easily made. When sections are stained only with the van Gieson mixture (with no prior nuclear stain), nuclei are coloured yellow by the picric acid. However, Mann's eosin–methyl blue method gives blue nuclei (Chapter 6). Thus, with one pair of dyes the nuclei of cells show affinity for the smaller anions, and with another pair they take up the larger anions. These observations cannot be explained by arguments based solely on control of staining by different rates of diffusion and dye binding in different parts of the tissue.

Lillie (1964) sought a chemical explanation for the differential dyeing of collagen and cytoplasm. He subjected sections to various pre-treatments before staining and found that:

(a)   Treatment with nitrous acid abolished all staining by ordinary anionic dyes such as eosin and biebrich scarlet but did not prevent the red coloration of collagen by van Gieson's method and some similar procedures. (Nitrous acid removes amino groups: $-NH_2$ is probably usually replaced by $-OH$; see Chapter 10.)

(b)   Treatment with a mixture of acetic anhydride, acetic acid, and sulphuric acid abolished all acidophilia, including the affinity of collagen for acid fuchsine in the van Gieson mixture. The formerly acidophilic structures became basophilic, a property attributable to the formation of $-NHSO_3^-$ groups with primary amines and of $-OSO_3^-$ groups with $-OH$ (Chapter 10). These changes could be reversed by hydrolysis (removal) of the sulphate esters in a methanol-sulphuric acid mixture.

The reagents used for deamination and acetylation–sulphation have small molecules and may reasonably be assumed to attack any parts of the tissue that are accessible to acid fuchsine ions. As the mechanism of collagen staining, Lillie (1964) tentatively suggested ionic attraction between the dye's sulphonate groups and arginine side-chains (which are not affected by nitrous acid), and hydrogen bonding of hydroxy groups of serine, threonine, and hydroxylysine, presumably to the nitrogen atoms of the dye. His contention was supported by Puchtler and Sweat (1964a), who found that many direct cotton dyes were effective substitutes for acid fuchsine in mixtures of the van Gieson type. Such dyes bind to cellulose and other materials by non-ionic mechanisms, though the occurrence of hydrogen bonding between dyes and substrates in an aqueous environment is questionable (Chapter 5 and Horobin, 1982). Simple adsorption of the dyes could account for their concentration in collagen, and closely apposed dye and protein molecules are likely to be held together by van der Waals forces and hydrophobic interactions (Puchtler, Meloan and Waldrop, 1988). Prento (1993, 2001) attributed collagen staining largely to hydrogen bonding because it could be blocked by adding urea to the dye mixture but not by prior or simultaneous treatment with sodium dodecyl sulphate (SDS), which suppresses hydrophobic interactions between large molecules.

There is also evidence that ionic attractions contribute significantly to the staining of collagen. Junqueira *et al.* (1979) found that deamination with nitrous acid reduced by about 30% the amount of sirius red F3B taken up by dermal collagen from a solution of the dye in picric acid. This apparently disagrees with Lillie's (1964) observation cited earlier. It is possible the dye uptake was not reduced enough to cause qualitatively less intense staining of collagen. However, Nielsen *et al.* (1998) noted that oxidative destruction of basic amino acid side chains greatly reduced the intensity of collagen staining, and Prento (1993) observed moderate suppression of both collagen and cytoplasmic staining by the van Gieson method in the presence of either sulphate or phosphotungstate anions, which were thought compete with anionic dyes for cationic binding sites.

The staining of cytoplasm and erythrocytes by picric acid has received less attention than the staining of collagen by acid fuchsine. Molecular size is significant because other dyes with small molecules, such as Martius yellow and tartrazine, are used as cytoplasmic stains in other techniques; these dyes have no groups capable of forming hydrogen bonds (Horobin and Flemming, 1988; Dapson, 2005a). The yellow component of van Gieson staining is prevented by SDS, indicating that hydrophobic interaction is a major factor serving to retain picric acid in cytoplasm (Prento, 1993).

8.2.2
van Gieson's method: instructions

This is the simplest method of its type, and works well after any fixative, but it does not demonstrate the thinnest collagen fibres. The water used for rinsing after application of the van Gieson stain (or similar mixtures) is slightly acidified. This ensures that amino groups of protein will be protonated, thereby minimizing extraction of bound dye anions from the tissue.

Solutions required

A. Weigert's iron–haematoxylin
This is made from two stock solutions, which can both be kept for 3–5 years. Lillie's modification of Weigert's iron haematoxylin (Chapter 6) may be used instead. See *Note 2* below for two alternatives to iron–haematoxylin.

Solution A
Haematoxylin (C.I. 75290):	5 g
95% ethanol:	500 ml

Solution B.
Ferric chloride ($FeCl_3.6H_2O$):	5.8 g
Water:	495 ml
Concentrated hydrochloric acid:	5 ml

Working solution
Mix equal volumes of A and B. Put A in the staining jar or tank first for more rapid mixing. The mixture should be made just before using. It may be re-used many times, and can be kept for 2 days at room temperature or for 10–14 days at 4°C. Older solutions stain nuclei brown or bluish-grey rather than black.

B. van Gieson's solution
Acid fuchsine (C.I. 42685):	0.5 g
Saturated aqueous picric acid:	500 ml

Optionally, add 2.5 ml of concentrated hydrochloric acid (See *Note 3* below).

This mixture can be reused many times, and it retains its staining power for more than 5 years.

C. Acidified water
Add 5 ml acetic acid (glacial) to 1 l of water (tap or distilled).

Procedure
(1) De-wax and hydrate paraffin sections.
(2) Stain in working solution of Weigert's haematoxylin for 5 min (may need 10 min if the solution is more than 4 or 5 days old).
(3) Wash in running tap water. Check the wet section with a microscope to ensure that nuclei are selectively stained. (See *Note 1* below.)

(4)   Stain in van Gieson's solution, 2–5 min. The time is not critical.
(5)   Wash in two changes of acidified water.
(6)   Dehydrate rapidly in three changes of 100% ethanol. This step also differentiates the picric acid.
(7)   Clear in xylene and mount in a resinous medium (see *Note 4* below).

Result

Nuclei black. Collagen red. Cytoplasm (especially smooth and striated muscle), keratin and erythrocytes yellow.

Notes

(1)   If a selective nuclear stain is not obtained, remedial action will be needed. See the more detailed account of iron-hematoxylin nuclear staining in Chapter 6.
(2)   An alternative nuclear stain is iron-alum–chromoxane cyanine R (Chapter 6). If this is used, the nuclei will be blue or greenish blue.
      A wider range of colours is obtained if Step 2 is replaced by a 5-min staining in toluidine blue (Chapter 6), followed by washing in water and insolubilization of the dye by immersion of the slides for 5 min in 5% aqueous ammonium molybdate. The toluidine blue colours nuclei and cytoplasmic RNA blue; cartilage, mast cell granules, and other metachromatic materials red-purple. A green colour is formed in the cytoplasms of many epithelial and secretory cells, presumably as a consequence of staining by both the blue and the yellow dyes.
(3)   Owing to the variable dye contents of different batches of acid fuchsine, a van Gieson mixture may perform unsatisfactorily. This should not be a problem with certified batches of the dye, which have been tested in van Gieson's and other techniques (Penney *et al.*, 2002).
      If stained sections are too red (e.g. orange muscle fibres), add 2.5 ml of concentrated hydrochloric acid to the 500 ml of van Gieson mixture (Solution B above). This nearly always corrects the colours, but if the red is still excessive throw away about one quarter of the mixture and top up the remaining three quarters to the original volume with saturated aqueous picric acid. If red is too weak (inadequate staining of collagen), add another 0.1 g of acid fuchsine. Once the mixture has been adjusted to give correct staining, it will retain its properties for several years.
(4)   Acid fuchsine and basic fuchsine have undeserved reputations for fading. In my experience sections stained by the van Gieson and Cajal trichrome methods show no deterioration after 15–20 years. Possibly the dyes fade in preparations mounted in Canada balsam, which contains reducing and acidic (albeit non-aqueous) substances (Chapter 4, and also Lillie and Fullmer, 1976).

8.2.3.
Other mixtures of two anionic dyes

The following mixtures are used in exactly the same way as the van Gieson's solution in the preceding method, except where otherwise indicated.

8.2.3.1. Picro-indigocarmine

Indigocarmine (C.I. 73015):	0.50 g
Saturated aqueous solution of picric acid:	200 ml

Keeps for 2 or 3 years, in a dark bottle.

This is used in the same way as van Gieson's stain. It gives yellow cytoplasm and blue or blue–green collagen. The most pleasing colours are obtained if the nuclei of cells have first been stained a strong red-purple with basic fuchsine (e.g. 0.2% in water or 1% acetic acid for 5–10 min). The method is then known as **'Cajal's** trichrome' (Gabe, 1976), but it should not be confused with the trichrome methods discussed later in this chapter. See also *Note 4* following the account of the van Gieson staining procedure.

8.2.3.2. Picro-aniline blue

Aniline blue (or methyl blue; see Chapter 5):	0.5 g
Saturated aqueous solution of picric acid:	500 ml

Keeps for more than 5 years. Sometimes the blue dye settles out as a precipitate; if this happens shake the bottle and filter the solution before using it.

This mixture, applied in the same way as van Gieson's stain, gives yellow cytoplasm and blue collagen, including basement membranes and reticulin, which are usually missed by indigocarmine or by the acid fuchsine of van Gieson's solution. If the periodic acid–Schiff technique (Chapter 11) is interposed between the nuclear staining with iron–haematoxylin and picro-aniline blue, basement membranes and many secretory products are coloured bright pink, and the whole procedure is then known as **Lillie's allochrome method** (see Luna, 1968; Lillie and Fullmer, 1976).

8.2.3.3. Picro-sirius red

The polyazo dye sirius red F3B has much larger molecules than acid fuchsine, indigocarmine or aniline blue, and it is also able to assume a planar configuration (Chapter 5). A solution in picric acid provides red staining of collagen and a yellow background. In ordinary light the sections resemble those stained by van Gieson's method. Picro-sirius red is used mainly in conjunction with polarized light microscopy: the natural birefringence of collagen is greatly enhanced by the binding of long, aligned molecules of sirius red (Puchtler *et al.*, 1973; Junqueira *et al.*, 1979). When examined through crossed polars, collagen fibres stand out brilliantly against a black background. Basement membranes are red but only slightly or not at all birefringent because their type IV collagen molecules are not aligned to form fibres.

Solutions required

A. Picro-sirius red

Sirius red F3B (C.I. 35780):	0.5 g
Saturated aqueous solution of picric acid:	500 ml

Add a little solid picric acid to ensure saturation. Keeps for at least 12 years and can be used many times.

B. Acidified water

Add 5 ml acetic acid (glacial) to 1 l of water (tap or distilled).

Procedure

(1) De-wax and hydrate paraffin sections.
(2) (Optional, and not usually done) Stain nuclei with Weigert's haematoxylin (as for the van Gieson method, Section 8.2.2, but for a longer time), then wash the slides for 10 min in running tap water. The staining should be excessive because the hour-long immersion in Solution A extracts most of the colour from selectively stained nuclei.)
(3) Stain in picro-sirius red (Solution A) for 1 h.
(4) Wash in two changes of acidified water (Solution B).
(5) Dehydrate in three changes of 100% ethanol.
(6) Clear in xylene and mount in a resinous medium.

Result

In ordinary bright-field microscopy collagen, including the finest fibres and basement membranes, is red on a yellow background. (Nuclei, if stained, are black.) The

intensity of the red colour can be measured by microdensitometry to provide esti-
mates of collagen content in different parts of a tissue (Malkusch et al., 1995;
Kratky et al., 1996). When examined through crossed polars the larger collagen
fibers are bright yellow or orange, and the thinner ones, including reticular fibers,
are green. According to Junqueira et al. (1979) the birefringence is highly specific
for collagen. A few materials, including keratohyalin granules and some types of
mucus, are stained red but are not birefringent.

It is necessary to rotate the specimen in order to see all the fibres, because in any
single orientation the birefringence of some will be extinguished. This minor incon-
venience can be circumvented by equipping the microscope for use with circularly
rather than plane polarized light (Whittaker et al., 1994; Whittaker, 1995).

Note
The dye benzo blue BB (C.I. 22610; Direct blue 6, see Chapter 5) can be substituted for sirius red F3B, at the same concentration. The birefringence colours are
blue–violet for thicker and yellow for thinner collagen fibres (Gitirana and Trindade,
2000).

8.2.4.
**Trichrome
methods:
principles**

The name 'trichrome' identifies staining techniques in which two or more anionic
dyes are used in conjunction with a heteropolyacid: either phosphomolybdic or
phosphotungstic acid. These acids are water- and alcohol-soluble crystalline compounds. They may be included in dye solutions or applied to the sections sequentially, between treatments with different dyes. Whatever technique is employed, the
result is a selective colouring of collagen by one of the dyes. Cartilage and some
mucous secretions acquire the same colour as collagen. but their intensity of staining is usually less. If one other dye is applied, it stains nuclei, cytoplasm and erythrocytes. If two other dyes are used, one imparts its colour to erythrocytes and the
other stains the cytoplasms of other types of cell and also cell nuclei. Secretory
granules are variously stained: sometimes the same colour as collagen, sometimes
the same colour as nuclei or erythrocytes.

The trichrome techniques reveal collagenous and reticular fibres, basement membranes and secretory granules, typically with stronger colour and greater clarity than
is possible with van Gieson's method. With most trichrome techniques the staining
is intense enough to obscure structural detail in sections more than than 5 μm
thick. van Gieson's and other two-dye methods work well on sections as thick as
15 μm.

8.2.4.1. The heteropolyacids and their effects on staining
Phosphomolybdic acid (PMA) and phosphotungstic acid (PTA) are known as heteropolyacids. They are formed by coordination of molybdate or tungstate ions with
phosphoric acid. They are sold as hydrated crystals, which are freely soluble in
water to give strongly acid solutions:

$$H_3PO_4 \cdot 12MoO_3 \cdot 24H_2O \longrightarrow 3H^+ + [PMo_{12}O_{40}]^{3-} + 24H_2O$$

phosphomolybdic acid   phosphomolybdate
(= *dodeca*-molybdophosphoric acid)   anion

$$H_3PO_4 \cdot 12WO_3 \cdot 24H_2O \longrightarrow 3H^+ + [PW_{12}O_{40}]^{3-} + 24H_2O$$

phosphotungstic acid   phosphotungstate
(= *dodeca*-tungstophosphoric acid)   anion

The oxidation number of Mo and W in these compounds is +6. The heteropoly-acids are decomposed by alkalis to give molybdate (MoO_4^{2-}) or tungstate (WO_4^{2-}) and dibasic phosphate ions (see Cotton *et al.*, 1999). In aqueous solutions, PTA forms complex anions, $[PO_4(WO_3)_{12}]^{3-}$ as shown above, but these decompose if the pH rises above 2.0, to give $[(PO_5)_2(WO_3)_{17}]^{10-}$ and $[PO_6(WO_3)_{11}]^{7-}$ (Rieck, 1967). The ionic weights of these inorganic anions (2877, 4163 and 2677 respectively) are all greater than those of dyes; the largest of 436 dye ions reviewed by Dapson (2005a) weighed in at 1681. The heteropolyacid ions have approximately spherical structures; different from the large anions of direct cotton dyes, which can assume planar configurations.

The heteropolyacids are able to bind to tissues from aqueous or alcoholic solutions. Baker (1958) called them 'colourless anionic dyes'. Sites of attachment of PMA are easily demonstrated by subsequent treatment of the sections with either ultraviolet radiation or a chemical reducing agent such as stannous chloride. A blue mixture of insoluble oxides of Mo(V) and Mo(VI), with compositions such as $MoO_2(OH)$ and $MoO_{2.5}(OH)_{0.5}$, is formed. It is known as molybdenum blue. A corresponding but less intensely coloured tungsten blue, formulated as $WO_{2.7}$ can also be produced. Sites of binding of PTA to tissues have been studied under the electron microscope, with which the electron-dense tungsten-containing deposits can be accurately localized.

The various studies of the binding of heteropolyacids to tissues (Baker, 1958; Puchtler and Isler, 1958; Bulmer, 1962; Puchtler and Sweat, 1964b; Everett and Miller, 1974; Hayat, 1975, 1993; Allison and Tanswell, 1993; Reid *et al.*, 1993) are not all in agreement, but the following facts appear to be undisputed:

(1) Chemical studies indicate that PTA binds to proteins and amino acids but not to carbohydrates. Both the heteropolyacids are used as precipitants for proteins, amino acids, and alkaloids. The heteropolyacid anions are held by ionic attraction to protonated amino and guanidino groups of proteins.

(2) Applied at pH <1.5, PTA imparts electron density to carbohydrate-containing structures, but at pH > 1.5 it binds to proteins. PTA can oxidase carbohydrate hydroxyl groups to aldehydes, so the electron-dense deposits resulting from staining at pH <1.5 may be insoluble compounds in which the oxidation state of the tungsten is less than +6.

(3) Collagen fibres bind large amounts of PMA. Cytoplasm binds smaller amounts. Nuclei of cells have very little affinity for PMA. PTA behaves similarly.

(4) Affinity for PMA and PTA is depressed or abolished if amino groups in the tissue are first removed by treatment with nitrous acid or esterified by reaction with acetic anhydride or benzoyl chloride. In light microscopy there is no evidence for binding of PMA or PTA to carbohydrates or to hydroxyl groups of amino acids.

(5) Methylation of sections results in increased attachment of PMA to all parts of the tissue, including erythrocytes. Methylating agents add methyl groups to amine nitrogen atoms (increasing their basicity) and to hydroxyl oxygen atoms (forming ethers or glycosides).

(6) Structures that have bound PMA or PTA become stainable by cationic dyes. [This change is exploited in Monroe and Frommer's (1967) variant of Twort's stain (See Chapter 6, Section 6.4.2).]

(7) Treatment with PMA or PTA affects stainability by anionic dyes. The effects are variable:

(a) There is considerable suppression of the staining of all parts of the tissue by some anionic dyes, including ones with small molecules, such as picric acid, Martius yellow, eosin, orange G, and biebrich scarlet. The amount of suppression is greater in collagen than in cytoplasm.

(b) There is similar suppression of cytoplasmic staining by dyes that have large molecules, including aniline blue, light green SF, fast green FCF, and acid fuchsine, but collagen is stained with only slightly reduced intensity by these dyes after treatment of the sections with a heteropolyacid.

(c) Treatment of sections with PMA or PTA either before or at the same time as staining with aniline blue, light green SF, or fast green FCF has the effect of preventing the attachment of these dyes to materials other than collagen, cartilage matrix, and certain carbohydrate-containing secretory products.

(d) If sections are treated with PTA, stained with aniline blue, and then exposed to 6 M urea, a reagent which disrupts hydrogen bonds, the dye is removed, but the PTA remains attached to the collagen in the tissue. The treatment with urea may not, however, be a specific test for hydrogen bonding.

(e) Freezing and thawing before fixation of a tissue changes the colours imparted by trichrome staining methods, such that the cytoplasms of some cells are atypically stained by the dye with the larger molecules.

8.2.4.2. How do trichrome methods work?

Three hypotheses have been advanced to account for the differential colouring of tissues by anionic dyes used in association with heteropolyacids.

In the **first theory**, championed by Baker (1958), and upheld by Horobin (1982, 1988) as an example of 'rate controlled' staining, it is held that the anions of the dyes and of the heteropolyacids compete with one another for cationic binding sites and that the textures of the various structural components of a tissue determine their penetration by molecules of different size. PMA and PTA anions are assumed to be intermediate in size between those of the dyes generally used as cytoplasmic stains and those which stain collagen. Large dye ions exist in solution as aggregates, so this is a reasonable supposition despite the ionic weights of PMA and PTA being greater than those of large dye ions. The smallest dye anions would enter and bind to the supposedly dense network of haemoglobin and other protein molecules forming the stroma of the erythrocyte, which would not be penetrated by the heteropolyacid. The collagen fibre is considered to be more porous, and able to accommodate the ions of PMA or PTA and those of a dye with large molecules such as aniline blue or light green SF. Small dye ions could also penetrate the collagen fibres but, because they diffuse rapidly, they would enter and leave freely. The larger, more slowly diffusing particles of the heteropolyacids and of such dyes as aniline blue would remain in the collagen and become attached to cationic sites there. Dyes with molecules of intermediate size (e.g. acid fuchsine) would compete with PMA or PTA for binding sites in the cytoplasm of muscle fibres and other cells. These dye molecules would be too big to enter erythrocytes in the presence of dyes with small molecules, but they would be small enough to escape from collagen fibres more quickly than the largest dye molecules. Bulmer (1962) demonstrated that heteropolyacids were bound to tissues only when the latter contained protonated amino groups, but agreed with Baker (1958) in attributing the trichrome staining effects to differential permeability of cytoplasm and collagen to large and small molecules.

A similar postulated mechanism was discussed earlier in relation to the differential staining of cytoplasm and collagen in van Gieson's and related methods. The objections raised there also apply to the application of this hypothesis to the trichrome techniques. Furthermore, it is difficult, in terms of this theory, to account for the fact that treatment with heteropolyacids induces basophilia, as well as selective though depressed affinity for certain anionic dyes, in collagen. Control of staining by different rates of diffusion receives some support from the atypical staining of cells by dyes of high molecular weight in previously frozen and thawed specimens (Allison and Tanswell, 1993). Tiny holes made by ice crystals can be expected to cause increased porosity in cytoplasm.

The **second hypothesis** accounts adequately for the basophilia produced by treatment of collagen with PMA or PTA. Puchtler and Isler (1958) proposed that cationic dyes were attracted by the free negatively charged groups of the collagen-bound ions of heteropolyacid. For example:

$$\boxed{\text{COLLAGEN}} -\!\!-NH_2 + H^+ + [PMA]^{3-} \longrightarrow \boxed{\text{COLLAGEN}} -\!\!-NH_2^{+\,-}[PMA]^{2-}$$

$$\boxed{\text{COLLAGEN}} -\!\!-NH_2^{+\,-}[PMA]^{2-} + 2\,\boxed{\text{DYE}}^{+}$$

$$\longrightarrow \boxed{\text{COLLAGEN}} -\!\!-NH_2^{+\,-}[PMA]^{-}_{-} \;{}^{+}_{+}\; \boxed{\text{DYE}}$$

Thus, a function similar to that of a classical mordant (Chapter 5) is attributed to the heteropolyacid. Puchtler and Isler noted that the dyes used to stain collagen in trichrome techniques were all amphoteric. They suggested that these dyes were bound by ionic forces to the PMA or PTA, which was itself attached electrovalently to protonated amino and guanidino groups of collagen. The cytoplasmic stains used in trichrome techniques are wholly anionic dyes, so they would not attach to the free negatively charged sites of the bound heteropolyacid molecules.

Several objections can be made to this hypothesis. The staining of collagen is attributed to its content of amino acids with basic side-chains: lysine, arginine, and histidine. Haemoglobin, the principal protein of erythrocytes, has a higher proportion of these basic amino acids than collagen but erythrocytes are not similarly stained in the trichrome procedures. Classical mordanting by PMA or PTA would be expected to result in intensification of staining by amphoteric dyes: two molecules of dye would attach to each of the bound (trivalent) anions of the heteropolyacid. All investigators agree, however, that pre-treatment with PMA or PTA reduces the intensity of staining by aniline blue and similar dyes, even in collagen (Baker, 1958). The matrix of cartilage and the granules of mast cells, although they are composed of strongly acid proteoglycans (Chapter 11), are not ordinarily stained strongly by amphoteric dyes such as acid fuchsine and aniline blue, so these dyes do not behave as if they were cationic. Finally, the effect of 6 M urea on trichrome-stained sections indicates that the dye is bound to collagen by non-ionic forces whereas the heteropolyacid is held in place by a different and stronger force, probably ionic attraction as proposed by Puchtler and Isler (1958).

A **third explanation** for the actions of PMA and PTA in trichrome procedures was offered by Everett and Miller (1974), who provided evidence of two different modes of binding of these acids to tissues. Ionic attraction of the heteropolyacid ions to cytoplasmic proteins was thought to inhibit there the binding of anionic dyes. The binding of the heteropolyacids to collagen was believed to be non-ionic, so that staining by anionic dyes was not prevented. The principal objections to this hypothesis are that it does not account for either the fact that PMA cannot be removed from collagen by 6 M urea or the fact that staining of collagen after treatment with PMA or PTA can be effected by some anionic dyes but not by others.

In summary, there is much evidence to support the idea that the stainability of tissues is determined by rates of diffusion within parts of the tissue that are differently permeable to large and small anions, but this proposed mechanism does not explain how the dyes and the PMA or PTA are bound to the cytoplasm and collagen. The second and third of the postulated mechanisms cannot fully account for the differential staining obtained with the trichrome methods, but they do shed some light of the action of heteropolyacids, which evidently are held to tissue proteins by electrostatic attraction, and on the attachment of larger dyes to collagen, which appears to be by way of non-ionic forces, which may include hydrogen bonds and van der Waals forces.

8.2.5.
Five trichrome methods: instructions

The techniques of Masson, Mallory, and Heidenhain are done in stages. This allows some control of the intensity of colour in cytoplasm and collagen. Two one-step procedures (Cason and Gabe) are also described here. They are technically simpler than the classical trichromes, but do not always work as well. See Luna (1968), Gabe (1976), Clark (1981) and Bancroft and Gamble (2002) for detailed technical instructions for these and other trichrome methods.

The **fixative** for tissues to be stained by any trichrome method should not be a simple formaldehyde solution with no other active ingredients, and it should not contain glutaraldehyde. Non-aqueous fixatives are not recommended. Mercury-containing mixtures such as SUSA give excellent results, and Bouin is also satisfactory. If you have used a mercury-containing fixative, do not forget to treat the sections with iodine and thiosulphate before staining (Chapter 4, Section 4.4.1). According to Churukian et al. (2000), zinc–formalin (Chapter 2) is also a satisfactory fixative for trichrome staining. The staining properties of neutral-formaldehyde-fixed tissue, especially of cytoplasm, can be improved by immersing hydrated paraffin sections overnight in fixative solutions such as Bouin, Zenker or zinc–formalin, either overnight at room temperature or for 10–15 min at 55–60°C. Saturated aqueous picric acid is as effective as Bouin (unpublished observations). Yu and Chapman (2003) pre-treated slides with either an iodine solution (0.33% I_2 in 0.67% aqueous KI) or a citrate buffer at pH 4 prior to staining by Masson's method. The mechanisms of action of pretreatments that enhance trichrome staining are in need of investigation.

Nuclei are stained by the dye with molecules of intermediate size (red in the methods that follow), but it is often desirable to stain them black instead, with an iron–haematoxylin (Chapter 6). This is always done with Masson's technique. Prior nuclear staining reduces the brilliance of the colours in cytoplasm and collagen, but it often improves the overall morphological clarity of the stained preparation.

8.2.5.1. Masson's trichrome
This is the simplest trichrome, because only two anionic dyes are used, after staining the nuclei with iron–haematoxylin. There are many variants of this method, using different dyes or a different heteropolyacid solution (see *Note* below). The following version is that of Luna (1968).

Solutions required
A. Iodine and sodium thiosulphate
For removing mercury deposits (Chapter 4).

B. Acid–alcohol
May be needed for differentiation of the nuclear stain.

Ethanol (95% or 100%):	140 ml
Concentrated hydrochloric acid:	1 ml
Water:	to make 200 ml

Mix before using and use only once.

C. Acidified water
This is water with about 5 ml of glacial acetic acid added to each litre.

D. Weigert's or Lillie's iron–hematoxylin
See Chapter 6.

E. Biebrich scarlet-acid fuchsine
Biebrich scarlet (C.I. 26905):	4.5 g
Acid fuchsine (C.I. 42685):	0.5 g
Water:	495 ml
Glacial acetic acid:	5 ml

Keeps for several months and may be used repeatedly. Filter before using.

F. PMA–PTA solution
Phosphomolybdic acid (also known as molybdophosphoric acid):	5 g
Phosphotungstic acid (also known as tungstophosphoric acid):	5 g
Water:	200 ml

Keeps for about 5 years, and goes on working despite a change in color from yellow to green.

G. Fast green FCF, 2%
Fast green FCF (C.I. 42053):	4.0 g
Water:	195 ml
Glacial acetic acid:	2.0 ml

Keeps for several years and may be used repeatedly.

Procedure
(1)   De-wax sections and bring to 70% alcohol. The next two steps are necessary if the fixative contained mercuric chloride. Otherwise they may be skipped.
(2)   Remove mercury deposits by immersion in Gram's iodine (1% I_2 in 2% aqueous KI) for 30 s. (Alternatively, use 0.5% iodine in 70% alcohol, which needs 3 min.)
(3)   Remove iodine stain by immersion in 5% sodium thiosulphate solution until sections are no longer yellow or brown (about 15 s). Proceed to Step 5.
(4)   If the fixative did not contain picric acid or mercuric chloride, place the slides in *either* saturated aqueous picric acid *or* Bouin's fluid *or* a zinc–formalin fixative solution. Duration of the pretreatment may be overnight at room temperature or 2 h at 55–60°C.
(5)   Wash in tap water (3 changes, or running water for 2 min), then in distilled water, 30–60 s. (If the fixative did not contain mercuric chloride, and the iodine-thiosulphate treatment was omitted, simply place in distilled water for 1 min with agitation for the first 30 s.)
(6)   Stain nuclei in a working iron–hematoxylin (Solution D) for 3 min. Rinse in tap water and check wet slide under a microscope. Only nuclei should be stained. See Chapter 6 for action to be taken if nuclear staining is unsatisfactory.
(7)   Wash in running tap water for 1 min.
(8)   Stain for 4 min in biebrich scarlet–acid fuchsine (Solution E).
(9)   Rinse in slightly acidified water (Solution C) to remove excess dye.
(10) Immerse in PMA–PTA (Solution F) for 10 min. Rinse in acidified water and check a slide under a microscope to ensure that the red dye has been removed from collagen. Return to the PMA–PTA solution for another 5 min if necessary.

(11) Stain for 4 min in 2% fast green FCF (Solution G).
(12) Immerse in 2 changes of slightly acidified water, each for about 30 s. (A longer time in the second change does no harm.)
(13) Dehydrate in 3 changes of 100% alcohol, clear in xylene and apply coverslips, using a resinous mounting medium.

Result
Nuclei black. Cytoplasm in shades of pink, red and brown. Erythrocytes, keratin and myelin scarlet. Collagen fibers strong bluish-green. Mucus lighter green.

Note
Masson (1929) used a more complicated iron–haematoxylin nuclear stain. For red dyes he used a mixture of acid fuchsine with an azo dye that was probably ponceau 2R (C.I. 16150). He used 1% PMA for the heteropolyacid and either aniline blue or light green for the collagen stain. In the present variant, following Lillie (1945), fast green FCF is used instead of light green because the latter fades with time (Chapter 5).

8.2.5.2. Mallory's trichrome
Mallory described at least three trichrome procedures. This one (Mallory, 1905) is the simplest.

Solutions required
A. Iodine and sodium thiosulphate
For removing mercury deposits (Chapter 4).

B. Acidified water
This is water with about 5 ml of glacial acetic acid added to each litre.

C. Acid fuchsine, 0.5%

Acid fuchsine (C.I. 42685):	1.0 g
Water:	200 ml

Keeps indefinitely and may be reused many times.

D. Aniline blue–orange G-PTA solution

Aniline blue (C.I. 42755):	1.0 g

Alternatively use methyl blue (C.I. 42780). These dyes are sometimes labeled soluble blue, water blue or aniline blue, water soluble. Aniline blue, alcohol-soluble (spirit blue; C.I. 42775) *cannot* be used in this solution.

Orange G (C.I. 16230):	4.0 g
Phosphotungstic acid (also called tungstophosphoric acid):	2.0 g
Water:	200 ml

Stable for about 2 years, but deteriorates with repeated use.

Procedure
(1) De-wax sections and bring to 70% alcohol. The next two steps are necessary if the fixative contained mercuric chloride. Otherwise they may be skipped.
(2) Remove mercury deposits by immersion in Gram's iodine (1% I_2 in 2% aqueous KI) for 30 s. (Alternatively, use 0.5% iodine in 70% alcohol, which needs 3 min.)
(3) Remove iodine stain by immersion in 5% sodium thiosulphate solution until sections are no longer yellow or brown (about 15 s). Proceed to Step 5.
(4) If the fixative did not contain picric acid or mercuric chloride, place the slides in *either* saturated aqueous picric acid *or* Bouin's fluid *or* a zinc–formalin fixative solution. Duration of the pretreatment may be overnight at room

temperature or 2 h at 55–60°C. (This option was not included in Mallory's original method.)

(5) Wash in tap water (3 changes, or running water for 2 min), then in distilled water, 30–60 s. (If the fixative did not contain mercuric chloride, and the iodine-thiosulphate treatment was omitted, simply place in distilled water for 1 min with agitation for the first 30 s.)

(6) Immerse in 0.5% acid fuchsine for 2 min.

(7) Shake off excess dye solution and transfer the slides directly into the aniline blue–orange G-PTA solution. Leave there for 30 min.

(8) Immerse in acidified water to wash off excess dye, shake the slides and transfer them to a clean, dry staining rack or Coplin jar.

(9) Dehydrate in 3 changes of 100% alcohol, clear in xylene and apply coverslips, using a resinous mounting medium.

Result
Nuclei red. Collagen blue. Cytoplasm in various shades of red, pink and orange. Erythrocytes and myelin yellow. Mucus and cartilage matrix blue.

Note
If Step 6 is omitted, blue and orange nuclei will be be seen in sections 6 μm and thicker, with the percentage of yellow nuclei increasing with section thickness. Lison (1955) deduced that aniline blue enters and stains only nuclei that have been cut by the microtome knife whereas orange G stains nuclei that are entirely contained in the section. Baccari et al. (1992a,b) found that treatment with RNase increased the proportion of orange nuclei and postulated that the blue nuclear staining occurred in cells with high rates of RNA synthesis.

8.2.5.3. Heidenhain's AZAN
This is the trichrome method that gives the user maximum control of the colours, because there are two destaining (differentiation) steps. AZAN (the acronym refers to *Azokarmin* and *Anilinblau*) is useful for showing cytoplasmic and extracellular structures, and it displays fine collagen and reticular fibers with brilliant clarity, even in sections as thick as 10 μm. The method takes 3 h, and is too troublesome for routine use with large numbers of slides.

For optimal staining of secretory products and other cytoplasmic components the tissue should have been fixed in a mixture containing mercuric chloride and either potassium dichromate or formaldehyde or both these compounds (Chapter 2). Treatment of sections of formaldehyde-fixed tissue with Bouin's fluid or saturated aqueous picric acid (as described for the Masson and Mallory techniques, in place of steps 2 and 3 of the procedure below) improves the colour contrast between cytoplasm and connective tissue but does not provide the sharply defined cytoplasmic detail that can be seen in well fixed cells stained by the AZAN method (my unpublished observations).

The most critical stage of the AZAN procedure is the first differentiation (in aniline–alcohol). The prescribed times for the other stages may be exceeded but cannot be shortened. This is the method as adapted by Gabe (1976).

Solutions required
A. Acidified water
This is water with about 5 ml of glacial acetic acid added to each litre.

B. Aniline–alcohol
70% ethanol:	400 ml
Aniline:	4 ml

Keeps for a few months. Can be reused even when pink from extracted azo-carmine, though there's little reason to keep the mixture for a long time. **Caution.** Aniline is poisonous and can pass through intact skin.

C. Acetic–alcohol
95% alcohol:	200 ml
Glacial acetic acid:	2 ml

Keeps for a few weeks.

D. Phosphotungstic acid, 5%
Phosphotungstic acid (also known as tungstophosphoric acid):	10 g
Water:	200 ml

Keeps for at least 2 years. Can be reused even when pink from extracted azo-carmine.

E. Azocarmine solution
Either azocarmine G (C.I. 50085) or azocarmine B (C.I. 50090) may be used. The latter is more soluble in water. Add 2 g of dye to 200 ml of water, heat to boiling, allow to cool to room temperature, filter to remove undissolved material, and add 2 ml of glacial acetic acid. Do not filter again, despite precipitation of some dye. This solution is stable for one year at room temperature (shake and heat to 55°C when needed), or for two weeks if it is kept all the time at 55°C.

F. Heidenhain's blue–orange: stock solution
Aniline blue (C.I. 42755):	1.0 g

Alternatively use methyl blue (C.I. 42780). These dyes are sometimes labeled water blue, soluble blue or aniline blue, water soluble. Aniline blue, alcohol-soluble (spirit blue; C.I. 42775) *cannot* be used in this solution.

Orange G (C.I. 16230):	4.0 g
Water:	200 ml
Glacial acetic acid:	16 ml

Stock solution is stable for at least 2 years. The blue component becomes weaker with age.

G. Heidenhain's blue–orange: working solution
Stock solution:	10 ml
Water:	20 ml

Working solution may be used repeatedly over the course of two or three weeks.

Procedure
(1) De-wax sections and bring to 70% alcohol. The next two steps are necessary if the fixative contained mercuric chloride. Otherwise they may be skipped.

(2) Remove mercury deposits by immersion in Gram's iodine (1% I_2 in 2% aqueous KI) for 30 s. (Alternatively, use 0.5% iodine in 70% alcohol, which needs 3 min.)

(3) Remove iodine stain by immersion in 5% sodium thiosulphate solution until sections are no longer yellow or brown (about 15 s).

(4) Wash in tap water (3 changes, or running water for 2 min), then in distilled water, 30–60 s. (If the fixative did not contain mercuric chloride, and the iodine-thiosulphate treatment was omitted, simply place in distilled water for 1 m with agitation for the first 30 s.)

(5) Put all the slides in a covered jar of pre-heated azocarmine solution (55°C) for 1 h. Make sure that the temperature does not rise above 60°C.

(6) Agitate the slides in running tap water for a few seconds to remove excess dye, including any insoluble red particles.

(7) Wash in two changes of deionized or distilled water.

(8) Put one slide into aniline–alcohol, and agitate gently. Keeping an eye on a clock with a second hand, watch the disappearance of much red color from the tissue. After about 1 min rinse this test slide in distilled water.

(9) Put the test slide onto the stage of a microscope. Nuclei should stand out sharply in red against a pink background. If necessary, return the slide to aniline alcohol for another minute, and re-examine. This checking may have to be done several times, and the time needed for this differentiation must be determined carefully for every batch of sections. Do not attempt to remove all the red dye from cytoplasm and collagen. The time needed for the aniline–alcohol differentiation is typically two to three min, but it may range from 30 s to more than 10 min. The end-point is reached when nuclei and some other components of the tissue (notably erythrocytes, the matrix of bone in decalcified specimens, and some cytoplasmic granules) are bright red and most other components are either pink or unstained. In smooth or striated muscle, nuclei should be easily visible against a more lightly stained background. When differentiation is judged to be correct, put the test slide into acetic–alcohol.

(10) Place the remaining slides in aniline–alcohol for the time found to give optimum differentiation, then move them into acetic–alcohol for about 1 min. (Longer times in acetic–alcohol do no harm).

(11) Transfer the slides to 5% phosphotungstic acid for 30 min.

(12) Rinse in slightly acidified water and check with a microscope. There should be no pink color in collagen. If any pink collagen is seen, return the slides to 5% phosphotungstic acid for another 30 min, and check again. (This stage may take 2 h. Impatience leads to poor results.)

(13) Immerse the slides in the working solution of Heidenhain's blue-orange for 60 min.

(14) Rinse in slightly acidified water, 15–30 s with agitation.

(15) Dehydrate in 3 changes of 100% alcohol, clear in xylene and apply coverslips, using a resinous mounting medium.

Result
Nuclei and erythrocytes bright red. Cytoplasm mostly orange or yellow, some red, some blue. Muscle cytoplasm ideally is orange–red. Secretory granules are strongly colored and stand out with great clarity after proper fixation. Collagen, reticular fibers and basement membranes dark blue. Cartilage matrix and mucus light blue. Matrix of decalcified bone red. Keratin and myelin orange. Gliotic areas in the central nervous system (fibrous astrocytes) red. Elastin is unstained.

Note
If the procedure must be interrupted during staining with azocarmine or differentiation in aniline–alcohol, transfer the slides to acetic- alcohol, in which they may remain for many hours. Rinse in distilled water before resuming the procedure. If there is to be an interruption in the treatment with phosphotungstic acid or Heidenhain's blue–orange, keep the slides in slightly acidified water.

8.2.5.1. Cason's trichrome
The one-solution method (Cason, 1950), which has aniline blue as the collagen stain, is for thin (less than 7 μm) sections. The prior staining of nuclei with iron–haematoxylin, not included in the original method, is optional.

Solutions required

A. Weigert's iron–haematoxylin (working solution)
See Chapter 6.

B. Cason's trichrome solution

Water:	200 ml

Dissolve in order stated:

Phosphotungstic acid:	1.0 g
Orange G (C.I. 16230):	2.0 g
Aniline blue (C.I. 42755):	1.0 g
Acid fuchsine (C.I. 42685):	3.0 g

Can be kept and used repeatedly for at least 5 years.

C. Acidified water
This is water with about 5 ml of glacial acetic acid added to each litre.

Procedure

(1–5) As for Masson's (Section 8.2.5.1) or Mallory's (Section 8.2.5.2) methods.
(6)   (*Optional*) Stain in Weigert's haematoxylin, 5 min.
(7)   Wash in running tap water, 2 min.
(8)   Immerse in Cason's trichrome solution, 5 min.
(9)   Wash in acidified water.
(10) Dehydrate rapidly in three changes of 100% ethanol.
(11) Clear in xylene and cover, using a resinous medium.

Result

Collagen blue. Cytoplasm, including muscle red. Keratin, and erythrocytes orange. Nuclei black to brown (but sometimes blue). The pre-staining with iron–haematoxylin makes the trichrome colours a little unpredictable with some material. If the nuclear stain with iron–haematoxylin is omitted, most nuclei are red: others may be blue or unstained.

8.2.5.2. Gabe's trichrome

This one-step technique (Gabe, 1976) can be applied to thicker sections, because fast green FCF colours the collagen less intensely than the aniline blue of Cason's mixture. An iron–haematoxylin nuclear stain (Step 6) does not interfere with the distribution of colours from the subsequently applied trichrome mixture.

Solutions required

A. An iron–haematoxylin
Such as that of Weigert or Lillie (Chapter 6).

B. One-step trichrome solution

Amaranth (C.I. 16185):	2.5 g
Phosphomolybdic acid:	2.5 g
Fast green FCF (C.I. 42053):	1.0 g
Water:	500 ml
Glacial acetic acid:	5.0 ml

Stir until all dissolved, then add:

Martius yellow (C.I. 10315):	0.5 g

Leave on magnetic stirrer for 1 h, then filter to remove undissolved Martius yellow. The solution is ready for use immediately, may be used repeatedly, and is stable for at least 5 years.

Naphthol yellow S (C.I. 10316), 0.05 g, may be used instead of Martius yellow. This dye dissolves completely and filtration is not needed.

C. Acidified water
Add 5 ml acetic acid (glacial) to 1 l of water.

Procedure
(1–5) As for Masson's (Section 8.2.5.1) or Mallory's (Section 8.2.5.2) methods.
(6) (*Optional*) Stain nuclei with an iron haematoxylin (Solution A).
(7) Wash in running tap water, 2 min.
(8) Immerse in Gabe's trichrome mixture (Solution B) for 10–15 min.
(9) Wash in two changes of acidified water.
(10) Shake off most of the water and dehydrate directly in 100% alcohol, 3 changes. (There is no need for speed in the washing or dehydration, because the colours are not extracted.)
(11) Clear in xylene and cover, using a resinous mounting medium.

Results
Nuclei black if stained with iron–haematoxylin; otherwise red. Cytoplasm pink, red or greyish purple. Erythrocytes yellow (ideally, but sometimes pink). Collagen fibres bluish green. Mucus, matrix of cartilage, and some secretory granules are also green.

8.3. Methods for reticulin

The methods for selective staining of reticulin, which are based on reduction of gold or silver salts, are explained in Chapter 18. Reticular fibres are also shown by the picro-sirius red method, with which they exhibit green birefringence. With benzo blue BB instead of sirius red F3B the birefringence colour of reticular fibres is yellow (Section 8.2.3.3).

8.4. Methods for elastin

There is no completely satisfactory explanation for the modes of action of the various staining methods for elastin.

8.4.1.
Binding of dyes to elastic fibres

Dyes are certainly not attracted to elastin by electrostatic forces (see Baker, 1958 and Horobin, 1982 for review of evidence). Thermodynamic studies, based on measurement of half-staining times with orcein at different temperatures, indicate that elastic fibres have low permeability to this dye (which stains them selectively), but that there are large numbers of weak (non-ionic) dye-binding sites per unit volume of substrate (Friedberg and Goldstein, 1969). It was once generally supposed that hydrogen bonding was primarily involved (see Pearse, 1968b). However, Horobin and James (1970) showed that elastic fibres could be coloured by dyes incapable of forming hydrogen bonds. These investigators found that the only feature held in common by all of a large number of dyes that stained elastin was the presence of at least five aromatic or quinonoid rings in the molecule. Chemical blocking methods for many reactive groups did not appreciably reduce the staining of elastin by such dyes, and the prevention of hydrogen bonding caused only slight inhibition. Horobin and James proposed that large dye molecules were bound to elastic tissue in the same way that they are thought to be bound to some textile fibres: namely by van der Waals forces or hydrophobic interactions. These types of intermolecular attraction have been explained in Chapter 5. Further evidence of hydrophobic bonding of dyes to elastin was obtained by Horobin and Flemming

(1980), who correlated several structural features of dye molecules with the ability to bind to elastic fibres. The most effective dyes were those whose molecules had the longest chains of conjugated bonds (alternating single and double bonds; see Chapter 5), and the greatest numbers of hydrophobic groups. It should be remembered that direct dyes are anionic, and they also colour all acidophilic components of a tissue, though not as intensely as elastin, when applied from aqueous solutions. Anionic dyes with smaller molecules, such as eosin, stain elastin lightly.

Synthetic dyes of known structure, such as those investigated by Horobin and colleagues, are not used in the traditional methods for elastin. The staining agents still most frequently employed are the following:

(a)   **Weigert's resorcin–fuchsine**, a compound made by boiling basic fuchsine with resorcinol and ferric chloride.
(b)   **Orcein**, a mixture of oxazine dyes, made by the action of oxygen and ammonia on orcinol (Chapter 5).
(c)   **Verhoeff's stain**, a mixture of haematoxylin, ferric chloride, iodine and potassium iodide. This also stains nuclei and the myelin sheaths of nerve fibres.
(d)   **Aldehyde–fuchsine**, made by reaction of pararosaniline with acetaldehyde. The resulting product colours elastic fibres and laminae and also binds to strong acid (sulphonic or sulphate–ester) groups, and aldehyde groups in the tissue.

Resorcin–fuchsine contains dimeric and trimeric compounds formed by oxidative coupling (Proctor and Horobin, 1983). The components of orcein contain 4 or 6 conjugated six-membered rings, with methyl and phenolic side-chains (see Beecken et al., 2003). It is probable that these large dyes stain elastin by virtue of van der Waals forces acting at multiple hydrophobic sites and hydrogen bonding to peptide linkages (Prento, 2001). Verhoeff's stain and aldehyde–fuchsine are considered in the next two sections of the chapter.

8.4.2.
Verhoeff's stain

Some of the Fe^{3+} in the staining solution oxidizes haematoxylin to haematein, which forms black complexes with iron ions. The actions of iodine and iodide remain obscure. Experiments with mixtures of varying composition were carried out by Puchtler and Waldrop (1979), who found that increasing the concentration of iodine increased the stability of the solution, but reduced the intensity of staining of elastin. The iodine in an aqueous solution containing iodide is present as triodide (I_3^-) ions. In some variants of Verhoeff's method (e.g. Clark, 1981) the iodine is omitted, though some must be formed from oxidation of iodide ions by Fe^{3+}. Puchtler and Waldrop suggest that the iodide ions serve as ligands that bind together those iron atoms that are complexed to haematein molecules. The resulting complexes would be large, coloured molecules and might be expected to bind to elastin by van der Waals forces.

As an iron–haematoxylin mixture, Verhoeff's stain imparts its black colour also to nuclei of cells, and to myelinated nerve fibres. Other components of the tissue are grey, unless a contrasting counterstain is applied.

The following method is that of Musto (1981). Any fixative may be used.

Solutions required
The stock solutions (A, B, C) are all stable for at least a year. The working solution (D) is made before using and used only once.

A. Haematoxylin
2% in 95% ethanol

B. Acidified ferric chloride:

FeCl$_3$.6H$_2$O:	12.4 g
Water:	495 ml
Concentrated HCl:	5 ml

C. Iodine

2% I$_2$ in 4% aqueous potassium iodide (KI)

D. Working solution

Solution A:	30 ml
Solution B:	20 ml
Solution C:	10 ml

E. Counterstain

If elastic laminae and fibres are the sole object of interest, no other stain is needed. Used alone, Verhoeff's haematoxylin also stains cell nuclei and gives a light grey background. If a more informative preparation is needed, apply a counterstain, following the principles explained in Chapter 6. The van Gieson method (Section 8.2.2) is also suitable.

Procedure

(1) De-wax and hydrate paraffin sections. (See *Note* below if the specimen was fixed in a solution that had formaldehyde as the only active ingredient.)

(2) Stain in the working solution (D) for about 45 min. The staining is progressive, and should be checked at intervals. To do this, rinse a slide in water and use a microscope to look for elastic laminae in the walls of arteries.

(3) (Optional) Apply a suitable counterstain.

Result

Elastic fibres, nuclei, and myelin sheaths (if present) black. Cytoplasm and collagen are coloured by the counterstain.

Note

Musto (1981) recommended a pretreatment with Bouin's solution for 10 min at 55°C (or overnight at room temperature) for sections of formalin fixed material. If this is done, the slides must be washed in running water until the sections are no longer yellow.

8.4.3. Aldehyde–fuchsine

Gomori's aldehyde–fuchsine reagent is made in the laboratory by treating pararosaniline with acetaldehyde (formed by acid-catalysed depolymerization of paraldehyde). The reaction occurs slowly, so that the solution matures and then deteriorates over the course of a few weeks. Alternatively, the product of the reaction may be precipitated, collected, and then dissolved when needed. This reagent provides one of the most easily used staining methods for elastin, but it is not entirely specific; it binds also to strong carbohydrate polyacids including heparin and the chondroitin sulphates (Chapter 11), and to the oxidation product of cystine (Chapter 10). The staining properties differ according to the way in which the stain is prepared (Mowry, 1978), but all variants are effective in colouring elastin. Redissolved and precipitated aldehyde–fuchsine stains less brightly than an optimally matured solution, and absorption spectra indicate that solutions have compositions that vary with the ways they are made (Nettleton, 1982).

Aldehyde–fuchsine is believed to contain condensation products of acetaldehyde with the amino groups of pararosaniline, with such structures as:

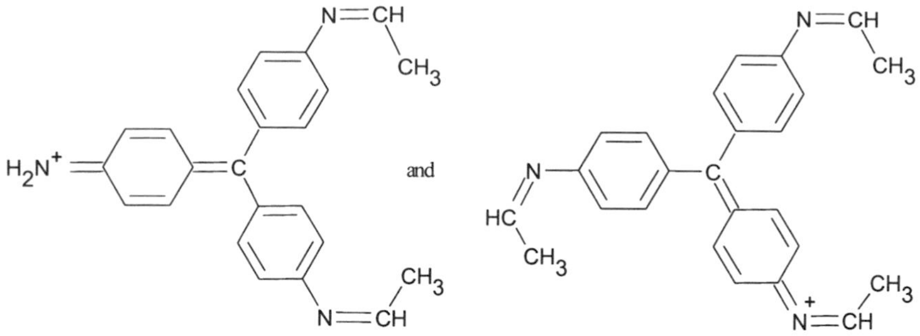

(Bangle, 1954; Buehner *et al.*, 1979; Lichtenstein and Nettleton, 1980; Proctor and Horobin, 1988). The binding to elastin is non-ionic (Goldstein, 1962), but extremely resistant to extraction. Such properties are to be expected of many dyes with large molecules (Chapter 5). Desmosine and isodesmosine structures are the most obvious chemically specific feature of elastin; they are formed in part from reactions of amines with aldehydes (Section 8.1.2). Free aldehyde groups in elastin could join covalently to aldehyde fuchsine.

In addition to elastic fibres and laminae, aldehyde–fuchsine stains the sites of half-sulphate esters (Chapter 11), and sulphonic acid or aldehyde groups artificially introduced into the tissue (Sumner, 1965; Gabe, 1976). If sections are treated with an oxidizing agent prior to staining, many carbohydrate components will be coloured (hydroxyls oxidized to aldehydes), as will sites of high concentration of disulphide groups (cystine oxidized to cysteic acid; see Chapter 10). The B cells of the pancreatic islets contain insulin, which is rich in cystine, but can be stained by fresh (not by reconstituted) solutions of aldehyde–fuchsine even without prior oxidation. The reason for this is unknown. In unoxidized sections, any sample of aldehyde–fuchsine stains elastin, the granules of mast cells and cartilage matrix.

Preparation of stain
There are many ways of preparing aldehyde fuchsine. The following (from Gabe, 1976) has the advantage of yielding a solid product which is stable for at least 10 years. It is important to use pararosaniline (C.I. 42500) or a sample of basic fuchsine consisting only of this dye (Mowry and Emmel, 1977).

Dissolve 1.0 g of pararosaniline in 200 ml of water (heat to boiling, then allow to cool to room temperature). Add 2.0 ml of concentrated hydrochloric acid and 1.0 ml of paraldehyde. Leave for 24 h, or for longer if a pink ring appears when the deep purple mixture is spotted onto filter paper. Filter. Discard the filtrate. Wash the residue with 50 ml of water. Dry the filter paper and its contents in an oven at 60°C. Collect and keep the aldehyde–fuchsine powder.

Working solution:
Aldehyde–fuchsine powder:	0.25 g
70% ethanol:	200 ml
Acetic acid (glacial):	2.0 ml

Leave overnight to dissolve. Filtration is not needed. The reconstituted solution is stable for 2 years.

Procedure
(1) De-wax and hydrate paraffin sections.
(2) Stain in aldehyde–fuchsine for 5 min.
(3) Rinse in running tap water to remove most of excess dye.

(4) Rinse in 95% ethanol containing 0.5% (v/v) concentrated hydrochloric acid until any remaining excess of dye is removed (usually 20–30 s; longer times do no harm.)

(5) Apply a counterstain if desired (alum–haematoxylin and fast green FCF make a suitable combination; see Chapter 6).

(6) Wash, dehydrate, clear, and cover.

Result

Elastic fibres and laminae purple. Oxytalan fibres (See Section 8.1.2) are stained by aldehyde–fuchsine only after treatment with an oxidizing agent (Lillie and Fullmer, 1976).

Note

Aldehyde–fuchsine is also used in methods for staining the endocrine pancreas, the adenohypophysis, mast cells, and neurosecretory material. The different techniques vary somewhat and are described by Luna (1968), Pearse (1968b, 1985), and Mowry (1978).

8.4.4.
Orcein

This is one of the oldest, and probably the easiest method for elastin, but the colour is less intense than that imparted by Verhoeff's method or by aldehyde–fuchsine. Bound orcein is not easily extracted, so it may be followed by almost any counterstain for nuclei, cytoplasm or collagen. If the nuclei are to be stained with an iron–haematoxylin, however, this should be done before staining the elastic fibres with orcein. Clark (1981) gives instructions for several multi-dye techniques that include orcein. As with the other methods for elastin, almost any fixation may be used.

Staining solution

Orcein:	1 g
70% alcohol:	100 ml

Heat to about 60°C, with stirring. Cool. Add 1 ml concentrated hydrochloric acid, and filter to remove any undissolved material. Keeps for several months. It is used at 37°C.

Procedure

(1) Take the sections to 70% alcohol.

(2) Stain in the orcein solution for 30–60 min at 37°C.

(3) Rinse in 70% alcohol and examine. If there is a brown background (in collagen and nuclei), differentiate in acid–alcohol (1 ml concentrated hydrochloric acid in 99 ml 70% alcohol). This usually takes only a few seconds.

(4) Wash in running tap water, at least 30 s

(5) Counterstain as required, dehydrate, clear and cover.

Result

Elastic fibres and laminae brown.

Note

For colour photographs of staining by various techniques using orcein, see Henwood (2003).

9 Methods for nucleic acids

9.1. Chemistry and distribution of nucleic acids

The nucleic acids are macromolecular compounds with the general repeating structure:

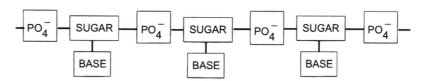

The phosphate and sugar moieties are shown in more detail in *Fig. 9.1*. The bases are pyrimidines or purines. These are heterocyclic aromatic compounds with 6- or 9-membered rings respectively. The two purine bases adenine and guanine and the pyrimidine base cytosine are present in DNA and RNA. The fourth base, a pyrimidine, is thymine in DNA, but uracil in RNA. The structural formulae of these bases are indicated in *Fig. 9.1* and are more fully explained in textbooks of biochemistry. The constituent units of a nucleic acid molecule are **nucleotides**, each consisting of a base, a sugar and a phosphate group. A **nucleoside** is formed from a base and a sugar only. In deoxyribonucleic acid (DNA) the sugar is deoxyribose (the full name is α-2-deoxyribofuranose), whereas it is ribose (α-ribofuranose) in ribonucleic acid (RNA). For a detailed account of the chemistry of nucleic acids, see Mainwaring *et al.* (1982).

In a **eukaryotic cell**, most of the DNA is in the chromosomes of the nucleus. There the molecules of DNA form paired strands, held in the famous double helical configuration discovered by Watson and Crick (1953). The chains of nucleotide units are held together by weak forces (hydrogen bonds and hydrophobic interactions) between **complementary bases**: guanine pairs with cytosine, and adenine pairs

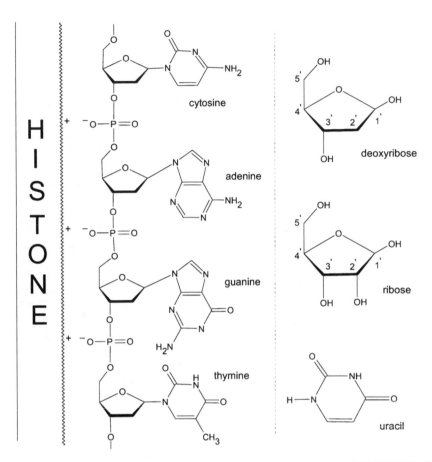

Figure 9.1. The left side of this diagram shows the structure of a tiny fragment of a single strand of DNA in a chromosome, associated with part of a basic nucleoprotein molecule, which neutralizes the phosphate groups of the DNA. On the right, the structure of 2-deoxyribose (of DNA) is shown alongside that of ribose (of RNA). Uracil (in RNA) differs from thymine only in the absence of one amino group. The numbers 1' to 5' identify the carbon atoms of the pentose sugars. Thickened lines indicate that the furanose rings lie perpendicular to the plane of the paper, with carbons 2' and 3' nearest to the reader. (See also Chapter 11 for structural formulae of sugars.) The aromatic rings of the bases are stacked in the centre of the double helix. The sugars, phosphoric acid groups and histones are on the outside.

with thymine. The backbone of the DNA helix consists of alternating phosphate and deoxyribose subunits, which form the outside of the spiral. The bases, which are hydrophobic, are directed into the centre of the helix. There they form a stack, with their planar aromatic rings perpendicular to the long axis of the macromolecule, and separated from one another by 0.36 nm. The external diameter of a DNA double helix is 1.8 nm. In eukaryotic cells the negative charges on the ionized free hydroxyl groups of the phosphoric acid residues are neutralized by the basic side-chains of the accompanying molecules of **nucleoproteins**: principally the strongly basic proteins known as **histones**, which are rich in lysine and arginine and have molecular weights in the range 12 000–20 000. The nucleoproteins also include species with very large molecules, of molecular weight 10^7 to 10^9.

In a **prokaryotic cell** such as a bacterium the DNA is in a single chain, not associated with a histone. The phosphate ions of the DNA are neutralized by small organic anions. Most of the DNA in a bacterium is concentrated in a central region, the **nucleoid**. Numerous loops of the DNA molecule extend from the nucleoid into the surrounding protoplasm, which contains ribosomes (see Robinow and Kellenberger, 1994).

The strands of DNA separate from one another immediately before they act as templates for the synthesis of new DNA (prior to mitosis) or of mRNA (transcription, prior to protein synthesis). In life, the separation is controlled by enzymes. The strands of DNA in dead tissue can be induced to separate by heating in the presence of a substance that disrupts hydrogen bonds; formamide (H_2NCHO) is used for this purpose in the technique of *in situ* hybridization (Section 9.6).

RNA has a more open structure than DNA. Most of it is in the ribosomes (ribosomal RNA or rRNA) and in the nucleolus, and most is in single-stranded form. Most of the messenger RNA (mRNA) in a cell is, at any one time, attached to the ribosomes. The much smaller transfer RNA (tRNA) molecules move between the ribosomes and the cytosol. Strands of RNA are folded in a complicated manner, owing to interactions between pairs of bases: guanine with cytosine, and adenine with uracil. The spacing between bases is 0.36 nm. During the process of transcription, similar base pairs are formed with chromosomal DNA and mRNA in the nucleus. The ribosomal and nucleolar RNA, like the chromosomal DNA, is associated with nucleoprotein. The nucleic acids of prokaryotic cells (organisms without nuclei in their protoplasm) have their phosphoric acid groups balanced by inorganic ions (Na^+, Mg^{2+}) and by certain amines.

The histochemical procedures discussed in this chapter demonstrate DNA only in the nucleus and RNA only in the nucleolus and ribosomes, although it is known that the nucleic acids are by no means confined to these situations. The nucleic acids of prokaryotes (such as bacteria) can also be stained. The Giemsa method (Chapter 7) displays the bacterial nucleoid with striking clarity, within the limits of resolution of ordinary light microscopy (Robinow and Kellenberger, 1994). This chapter also contains a brief introduction to hybridization histochemistry, in which a particular species of nucleic acid (such as the mRNA for a known protein) can be demonstrated by virtue of its affinity for suitably labelled complementary RNA or DNA molecules. Techniques known as end labelling, used to recognize the DNA of certain types of dying cell, are also discussed.

Both the nucleic acids can be stained with cationic dyes, and DNA can be demonstrated selectively by the Feulgen reaction. The specificity of a histochemical method for DNA or RNA can be confirmed by specific removal of either of these substances by enzymatic hydrolysis or chemical extraction.

9.2. Demonstration of nucleic acids with dyes and fluorochromes

The chemistry of the staining of nucleic acids by cationic dyes has already been discussed in Chapter 6. The process is considered to be histochemical when conditions are carefully standardized and suitable control procedures are carried out. Any basic dye may be used for the purpose, but the specificity of staining of nucleic acids in any structure must be confirmed by chemical or enzymatic extraction, because nucleic acids are not the only substances capable of binding coloured cations. Controls are particularly important in the case of cytoplasmic RNA, which cannot easily be distinguished from the basophilic secretory products of some cells. The dye–metal complex formed from gallocyanine and chromic ions (Chapter 5) is a cationic dye and is also used to stain DNA and RNA. The chrome alum–gallocyanine method of Einarson (1951) is used in quantitative micro-photometric studies of the nucleic acid contents of cells because the bound dye–metal complex is more stable towards light, water, and organic solvents than are ordinary cationic dyes.

Some simple fluorescent or coloured compounds have molecules that fit tightly into the hydrophobic domains of nucleic acids, and provide quite specific staining (see Gurr et al., 1974). Some of these are now considered.

9.2.1.
Intercalation and other staining mechanisms

A planar aromatic ring of suitable dimensions that bears at least one polar group is able to fit, like the filling of a sandwich, between the stacked base pairs of a nucleic acid molecule. The phenanthridine fluorochromes ethidium and propidium fulfil this structural requirement, as do some common cationic dyes, including acridines, phenothiazines, and oxazines, though they can also bind to macromolecular anions by electrostatic attraction. The mechanism of intercalation into DNA requires transient opening of the helix to admit the coloured or fluorescent molecule. This opening does not involve unwinding of the helix, because hinge-like bending can occur at certain sites (Sobell et al., 1977; see Fig. 9.2). The fluorescence efficiency is increased by binding to nucleic acid, and there is sometimes a change in the colour of the emitted light (Morthland et al., 1954; Burns, 1972; Hilwig and Gropp, 1972). With some of these reagents, it is possible to distinguish between the two nucleic acids by the colour of the fluorescence (Bertalanffy and Bickis, 1956) or by adjusting the pH of the solution to favour selective staining (Hilwig and Gropp, 1975). For several dyes, the binding is to adenine–thymine base pairs of DNA or to adenine-uracil pairs of RNA, and intercalation greatly increases the fluorescence (Kapuscinski, 1990)

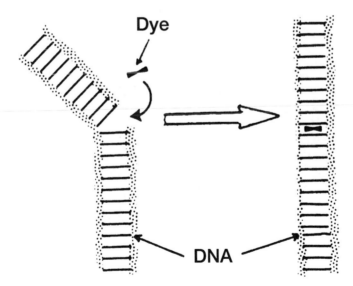

Figure 9.2. Transient bending of a DNA helix to admit a planar dye or fluorochrome ion, which intercalates between base pairs in the hydrophobic centre of the macromolecule.

Another cationic fluorochrome is **quinacrine** (also known as atebrine and mepacrine; MW 472.9). This exhibits enhanced fluorescence when it is intercalated into an adenine–thymine pair, but the fluorescence is suppressed by guanine (Weisblum and de Haseth, 1972). Consequently, regions of DNA rich in adenine–thymine pairs fluoresce brightly, and regions in which guanine–cytosine pairs predominate appear darker. This is the reason why mitotic chromosomes stained with quinacrine exhibit patterns of bright and dark transverse bands, which are useful for identification, description, and the recognition of abnormalities.

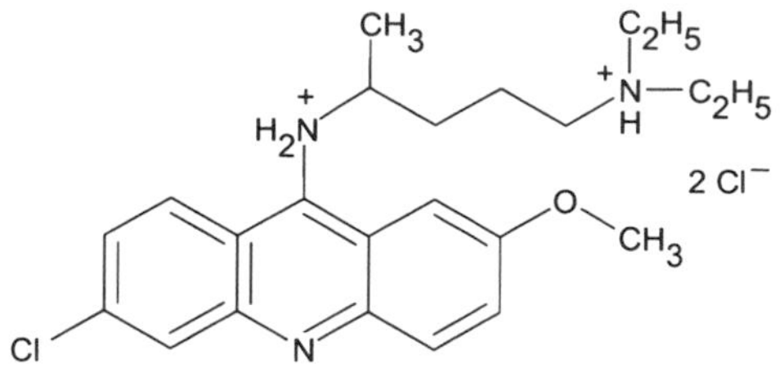

There are other cationic fluorochromes that are attracted to the phosphate of DNA by ionic forces and are then attached to regions on the outside of the double helix that are rich in adenine–thymine, by non-ionic forces but without intercalation. These substances are conspicuously fluorescent only when bound by DNA. Examples of this type include bisbenzimidazoles (also called Hoechst dyes), and 4'-6-diamidino-2-phenylindole (DAPI) (Kapuscinski, 1990, 1995).

The cyanine dyes known as TOTO-1 and YOYO-1 can bind to DNA both externally and by intercalation. They fade more slowly than the other fluorochromes and are extremely sensitive and specific, though expensive reagents (Tekola *et al.*, 1994; Haugland, 2002; Gurrieri *et al.*, 1997).

Three popular intercalating fluorochromes used for staining nucleic acids are **acridine orange** (Chapter 5), **ethidium bromide** and **propidium iodide**

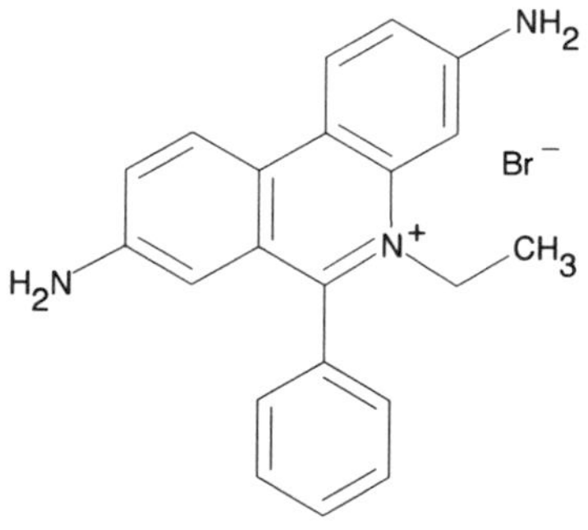

ethidium bromide (MW 394.3) 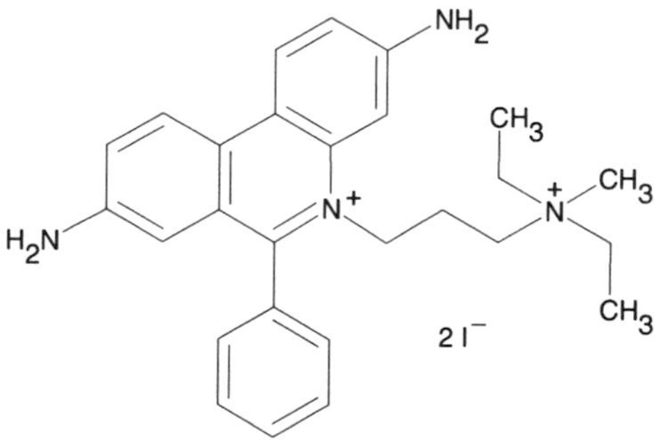   propidium iodide (MW 668.4)

Of the non-intercalating reagents that bind specifically to DNA, **Hoechst 33258**, also called **bisbenzimide**, is available as its pentahydrated trihydrochloride salt (MW 624):

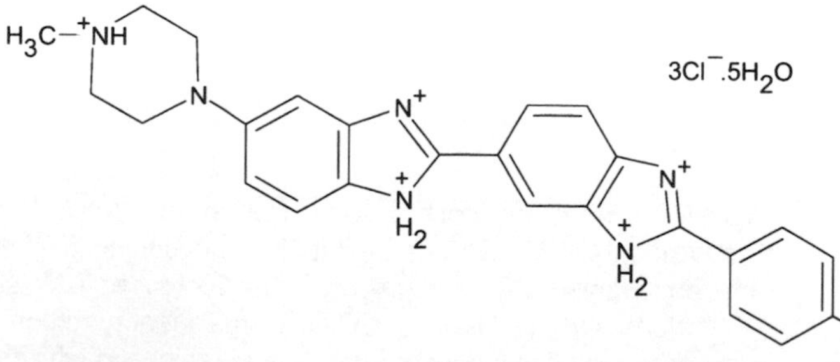

Several similar compounds (with other numbers) are also made by the Hoechst company. **DAPI** is sold as its dichloride (MW 350) and dilactate (MW 457):

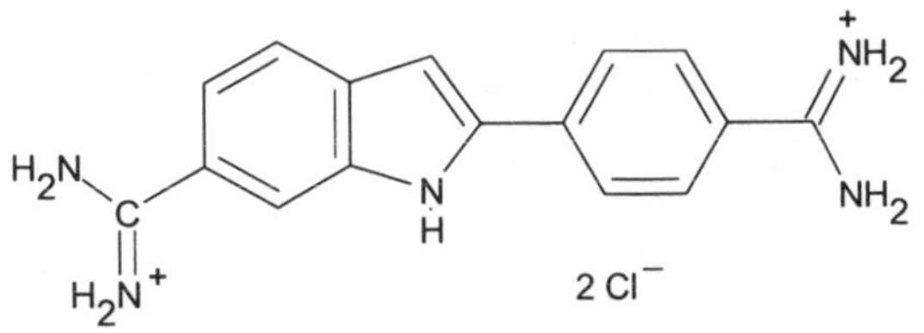

The iodides of **TOTO-1** and **YOYO-1** are sold as 1 mM solutions in DMSO:

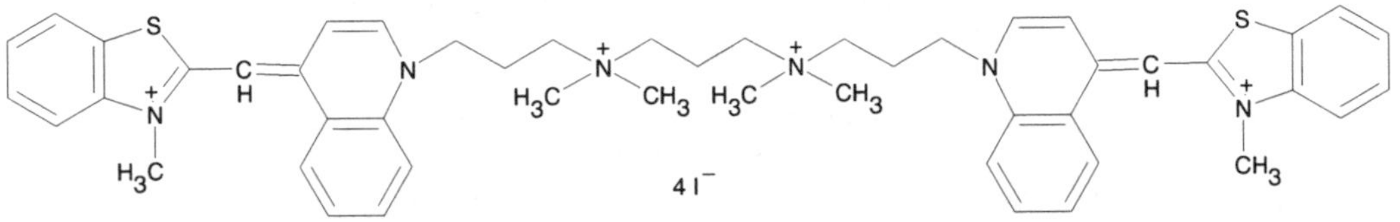

TOTO-1 (MW 1250.7)

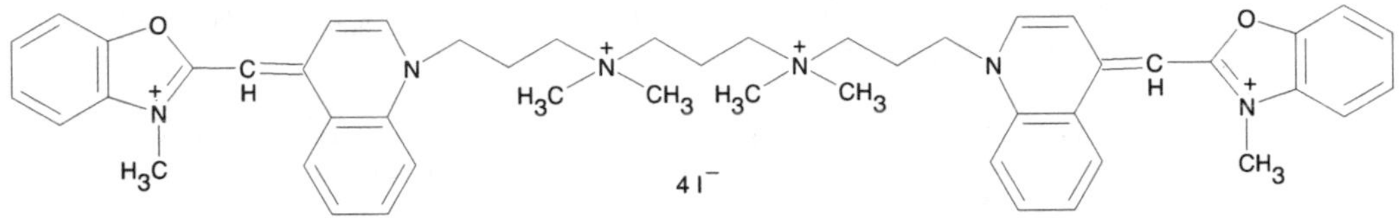

YOYO-1 (MW 1218.6)

9.2.2.
Fluorescent
demonstration
of nucleic acids

The procedures are simple, and vary only in details of the composition of the staining solutions. The concentrations of fluorochromes are not critical, and those recommended by different authors often vary by 3 orders of magnitude. After staining, the preparations are washed in a solution (water. buffer, culture medium, etc.) identical to that in which the fluorochrome was dissolved.

Fluorochrome solutions
Use one of the following. See below for the results that can be expected. The stock solutions are stable for months if kept in dark bottles, or in a dark cupboard. Refrigeration (4°C) retards microbial contamination.

Acridine orange. A stock solution of acridine orange (C.I. 46005), 1.0 mg/ml in water, is diluted 10-fold, immediately before use, with 0.1 M phosphate buffer, pH 6.0 (Chapter 20).

Ethidium bromide. 1.0 µg/ml, in 0.1 M phosphate buffer, pH 7.2. This solution (Franklin and Locker, 1981) will stain both nucleic acids. See also *Note 1* below.

Propidium iodide. 1.0 µg/ml, in 0.1 M phosphate buffer, pH 7.2

Quinacrine hydrochloride. 0.25 µg/ml, in 0.1 M phosphate buffer, pH 7.2

Hoechst 33258 (also known as **bisbenzimide** though the latter name has also been applied to Hoechst 33342, a closely related fluorescent bisbenzimidazole dye): 0.5 µg/ml in a balanced salt solution (Chapter 20), pH 7.0–7.4. At this pH, the fluorochrome is selective for DNA. To stain both nucleic acids, add HCl to lower the pH to 2. *If staining is done at pH 2, the preparation must be washed afterwards at pH 7*, to avoid loss of the fluorescent reagent (Hilwig and Gropp, 1975).

DAPI (4′,6-diamidino-2-phenylindole dichloride): 1.0 µg/ml in a balanced salt solution (Chapter 20), pH 7.0–7.4. The solution keeps for 1 month, in the dark. This is selective for DNA. A mixture of equal volumes of glycerol and a buffer at pH 4.2 is recommended for mounting (Bilinski and Bilinska, 1996).

TOTO-1 and **YOYO-1**: A tiny drop of the 1 mM stock solution in DMSO is diluted 2000 times in a balanced salt solution (e.g. 10 μl stock into 20 ml). The dilution should be done in a plastic container because glass adsorbs these dyes from aqueous solutions.

Procedure

(1) Fix specimens, suspended cells, or cultured monolayers in any fluid that preserves nucleic acids (Chapter 2). Acetic–alcohol mixtures are recommended.
(2) Rinse the preparation in the buffer or salt solution used as solvent for the fluorescent reagent.
(3) Stain for 15–60 min at room temperature.
(4) Wash in three changes of the buffer or salt solution.
(5) Apply a coverslip, using a mixture of equal volumes of glycerol and buffer (or balanced salt solution) as the mounting medium. Examine immediately.

Instructions for fluorescence microscopy are summarized in *Table 9.1*. These fluorochromes are easily seen even if the equipment cannot provide illumination at the optimum wavelength.

Table 9.1. Absorption and emission maxima of some fluorochromes that bind to nucleic acids

Fluorochrome	Absorption	Emission
Acridine orange	500 nm (blue)	530 nm (DNA green); > 600 nm (RNA red-brown)
DAPI	358 nm (near UV)	461 nm (blue)
Ethidium bromide	520 nm (green)	610 nm (orange)
Hoechst 33258	365 nm (near UV)	480 nm (blue)
Propidium iodide	535 nm (green)	617 nm (orange-red)
Quinacrine	440 (UV or blue)	530 (blue, green)
TOTO	514 nm (blue)	533 nm (green-yellow)
YOYO	491 nm (blue)	509 nm (green)

Results

Fluorescence due to DNA is seen in nuclear chromatin. Fluorescence due to RNA is seen in nucleoli and cytoplasm.

Notes

(1) If ethidium bromide is applied from a strongly acid solution (0.25 M HCl, pH 0.6), RNA is destroyed by hydrolysis and the method becomes specific for DNA. The staining of DNA is prevented by prior methylation (Chapter 10) for 3 h at 55°C in 0.1 M HCl in absolute methanol. After this treatment, the reagent binds only to RNA (Cox et al., 1982). If ethidium bromide is added to a culture medium for 2 h, the fluorescence of the living cells is due almost entirely to RNA (Burns, 1972).
(2) The preparations are not permanent, so they should be examined and photographed immediately. If the washed slides are thoroughly air-dried, rinsed in xylene, and then coverslipped with a non-fluorescent resinous mounting medium, some fluorescence is preserved, though with reduced brightness.
(3) In spermatozoa, which have highly condensed nuclei, red fluorescence with acridine orange is not due to RNA but possibly to certain domains in the nuclear DNA (Lewin et al., 1999).

(4) Cationic fluorochromes can be applied to sections as counterstains, in conjunction with fluorescent immunohistochemical procedures (Jones and Kniss, 1987). In critical histochemical work, however, it is always necessary to use extracted or enzyme-treated control sections (Sections 9.4, 9.5) to check the specificity of staining of DNA or RNA.

9.2.3.
Cuprolinic blue
for selective
RNA staining

Alcian blue, a basic dye in which large cationic side-chains are attached to copper phthalocyanine, stains carbohydrate polyanions but not nucleic acids (Chapter 11). While investigating this useful property, Scott (1972b) synthesized a compound with molecules similar in shape and size to copper phthalocyanine, but with positively charged nitrogen atoms within the chromophore, and no side-chains. He called this substance **quinolinic phthalocyanine**. When the new dye became available commercially, with the name **cuprolinic blue**, Mendelson et al. (1983) exploited its properties in a method for selective staining of single-stranded RNA. (Most of the RNA in the nucleolus and cytoplasm is single-stranded, whereas DNA is double-stranded, except transiently at sites of transcription or replication.) The structural formulae of cuprolinic blue and alcian blue are shown in Chapter 5 (Section 5.9.14).

The dye is used as a solution in aqueous 1.0 M magnesium chloride, and the sections are treated with 1.0 M $MgCl_2$ after staining. Magnesium ions, being smaller and more mobile than those of the dye, quickly enter the double helix of DNA and neutralize its phosphate groups, but the more open structure of single-stranded RNA allows the dye to compete with Mg^{2+} for anionic sites. Once attracted and brought into contact with the RNA molecule, the cuprolinic blue ions are held in place by van der Waals forces, which are effective even in the presence of Mg^{2+}. The specificity of the method for RNA has been established in studies with pure compounds and by histochemical extraction and blocking tests (Tas et al., 1983). Other than RNA, the only substances stained in the presence of 1.0 M $MgCl_2$ are sulphated mucosubstances, and these are coloured metachromatically (Chapter 11) red–purple rather than greenish blue. Once a tissue has been stained with cuprolinic blue, the dye resists extraction by aqueous washing and alcoholic dehydration. Selective RNA staining is possible only after coagulant fixation, which makes spaces through which dye molecules can diffuse. After a cross-linking fixative like formaldehyde, the selectivity is sometimes lost. Tissue porosity is clearly an important factor for this technique.

Cuprolinic blue is useful for picking out cells with abundant ribosomes. Neurons (with much RNA in the Nissl substance) are prominently displayed. Small neurons are not confused with the nuclei of neuroglial cells, which are equally or more strongly coloured by other basic dyes. The greenish-blue colour imparted to RNA is never very dark, and it does not interfere with other staining methods. For example, cuprolinic blue can be applied to sections before staining by immunohistochemical procedures that generate brown products (Holst and Powley, 1995). Disadvantages of cuprolinic blue are its high price, its availability from only a few suppliers, and the dependence of the specificity on suitable fixation.

Solutions required
A. Buffered magnesium chloride

Sodium acetate: either CH_3COONa:	1.48 g
or $CH_3COONa.3H_2O$:	2.46 g
Glacial acetic acid:	1.08 ml
Magnesium chloride ($MgCl_2.6H_2O$):	40.6 g
Water:	to make 200 ml

The pH of this solution is approximately 4.5 (even though the acetate buffer ingredients alone make a pH of 5.6). Unused solution can be kept indefinitely at 4°C but should be replaced if there are signs of bacterial or fungal growth.

B. Cuprolinic blue staining solution

Cuprolinic blue:	20 mg
Buffered MgCl$_2$ (Solution A):	20 ml

This solution may be used repeatedly, and it retains its staining properties for 4 years at 4°C. Some weakening of the colour is evident with solutions stored for 8 years.

Procedure

(1)   Specimens are fixed in **modified Carnoy's fluid** (Chapter 2). Paraffin sections are prepared and mounted in the usual way.
(2)   De-wax and hydrate the sections.
(3)   Stain in cuprolinic blue (Solution B) for 60 min at room temperature. (A drop of dye may be placed over each section, and the slides placed in a humid atmosphere to prevent drying.)
(4)   Recover the dye solution for reuse, then rinse the slides in water.
(5)   Immerse slides in buffered 1.0 M magnesium chloride (Solution A) for 30 min.
(6)   Discard the MgCl$_2$ solution and wash in 3 changes of water.
(7)   Dehydrate through graded alcohols, clear in xylene, and apply coverslips, using a resinous mounting medium.

Result

Sites of single-stranded RNA (nucleoli and cytoplasmic regions rich in ribosomes) are a blue-green colour. Nuclei (other than in nucleoli) are unstained. Sites of high proteoglycan or sulphated glycoprotein concentration (cartilage matrix, mast cell granules, goblet cells, etc.) are metachromatically stained (red–purple).

Notes

(1)   A variant of this method for staining neurons in whole-mounts is described by Heinicke *et al.* (1987).
(2)   To check the specificity of the method, treat some control sections with either ribonuclease (Section 9.4) or perchloric acid (Section 9.2), to extract RNA before staining.

**9.2.4.
Ethyl green–pyronine and related methods**

With these techniques two cationic dyes are applied simultaneously under carefully controlled conditions of concentration and pH. This results in differential colouring of DNA (bluish green with ethyl green) and RNA (pink to red with pyronine Y). There has been much speculation and disagreement on the mechanism of this staining (Baker and Williams, 1965; Scott, 1967; Lyon, 1991), but all agree that the shapes and sizes of the dye molecules (Chapter 5) determine which colour will be imparted to each nucleic acid.

It seems probable that the large, hydrophilic, propeller-shaped cation of ethyl green is attracted electrostatically to the phosphate groups on the outside of the DNA helix. Non-ionic bonds to the sugar units of DNA and to the associated nucleoprotein may help to hold the dye in position. Pyronine Y ions are smaller and planar, and could be expected to intercalate between the base pairs of a nucleic acid. Pyronine does not enter the DNA molecule, however, because its ions are excluded by the ethyl green on the outside of the helix. Ribosomes and nucleoli admit pyronine cations, which are attracted by the phosphate groups of RNA and then held in place by hydrophobic interaction of the ring system of the dye with those of the purine and pyrimidine bases.

Support for the mechanism summarized above comes from the observation that pyronine Y can be replaced by thionine (Roque *et al.*, 1965), whose planar cations are much the same size and are comparably hydrophobic. It is also possible to replace the ethyl green with a cationic surfactant, so that RNA is the only nucleic acid stained (Bennion et al., 1975).

Ethyl green–pyronine is traditionally used to detect plasma cells. The method is also valuable as a general histological stain, especially for nervous and lymphoid tissues. Basophilic materials other than nucleic acids are stained mainly by the pyronine Y.

9.2.5.
An ethyl green–pyronine procedure

The simple method given below (Hoyer et al., 1986) is for use with pure samples of both dyes, which have become available in recent years (Chapter 5; also Lyon et al., 1987). Older samples of the dyes may not work with the quantities given below. Detailed instructions for getting the method to work with impure dyes were given in the first edition of this book. Techniques can also be found in Pearse (1968b or 1985), Bancroft and Cook (1984) and Bancroft and Gamble (2002).

Solutions required
A. 0.01 M phthalate buffer, pH 4.0

Potassium hydrogen phthalate ($KHC_8H_4O_4$):	1.02 g
Water:	490 ml
0.01 M HCl:	approximately 1.0 ml
Check the pH, then add water to make volume up to:	500 ml

See also *Note 1* below.

B. Dye mixture

Pyronine Y (C.I. 45005; dye content >90%):	0.03 g
Ethyl green (C.I. 42590):	0.15 g
Buffer, pH 4.0 (Solution A):	100 ml

Procedure
(1) De-wax and hydrate paraffin sections of material fixed in Carnoy or aqueous formaldehyde.
(2) Stain in the dye mixture (Solution B) for 5 min.
(3) Rinse in two changes of water, 5 s in each. Shake to drain off most of the water.
(4) Dehydrate by agitating vigorously in each of 3 changes of n-butanol, about 1 min in each. The volume of butanol must be adequate (about 300 ml for a rack of 10–12 slides, or 50 ml for 1 or 2 slides in a coplin jar).
(5) (Optional) Clear in xylene.
(6) Apply coverslips, using a resinous mounting medium.

Results
DNA green or bluish–green. RNA bright pink or red. Sulphated carbohydrates (mast cell granules, cartilage matrix, some types of mucus) are coloured metachromatically (orange) by the pyronine Y.

Microdensitometric measurements of the DNA staining show a linear correlation with figures obtained from sections stained by the Feulgen technique; standardized ethyl green–pyronine staining can be used for quantitative histochemical studies of DNA and RNA (Lyon et al., 1989).

Notes
(1) The pH of the staining solution may be varied within the range 4.0–4.6. pH 4.0 has been found optimal for most material (Hoyer et al., 1986).
(2) The histochemical specificity of staining, especially of RNA, should be checked by selective enzymatic or chemical extraction as described later in this chapter.
(3) Detailed troubleshooting instructions are given by Horobin and Bancroft (1998) who emphasize the need for pure dyes. Pyronine Y has been a cause of trouble in the past, being sometimes incorrectly labelled or of low dye content.

(4)   The Biological Stain Commission's testing procedure for ethyl green and pyronine is similar to the one given here but uses a more concentrated staining solution, with 1% ethyl green and 0.1% pyronine Y in 0.2 M acetate buffer, pH 4.2 (Penney et al., 2002).

9.3. The Feulgen method for DNA

**9.3.1.
Chemical
principles**

When sections are treated with 1.0 M hydrochloric acid at 55–60°C for 5–20 min (according to the fixative used, see below), most of the RNA is broken down to soluble substances and lost from the tissue, but DNA is only partly hydrolyzed. The purine and pyrimidine bases of the DNA are removed from the deoxyribose residues, which remain in their original positions and are capable of reacting as aldehydes (Overend and Stacey, 1949). The Feulgen hydrolysis does not break the ester linkages between the phosphoric acid and sugar units of the DNA.

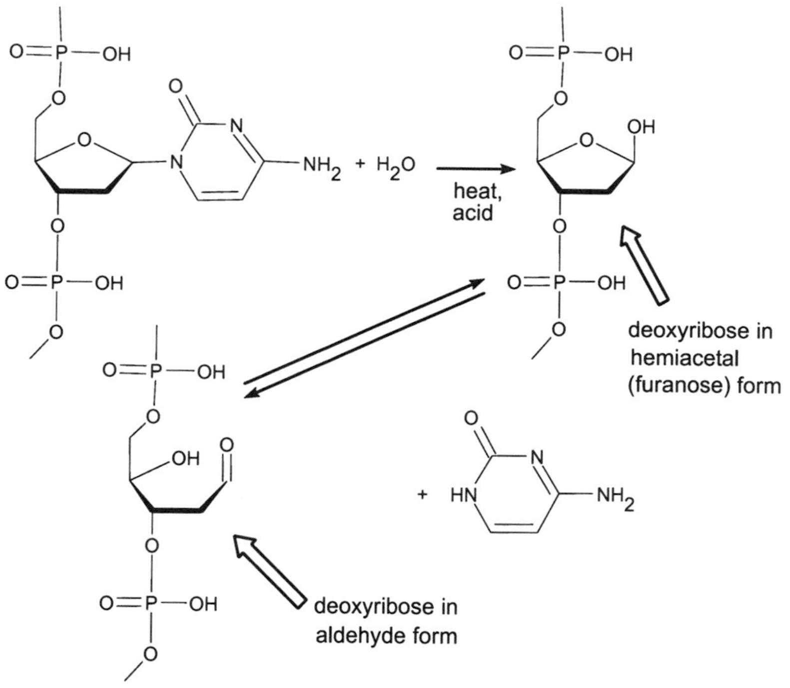

Reasons for the different effects of acid hydrolysis on RNA and DNA are discussed at some length by Pearse (1968b, 1985). The ribosyl residues of any RNA that is not removed during the hydrolysis do not react as aldehydes, probably because there is a hydroxy group at position 2′ of ribose. The aldehyde groups liberated by the Feulgen hydrolysis are stained with Schiff's reagent; the chemistry of this latter process is considered in Chapter 10. Other reagents, notably silver diammine and naphthoic acid hydrazide, can also be used to detect aldehydes formed from partly hydrolyzed DNA. The Feulgen reaction is a highly specific method for DNA. Any free aldehydes initially present in the tissue (i.e. introduced by fixative or present in immature elastic tissue and some lipids) will give false positive staining, but this will be obtained when the acid hydrolysis is omitted (except, rarely, in the case of some lipids), so it is unlikely to cause confusion.

Pre-existing aldehydes are easily destroyed before staining by treating the sections with sodium borohydride. This manoeuvre (Chapter 10) is always necessary with tissue fixed in glutaraldehyde (Kasten and Lala, 1975). It should be noted that Bouin's fluid and acid decalcifying agents can attack DNA and with prolonged contact they may hydrolyze it excessively with consequent loss of stainability by the Feulgen method. For the histochemistry of nucleic acids it is desirable to avoid the use of fixatives containing picric acid, and chelating agents are preferred to acids when decalcification is necessary (Chapter 3).

The intensity of staining by the Feulgen method is proportional to the concentration of DNA. Thus it is possible to make micro-photometric and morphometric observations and determine the quantities of DNA in the nuclei of cells. Important studies of the cell cycle have been carried out in this way. A valuable application of the Feulgen reaction in pathology is the quantitation of cells that contain abnormal quantities of DNA in malignant tumours (Motherby et al., 1998).

9.3.2.
Feulgen staining in practice

The optimum time of hydrolysis by 1.0 M HCl at 55–60°C varies with the fixative:

Bouin:	12 min
Carnoy:	8 min
Flemming:	16 min
Formaldehyde:	8 min
Helly:	5 min
SUSA:	18 min
Zenker:	5 min

(Data summarized from McManus and Mowry, 1960 and Pearse, 1968b.)

This is the most critical component of the Feulgen reaction. Currently it is fashionable to use a more concentrated HCl solution, at room temperature (See *Note 4c* below).

Preparation of Schiff's reagent
This is not the only way to make Schiff's reagent. For other methods, see Pearse (1968b), Lillie and Fullmer (1976) or Presnell and Schreibman (1997). It is important to use certified basic fuchsine or pure pararosaniline. Some products are designated 'special for DNA'. Schiff's reagent can also be bought ready-made from a chemical supplier.

Boil 400 ml of water, add 1.0 g of basic fuchsine, cool to room temperature, and filter. Add 1.0 ml of thionyl chloride (**cautiously:** the reaction $SOCl_2 + H_2O \rightarrow SO_2(g) + 2HCl$ is very rapid. Use a fume hood.) If thionyl chloride is not available, add 1 g sodium metabisulphite to the cooled, filtered dye solution, followed by 2 ml concentrated hydrochloric acid. Allow to stand in a stoppered bottle overnight, then shake with about 2 g of activated charcoal, which should remove all residual colour. A slight yellowish–brown tinge does not matter, but the solution must not be pink. Filter to remove charcoal and store in a tightly closed brown glass bottle.

A new bottle of Schiff's reagent is stable for years. Once started it will keep for about 6 months, but it must be discarded if a pink colour develops or if it no longer smells strongly of sulphur dioxide. Schiff's reagent is commonly kept at 4°C but this is not necessary. See *Note 3* below for an alternative to Schiff's reagent.

Other solutions required
A. 1.0 M hydrochloric acid
Alternatively, 5.0 M hydrochloric acid. See Chapter 20 for information about diluting concentrated HCl.

B. Bisulphite water
Dissolve approximately 5 g of sodium or potassium metabisulphite (anhydrous) in 1 l of water and add 3–5 ml of concentrated hydrochloric acid. This solution must be freshly made. Put it into three staining tanks.

C. A counterstain
This can be used, if desired. Fast green FCF gives a suitable background colour (Chapter 6).

Procedure
(1)   If 1.0 M hydrochloric acid is to be used for the hydrolysis, pre-heat it to 60°C in a covered container (see also *Note 1*). If the Schiff's reagent has been refrigerated, allow it to warm to room temperature.
(2)   De-wax and hydrate paraffin sections.
(3)   Immerse in 1.0 M HCl at 60°C for the optimum time. *Alternatively* use 5.0 M HCl for 30 min at room temperature (see *Note 4c* below).
(4)   Rinse in water (two changes).
(5)   Immerse in Schiff's reagent, at room temperature, for 15–30 min (until nuclei are stained; the sections should be pale pink to the unaided eye).
(6)   Transfer slides directly to bisulphite water: three changes, each 10–15 s with agitation (see *Note 2*).
(7)   Wash in running tap water for 2 min.
(8)   Counterstain (if desired). Wash briefly in water (which also differentiates fast green FCF) or in slightly acidified water (which does not extract anionic dyes).
(9)   Dehydrate, clear, and mount in a resinous medium.

Result
DNA (nuclear chromatin; chromosomes) deep pink to purple.

Notes
(1)   Do not allow water vapour to contaminate any melted wax that is also in the 60°C oven. A microwave oven is convenient for pre-heating.
(2)   The purpose of the bisulphite rinse is to prevent the re-colorization of Schiff's reagent, which occurs on dilution with water alone and can cause artifactual background staining. Demalsy and Callebaut (1967) recommend omission of this rinse and prescribe washing in copious running tap water instead.
(3)   Horobin and Kevill-Davies (1971a) have shown that an acidified alcoholic solution of basic fuchsine (not decolorized with SO_2) will stain aldehyde groups. This solution is made as follows:

Basic fuchsine:	1 g
Ethanol:	160 ml
Water:	40 ml
Concentrated hydrochloric acid:	2 ml

Keeps for a few weeks. Without the hydrochloric acid, it is indefinitely stable. The HCl can be added before use. Store in a tightly closed bottle. After staining for 20 min in this solution, the slides are washed in absolute or 95% alcohol to remove all excess dye, cleared, and covered. (See Chapter 10 for discussion of histochemical detection of aldehydes.)

(4)   **Controls.** The specificity of Feulgen staining may be checked in various ways:
(a) Omit the acid hydrolysis (step 3). Nothing should be stained. A positive result may indicate pre-existing aldehyde groups derived from the fixative (especially glutaraldehyde) or hydrolysis of DNA during fixation (picric acid can do this) or decalcification. Elastin of immature animals normally has free aldehyde groups (Chapter 8), but is unlikely to be mistaken for DNA. The pseudo-plasmal reaction of some lipids (Chapter 12) can be a cause of direct reactivity with Schiff's reagent in frozen sections, especially after fixation and storage in formaldehyde solutions.
(b) The times for hydrolysis given above are only approximate. In critical work the optimum time must be determined experimentally for each batch of sec-

tions. The optimum hydrolysis is that which yields the most darkly stained nuclei. If an unexpected negative result is obtained, stain a hydrolyzed section with a basic dye: the DNA may have been completely depolymerized and extracted.

(c) In a chemical study of the acid-catalyzed hydrolysis of DNA Kjellstrand (1977) obtained the highest yields of aldehydes by using concentrations of HCl considerably higher than 1.0 M, at or only slightly above room temperature. It is now a common practice to use 5.0 M hydrochloric acid at room temperature for 30 min. The time is less critical than when the hydrolysis is carried out at 60°C (Churukian, 2000; Presnell and Schreibman, 1997).

(5)   If staining seems to be too weak, even with an optimum hydrolysis, the Schiff's reagent is probably unsatisfactory.

9.4. Enzymatic extraction of nucleic acids

9.4.1.
Enzymes as regents in histochemistry – general considerations

Sections of tissue can be treated with the pancreatic enzymes ribonuclease (RNase) and deoxyribonuclease (DNase) in order to remove, selectively, the two nucleic acids. Other enzymes are also used in histochemistry to remove (or prevent the staining of) such substances as collagen, glycogen, and various carbohydrate constituents of mucosubstances. Some caution is required in interpreting the results of enzymatic treatments, and the following conditions must always be satisfied in order to draw valid conclusions:

(1)   The substrate must be present in a suitable state for being attacked by the enzyme. Fixatives containing picric acid, mercury, or chromium should be avoided because these substances are inhibitory to many enzymes. Fixation in formaldehyde prevents the subsequent digestion of collagen and reticulin by collagenase. For most other enzymes the least objectionable fixatives are formaldehyde (aqueous or alcoholic) and mixtures of alcohol with acetic acid.

(2)   The enzyme used must be free from contamination by other enzymes that might produce confusing effects. The presence of proteolytic enzymes in a specimen of RNase, for example, would be undesirable. Similarly, DNase must be free of RNase.

(3)   The conditions of incubation must be adequate for complete action of the enzyme upon all of the substrate present in the section. The use of an identically fixed and processed control section known to contain the substrate is recommended.

(4)   Non-specific extraction of the substrate should not occur and should be sought in control sections incubated only in the buffer or water used as solvent for the enzyme. Buffer solutions alone sometimes extract appreciable quantities of RNA and glycogen from sections. In some circumstances it is preferable to dissolve the enzyme in plain water, even if this does not provide the optimum pH for the reaction.

(5)   Any necessary co-factors must be provided. Neuraminidase, for example, will function only in the presence of calcium ions, and DNase requires magnesium.

Ribonuclease, labelled with colloidal gold, has been used to detect RNA in electron micrographs (Bendayan, 1981a), but this reagent adheres also to sulphated carbohydrate-containing structures (Dvorak and Morgan, 1998).

9.4.2.
Ribonuclease and deoxyribonuclease

Enzymes from various animal and plant sources catalyze the decomposition of nucleic acids. In histochemical practice, enzymes extracted from the bovine or porcine pancreas are usually used. The enzymes should be of the highest available purity, regardless of expense, for the reasons given in the preceding section. Cruder preparations are cheaper and will work, but when they are used there can be no certainty that the observed alterations in stainability of the tissue are due solely to removal of RNA or DNA. The reason for using an enzyme is that it acts with high specificity upon its substrate. With a mixture of enzymes, this specificity is lost.

Ribonuclease (systematic name: polyribonucleotide 2-oligonucleotido-transferase (cyclizing); E.C. 2.7.7.16) acts on the phosphate group attached to position 3′ of those ribose units of RNA that bear pyrimidine bases at position 1′. The phosphate–ester linkage to position 5′ of the adjacent sugar residue is transferred to position 2′ of the first ribose unit: the one bearing the pyrimidine base. (Systematic names and E.C. numbers of enzymes are explained in Chapter 14.)

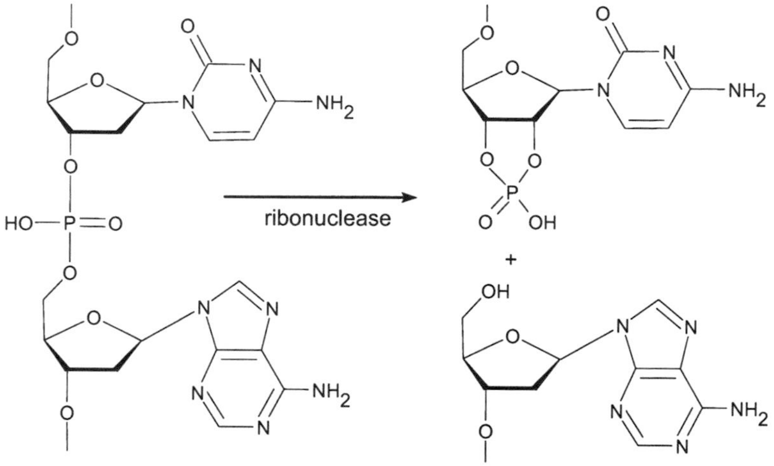

The long molecule of RNA is thus broken into small, soluble oligonucleotides. These products are lost from the tissue by diffusion into the RNase solution and the water used for subsequent washing.

Ribonuclease is present in sweat, saliva and other human secretions, and can attack RNA in sections of tissue. This enzyme is not easily inactivated by heating.

Deoxyribonuclease (systematic name: deoxyribonucleate oligonucleotido-hydrolase; E.C. 3.1.4.5) of pancreatic origin catalyzes the attack of water upon multiple phosphoric acid ester linkages to position 5′ of deoxyribose. The DNA is thus hydrolyzed to yield soluble oligonucleotides. A related enzyme is deoxyribonuclease II (systematic name: deoxyribonucleate 3′-nucleotidohydrolase; E.C. 3.1.4.6), extracted from spleen and from various micro-organisms, which brings about hydrolysis at position 3′ of deoxyribose. The latter enzyme has been used less often in histochemistry than pancreatic DNase.

9.4.3.
Techniques of application

DNase and RNase are expensive, so they can be used only in small quantities, applied as drops to individual sections. This is conveniently done in a closed petri dish containing damp gauze or filter paper to saturate the atmosphere inside with water vapour and prevent evaporation of the drop of enzyme solution. The dish containing the slide is placed in an incubator at 37°C. One section on a slide can be treated with enzyme while another is treated only with the solvent. Any other sections on the slide remain dry. In this way the effects of both the enzyme and its solvent can be examined on adjacent serial sections.

Enzyme solutions
The enzymes should be free of other interfering enzymes. Very small quantities may be weighed with a torsion balance. The solutions of the enzymes can be

recovered after use (by sucking off the slide with a syringe and needle) and stored frozen at −20°C, but the potency declines with such storage.

Ribonuclease is used as a solution containing 0.2–0.5 mg of enzyme per ml of water. Incubate for 1 h at 37°C.

Deoxyribonuclease is used as a solution containing 0.05 mg of enzyme per ml in TRIS buffer (pH 7.5) containing 0.001 M $MgSO_4$. The usual 0.2 M TRIS buffer (Chapter 20) should be diluted fivefold with water. Incubate for 3–6 h at 37°C.

Sections of central nervous tissue are valuable for determining the adequacy of extraction of nucleic acids. The Nissl substance of neurons (stainable by cationic dyes) should be completely removed by an adequate RNase treatment. The nuclear chromatin (but not the nucleoli) of all cells should fail to stain with cationic dyes or by the Feulgen method after adequate treatment with DNase. The control sections of central nervous tissue should have been fixed and processed in parallel with other specimens being studied.

9.5. Chemical extraction of nucleic acids

It is possible to extract nucleic acids non-enzymatically from sections of tissue. **Trichloroacetic acid** (4% aqueous, 80°C, 15 min) removes both DNA and RNA. **Perchloric acid** (10% aqueous $HClO_4$, at 4°C, overnight) removes RNA but not DNA. A more drastic treatment (5% aqueous $HClO_4$, 30 min, 60°C) extracts both nucleic acids. Perchloric acid also extracts some protein from sections (Kasten, 1965). These chemical procedures are based on the catalysis by acids of the hydrolysis of the bonds between the sugars and the bases and between the sugars and phosphoric acid. The phosphate–ester bonds of RNA are more labile to hydrolysis than those of DNA. It is also possible to remove RNA by treatment with hot 1.0 M **hydrochloric acid**, as in the Feulgen hydrolysis. Extraction of RNA by perchloric or hydrochloric acid removes the purine and pyrimidine bases from DNA, thus engendering stainability of this nucleic acid by Schiff's reagent. The reagents used for chemical extraction are less expensive than RNase and DNase, but they are also less specific for the nucleic acids, and their actions are more difficult to control.

Caution. The concentrated acids (60% perchloric and 100% trichloroacetic) are highly caustic and must be handled carefully. Small quantities may be discarded by neutralizing and then flushing down the sink with copious tap water.

9.6. Hybridization histochemistry

The affinities between the purine and pyrimidine bases of nucleic acids were mentioned in Section 9.1. It is possible to synthesize polynucleotides or oligonucleotides in which the sequences of bases are complementary to those in fragments of naturally occurring DNA or RNA. These are known as **cDNA** or **cRNA probes**. (The 'c' is for 'complementary'.) A cDNA or cRNA probe will adhere to a molecule of messenger RNA (mRNA) containing the complementary sequence of nucleotides. The specific joining (often called annealing) of a natural nucleic acid strand and a complementary probe strand is known as base-pairing or **hybridization**. The term '*in situ*' is used when the nucleic acid probes are applied to whole cells or sections of tissue, rather than to solutions or other cell-free preparations.

Only a few aspects of *in situ* hybridization are considered here. Detailed accounts, with practical instructions for the production, labelling, application and detection of nucleic acid probes, can be found in Sambrook *et al.* (1989), Mitchell *et al.* (1992), Sharif (1993), Leitch *et al.* (1994), Thiry (1995) and Polak and McGee (1998).

9.6.1.
Reasons for doing *in situ* hybridization

There are three reasons for wanting to identify the sites of hybridization of nucleic acid probes:

(1)   A cDNA or (more commonly) a cRNA probe identifies the mRNA for the protein encoded by a specific nucleotide sequence (or gene) of chromosomal DNA. The presence of the mRNA is revealed in interphase nuclei and in cytoplasm. Thus, it is possible to determine whether a cell is actively transcribing the gene and thus presumably synthesizing the encoded protein. This can be important, because protein molecules are often degraded or expelled from cells (secreted) soon after they have been assembled. Immunohistochemical staining in these cases may be negative, but binding of cDNA can identify the cells that produce such proteins. Conversely, a positive immunohistochemical reaction may be obtained in a cell that has taken up a protein that was synthesized and secreted by another cell. *Nucleic acid hybridization reveals the site of origin, as distinct from the site of binding or storage of a protein.*

(2)   A cDNA probe may hybridize with a gene, which is the nucleotide sequence of DNA encoding the amino acid sequence of a particular protein. For this to occur, the two DNA strands of the chromosome at the site of the gene must be separated, either as part of the mitotic or meiotic cycle or by artificial denaturation. It is thus possible to detect the presumptive positions of some genes on some types of chromosome.

It is also possible to prepare a mixture of large cDNA molecules known as a **genomic probe** that can hybridize with all the chromosomes of a particular species. Genomic probes are used in the study of hybrid plants and animals. Similarly, probes can be made that recognize whole individual chromosomes; these are applied in a technique known as **chromosome painting**, which can be used in the diagnosis of diseases due to abnormal structure or complement of particular chromosomes.

(3)   Infection by a **virus** introduces into cells nucleotide sequences that they normally do not contain. The viral genetic material may exist as DNA or RNA, and it may be present in the cytoplasm or integrated into chromosomal DNA. Hybridization histochemistry provides an important technique in the diagnosis of diseases due to viruses.

9.6.2.
Labelled nucleic acid probes

A nucleic acid probe can be labelled in various ways. A radioactive tag, such as ^{3}H, ^{125}I or ^{35}S is often used, and is eventually detected by autoradiography. Alternatively, the probe can be labelled by joining some of its nucleotide units covalently to an organic molecule that can be detected histochemically. The method of detection must involve **amplification**: that is, many visible molecules must be generated in close proximity to each labelled molecule. Autoradiography brings about considerable amplification, because a beta particle from a single atomic disintegration can result in a visible silver grain in the developed emulsion. Histochemical amplification methods are discussed in connection with enzyme histochemistry (Chapters 14–16) and immunohistochemistry (Chapter 19). An example of a label used for *in situ* hybridization is a reactive derivative of **digoxigenin**:

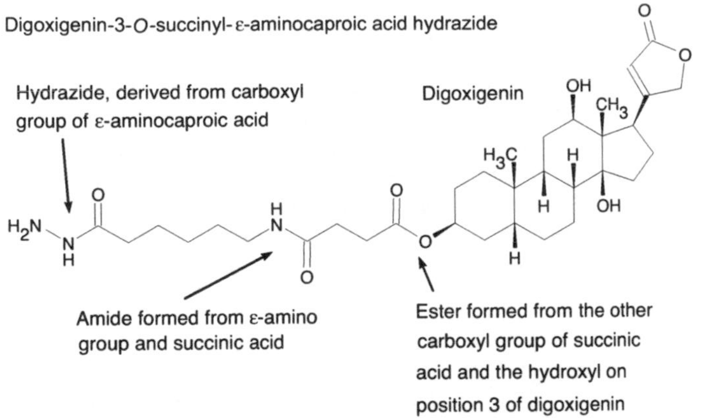

Digoxigenin-3-O-succinyl-ε-aminocaproic acid hydrazide

Hydrazide, derived from carboxyl
group of ε-aminocaproic acid

Digoxigenin

Amide formed from ε-amino
group and succinic acid

Ester formed from the other
carboxyl group of succinic
acid and the hydroxyl on
position 3 of digoxigenin

The hydrazide group shown at the left-hand side of the formula can combine with the aldehyde group of the deoxyribose in deoxyuridine triphosphate (dUTP). The reaction of hydrazides with aldehydes has other uses in histochemistry, and is discussed in Chapter 10. The digoxigenin-labelled deoxyuridine can be incorporated into RNA (in place of some of the uridine units) or DNA (in place of some of the thymidine). A digoxigenin-labelled polynucleotide is hybridized with complementary strands of DNA or RNA in a section of tissue, and the label is detected immunohistochemically, using an antibody that specifically recognizes and binds to digoxigenin (Arnold *et al.*, 1992). Immunohistochemical methods typically include at least two successive amplifications (Chapter 19). Digoxigenin does not occur naturally in animals or most plant species, so its presence in a tissue reliably indicates sites of incorporation of the labelled nucleotide. Digoxigenin labelled dUTP is used also in methods for detecting cells with fragmented DNA (Section 9.7.1).

9.6.3.
Pre-treatments
and conditions
for hybridization

Although the affinity between matched base pairs of nucleic acids is high, the conditions required for *in situ* hybridization are far from physiological. Fortunately, nucleic acids have considerable chemical stability. The following comments apply principally to the use of a cRNA probe for the detection of a specific mRNA.

The tissue must be permeable to the large molecules of the probe. This could be achieved by coagulant fixation, and predictably Urieli-Shoval *et al.* (1992) found that Carnoy's fluid was superior to formaldehyde for blocks of tissue, and Kapranos *et al.* (1997) found acetone superior to formaldehyde for smears of cells. In contrast, Tournier *et al.* (1987), preferred perfusion of buffered formaldehyde to coagulants, and Uehara *et al.* (1993) favoured a glutaraldehyde-containing mixture. Aldehydes do not react chemically with nucleic acids (Chapter 2), so mRNA is probably immobilized by being trapped among cross-linked protein molecules, and DNA by the insolubilization of chromosomal proteins. Some mRNAs are quite quickly degraded after death (Pardue *et al.*, 1994), so prompt fixation of specimens is advisable. If a specimen must be **decalcified** before sectioning, EDTA should be used, not an acid (Chapter 3 and Alers *et al.*, 1999).

The fixed section or smear is often treated with a **proteolytic enzyme** after fixation but before application of the probe. This is reputed to enhance penetration, especially after formaldehyde fixation (Guiot and Rahier, 1995). The bacterial enzyme proteinase K is effective for removing histones, thereby exposing nuclear DNA, and it also destroys any nucleases in the preparation that were not inactivated by the fixative. RNase, for example, might destroy endogenous mRNA or an applied cRNA probe. Sections are sometimes treated with 0.2 M HCl or 0.07 M NaOH to enhance pentration and to separate the paired strands of nuclear DNA, but these harsh treatments can usually be omitted. An acid treatment must not be severe enough to hydrolyse nucleic acids (Section 9.3.2).

A cDNA probe must be **denatured** or 'melted' before and during exposure to the tissue, to make it single-stranded. This is achieved by incubating in the hybridization mixture at a temperature about 30°C higher than the estimated melting temperature for the hybridization (for example, at 70°C for about 5 min). If the target of the probe is DNA in the tissue, this DNA must also be denatured. The hybridization is therefore started at an even higher temperature (such as 90°C), at which no annealing of DNA strands can occur, and then slowly lowered, allowing the formation of stable hybrid DNA strands.

RNA probes are also briefly heated (e.g. 80°C for 2 min) before use, to break up nonspecific associations within and between molecules. If the target is RNA in the tissue, this is already single-stranded and does not need to be denatured. Single-stranded RNA in the probe or tissue is in danger of being digested by RNase, an enzyme present in saliva and sweat, and likely to be present in water and on glassware. Glassware must be strongly heated (180°C, 2 h) to destroy the enzyme, or disposable plastic containers should be used. The water used for making up all reagents must be made RNase-free by adding diethyl pyrocarbonate (DEPC; 1 g for each liter of water). The DEPC is then removed by autoclaving for 15 min at 120°C or boiling for 30 min. (It is hydrolysed, yielding ethanol and carbon dioxide) Lu *et al.* (1996) added DEPC to the saline used to wash out the vascular system prior to perfusion of the fixative, to inhibit endogenous RNase in the tissue.

During (and sometimes also before) hybridization, the preparation is exposed to **blocking DNA**, which contains single-stranded nucleic acids that would not be expected to hybridize with the mRNA or DNA being sought by the specific probe. DNA from salmon sperm or tRNA from yeast are used with mammalian tissues. These substances will bind invisibly to any sites that bind nucleotides non-specifically, excluding the probe. Their function is comparable to that of non-immune serum included in immunohistochemical incubation media (Chapter 19). The affinity of the blocking DNA is too weak to interfere with appropriate annealing of the probe to a complementary nucleic acid strand in the tissue.

The conditions for hybridization include the presence of a fairly high concentration of a **salt** of a monovalent cation (typically 0.3 M Na$^+$) in a solvent consisting of 50% formamide and 50% water. The **formamide** reduces hydrogen-bonding of nucleic acids to water, thereby increasing the probability of union between complementary base pairs, but it also destabilizes the hybrid nucleic acid that has formed. This latter effect is opposed by the high salt concentration. Formamide may also destroy the activity of any RNases that have survived fixation and other pretreatments. **Dextran sulphate** can also be included in the medium, to displace water and effectively increase the concentration of the probe. The **temperature** is critical, and should be some 10°C below the melting temperature of the nucleic acid hybrid that is to be formed. It may vary between 20°C and 70°C. according to the hybrid and the other ingredients of the medium. The **melting temperature**, T_m is that at which the complementary nucleic acid strands are half-disassociated or denatured. It is estimated (in °C) from the formula:

$$T_m = 0.41(\%GC) + (16.6\log M - 500)/n - 0.61(\%F) + 81.5$$

where %GC is the percentage of guanine and cytosine in the probe (assume 40% if unknown); M is the molarity of monovalent cations (Na$^+$) in the solution; n is the number of base pairs in each molecule of probe; %F is the percent concentration of formamide.

After several hours, the preparations are washed. It is necessary to remove all unbound or non-specifically bound probe, and this is done in water containing less formamide (e.g. 20–30%) and much less salt (e.g. 0.03 M Na^+) than the hybridization mixture. In the case of a cRNA, the removal can be accelerated by treatment with ribonuclease A. The molecules of probe that have hybridized with nucleic acids in the specimen are not attacked by this enzyme, which catalyses the hydrolysis only of single-stranded RNA.

The specificity of annealing of a probe to a complementary strand of RNA or DNA is determined by the number of mismatched pairs of nucleotides that remain annealed after hybridization and subsequent washing. The approximate percentage of correctly matched nucleotides, known as the **stringency** of the procedure, increases with the length of the probe. Stringency is increased by higher concentrations of formamide in the hybridization mixture and washing solution, and by a small difference between the melting temperature and the temperature at which the hybridization was carried out. Conditions favouring the highest stringency can also reduce the specific binding of the probe, thereby reducing the sensitivity of the technique. Stringency is calculated from the formula:

$$\text{Stringency (\%)} = 100 - M_i(T_m - T_h)$$

where M_i is a 'mismatch factor' ranging from 1 (for probes of more than 150 base pairs) to 5 (for probes of fewer than 20 base pairs); T_m is the estimated melting temperature, and T_h is the temperature at which hybridization is carried out.

Finally, sites at which the probe has been bound must be made visible. **Autoradiography** provides high sensitivity, and the silver grains can be counted to provide quantitative data. The autoradiographic background is often high, however, and the accuracy of microscopic localization is poor. Superior resolution can be obtained with a chemically labelled probe. The use of **digoxigenin** for this purpose has already been mentioned. Many other labels, including **biotin** (McQuaid and Allen, 1992) and a variety of fluorescent compounds, are also suitable. (Most are used also in immunohistochemistry, and are discussed in Chapter 19.) Fluorescent labels are much used in probes that hybridize to chromosomes, and it is possible to make fluorescent *in situ* hybridization (**FISH**) preparations in which different chromosomes or DNA sequences are simultaneously demonstrated in separate colours, by using different fluorescent labels (see Leitch *et al.*, 1994; van Gijlswijk *et al.*, 1996; Nath and Johnson, 1998, 2000).

From the foregoing summary, it will be appreciated that several potentially destructive steps are involved in techniques of *in situ* hybridization. Sections of tissue that have been subjected to all the procedures mentioned above are often in a condition that would be considered unsatisfactory with other histochemical procedures. Hybridization is less damaging to chromosomes than to histological sections, and the appearances are similar to those of conventional cytological preparations. Damaging pretreatment of sections with acids and proteolytic enzymes is often unnecessary, and in recent years *in situ* hybridization has provided more satisfactory morphological images in the past. It is also possible to combine *in situ* hybridization with immunohistochemical staining of the same section (Mullink *et al.*, 1989).

9.7. Detection of apoptotic cells

When a cell dies, it may undergo **necrosis**, in which components of the cytoplasm are released directly into the extracellular space, or **apoptosis**, which is a series of events in which nucleic acids and proteins are degraded by enzymes and encapsulated in tiny membrane-bound bodies. In animals, necrosis causes an inflammatory reaction, whereas the products of apoptosis are inconspicuously taken up into neighbouring cells (Kerr *et al.*, 1972; Wyllie *et al.*, 1980). Apoptosis is also known as **programmed cell death** because the biochemical events follow an orderly sequence. This type of cell death occurs extensively in developing organisms, and is a major factor determining shapes, sizes and cell populations of organs. In adults, cells with limited life spans, such as lymphocytes and intestinal epithelial cells, die by apoptosis. Malignant cells divide frequently but do not undergo apoptosis.

During the course of apoptosis, proteolytic enzymes and nucleases are synthesized and used to break down proteins and nucleic acids. An endonuclease cuts the DNA into short segments, each about 180 base pairs in length (Sen, 1992; Bosman *et al.*, 1996). A series of calcium-activated enzymes, the **caspases**, are the principal proteolytic enzymes in apoptotic cells.

There are four methods for identification of apoptotic cells:

(1) **Simple nuclear staining**, usually with either a cationic dye or an alum–haematoxylin (Chapter 6). This stains the chromatin of normal nuclei. Shrunken (pyknotic) nuclei are more darkly coloured, and at later stages the apoptotic bodies appear as tiny dots, intensely stained because they contain condensed nuclear material. (Necrotic cells may also have small, fragmented nuclei, but these are surrounded by remnants of the cytoplasm, and the tissue is infiltrated with inflammatory cells.) For coloured micrographs of apoptotic cells, see Merritt *et al.* (1996). Dark-field illumination facilitates the detection of stained apoptotic cells at lower magnifications (Lange *et al.*, 1999). Alternatively, a stain for DNA may be used. Acridine orange (Magrassi and Graziadei, 1995; Mpoke and Wolfe, 1997; Tatton and Kish, 1997) and DAPI (Collins *et al.*, 1997) are suitable. With some cationic fluorochromes, notably acridine orange, shrunken apoptotic nuclei and apoptotic bodies fluoresce less brightly than normal nuclei. This is attributed by Erenpreisa *et al.* (1997) to self-quenching as a result of aggregation of dye molecules in the condensed chromatin.

(2) The many cut ends of the fragmented DNA can be identified by *in situ* **end labelling (ISEL)** methods, which are discussed in the next section (9.7.1).

(3) Phosphatidyl serine is a phospholipid that normally occurs on the inner surface of the cell membrane (Chapter 12). An early event in apoptosis is movement of this lipid to the external surface (Fadok *et al.*, 1992). Whole cells in suspension or in cultures can be labelled from the medium with **fluorescently labelled annexin V**. In the presence of calcium ions, this protein has high affinity for phosphatidyl serine (Martin *et al.*, 1996). Kits containing fluorescently labelled annexin V are commercially available; the method is not appropriate for sections.

(4) Immunohistochemical methods can be used to detect proteins that are synthesized only in apoptotic cells (Grand *et al.*, 1995). The enzyme poly(ADP-ribose) polymerase-1 (PARP-1; E.C. 2.4.2.30), which is activated by free ends of DNA, is one such protein (Negri *et al.*, 1997; Soldani *et al.*, 2005); The product of the action of PARP-1, poly(ADP-ribose), can be detected immunohistochemically in nuclei as soon as 4 h after initiation of apoptosis, before ISEL tests are positive (Chang *et al.*, 2002). Products released from proteins attacked by proteolytic enzymes in apoptotic cells are stained immunohistochemically. An example is **fractin**, a product derived from actin (Suurmeijer *et al.*, 1999; see also Willingham, 1999). Antibodies that recognize the cleaved (activated) form of caspase-3 were introduced by Urase *et al.*

(1998) in a study of programmed cell death in the developing nervous system and soon came to be widely used for the demonstration of apoptosis. Immunohistochemistry with **anti-(cleaved caspase-3)** is a simple, reliable way to stain apoptotic cells (Gown and Willingham, 2002) and is often used instead of the ISEL methods.

9.7.1. *In situ* end labelling (ISEL) methods

In these techniques enzymes are used to add labelled nucleotides to the many loose ends of fragmented DNA. The two procedures differ in the choice of enzymes. Both methods demonstrate DNA in nuclei of apoptotic cells and in apoptotic bodies, and also in nuclei of necrotic cells that are in an advanced state of degeneration. TUNEL is the more popular ISEL method, and Nakamura *et al.* (1995) found it more reliable in practice than *in situ* nick translation.

Fixation is generally not critical for these methods. Brief fixation in buffered formaldehyde is most frequently used, but an alcohol-based mixture is probably preferable to avoid masking of DNA by cross-linked nucleoprotein. Of three fixatives tested on cultured cells by Kishimoto *et al.* (1990), 70% ethanol was considered the best, but this would give poor structural preservation in blocks of tissue. Fixation in 1:3 acetic acid-ethanol (Clarke's fluid, which preserves structure well; see Chapter 2) damaged DNA so that normal nuclei were stained by *in situ* nick translation. Merritt *et al.* (1996) recommend Carnoy's or Clarke's fixative, or buffered aqueous formaldehyde. ISEL methods fail when applied to tissue that has been kept for several months in aqueous formaldehyde (Davison *et al.*, 1995). It is probably wise to avoid mercury- or dichromate-containing mixtures, which might interfere with the actions of the enzymes used in ISEL techniques.

It is important to recognize that these procedures are not specific for apoptosis. Some normal nuclei become TUNEL-positive when they are cut by the microtome knife. such false-positive nuclei are more numerous in thin (5 μm) than in thick (15 μm) sections (Sloop *et al.*, 1999). Cells in an advanced state of necrosis contain damaged DNA and are stained by both methods. The nick translation method is positive with necrotic cells that are not yet detectable by TUNEL, and is therefore a more sensitive test for the early nuclear changes of apoptosis (Gold *et al.*, 1994). False-positive artifacts, often seen in biopsies, are discussed by Tsutsumi and Kamoshida (2003). The earliest changes in apoptosis are in the cytoplasm and cell membrane, and these are not detectable by ISEL methods or by fluorescent staining of DNA (Collins *et al.*, 1997).

In situ nick translation is more sensitive than terminal uridine nick end labelling for detecting the early stages of apoptosis (Yamadori *et al.*, 1998). Comparative, quantitative studies indicate that ISEL methods offer no advantages over simple nuclear stains for detecting cells that have reached the stage of nuclear pyknosis or fragmentation (Drachenberg *et al.*, 1997; Hawkins *et al.*, 1997).

9.7.1.1. Terminal uridine nick end labelling (TUNEL)

This technique, also called 'tailing', has three stages. In the first, which is necessary after aldehyde fixation but probably not after a simple coagulant, the fragmented DNA is made accessible to the reagents by degrading or denaturing the associated nucleoprotein. This is usually done with proteinase K (E.C. 3.4.21.14), a proteolytic enzyme of fungal origin that also attacks nucleases and prevents further degradation of DNA. A cheaper alternative is to heat to 86°C in citrate buffer, pH 6.0 in a microwave oven. Negoescu *et al.* (1996) preferred this treatment to proteinase K, but Lucassen *et al.* (1995) noted that it induced false-positive labelling of nuclei if there had been a post mortem delay of several hours before fixation of the tissue. The optimum procedure also varies with the fixative (Labat-Moleur *et al.*, 1998).

In the next step the sections are exposed to a buffered solution containing the terminal deoxynucleotidyl transferase (E.C. 2.7.7.31; often called terminal transferase or TdT), labelled deoxyuridine triphosphate (dUTP), and cobalt ions. The enzyme, which needs Co^{2+} as a cofactor, catalyses the addition of labelled nucleotide molecules to nucleotides in DNA that have a hydroxyl group at position 3' of deoxyribose in DNA. The 3' carbon atom is normally joined to a phosphate (see Fig. 9.1), and bears a hydroxyl group only where there is a break in the DNA strand. Apoptotic cells incorporate the labelled nucleotide at one end of every segment of their greatly fragmented DNA.

In the final stage of the method, the label is made visible. A fluorescent label such as fluorescein can be observed directly by fluorescence microscopy. Another common label is biotin, which is made visible by virtue of its affinity for avidin (Chapter 19 for more information); this was used in the original procedure of Gavrieli *et al.* (1992). A slightly different approach is to use 5-bromo-2'deoxyuridine (BrDU) as the thymidine analogue (Aschoff *et al.*, 1996). This is less expensive than the biotinylated nucleotide, and it can be detected immunohistochemically with commercially available antibodies that recognize BrDU. Detailed instructions for a fluorescent TUNEL procedure are given by Darzynkiewicz and Li (1996).

9.7.1.2. *In situ* nick translation

This procedure differs from TUNEL in the enzymes used to catalyze the incorporation of the labelled nucleotide into fragmented DNA. As with TUNEL, pre-treatment with proteinase K is usually needed to expose the DNA in formaldehyde-fixed material.

The nick translation reaction mixture contains labelled dUTP, together with the unlabelled nucleotides of DNA (dATP, dCTP, dGTP, and dTTP) and DNA polymerase I (E.C. 2.7.7.7), together with Mg^{2+} ions and a sulphydryl protecting compound such as 2-mercaptoethanol or dithiothreitol (Chapter 10), which are needed by the enzyme. DNA polymerase I has two synergistic actions. DNA polymerase I adds a nucleotide to the 3' end of a break (or nick) in one strand of DNA, and it breaks the next 5' linkage. Nucleotides, complementary to those of the other strand, are added sequentially as the nick moves along the DNA molecule. The newly generated strand incorporates some labelled deoxyuridine instead of thymidine. The nuclei of apoptotic cells contain DNA molecules with many free 3' ends at which nick translation can be initiated, so the nuclei incorporate large numbers of labelled deoxyuridine molecules. The label is detected histochemically.

Labels used for *in situ* nick translation include biotin (Kishimoto *et al.*, 1990, Fensel *et al.*, 1994), digoxigenin and fluorescein (Gold *et al.*, 1993). Detailed instructions for a method using digoxigenin labelling are given by Merritt *et al.* (1996).

9.7.1.3. Controls for ISEL methods

With both techniques, there is the risk of false-negative results (due to failure of the enzymatic reaction or of the procedure for detecting the label) or false-positive nuclei (due to DNA damage during fixation, or to excessive incubation in the enzyme-nucleotide mixture.

A pre-treatment with DNase I will determine that an ISEL procedure is capable of detecting fragmented DNA. Before staining, some control sections are incubated for 10 min in a solution containing deoxyribonuclease I (E.C. 3.1.21.1; deoxyribonucleate-5'-oligonucleotidohydrolase; commonly called DNase I). The solution contains 0.1–1.0 μg/ml of enzyme, in a buffer containing 4 mM $MgCl_2$. This enzymatic treatment is much milder than when a DNase is used to extract DNA from a section (Section 9.4.3.). DNase I makes breaks in the DNA strands throughout the tissue, and all nuclei will incorporate labelled nucleotides.

False-positive staining should be suspected if large numbers of labelled nuclei are encountered in a normal tissue in which there is not a rapid turnover of cells. A section of normal brain, liver, muscle, or kidney should contain hardly any apparently apoptotic cells. Moderate numbers of ISEL-positive cells are seen in lymphoid tissues and in the intestinal epithelium.

9.8. Nucleolar organizer regions

Ribosomal RNA is transcribed and assembled into ribosomes on certain chromosomes at sites known as nucleolar organizer regions or **NORs**. The method for staining them is included in this chapter for convenience, even though NORs are not themselves composed of a nucleic acid.

These sites can be made visible by staining with silver nitrate, either in smears containing metaphase chromosomes (Goodpasture and Bloom, 1975) or in paraffin sections (Ploton et al., 1986). Black colloidal silver is deposited in the stained objects. The use of silver nitrate has led to the widespread use of the term **AgNOR** to identify both the methods and the NORs themselves. In proliferating cells NORs are smallest and most numerous in early prophase and late telophase. They come together to form one or two nucleoli in the G1, S and G2 phases (interphase) of the cell cycle (see Jewell and Cordial, 1996). The size and number of NORs are increased in malignant tumours, and have prognostic value (Derenzini et al., 1988; Raymond and Leong, 1989; Derenzini, 2000). Quantitative data from AgNOR-stained tissues have been used also as an indicator of the general level of RNA and protein synthesis (Jewell and Cordial, 1996; Moreno et al., 1997). There are instances, however, of conspicuous AgNORs in cells known to be metabolically inactive (Morales et al., 1996).

The objects stained by an AgNOR method are the proteinaceous fibrillary cores of developing and mature nucleoli. The protein is not a histone, and the argyrophilia has been attributed to peptide sequences rich in aspartic acid (Valdez et al., 1995). Argyrophilic NOR proteins occur at the same chromosomal sites as their encoding genes (Zurita et al., 1998), and move into nucleoli in response to cellular stress (Zhu et al., 1997). The staining with silver depends on the presence of reduced cysteine (De Capoa et al., 1982), and NORs can be stained by a fluorescent reagent that combines specifically with the sulphydryl group of this amino acid (Mehes et al., 1993). In plants, AgNOR staining is associated with tyrosine-rich proteins.

The chemistry of silver staining is not simple (Grizzle, 1996; see also Chapter 18), and results are strongly influenced by fixation and the composition of the solutions used. Conspicuous features of the AgNOR methods are the high concentration of $AgNO_3$ used, and the presence in the solution of formic acid and a substance of high molecular weight such as gelatin or polyethylene glycol (Rowlands et al., 1990). The formic acid produces a low pH, which discourages the binding of silver ions to most tissue components (see Peters, 1955a). It is also a reducing agent, so it can be expected to reduce Ag^+ to Ag^0. This reaction is catalyzed by tiny particles of metallic silver or silver sulphide, which are probably formed initially at sites of high cysteine concentration in the NOR. The macromolecular ingredient is a 'protective colloid', which delays the reduction of silver ions in the solution. AgNOR staining is usually performed on smears of cells fixed in alcoholic liquids such as Clarke's fluid, or on paraffin sections of formaldehyde-fixed tissue. Oxidizing fixatives should be avoided because they cause excessive background staining (Lindner, 1993).

9.8.1.
AgNOR method

This is the procedure recommended by Jewell and Cordial (1996) for paraffin sections of formaldehyde-fixed material, incorporating also some of the improvements made by Lindner (1993). The method may also be applied to smears or preparations made from suspended cells. If AgNORs are to be assessed quantitatively, it is necessary for all the sections to be cut at the same thickness setting, ideally 4 μm, on the same microtome. All glassware must be perfectly clean, and the water must be the purest available.

The silver staining reagent is applied as drops that lie on horizontal slides, in a dark, humidified container. A plastic box containing some wet filter paper or gauze is suitable.

Solutions required
Staining solution
This is made up immediately before using, from two components:

Formic acid–gelatin
Formic acid (88%):	0.3 ml
Water:	24.7 ml
Gelatin:	500 mg

Leave at room temperature until the gelatin dissolves (takes at least 30 min). This solution is made on the day it is to be used. Filter before using.

50% silver nitrate
Silver nitrate:	25 g
Water:	50 ml

This can be kept for many years in a dark glass bottle. Be careful to avoid contamination of this stock solution.

Working silver solution
This is mixed immediately before using. The quantities below are for staining just one slide.
Formic acid–gelatin:	0.1 ml
50% silver nitrate:	0.2 ml

5% sodium thiosulphate
Sodium thiosulphate ($Na_2S_2O_3.5H_2O$):	20 g
Water:	400 ml

This can be kept indefinitely, but should be used only once. Replace if it is cloudy or contains a precipitate.

A counterstain
Ethyl green is recommended, but other cationic dye counterstains may also be used (Chapter 6 for instructions). Avoid dark colours, especially blue. The Feulgen reaction (Section 9.3.2) is also suitable, but it should be done before the AgNOR method.

Procedure
(1) De-wax and rehydrate paraffin sections and wash in three changes of pure water. (Pass smears through graded alcohols to water.)
(2) Shake off excess water, and place the slides horizontally in the humidified staining container.
(3) Mix the working silver solution and put a large drop of it on each section. Cover the container and put it in a dark place. The ideal staining time varies with the material: 10–20 or occasionally as long as 45 min.
(4) Wash the slides in 3 changes of water.

(5) Immerse in 5% sodium thiosulphate, 5 min.
(6) Wash in running tap water for 10 min.
(7) (Optional) Apply a counterstain.
(8) Dehydrate, clear and mount in a resinous medium.

Result

Nucleolar organizer regions are black dots. Ideally there should be no brown background staining from the silver solution. Other structures are coloured according to the counterstain used.

9.9. Detection of DNA synthesis, mitosis and meiosis

9.9.1.
DNA synthesis

DNA replicates in the S phase of the cell cycle, before mitosis. The tradition way to label newly synthesized DNA is to administer [^{3}H]thymidine, which is incorporated into DNA but not into RNA. A single dose is available in an animal for about 1 h (Nygaard and Potter, 1959), whereas repeated injections or continuously infused thymidine will label DNA that is newly replicated over a longer time (Messier and Leblond, 1960; Bertalanffy, 1964). The incorporated tritium in the nuclei of labelled cells is easily demonstrated by autoradiography (Kopriwa and Leblond, 1962). Later cell divisions halve the amount of label in each nucleus. It is possible to recognize second and third generation cells in this way, and also to determine the life spans of cells that do not divide again. Major limitations of autoradiography include limited accuracy of resolution (though there is no difficulty recognizing a heavily labelled nucleus), the high price and short shelf life of the emulsion, and the the long duration of the exposure (often a month or more).

If living cells that are about to divide are exposed to **5-bromo-2'-deoxyuridine** (BrDU), this synthetic compound is incorporated into their DNA and passed on to the daughter cells. Monoclonal antibodies are available that recognize BrDU, and these can be used for the immunohistochemical identification of cells that contain the tracer (Morstyn *et al.*, 1986; de Fazio *et al.*, 1987). The method gives results similar to those obtained with [^{3}H]thymidine, but autoradiography is not needed. BrDU is therefore useful in studies of cell kinetics. (The same compound is used in the TUNEL method, see Section 9.7.1.1.) For recognition of later generations of cells, the grain count over a labelled nucleus is probably a more accurate indicator than a measurement of colour intensity in an immunostained preparation.

9.9.2.
Mitosis and meiosis

The appearances and movements of chromosomes were described in mitotic cells by Flemming in 1879 and in meiotic cells by Van Beneden in 1887. In the latter year also, Weismann postulated that the material of heredity was linearly arrayed in the chromosomes (see Mason, 1956). These discoveries were made in fragments of fixed tissue that had been squashed or sectioned and then stained with a variety of dyes. The number of available fixatives, dyes and fluorochromes has increased greatly since the original observations were made, and the use of cultured cells has simplified and improved the accuracy of the examination of animal chromosomes.

For fixatives that preserve the spindle apparatus and/or chromosomes, see Chapter 2. Some methods for handling suspended cells are described in Chapter 7. Chromosomes can be made visible with many staining methods, including those used for cell nuclei (Chapter 6), the Romanowsky–Giemsa methods (Chapter 7) and histochemical techniques for DNA such as the Feulgen reaction (Section 9.3 of this chapter). The field of **cytogenetics** also embraces many other techniques that are outside the scope of this book.

10 | Organic functional groups and protein histochemistry

This chapter is devoted to the histochemistry of the side-chains of some amino acids and the reactions of a few functional groups artificially produced by the action of reagents upon tissues. The histochemical reactions of other organic compounds such as carbohydrates, lipids, nucleic acids, and amines are described in other chapters.

As elsewhere in this book, no attempt is made to describe more than a small selection of the methods available for the various organic functional groups. **For seldom used techniques, the theory is explained briefly, but practical instructions are not given.** Functional group histochemistry is treated at length by Lillie and Fullmer (1976), and much information can also be found in the works of Gabe (1976), James and Tas (1984) and Pearse (1985).

Blocking reactions common to many methods are given at the end of the chapter, in Section 10.11.

10.1. General considerations and methodology

Functional groups are detected histochemically by making use of their characteristic chemical reactions to produce coloured compounds. The techniques can be properly understood and intelligently used only when the underlying organic chemistry is constantly kept in mind. For more information the reader should consult a textbook of organic chemistry. Those of Noller (1965), Smith and March (2001), and Morrison and Boyd (1992) are recommended. Some histochemically valuable reactions are not included in general texts, but many of them are described by Feigl (1960) and Glazer (1976).

The methods discussed in this chapter are for functional groups that form part of the macromolecular structure of the tissue. Diffusion and extraction by solvents prior to staining cannot, therefore, give rise to false localizations. The reactions can all be carried out on frozen or paraffin sections of suitably fixed material. It is necessary, however, to take into account the chemical reactions of fixation. The non-additive coagulant fixatives do not cause chemical changes in tissues, so alcohol-based mixtures such as Carnoy's fluid or methacarn are ideal for the histochemical study of proteins (except for a few secretory products not fixed by alcohol). Formaldehyde is also acceptable, because most of its reactions with the side-chains of amino acids are reversed when the fixative is washed out (Chapter 2). The same is true of picric acid and, except when sulphydryl groups are to be demonstrated, of mercuric chloride. Chromium trioxide, potassium dichromate, osmium tetroxide, and glutaraldehyde are best avoided: they all produce irreversible chemical changes in proteins.

Often a chromogenic reaction for a functional group is not as specific as we would like it to be. It is then necessary to examine control sections in which the group has been chemically altered (i.e. 'blocked') so that it can no longer take part in the reaction that yields a visible deposit. Many of the blocking reactions are also of low specificity, however, so it is frequently necessary to use more than one of them in order to discover, by elimination, the sites at which a single functional group is present in the tissue. Sometimes it is possible to undo the effect of blockade of a functional group by judicious application of a second reagent. This strategy is valuable when the blocking of one functional group is reversible but that of another is not.

Despite the intrinsic interest and great instructional value of functional group histochemistry, the methods derived from this branch of the science are used only on rare occasions in routine histological and pathological practice and in the investigation of biological problems. This is unfortunate because the techniques are often valuable for displaying structural features of tissues and have the added advantage of providing some chemical information.

The major histochemically demonstrable organic functional groups present in animal tissues are listed in *Table 10.1*.

10.2. Alcohols

Aliphatic hydroxy groups occur in carbohydrates, and also in the widely distributed amino acids serine, a primary alcohol, and threonine, a secondary alcohol. Hydroxylysine and hydroxyproline, which occur principally in collagen, are also secondary alcohols. Some lipids are alcohols of high molecular weight, but in tissues they are usually esterified.

10.2.1.
Histochemical detection

Hydroxy groups in tissues can be detected by converting them to sulphate esters and then staining with a cationic dye at pH 1.0 or lower (Chapter 6). This procedure demonstrates all hydroxy groups. Those of proteins cannot be distinguished from those of carbohydrates, which are generally more abundant. The dye will also bind to preexisting sulphate–ester groups in the tissue, such as those of some proteoglycans, glycoproteins and sulphatide lipids. The native sulphate esters are recognized by staining control sections that have not been subjected to the sulphation

Table 10.1. Histochemically demonstrable functional groups

Functional group	Occurrence
Aliphatic hydroxyl	Proteins: serine, threonine, hydroxyproline, hydroxylysine. All carbohydrates (Chapter 11). Some lipids (Chapter 12).
Phenol	Proteins: tyrosine. In plants: tannins. Small molecules: serotonin, catecholamines (Chapter 17).
Carboxyl	Proteins: C-termini of all peptide chains; side chains of glutamic and aspartic acids. Carbohydrates: most glycoproteins and proteoglycans (Chapter 11). Lipids: free fatty acids (Chapter 12).
Amino	Proteins: N-termini of all peptide chains; side-chain of lysine. Some carbohydrates, lipids and small molecules (Chapters 11, 12, 17).
Guanidino	Proteins: side-chain of arginine.
Indolyl	Proteins: side chain of tryptophan. Small molecules: serotonin (Chapter 17).
Sulphydryl (thiol)	Proteins: side-chain of cysteine; also by reduction of cystine.
Disulphide	Proteins: cystine bridges between peptide chains.
Sulphate ester	Carbohydrates: most proteoglycans and many glycoproteins (Chapter 11). Lipids: sulphatides (Chapter 12). Also introduced by artificial sulphation of $-OH$, $-NH_2$.
Sulphonic acid	Produced or artificially introduced in various histochemical procedures.
Phosphate esters	Nucleic acids (Chapter 9). Some lipids (Chapter 12). Some proteins (e.g. casein in mammary gland and vitellin in egg yolk have many serines esterified by H_3PO_4).
Aldehyde	Proteins: elastin of immature animals (Chapter 8). Lipids, when oxidized by air (Chapter 12). Produced artificially in many histochemical methods.
Ketone	Lipids: some steroids (Chapter 12). Produced artificially in a few histochemical procedures.
Olefinic bonds	All lipids (Chapter 12).

treatment. Both natural and artificially produced sulphate esters are hydrolysed, with loss of the sulphate group, by exposure to hot acidified methanol (Section 10.11.4).

Various reagents are available for sulphation of hydroxy groups in sections. Concentrated sulphuric acid is the simplest, but is physically injurious. It works well, however, with semi-thin sections (0.5–1.0 μm) of plastic-embedded material. A mixture of sulphuric acid and diethyl ether is milder. An even more gentle reagent is 0.25% sulphuric acid in a mixture of acetic acid and acetic anhydride (Lillie, 1964), but this also brings about *N*-sulphation of amino groups (Section 10.11.3).

10.2.2
Blocking
procedures

The reactivity of hydroxy groups is blocked by base-catalysed acylation with either acetic anhydride:

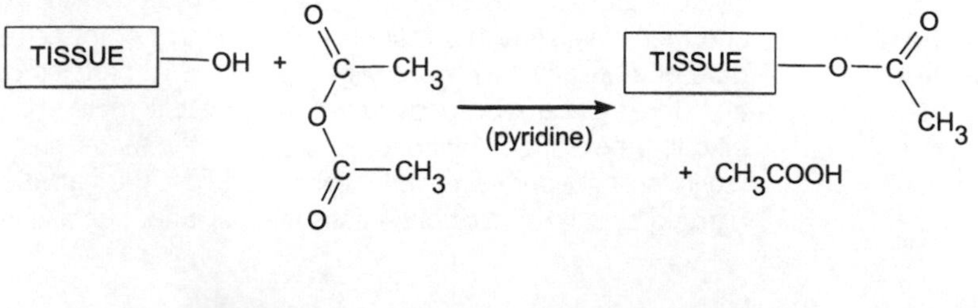

or benzoyl chloride. These reactions generate esters at the sites of hydroxy groups. Acetic anhydride also produces N-acetylation of some amino groups. Benzoyl chloride causes benzoylation of almost all amino groups. The acylation reactions also block the reactivity of tyrosine, tryptophan, and histidine residues. The histochemical reactivity of arginine, however, is only slightly depressed by acylation. Esters formed with hydroxy groups and amides formed by N-acylation of amines are hydrolysed. with reversal of the blockade, by exposure of the sections to alkaline ethanol, a procedure known in histochemical parlance as 'saponification'.

Diisopropyl fluorophosphate (DFP) and related organophosphorus compounds combine irreversibly with the hydroxy group of serine, but not in all proteins. The value of these reagents in histochemistry is therefore limited to their uses as inhibitors of certain serine-containing enzymes (Chapter 15).

10.3. Carboxylic acids

Free carboxyl groups occur in glycoproteins and proteoglycans (Chapter 11), in fatty acids (Chapter 12), and in proteins. Every protein molecule has a terminal carboxyl group, but this is usually outnumbered by the side-chain carboxyls of glutamic and aspartic acids.

10.3.1.
Histochemical detection

Cationic dyes will bind to carboxylic acids when the latter are ionized. For this to be so, the pH of the dye solution must usually be 4.0 or higher, so sulphate esters of proteoglycans and phosphoric acid groups of nucleic acids are also stained (Chapter 6). Dyes are therefore of limited use for the identification of sites of carboxyl groups in tissues.

The **acid anhydride method** supposedly demonstrates only the carboxyl groups of proteins. Sections are first treated with a solution of acetic anhydride in pyridine at 60°C. This reagent is thought to react in different ways with C-terminal and with side-chain carboxyl groups:

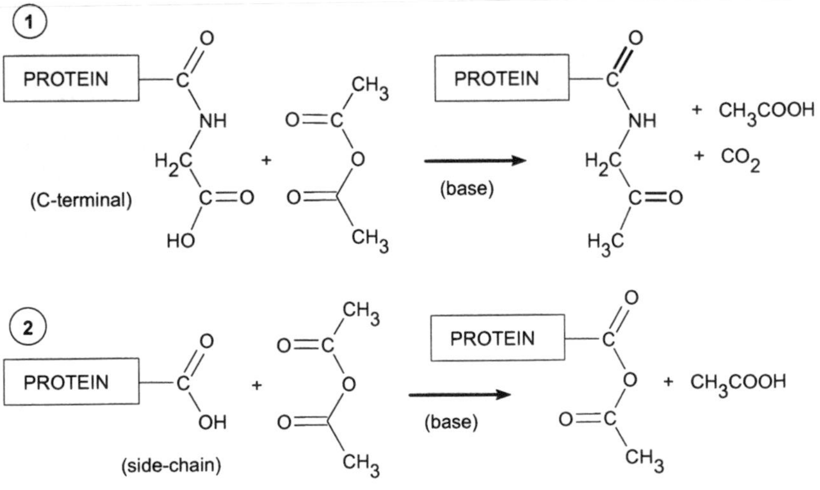

The product of the first reaction (Barrnett and Seligman, 1958) is a ketone and it combines with the next reagent to be applied to the sections, 2-hydroxy-3-naphthoic acid hydrazide (HNAH) as described in Section 10.10.2. The second reaction of acetic anhydride with side-chain carboxyls yields a mixed anhydride (Karnovsky and Fasman, 1960). This also combines with HNAH. The reaction is analogous to the acylation of an amine:

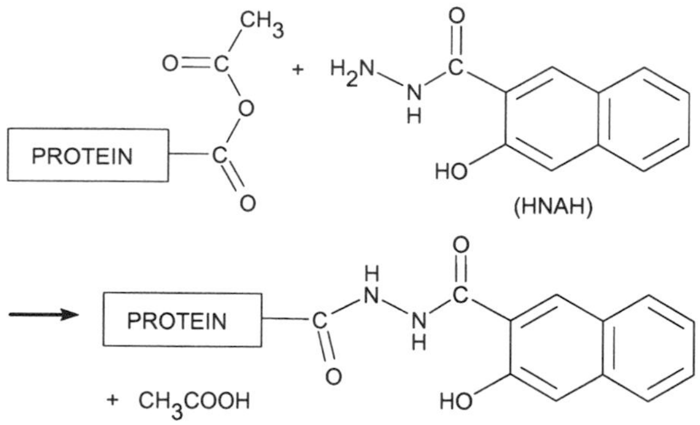

Both reactions result in the covalent binding of a naphthol group at the site of the carboxyl of the protein molecule. The naphthol can easily be made to couple with a diazonium salt to yield a coloured product (Chapter 5).

The carboxyl groups of carbohydrates do not react with acetic anhydride to give mixed anhydrides (Karnovsky and Mann, 1961), though there is no obvious reason why they should not behave in the same way as those of protein side-chains. A chemical study by Stoward and Burns (1971) indicated that the principal effect of hot acetic anhydride in pyridine was the formation of ketones at the sites of C-terminal carboxyl groups and that the side-chains of glutamic and aspartic acids formed mixed anhydrides only to a very slight extent. The histochemistry of carbohydrates with free carboxyl groups is discussed in Chapter 11.

10.3.2.
Blocking procedures

Carboxyl groups are easily blocked by converting them to their methyl esters. This may be accomplished with a variety of reagents. The simplest is 0.1 M HCl in methanol:

Other methylating agents occasionally used by histochemists are methyl iodide, diazomethane, and a solution of thionyl chloride in methanol.

Methylation also blocks amino groups, sulphydryl groups, and the phosphoric acid moieties of nucleic acids. The reagent brings about hydrolysis of sulphate esters. It is a blocking reaction of greater importance in carbohydrate histochemistry than in the examination of carboxyl groups of proteins. Methyl esters of carboxylic acids are hydrolysed by saponification with alkaline ethanol.

10.4. Amino groups

This section is concerned with primary amino ($-NH_2$) groups of proteins. Some important soluble amines are also detectable histochemically (Chapter 17), but these are no longer present in sections of tissues prepared by ordinary techniques. The most numerous amino groups of proteins are those in the ε-position on the side-chain of lysine. N-terminal amino groups are less abundant because there is only one for each peptide chain.

Fixatives that combine covalently with amines, such as aldehydes, should be avoided if possible. They always impair staining of amino groups and sometimes prevent it completely. Strong oxidizing agents are also unsuitable for fixation, because they can cause oxidative deamination of proteins.

10.4.1.
Histochemical detection

There are two main groups of methods for the demonstration of the amino groups of proteins. The first group consists simply of staining the tissue with a suitable anionic dye. This must be a dye that binds to its substrate exclusively by ionic attraction: usually one with fairly small molecules. Anionic dyes of high molecular weight, which are bound to tissues by forces other than electrostatic ones, are unsuitable. The mechanisms of staining by anionic dyes have already been discussed in Chapters 5, 6, and 8. Staining is to be expected at the sites of all tissue-bound cations, including amino and guanidino groups of proteins and organic bases such as choline that occur in some lipids. Blocking reactions (Section 10.4.2) and extraction of lipids (Chapter 12) must be used in order to establish that the acidophilia of a structure is due to the presence of amino groups.

The methods of the second group depend upon the formation of coloured deposits as the result of covalent combination of reagents with either intact or chemically modified amino groups. Many techniques are available. A typical one is the hydroxynaphthaldehyde method. The reagent, 2-hydroxy-3-naphthaldehyde, condenses with the protein-bound amino group to form an imine (also known as an azomethine or Schiff's base):

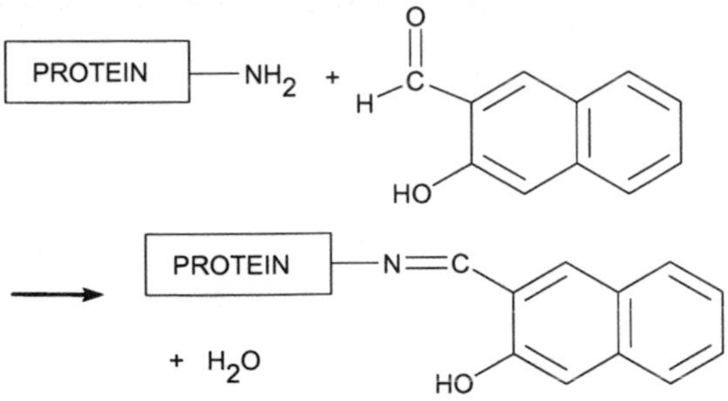

PROTEIN —NH$_2$ + (2-hydroxy-3-naphthaldehyde)

⟶ PROTEIN —N=C (naphthol) + H$_2$O

Thus, a naphthol becomes covalently bound at the site of the original –NH$_2$ group. In the second stage of the method, the naphthol is made to couple with a diazonium salt to form an azo dye. The diazonium salt will, of course, also couple with the aromatic ring of tyrosine and with some other amino acids (Section 10.9.2). However, the colours produced with these amino acids are different from and paler than that of the naphtholic azo dye. In any case they are easily allowed for in control sections that have not been treated with hydroxynaphthaldehyde.

A more recent method for the amino group is the **dithiocarbamylation reaction** (Tandler, 1980), in which small pieces of fixed tissue are immersed in a mixture of carbon disulphide and a strong base, triethylamine. Dithiocarbamyl derivatives of primary amino groups are formed:

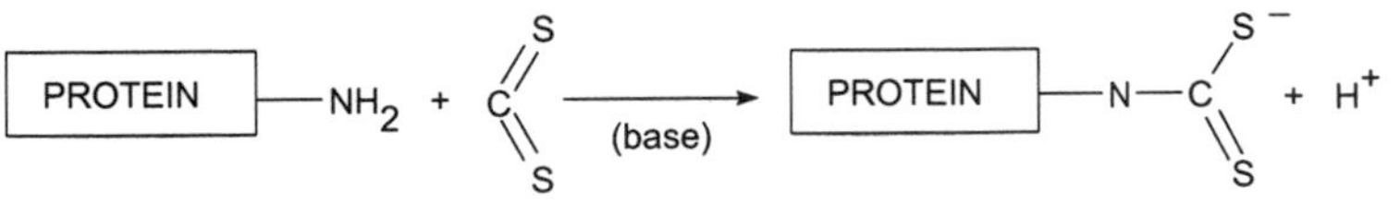

PROTEIN —NH$_2$ + CS$_2$ —(base)→ PROTEIN —N—C(=S)S$^-$ + H$^+$

After washing out excess carbon disulphide, the tissue is exposed to lead acetate. A lead dithiocarbamate complex is first formed, but it decomposes and yields lead sulphide, which is insoluble, brown–black in colour, and also dense enough to impart contrast in the electron microscope.

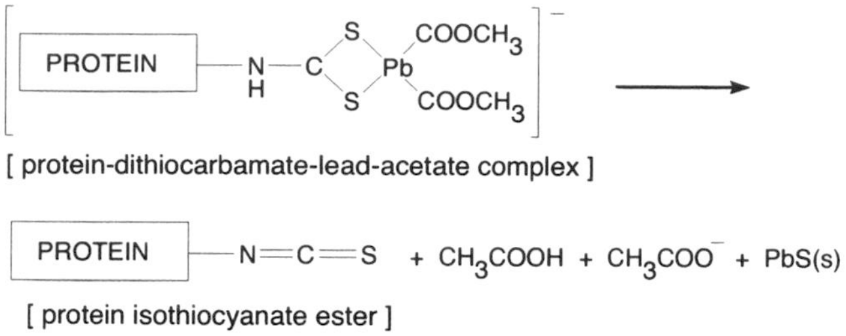

$$\left[\boxed{\text{PROTEIN}} - \underset{\text{H}}{\text{N}} - \text{C} \underset{\text{S}}{\overset{\text{S}}{\diagdown}} \text{Pb} \underset{\text{COOCH}_3}{\overset{\text{COOCH}_3}{\diagup}} \right]^- \longrightarrow$$

[protein-dithiocarbamate-lead-acetate complex]

$$\boxed{\text{PROTEIN}} - \text{N} = \text{C} = \text{S} \ + \text{CH}_3\text{COOH} \ + \ \text{CH}_3\text{COO}^- \ + \ \text{PbS(s)}$$

[protein isothiocyanate ester]

The guanidino group of arginine does not react with carbon disulphide, which is a reagent of high specificity for the –NH$_2$ group. The sensitivity of the method is not high, however, so dithiocarbamylation can be used for histochemical localization of proteins that owe their basicity to lysine.

10.4.2.
Blocking reactions

Primary amines may be blocked either by removing them or by converting them to amides or sulphoamino compounds.

Deamination is most easily accomplished by treating the sections with nitrous acid, which is usually applied as a solution of sodium nitrite in aqueous acetic acid, known as van Slyke's reagent. The reaction is most simply expressed as:

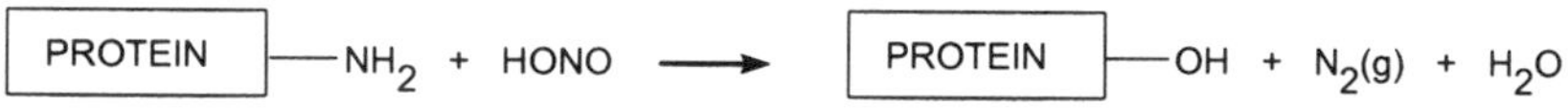

$$\boxed{\text{PROTEIN}} - \text{NH}_2 \ + \ \text{HONO} \ \longrightarrow \ \boxed{\text{PROTEIN}} - \text{OH} \ + \ \text{N}_2\text{(g)} \ + \ \text{H}_2\text{O}$$

but is much more complicated in reality (White and Woodcock, 1968). Nitrous acid also reacts with tyrosine (Section 10.7.1) and with sulphur containing amino acids, but these reactions are unlikely to cause confusion in the testing of histochemical methods for amino groups. The guanidino group of arginine is not removed by treatment with nitrous acid (Lillie et al., 1971). Strong oxidizing agents such as osmium tetroxide and potassium permanganate also bring about deamination of lysine side-chains, but their actions are rather unpredictable.

Acylation of amines is brought about by reaction with either acetic anhydride or benzoyl chloride:

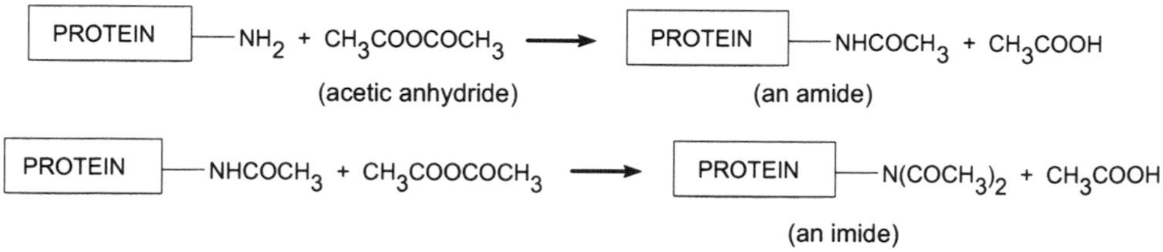

$$\boxed{\text{PROTEIN}} - \text{NH}_2 \ + \ \text{CH}_3\text{COOCOCH}_3 \ \longrightarrow \ \boxed{\text{PROTEIN}} - \text{NHCOCH}_3 \ + \ \text{CH}_3\text{COOH}$$

(acetic anhydride)   (an amide)

$$\boxed{\text{PROTEIN}} - \text{NHCOCH}_3 \ + \ \text{CH}_3\text{COOCOCH}_3 \ \longrightarrow \ \boxed{\text{PROTEIN}} - \text{N(COCH}_3)_2 \ + \ \text{CH}_3\text{COOH}$$

(an imide)

Equivalent reactions occur with benzoyl chloride. The reaction of acylation is catalysed either by a weak base such as pyridine or by a strong acid such as perchloric acid. *Longer times and higher temperatures are needed for the base-catalysed acetylation and benzoylation of amines than for the esterification of hydroxy groups by the same reagents.* The amides and imides produced by these reactions are hydrolysed, with regeneration of the amines, by 'saponification' with an alcoholic solution of potassium hydroxide. For example:

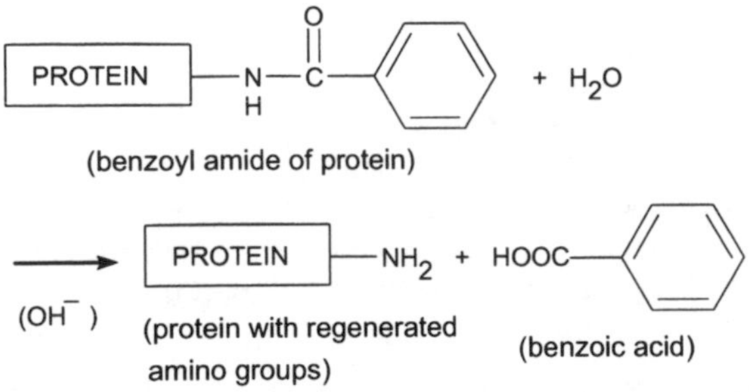

(benzoyl amide of protein)

(OH⁻) (protein with regenerated
amino groups) (benzoic acid)

When sections are treated with acetic anhydride in the presence of a little sulphuric acid, amino groups are blocked in a few minutes and their sites become strongly basophilic. Although some acetylation may occur, the principal reaction is probably N-sulphation:

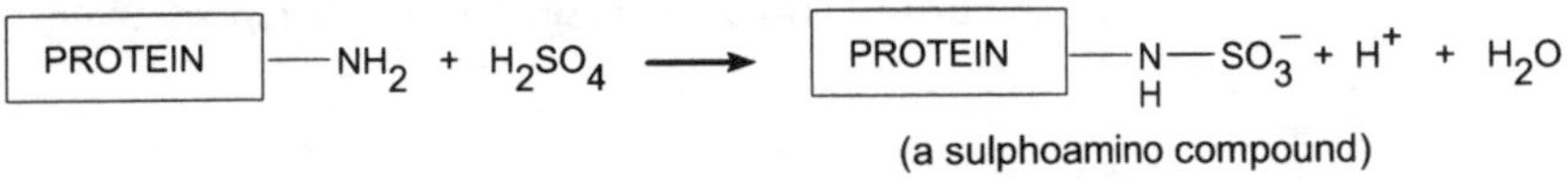

PROTEIN $-$NH$_2$ + H$_2$SO$_4$ $\longrightarrow$ PROTEIN $-$N$-$SO$_3^-$ + H$^+$ + H$_2$O
$\quad$ H

(a sulphoamino compound)

The product ionizes as a strong acid, thus accounting for the induced basophilia. This blockade is not reversible by saponification, but it is reversed by treatment with hot acidified methanol, which presumably causes breaking of the nitrogen-sulphur bond. It should be noted that the chemistry of this sulphation-acetylation procedure (Lillie, 1964) is still poorly understood, though the technique is useful on account of the rapidity and completeness of the reaction. The reagent also brings about O-sulphation of hydroxy groups, as has already been described (Section 10.2.2).

Primary amines are converted to secondary and tertiary amines by **alkylation** with reagents such as methanolic hydrogen chloride:

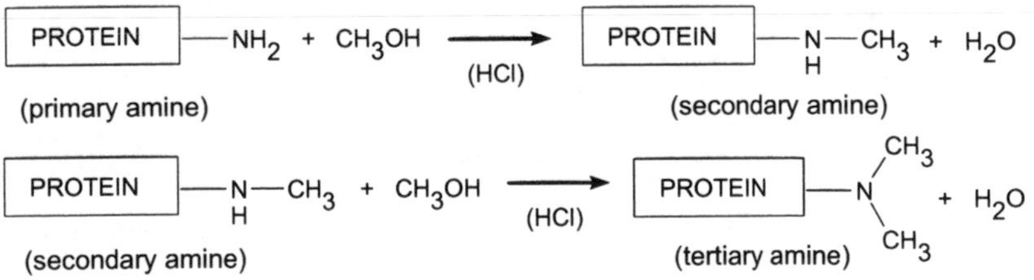

PROTEIN $-$NH$_2$ + CH$_3$OH $\longrightarrow$ PROTEIN $-$N$-$CH$_3$ + H$_2$O
$\qquad\qquad\qquad\qquad$ (HCl) $\qquad\qquad\qquad\qquad$ H

(primary amine) $\qquad\qquad\qquad\qquad$ (secondary amine)

PROTEIN $-$N$-$CH$_3$ + CH$_3$OH $\longrightarrow$ PROTEIN $-$N$\big\langle{}^{CH_3}_{CH_3}$ + H$_2$O
$\qquad$ H $\qquad\qquad$ (HCl)

(secondary amine) $\qquad\qquad\qquad\qquad$ (tertiary amine)

This reaction, which is slower than the methylation of carboxyl groups, does not prevent the binding of anionic dyes because the products are more strongly basic than primary amines. Arylation of amino groups can be achieved by reaction with 2,4-dinitrofluorobenzene, but this reagent also combines with the side-chains of cysteine, histidine, and tyrosine.

10.5. Arginine

Most proteins contain some arginine, but the highest concentrations are found in the histones associated with DNA and in certain cytoplasmic granules. The side-chain of this amino acid is strongly basic, owing to its guanidino group:

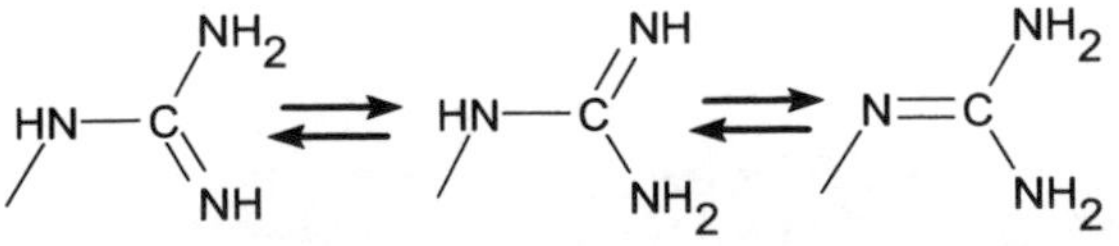

One proton, which may be shown attached to any of the nitrogen atoms, transforms the guanidino group into a guanidinium ion, and this is the condition even at high pH. The easiest way to stain sites of high concentration of arginine is to use an **alkaline solution of an anionic dye**. Biebrich scarlet (Spicer and Lillie, 1961) or fast green FCF (see James and Tas, 1984), at pH 8–9, are commonly used. Amino groups are not protonated at high pH, and they do not attract the dye anions. To stain the histone proteins of chromatin it is necessary first to remove the DNA by chemical or enzymatic extraction (Chapter 9), because the phosphate groups of the nucleic acid compete with and exclude dye anions.

Highly specific histochemical tests are also available for arginine. In the **Sakaguchi reaction** sections are treated with a solution containing sodium hypochlorite and α-naphthol, made strongly alkaline by addition of sodium hydroxide. A pink or red colour develops at the sites of arginine residues. It is unstable, so permanent preparations cannot be made. Baker (1947) tested the Sakaguchi reaction with several pure compounds of known structure and concluded that coloured products were formed by reaction of the reagent with substances containing the arrangement:

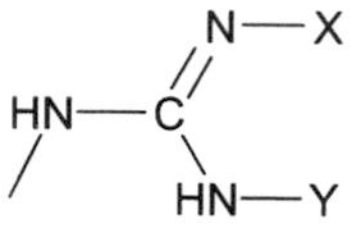

in which X and Y were –H or –CH$_3$. Arginine probably is the only component of fixed tissues to conform to this structural requirement. Lillie *et al.* (1971) discovered an identical pattern of staining with an alkaline solution of the sodium salt of 1,2-naphthoquinone-4-sulphonic acid (NQS):

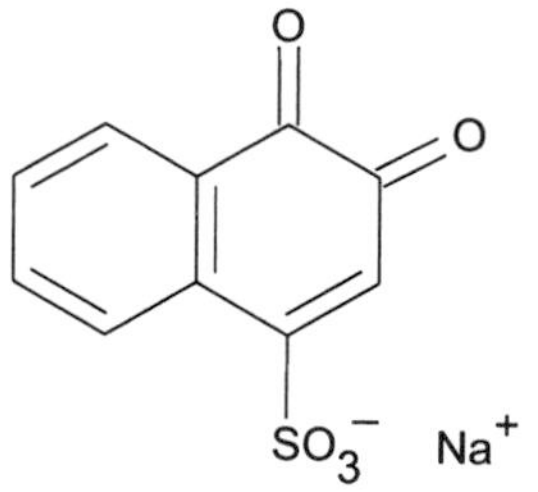

The alkalinity was produced by barium or strontium hydroxide. (The hydroxides of sodium, calcium, and magnesium did not permit full development of the colour.) The product of the reaction with NQS, unlike that formed in the Sakaguchi reaction, resisted extraction by organic solvents, and was permanent in resinous mounting media. Studies with blocking reactions indicated that NQS stained arginine specifically. Lillie *et al.* (1971) speculated that the coloured product of the reaction of the guanidino group with NQS was:

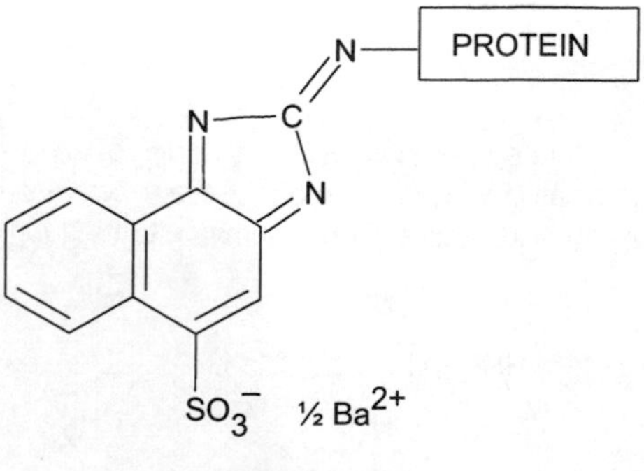

Cleavage of the chromogenic part of the structure from the remainder of the arginine residue might occur during the course of staining to give a closely similar anion (with a hydrogen atom in place of protein in the above formula). This compound has a soluble sodium salt but an insoluble barium salt (Lillie and Fullmer, 1976). Lillie *et al.* (1971) suggested that in the Sakaguchi reaction α-naphthol was oxidized by hypochlorite and the resulting 1,2-naphthoquinone condensed with guanidino groups to give an unstable coloured substance similar to the NQS product but lacking the sulphonic acid group.

The histochemical specificity of the Sakaguchi and related reactions is so high that blocking reactions are rarely considered necessary, though several are available. Lillie *et al.* (1971) and Montero *et al.* (1991) used alkaline alcoholic solutions of **benzil** to convert the guanidino group to an unreactive imidazole. By analogy to the well studied reactions of benzil with urea (Dunnavant and James, 1956) and with guanidine and *n*-butylguanidine (Lempert-Sreter *et al.*, 1963) the resulting compound can be expected to have the structure shown (Gutierrez, 1991), in which one of the phenyl groups of benzil migrates to the adjacent carbon atom:

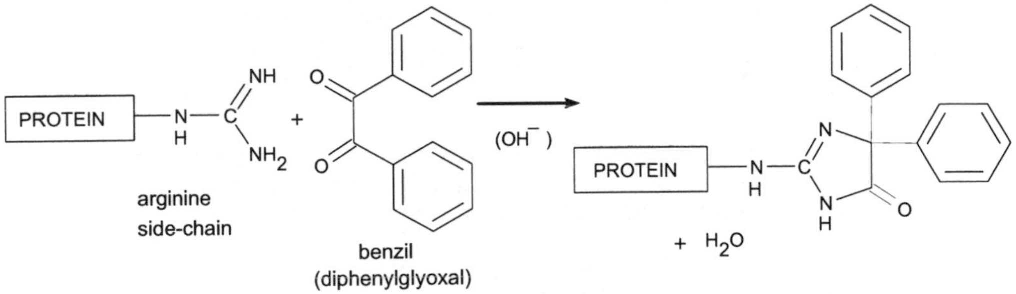

arginine
side-chain

benzil
(diphenylglyoxal)

An arginine-blocking reagent used by biochemists is the trimer of 2,3-butanedione (also called diacetyl trimer), which reacts with arginine in neutral solution. Monomeric diacetyl (dimethylglyoxal) is preferred for histochemical blockade of arginine (Segura *et al.*, 1994).

10.6. Tryptophan

Tryptophan is a ubiquitous component of proteins, so histochemical methods are employed only for the study of sites of high concentration of this amino acid, such as the Paneth cells of the intestine, the zymogen granules of the exocrine pancreas and several other secretory products. Amyloid (Chapter 11) also contains much tryptophan.

Histochemical techniques are based on the reactions of the indole ring, which remains free to react when the carboxyl and amino groups of tryptophan are incorporated into peptide linkages. Other naturally occurring indole-containing compounds are soluble and are therefore unlikely to be confused with tryptophan in paraffin sections. A possible exception is the serotonin of argentaffin cells and of mast cells of rodents (Chapter 17). Reactions for tryptophan can be obtained after almost any fixation but are strongest following formaldehyde or an alcoholic fixative. Picric acid, mercuric chloride, and potassium dichromate partly inhibit staining.

The most popular histochemical method for tryptophan is based on the addition of *p*-dimethylaminobenzaldehyde (DMAB) to the indole ring, which occurs at the position adjacent to the nitrogen atom. Sections are first treated with a solution of DMAB in acetic acid to which a strong acid (perchloric, hydrochloric, or a mixture of the two) has been added. The DMAB combines with the indole ring in an acid-catalysed hydroxyalkylation reaction:

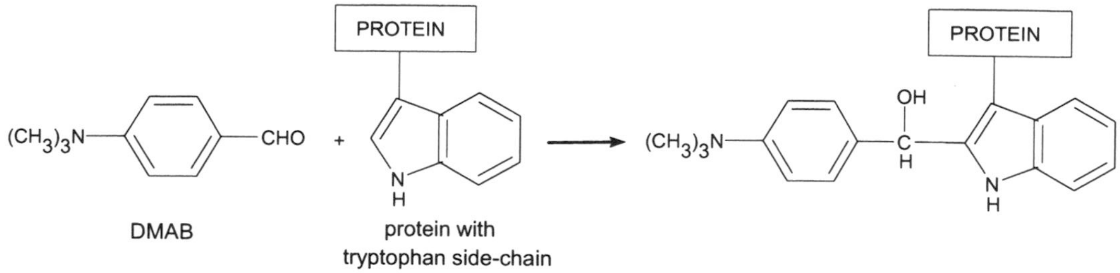

DMAB   protein with
              tryptophan side-chain

The product resembles a leuko-compound of a diarylmethane dye (See Section 5.9.5.2). In the second stage of the method an oxidizing agent, usually a strongly acidified solution of sodium nitrite, is applied. A blue colour develops due to the formation of a product that may have a structure such as:

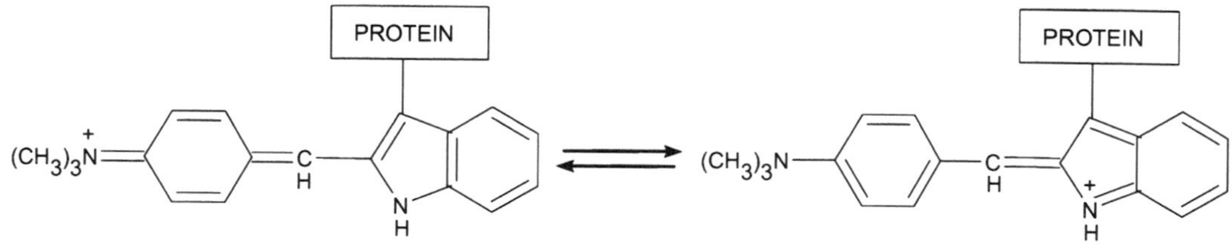

The resonance structure of such a compound shows similarity to those of diphenyl-methane and cyanine dyes (Chapter 5). Glenner (1957) suggested the product of the reaction was a 'rosindole' triarylmethane dye:

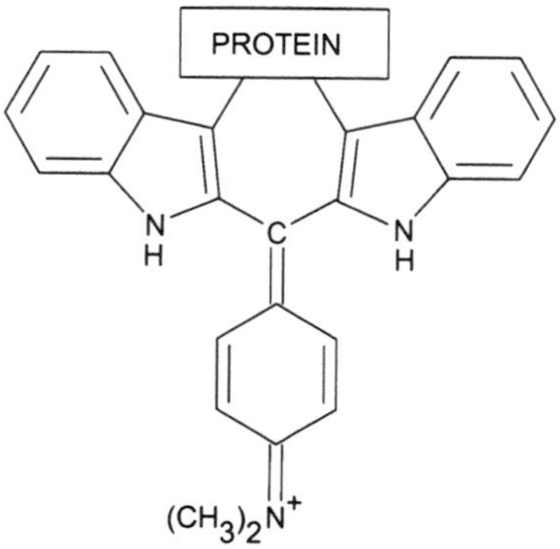

Such a compound could be formed with fixed proteins only where two indole rings are exactly the right distance apart to be able to combine with one molecule of DMAB. A triarylmethane dye is a likely product of the reaction of DMAB with solutions of indole-containing compounds but probably an infrequent one under the conditions of the histochemical procedure.

There is no reaction of high specificity for preventing the characteristic reactions of the indole group of tryptophan. Strong oxidizing agents cause opening of the heterocyclic ring; an alkaline solution of potassium persulphate is suitable for this purpose. The products of the reaction have not been identified and the blockade is irreversible. Performic and peracetic acids may also be used.

10.7. Tyrosine

Tyrosine is another ubiquitous amino acid. Its histochemical demonstration may be considered indicative of the presence of proteins. Several techniques for the detection of the simple phenolic side-chain are available. Other phenols such as serotonin, the catecholamines, and tannins will give the same reactions, but protein-bound tyrosine and the serotonin of argentaffin cells are the only reactive compounds likely to be present in fixed animal tissues.

Millon's classical test for protein was adapted for histochemical use by Baker (1956). A red colour develops when tissues are treated with an acid solution containing mercuric and nitrite ions. All investigators agree that the reaction is specific for phenolic compounds.

In the first stage of the Millon reaction, nitrous acid reacts with the phenolic ring causing C-nitrosation, principally *ortho* to the hydroxyl group:

protein with tyrosine side-chain

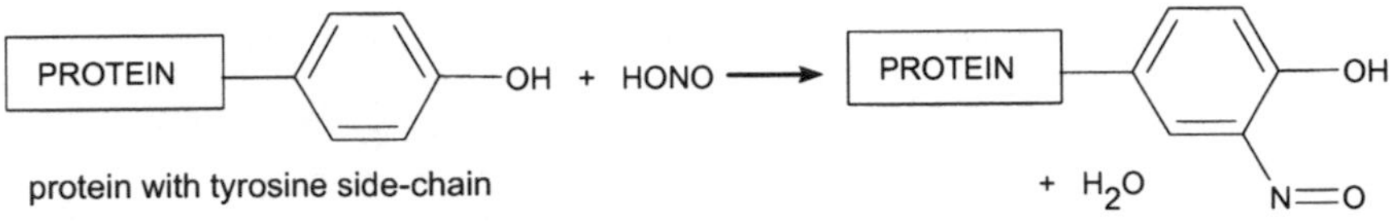

The nitroso compound forms with mercuric ions a stable chelate, which is red and may have a structure such as

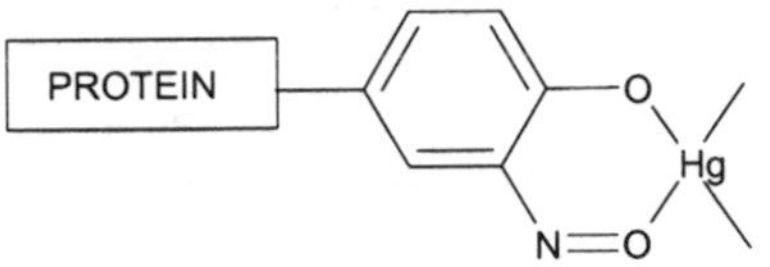

The other two coordination positions of the mercury atom may be satisfied by another nitrosophenol molecule (if one is suitably positioned in the fixed tissue) or by an inorganic ligand such as water.

In the absence of a metal such as mercury, further reaction of tyrosine with nitrous acid results in the formation of a diazonium salt:

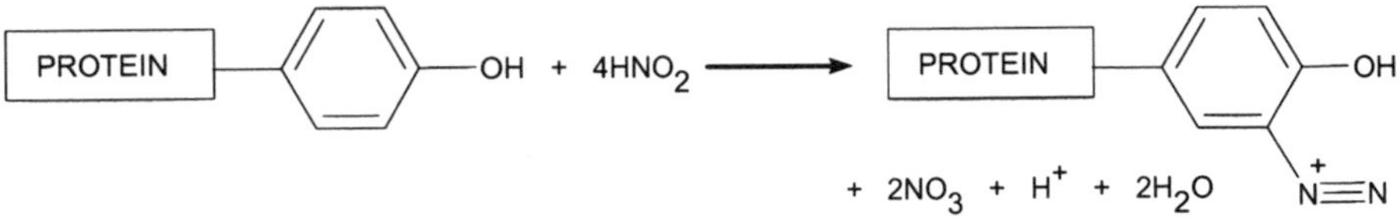

This product is rapidly decomposed by light, but in darkness it is stable enough to be coupled with a naphthol to form an azoic dye. These reactions form the basis of another histochemical technique for tyrosine.

As a phenol, tyrosine can couple with an exogenous diazonium salts to form an azo dye (see Section 5.9.4.1), but a similar reaction occurs with the imidazole ring of histidine (Section 10.9.2) and probably also with the indole ring of tryptophan. Diazonium salts detect proteins but lack specificity for any individual amino acid side-chains.

The phenolic hydroxy group of tyrosine can be blocked by **acylation** with acetic anhydride or benzoyl chloride. The aromatic rings of the resultant esters no longer possess the reactivity of phenols towards nitrous acid and other reagents. Aliphatic hydroxy and amino groups are also acylated.

The hydrogen atoms of phenolic rings are quite easily replaced by iodine atoms, so adequate treatment with a solution of **iodine** will prevent the histochemical reactions of tyrosine. Iodination can also cause oxidation of free sulphydryl groups of cysteine and partial inhibition of the reactions of tryptophan. Blockade of tyrosine can also be achieved with **tetranitromethane**, which introduces a nitro group *ortho* to the hydroxy group. This reagent, however, also decomposes tryptophan and the sulphur-containing amino acids.

10.8. Cysteine and cystine

10.8.1.
Some properties of cysteine and cystine

In ordinary paraffin sections, sulphydryl (thiol) groups are demonstrable only if an unreactive fixative has been used and if exposure of the tissue to atmospheric oxygen has been kept to a minimum at all stages of processing. Fixatives that react with the –SH group, such as mercuric chloride, oxidizing agents, and, to a lesser extent, aldehydes, must be avoided.

Suitably positioned sulphydryl groups may be oxidized in pairs to yield disulphides:

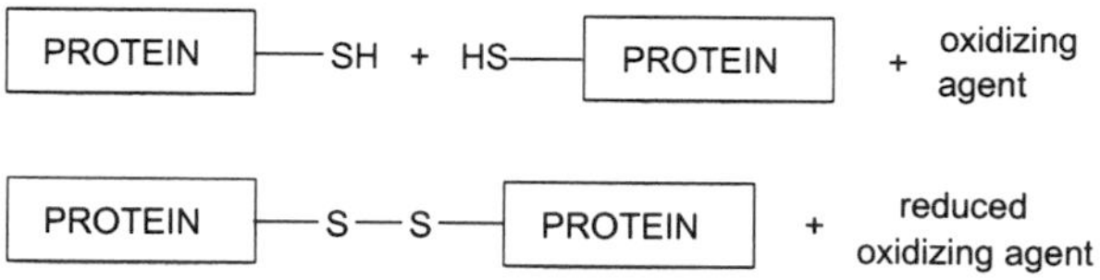

This is the normal mode of formation of **cystine**, the predominant sulphur-containing amino acid in both living and fixed tissues. Strong oxidizing agents, such as the permanganate ion and performic and peracetic acids, will cleave the disulphide bridge of cystine to yield two molecules of cysteic acid, which is an aliphatic sulphonic acid:

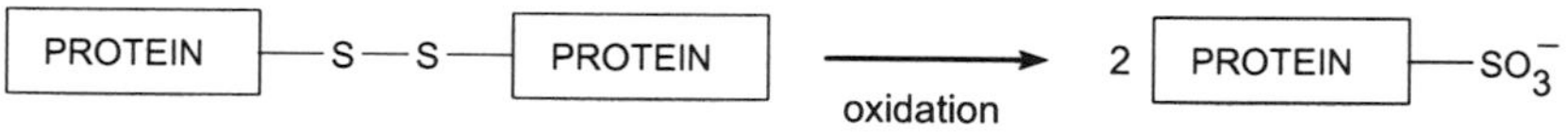

Cystine is easily reduced to cysteine. The reducing agents used in histochemistry include the alkali metal cyanides:

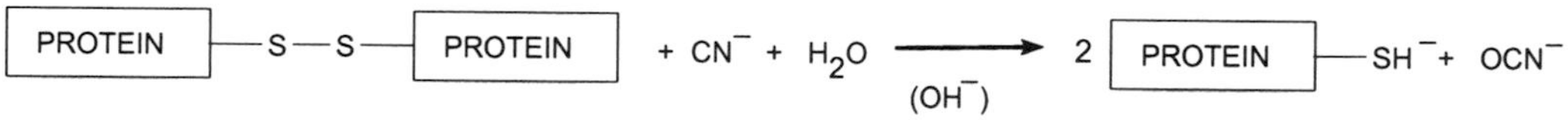

and a variety of compounds containing the sulphydryl group. For example:

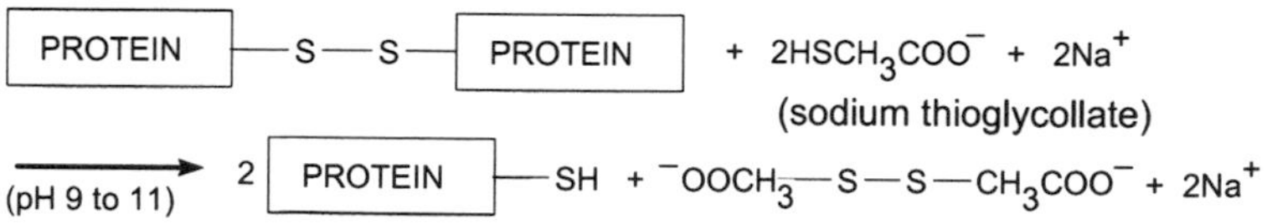

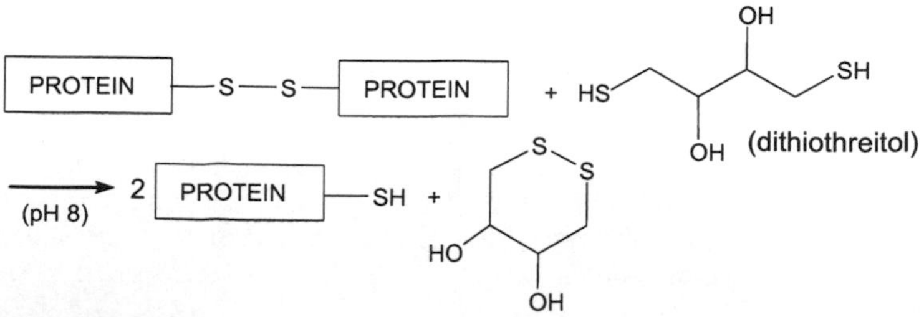

Dithiothreitol (Cleland, 1964) is more expensive than sodium thioglycollate, but can be used in a less strongly alkaline solution. As a reducing agent, the –SH group in proteins can convert iron(III) to iron(II).

The other histochemically important property of the sulphydryl group is its ability to combine with both inorganic and organic compounds of metals. Strong bonds are formed between sulphur and mercury. For example:

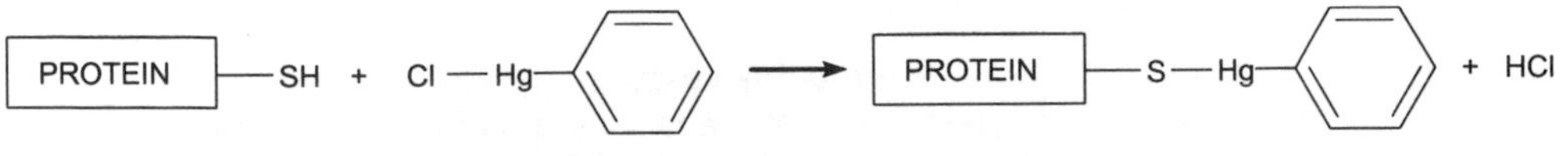

phenylmercuric chloride

There are also many metals other than mercury that form complexes with thiols.

**10.8.2.
Histochemical
methods for
cysteine**

It is possible to demonstrate sulphydryl groups either by virtue of their reducing properties or by the binding of chromogenic mercury-containing reagents. These methods may be applied directly to sections, to detect any cysteine that has survived fixation, or they may be applied to sections previously treated for the reduction of −S−S− to −SH. In the latter case, cysteine and cystine will both be demonstrated.

The simplest and probably the most sensitive technique based on the reducing properties of the sulphydryl group is the **ferric ferricyanide method**. A solution containing the ions Fe^{3+} and $[Fe(CN)_6]^{3-}$ yields an insoluble blue pigment when it is acted upon by a reducing agent. According to Lillie and Donaldson (1974) it is the ferric ion rather than the ferricyanide which is reduced by −SH, so the pigment would be expected to be ferrous ferricyanide, also known as Turnbull's blue. This substance, however, is known to be chemically identical to Prussian blue, the pigment precipitated when ferric and ferrocyanide ions meet one another. Prussian blue is ferric ferrocyanide, $Fe_4[Fe(CN)_6]_3$, but its crystals also include ions of sodium or potassium and molecules of water (see Cotton et al., 1999).

The ferric ferricyanide reaction is positive with reducing agents other than cysteine, including serotonin, catecholamines, and some of the metabolic precursors of melanin. The reagent is also reduced by lipofuscin pigment and (sometimes) by elastin, for reasons that are incompletely understood. In the histochemical study of cysteine and cystine, blocking reactions must be used to confirm the specificity of staining.

Several organic compounds of mercury are used as histochemical reagents for the sulphydryl group (see Cowden and Curtis, 1970; Lillie, 1977). Examples are:

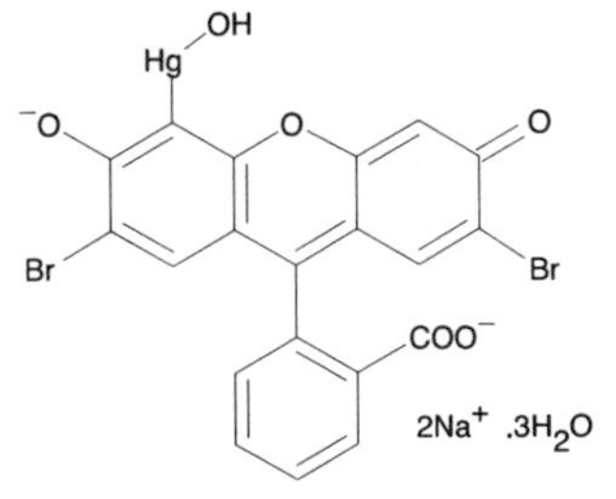

mercurochrome (merbromin)

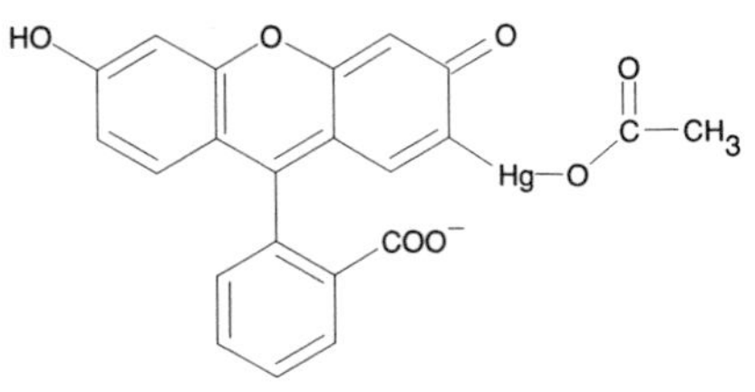

fluorescein mercuric acetate

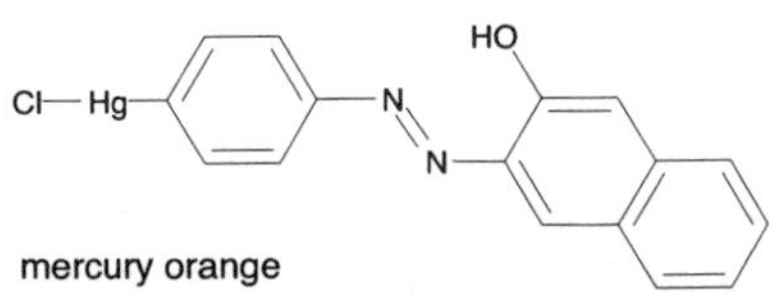

mercury orange
(p-chloromercuriphenylazo-2-naphthol)

These and other mercurials react rather slowly with sulphydryl groups to give covalent coloured adducts. Reaction is favoured by an aprotic polar solvent such as N,N-dimethylformamide, in which the active anion of the reagent is not hindered by dipole-dipole attractions to the solvent molecules, as would occur in water.

10.8.2.1. Ferric ferricyanide reaction

This, as explained, is a rather general reaction for reducing groups. If the sections are treated for conversion of disulphide to sulphydryl groups (Sections 10.8.1 and 10.11.9) between stages 1 and 2 of the procedure, −SH generated from −S−S− will react. Controls with sulphydryl blockade are necessary if any demonstrated site of reduction is to be attributed to cystine or cysteine. Free sulphydryl groups naturally present in tissues are seen to best advantage after fixation in Carnoy or a similar non-reactive coagulant fixative.

Solutions required

A. Ferric ferricyanide reagent
This is made from two stock solutions, both of which are stable for about 3 years:

(i)	Potassium ferricyanide, $K_3Fe(CN)_6$:	80 mg
	Water:	200 ml
(ii)	Ferric chloride ($FeCl_3.6H_2O$):	5.0 g
	Water:	500 ml

The working solution, prepared immediately before use and used only once, is made by mixing 10 ml of (i) with 30 ml of (ii).

B. 1% acetic acid

Glacial acetic acid:	1.0 ml
Water:	to 100 ml

Procedure

(1) De-wax and hydrate paraffin sections. If desired apply a reaction for conversion of cystine to cysteine (Section 10.11.9). Blocking reactions for −SH (Sections 10.8.4 and 10.11.8) may be carried out after or instead of the reduction, with control sections.
(2) Immerse in Solution A for 10 min.
(3) Rinse in 1% acetic acid (Solution B). See *Notes 1* and *2* below.
(4) Dehydrate through graded alcohols, clear in xylene, and mount in a resinous medium.

Results

Sites of strong reduction blue. Sites of weak reduction (most of the 'background') yellow–green. See Lillie and Burtner (1953) for a long list of positively reacting substances.

Notes

(1) The wash in dilute acetic acid is probably unnecessary. The idea is to preserve as much as possible of the Prussian blue, which is soluble in alkalis and might be slightly extracted by a neutral liquid such as tap water.
(2) A counterstain may be applied after stage 3 if considered necessary. A pink or red nuclear stain (Chapter 6) is convenient, but usually the background coloration is adequate for recognition of the architecture of the tissue.

10.8.2.2. Mercurochrome method for cysteine

This technique (Cowden and Curtis, 1970) is for paraffin sections of tissue fixed in Carnoy.

Solutions required

A. Mercurochrome reagent

Mercurochrome (merbromin):	20 mg
Water:	0.5 ml

Dissolve, then add:

N,N-dimethylformamide:	100 ml

B. N,N-dimethylformamide (required for washes)

Procedure

(1) De-wax and hydrate paraffin sections. If desired, apply a reaction for the conversion of cystine to cysteine (Section 10.11.9). Wash in water, drain, and proceed to stage 2.

(2) Immerse in mercurochrome reagent (Solution A) for either 1 h or 48 h (for fluorescence or conventional microscopy, respectively).

(3) Wash in two changes of N,N-dimethylformamide, each 3 min.

(4) Dehydrate in absolute ethanol (two changes), clear in xylene, and cover, using a non-fluorescent resinous mounting medium.

Result

Bright green fluorescence (excitation by blue or ultraviolet) at sites of sulphydryl groups, after 1 h at stage 2. Red to pink staining of sulphydryl sites after 48 h at stage 2.

Notes

(1) The specificity of staining may be confirmed in control sections by applying a sulphydryl-blocking procedure (Section 10.11.8) before stage 2 of the technique. If non-specific background staining is troublesome (mercurochrome is an anionic dye, but has little staining power in the solvent used), try washing it out with water or 70% alcohol.

(2) Some batches of mercurochrome are unsatisfactory for this method (Lillie, 1977) for unknown reasons.

10.8.3. Cysteic acid methods for cystine

Cystine may be demonstrated without prior reduction to cysteine by oxidizing it to cysteic acid (Section 10.8.1). This sulphonic acid is ionized even at very low pH and can therefore bind cationic dyes from strongly acid solutions. Alcian blue (even at pH 0.2), thiazine dyes (at pH 1.0), and aldehyde–fuchsine (Chapter 8) are often used for the staining of cysteic acid.(see Gabe, 1976; Lillie and Fullmer, 1976). The other properties of these dyes, especially their attachment to sulphated carbohydrates, must, of course, be allowed for in suitable control sections.

Several other methods for cysteine and cystine are described in the larger textbooks of histochemistry. No histochemical method is yet available for methionine, the third sulphur-containing amino acid.

10.8.3.1. Cysteic acid method for cystine

This is a slightly modified version of the performic acid–alcian blue technique of Adams and Sloper (1955). If the method is to be used simply to allow the morphological study of structures that happen to be rich in cystine, I recommend the substitution of acid permanganate for performic acid (*Note 5*) and of aldehyde fuchsine for alcian blue (*Note 6*).

Fixation is not critical for most cystine-rich proteins, but classical neurosecretory material is poorly preserved by alcoholic fixatives. An aqueous fixative containing formaldehyde and mercuric chloride is optimal. Paraffin sections must be firmly stuck to slides, especially if performic acid is used as the oxidizing agent.

Solutions required
A. Performic acid
This reagent should be prepared in a 150–200 ml conical flask. A magnetic stirrer should be used, but if one is not available, mix the ingredients in a 200 ml beaker and stir with a glass rod, taking great care to avoid splashing and spillage. See *Note 4* below.

Formic acid (the 98% acid is recommended, but the 88% acid is suitable):	80 ml
Hydrogen peroxide (30%; '100 volumes available oxygen'):	8.0 ml
Concentrated sulphuric acid (96%):	1.0 ml

Stir vigorously at intervals for 1 h. This solution is highly corrosive. It should be free of bubbles when used. It keeps for 24 h. Dilute with at least 1 l of tap water and neutralize before discarding. See *Note 5* below for alternatives to performic acid.

B. Alcian blue

Alcian blue 8G (C.I. 74240):	6.0 g
Water:	200 ml
Concentrated sulphuric acid (96%):	5.5 ml

Heat to 70°C, cool to room temperature and filter. With some batches of alcian blue it is impossible to obtain a 3% solution, but this does not matter. See *Note 6* below for some alternatives to alcian blue.

Procedure
(1) De-wax and hydrate paraffin sections. Coating with a film of nitrocellulose (Chapter 4) is advisable, though not always necessary. Blot dry with filter paper.

(2) Immerse in performic acid (Solution A) or an alternative (see *Note 5* below) for 5 min.

(3) Rinse in four changes of tap water, without agitation, for a total of 10 min.

(4) Transfer to 70% and then to absolute alcohol. Blot the sections with wet filter paper to flatten creases and return to water. Place slides on a hotplate until just dry.

(5) Stain in alcian blue (Solution B) for 1 h.

(6) Wash in three or four changes of tap water until all excess dye is removed.

(7) Counterstain if desired (see *Note 1* below).

(8) Wash in water, blot dry, dehydrate in two changes (each 5 min) of *n*-butanol, clear in xylene, and cover. See *Note 2* below.

Result
Sites of high cystine concentration (more than 4% of total amino acid content of protein) blue. Keratin (of epidermis etc.), insulin (in B-cells of pancreatic islets) and classical neurosecretory material (in the posterior lobe of the pituitary gland, and in many invertebrate endocrine organs) are among the substances conspicuously stained by this method. Sulphated carbohydrates are also blue. (See *Note 3* for controls.)

Notes
(1) Suitable counterstains (Chapter 6) are: 0.5% aqueous neutral red or safranine (for nuclei, etc.); 0.5% aqueous eosin (for general pink background). Alcian blue resists extraction by most of the commonly used histological reagents, so almost any method can be used.

(2) If the sections look as if they will come off the slides, mount into a resinous medium directly from the second change of *n*-butanol.

(3) To control for the specificity for cystine, omit the oxidation (step 2). Sulphate esters (Chapter 11) are stained in oxidized or unoxidized sections. Their stainability can be prevented by prior methylation (Section 10.11.4).

(4) Performic and peracetic acids can react explosively with copper and its salts. Use clean glassware and remember to dilute the reagent before pouring it down the sink.

(5) An alterative oxidizing agent is **peracetic acid**,

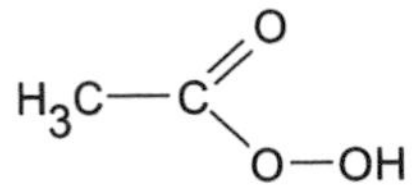

$$H_3C-C(=O)(O-OH)$$

This is much more stable than performic acid and is available commercially as a 40% solution. Peracetic acid can also be made in the laboratory: Thoroughly mix 40 ml of acetic anhydride with 10 ml of 30% hydrogen peroxide; leave to stand for 24 h and then add an equal volume of water.

A less noxious but also less specific oxidizing agent is an **acidified permanganate** solution (Pasteels and Herlant, 1962; see Adams, 1965, and Gabe, 1976, for discussion). Sections are immersed for 5 min in a freshly prepared 0.5% solution of potassium permanganate ($KMnO_4$) in 2% sulphuric acid and then rinsed in 1% aqueous oxalic acid ($H_2C_2O_4.2H_2O$) to remove the brown stain of manganese dioxide from the sections. A further wash in water precedes staining with alcian blue (or an alternative). Oxidation with permanganate is acceptable when the cysteic acid method is being used for histological purposes such as the study of cell types in the hypophysis or endocrine pancreas. Performic or peracetic acid must be used for critical histochemical identification of cystine-containing proteins.

(6) Other cationic dyes in acid solution (pH <1.0) may be substituted for alcian blue, but they will be less resistant to extraction during counterstaining and dehydration. **Aldehyde fuchsine** (see also Chapter 8, Section 8.4.3) gives a strong purple colour that resists any attempted extraction by acids or organic solvents.

10.8.4. Sulphydryl blocking reagents

Two convenient blocking agents for the sulphydryl group are *N*-ethylmaleimide and iodoacetic acid:

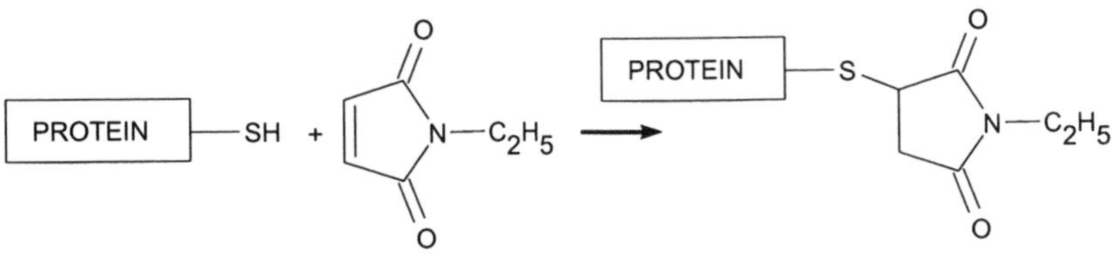

N-ethylmaleimide

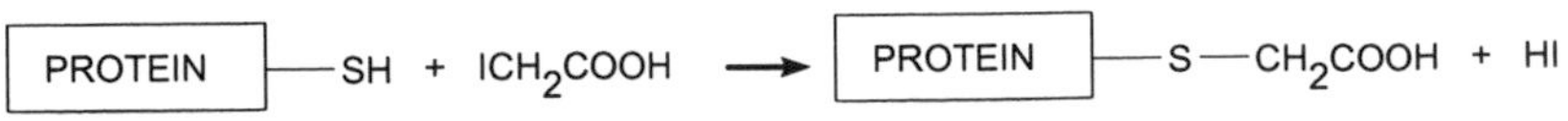

iodoacetic acid

Both these reagents completely block the reactivity of SH groups. See Section 10.11.8 for technical details. Other blocking agents, including iodine and various compounds of mercury, are likely to give incomplete or easily reversible blockades.

10.9 Methods for proteins in general

The histologist or pathologist often wants to know whether or not an intracellular inclusion or an extracellular material is composed largely of protein. For the simple staining of protein, techniques are available that do not depend upon the presence of individual amino acids. Two will be considered here.

10.9.1.
Demonstration of proteins with dyes

Staining by anionic dyes, especially those with small molecules, is due largely to electrostatic attachment to the basic side-chains of lysine and arginine. Such staining has already been discussed in Chapters 5 and 6 and in Section 10.4.1 of this chapter. Anionic dyes with large, long molecules (especially those used industrially for the direct dyeing of cotton) are bound principally by non-ionic forces (Chapter 5).

An anionic dye is useful for the demonstration of protein only if the intensity of the colour produced at any site in the tissue is proportional to the local concentration of protein there. A triphenylmethane dye that binds stoichiometrically to proteins under histochemical conditions is **coomassie blue R250**, also called **brilliant blue R** and **brilliant indocyanine 6B**. It is used by biochemists for staining proteins in acrylamide gels. The dye is almost insoluble in cold water. Sections are stained from a solution of the dye in a mixture of ethanol and acetic acid, and rinsed in an acetic–ethanol mixture to remove unbound dye. The chemical specificity of the staining and the mode of binding of the dye are in need of more investigation. The structural formula of the dye (Chapter 5) indicates a large non-planar zwitterion with hydrophilic and hydrophobic parts. There is no obvious reason why this dye should not attach to substances other than proteins. Nevertheless, staining of plastic-embedded sections is prevented by prior treatment with proteolytic enzymes (Cawood *et al.*, 1978).

10.9.1.1. Coomassie blue R250 for proteins

This technique is suitable for paraffin sections of tissues fixed in formaldehyde, Carnoy or Bouin. See *Note* below.

Solutions required
A. Acetic–ethanol

Glacial acetic acid:	100 ml
Absolute ethanol:	300 ml

Can be kept for several months. It is used to dissolve the dye and to remove unbound dye from the stained sections.

B. Dye solution

Coomassie blue R250 (C.I. 42660):	40 mg
Acetic–ethanol (Solution A above):	200 ml

The dye dissolves completely and filtration is not needed. The solution is stable for at least 5 years.

Procedure
(1) De-wax and hydrate paraffin sections and take to absolute ethanol.
(2) Stain in the dye solution (B) for 30 min.
(3) Drain slides and immerse in acetic–ethanol (solution A) for 5 min with occasional agitation.
(4) Rinse in 95% ethanol, dehydrate in absolute ethanol, clear in xylene, and cover, using a resinous mounting medium.

Result
Proteins are stained a bright royal blue. The intensity of colour is proportional to the local concentration of protein. See also *Note* below.

Note

In the original description of this technique (Cawood *et al.*, 1978), plastic-embedded sections were stained for 24 h and stage 3 lasted 20 min. When paraffin sections are used, there is no increase in intensity of staining after 15–20 min and subsequent washing in acetic–ethanol removes hardly any dye from the sections.

The specificity for proteins is not fully established. Carbohydrate-rich components of tissues, such as the matrix of cartilage, are very weakly stained by comparison with cytoplasm and collagen. Nuclei are recognizable in the stained sections but are no more strongly coloured than the surrounding cytoplasm. Carri and Ebendal (1989) found this method useful for staining tissue cultures of chick retina: neurites (axons and dendrites) stained dark blue, whereas neuronal cell bodies were only faintly coloured. The method is much used for recognizing proteinaceous inclusions in plant tissues.

10.9.2. The coupled tetrazonium reaction and related methods

Alkaline solutions of diazonium salts combine with proteins in at least three different ways. Thus, the expected coupling reaction occurs with the phenolic side-chains of tyrosine:

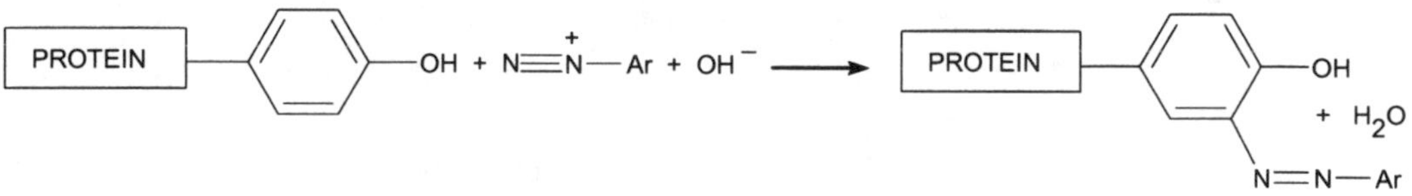

PROTEIN—⟨ ⟩—OH + $N{\equiv}\overset{+}{N}$—Ar + OH⁻ ⟶ PROTEIN—⟨ ⟩—OH + H_2O, with N=N—Ar substituent

A similar coupling reaction occurs with the imidazole ring of histidine. The nitrogen atoms of this aromatic heterocycle confer some of the properties of an aromatic amine to the ring:

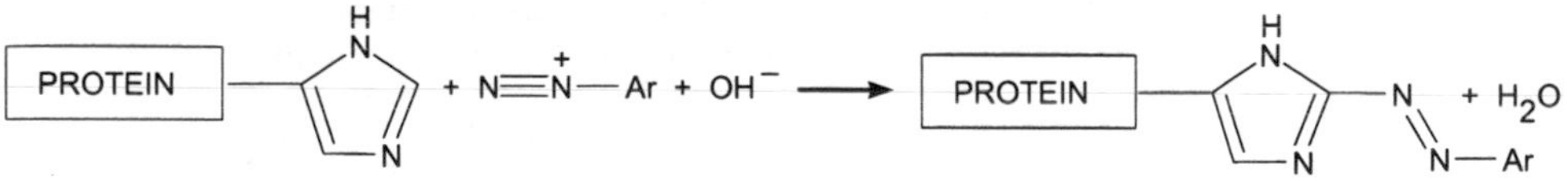

PROTEIN—(imidazole) + $N{\equiv}\overset{+}{N}$—Ar + OH⁻ ⟶ PROTEIN—(imidazole)—N=N—Ar + H_2O

Coupling probably also occurs ortho to the nitrogen atom in the indole ring of tryptophan.

A different reaction takes place with the ε-amino group of lysine:

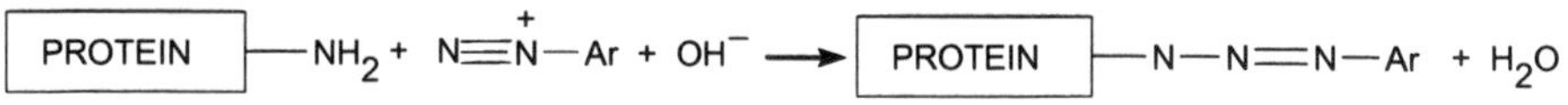

PROTEIN—NH_2 + $N{\equiv}\overset{+}{N}$—Ar + OH⁻ ⟶ PROTEIN—N—N=N—Ar + H_2O

The product is a **triazene**. Similar reactions may occur with the secondary amine nitrogen atoms of proline and hydroxyproline and with the guanidino and sulphydryl groups of arginine and cysteine respectively. The nitrogen atoms of the purine and pyrimidine bases of the nucleic acids almost certainly do not couple with diazonium salts (see Lillie and Fullmer, 1976). Thus, a diazonium salt applied to a section of tissue will be covalently bound to several organic functional groups, all of which are found principally in proteins. Exceptions are certain phenols: the catecholamines of chromaffin cells and serotonin in argentaffin cells (Chapter 17), but these substances are absent from most tissues and their presence can be detected by other methods. Phenolic compounds of plants, such as tannins, may also be expected to couple with diazonium salts.

In the original coupled tetrazonium reaction (Danielli, 1947), the diazonium salt used is tetraazotized benzidine, which has to be freshly prepared in the laboratory from benzidine and nitrous acid:

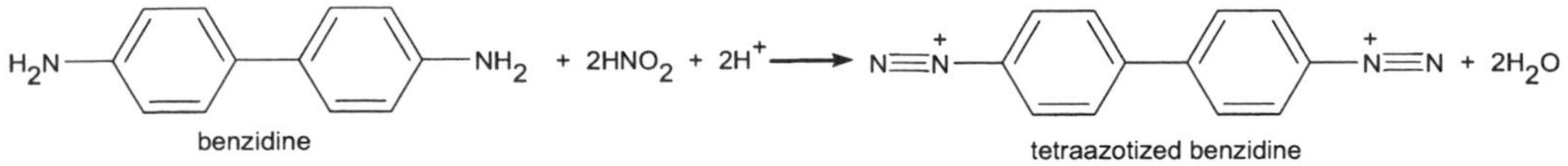

benzidine   tetraazotized benzidine

An alternative, more convenient reagent is the stabilized tetrazonium salt derived from o-dianisidine, known as **fast blue B salt** (see Chapter 5 for formula). It will be noticed that each of these compounds bears two diazonium groups per molecule. Usually only one of these will couple with a reactive site in a section, because not often will two coupling sites in the fixed tissue be exactly the right distance apart to react with the same molecule of reagent.

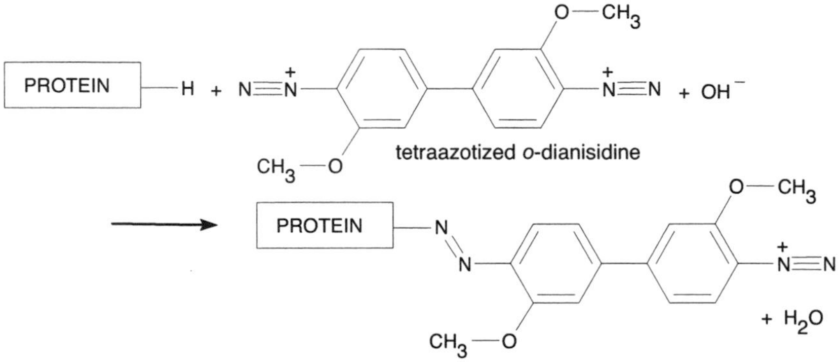

tetraazotized o-dianisidine

Azo compounds formed by coupling of simple diazonium salts with proteins are only feebly coloured. However, the free −N≡N⁺ group of a bound tetrazonium salt is able to couple with any phenol or aromatic amine subsequently applied to the section, to give a strongly coloured dye containing two azo linkages. **H-acid** (Chapter 5) is a suitable azoic coupling component for this purpose:

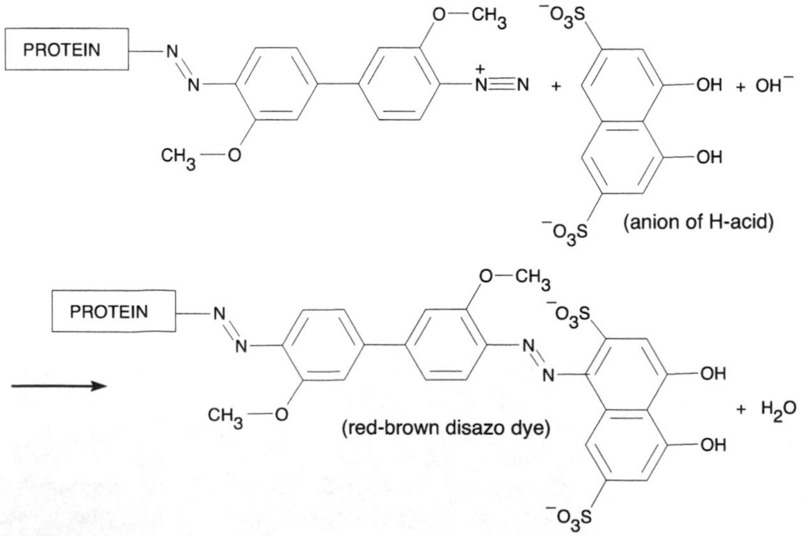

(anion of H-acid)

(red-brown disazo dye)

As an alternative to the coupled tetrazonium reaction, one may use a diazonium salt (with only one −N≡N⁺ group) that is itself an azo dye. Such a salt couples with proteins to give disazo dyes in a single-step reaction. A coloured stabilized diazonium salt suitable for staining proteins is **fast black K salt** (Chapter 5). Freshly diazotized safranine can also be used (Lillie *et al.*, 1968a).

In attempts to make the coupled tetrazonium reaction specific for aromatic amino acids, sections are commonly treated with dilute hydrochloric acid after the first coupling, to destroy triazenes, but the efficacy of this manoeuvre is questionable.

10.10. Aldehydes and ketones

Free aldehyde groups occur naturally in immature elastin (Chapter 8), in lignin, in lipids that have been oxidized by air (Chapter 12), and in specimens fixed in glutaraldehyde (Chapter 2), but otherwise are largely absent from animal tissues. They are often produced in the course of histochemical manipulations. The Feulgen reaction (Chapter 9) and the PAS reaction (Chapter 11) are the most commonly used methods of this type. Ketones occur naturally as ketosteroids, for which histochemical techniques have been described, and as intermediate products in some staining methods (e.g. see Section 10.3.1), but are generally less important to the histochemist than are aldehydes.

10.10.1.
Schiff's reagent

Before reading this section the reader may wish to review the chemistry of pararosaniline and related triphenylmethane dyes (Chapter 5). In this account it is assumed that Schiff's reagent is prepared from pararosaniline, but equivalent chemical reactions occur with the other components of basic fuchsine. This traditional reagent for detecting aldehyde groups is made by treating a solution of basic fuchsine with sulphurous acid. This weak acid is formed when sulphur dioxide combines with water:

$$H_2O + SO_2 \rightleftharpoons H_2SO_3 \rightleftharpoons H^+ + HSO_3^- \rightleftharpoons 2H^+ + SO_3^{2-}$$

These equilibria are displaced to the left when [H$^+$] rises. Sulphurous acid, containing free sulphur dioxide, is prepared in the course of making Schiff's reagent, either from the reaction of a bisulphite (sodium metabisulphite, $Na_2S_2O_5$, is usually used) with a mineral acid, or of thionyl chloride with water (Chapter 9, Section 9.3.2), or by bubbling gaseous sulphur dioxide through an aqueous solution of the dye.

The reaction with sulphorous acid adds a sulphonic acid group to the central carbon of the triphenylmethane structure:

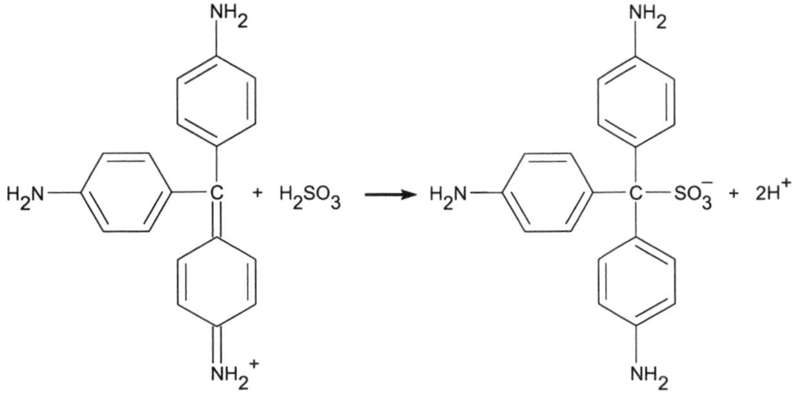

Schiff's reagent therefore consists of a solution of this colourless derivative of the dye in water, which contains an excess of sulphurous acid.

Schiff's reagent reacts with aldehydes, but not with ketones, to form brightly coloured products. This is not simply a matter of recolorizing the dye. New compounds are formed with colours somewhat different from that of basic fuchsine. The results of three investigations (Dujindam and van Duijn, 1975; Gill and Jotz, 1976; Nettleton and Carpenter, 1977) concur in attributing the structure:

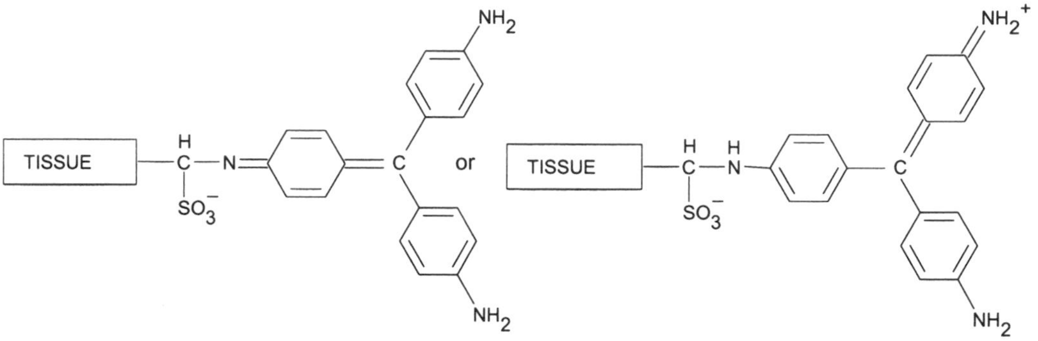

to the principal coloured compound formed when Schiff's reagent reacts with tissue-bound aldehyde groups. Both these compounds are alkylsulphonic acid derivatives of pararosaniline, and the two structures would be expected to exist in tautomeric equilibrium. There is still some uncertainty as to whether the aldehyde group first reacts with sulphurous acid to form a bisulphite compound, which then condenses with an amino group of Schiff's reagent, or whether the amino group of the reagent first reacts with the aldehyde to form an imine (Schiff's base, anil, or azomethine), which is subsequently sulphonated. The second stage of either scheme must involve removal of the sulphonic acid group from the dye molecule and re-establishment of the triphenylmethane chromophore.

Several dyes and fluorochromes other than basic fuchsine will serve as substitutes for Schiff's reagent if their solutions are treated with sulphur dioxide, but usually these **'pseudo-Schiff'** reagents are coloured (see Kasten, 1960). The most widely used ones are derived from thionine with bisulphite (van Duijn, 1956) and from acriflavine with thionyl chloride (Ornstein et al., 1957). The latter is useful for the demonstration of aldehyde-containing components of tissues by fluorescence microscopy. The traditional Schiff's reagent also gives a fluorescent product with aldehydes, but its orange-brown emission is rather weak, and contrasts poorly with a dark background.

A method for the **preparation of Schiff's reagent** is described in Chapter 9 (Section 9.3.2), in conjunction with the Feulgen technique. The reagent can also be bought as a ready-made solution. Technical details for its use in various procedures can be found in Chapters 9, 11 and 12.

10.10.2.
Hydrazines and hydrazides

Organic hydrazines are compounds in which one hydrogen atom of hydrazine, $H_2N–NH_2$, is replaced by an organic radical. They have the general structure:

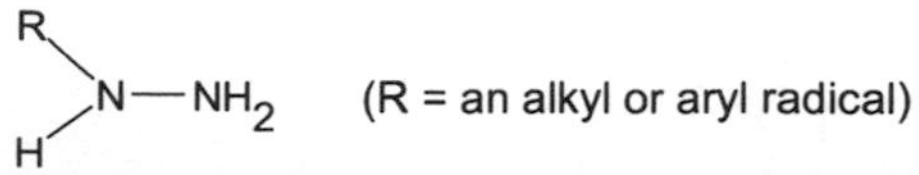

(R = an alkyl or aryl radical)

Hydrazides are similar but with an acyl in place of R in the above general formula. Hydrazines and hydrazides condense readily with both aldehydes and ketones:

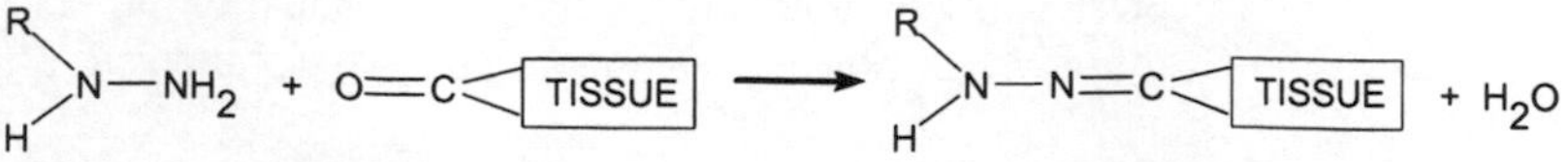

The reagent RNHNH$_2$ in this equation will be potentially useful for the demonstration of tissue bound carbonyl groups if R is either coloured or able to form a coloured compound by reaction with another reagent. Several hydrazines and hydrazides serve as histochemical reagents in this way. They include the following:

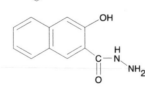

Phenylhydrazine-4-sulphonic acid (Shackleford, 1963): Confers affinity for cationic dyes at low pH on sites of aldehydes.

Dansylhydrazine (Weber et. al., 1975): Forms fluorescent adducts, which can be made chemically more stable by reduction of the C=N bond to C-NH, to give a secondary amine.

Salicylhydrazide (Stoward, 1968): forms fluorescent adducts. Chelation with certain metals (Zn^{2+}, Al^{3+}) results in emission of different colours by aldehydes and ketones.

2-hydroxy-3-naphthoic acid hydrazide (HNAH): This is the most popular reagent of its type. Sites of attachment are made visible by coupling with a diazonium salt.

Phenylhydrazine (C$_6$H$_5$NHNH$_2$) is another useful reagent for blocking the reactivity of carbonyl compounds.

10.10.2.1. Hydroxynaphthoic acid hydrazide (HNAH)
The HNAH reagent is made up as follows:

2-hydroxy-3-naphthoic acid hydrazide:	200 mg
Absolute ethanol:	100 ml
Glacial acetic acid:	10 ml
Water:	90 ml

Dissolve with aid of gentle heat (up to 70°C) and vigorous stirring. The solution can be kept for a few weeks.

Sections of tissue in which aldehyde or ketone groups have been produced are immersed in the HNAH reagent for 1 h at 60°C or for 3 h at room temperature. They are then washed in three changes (each 10 min) of 50% ethanol, taken to water, and reacted at 0°C with a freshly made solution of **fast blue B salt** (1 mg/ml, pH 7.5, 3 min). The sections are then washed, dehydrated, cleared, and mounted in a resinous medium. Sites of aldehydes and ketones are shown in blue and purple. There is also a pink to light brown background staining, which has no histochemical significance.

10.10.3.
Aromatic amines

The simplest reaction of a primary amine with an aldehyde is

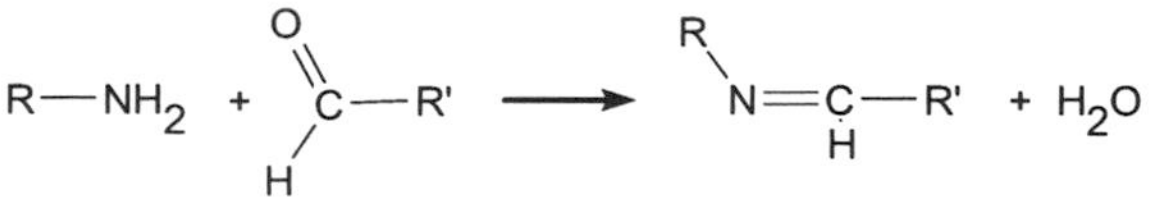

$$R-NH_2 \; + \; \underset{H}{\overset{O}{\underset{|}{\overset{\|}{C}}}}-R' \longrightarrow \underset{H}{\overset{R}{\underset{|}{N=C}}}-R' \; + \; H_2O$$

The product, containing the –C=N– linkage, is variously known as an **imine**, an azomethine, a Schiff's base, or an anil. It is stable only when R or R' is an aromatic ring. If the amine is present in excess, as it must be when it is a reagent applied to a section of a tissue, two of its molecules may react with one aldehyde group:

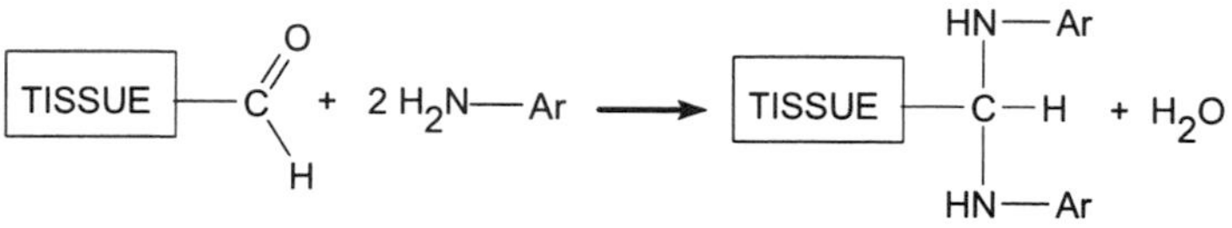

$$\boxed{\text{TISSUE}}-\underset{H}{\overset{O}{\overset{\|}{C}}} \; + \; 2\,H_2N-Ar \longrightarrow \boxed{\text{TISSUE}}-\underset{HN-Ar}{\overset{HN-Ar}{\underset{|}{C}-H}} \; + \; H_2O$$

The product is known as an **aminal** (Smith and March, 2007). Its formation is favoured when the group Ar in the above equation carries an electron-withdraw-ing substituent (see Sollenberger and Martin, 1968). In an elegant study of the reaction of *m*-aminophenol with tissue-bound aldehydes, Lillie (1962) provided convincing evidence that aminals were the principal products of the reaction, which was acid-catalysed and occurred in the absence of water. Sites of attach-ment of *m*-aminophenol could be demonstrated by coupling with a diazonium salt to give coloured products with structures such as

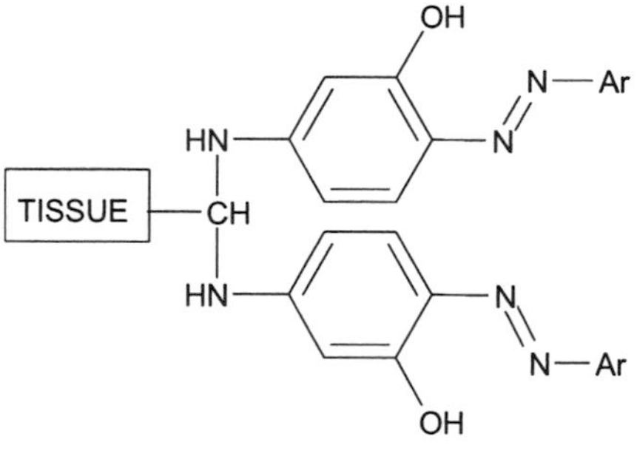

In earlier histochemical literature aminals have also been termed diphenamine bases and, wrongly, secondary amines. Aromatic amines are also used as blocking agents for aldehyde groups. Blockade is achieved more rapidly with *m*-aminophe-nol than with aniline. Both reagents are used as solutions in glacial acetic acid (Section 10.11.10).

Many dyes are primary aromatic amines. An acidified alcoholic solution of basic fuchsine (Horobin and Kevill-Davies, 1971a) is a useful substitute for Schiff's reagent. The dye in this solution almost certainly condenses with aldehydes to form aminals in the same way as does *m*-aminophenol (Horobin and Kevill-Davies, 1971b). A solution of acriflavine in ethanol, used similarly, serves as a fluorescent reagent for aldehydes and has some advantages over the 'pseudo-Schiff' reagent prepared by treatment of the same dye with sulphurous acid (Levinson *et al.*, 1977). Fluorescent products are formed when DAB (3,3'-diaminobenzidine), which is not itself fluorescent, reacts with aldehyde groups formed by atmospheric oxida-tion of lipids (Chapter 12). A fluorescent background is present in lipid-containing sections that have been exposed to DAB for other purposes, notably the localization of peroxidase-labelled antibodies (Chapters 16, 19). This can provide a simple fluorescent counterstain, but in the experimental tracing of neuronal connections it may interfere with the detection of other fluorescent labels (von Bohlen und Halbach and Kiernan, 2000).

10.10.4.
Ammoniacal
silver nitrate

An aqueous solution of ammonia contains the dissolved gas in equilibrium with ammonium hydroxide:

$$NH_3 + H_2O \rightleftharpoons NH_4OH$$

Ammonium hydroxide ionizes as a weak base, so the solution is alkaline:

$$NH_4OH \rightleftharpoons NH_4^+ + OH^-$$

When an ammonia solution is added in small aliquots to aqueous silver nitrate, a black or brown precipitate of silver oxide is first formed:

$$2Ag^+ + 2OH^- \longrightarrow Ag_2O(s) + H_2O$$

With further addition of ammonia the precipitate dissolves. The solution contains the silver diammine ion, $[Ag(NH_3)_2]^+$:

$$Ag_2O(s) + 4NH_3 + H_2O \longrightarrow 2[Ag(NH_3)_2]^+ + 2OH^-$$

The silver diammine ion rapidly oxidizes aldehydes (but not ketones) and is itself reduced to metallic silver:

$$\boxed{\text{TISSUE}}-CHO + 2[Ag(NH_3)_2]^+ + H_2O \longrightarrow \boxed{\text{TISSUE}}-COOH + 2Ag(s) + 4NH_3 + 2H^+$$

The precipitated silver is black, and the deposits can be further intensified by gold toning or by physical development (Chapter 18), making the test very sensitive. The silver is electron opaque, so ammoniacal silver nitrate solutions are sometimes used as substitutes for Schiff's reagent in ultrastructural histochemical studies. Other complexes of silver, notably that formed with hexamethylenetetramine (also known as methenamine or hexamine), may be used instead of silver diammine.

Unfortunately the histochemical specificity of this method is low. The silver complexes are also reduced by sulphydryl groups and by o-diphenols (Chapter 17). The staining method for reticulin described in Chapter 18 is an example of a useful histological technique based on the detection of artificially produced aldehyde groups.

10.10.5.
Other methods
for aldehydes

Three other methods for the localization of aldehydes are worth mentioning, but none are much used.

(a) Aldehydes have a peroxidase-like property (see Feigl, 1960) in that they catalyse the oxidation of p-phenylenediamine by hydrogen peroxide. This reaction is also used as a spot-test in analytical chemistry.

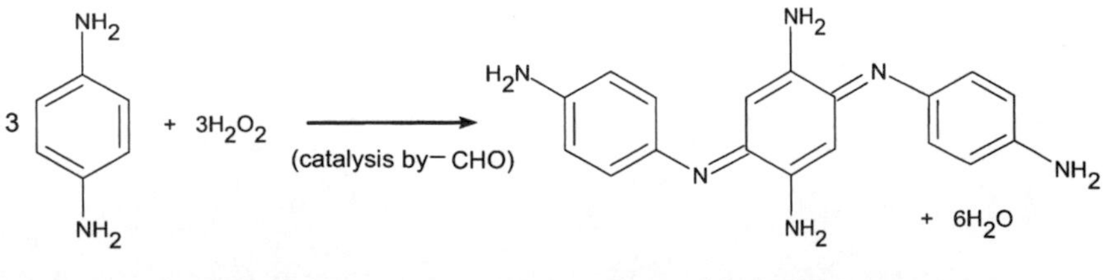

The product, which is known as Bandrowski's base, is darkly coloured and unstable, but is said to be stabilized by treatment with a solution of gold chloride (Scarselli, 1961). The structure of Bandrowski's base and the reactions involved in its formation are discussed by Corbett (1971).

(b) Another reagent used in spot-tests is 3-methyl-2-benzothiazolone hydrazone (MBTH) (Sanwicki *et al.*, 1961). It combines with aldehydes to form blue and green dyes and is a sensitive and specific histochemical reagent. The coloured product can be stabilized for a few days by treatment of the stained sections with ferric chloride or phosphomolybdic acid (Davis and Janis, 1966; Nakao and Angrist, 1968), but permanent preparations cannot be made.

(c) The aldehyde may be converted to its bisulphite addition compound:

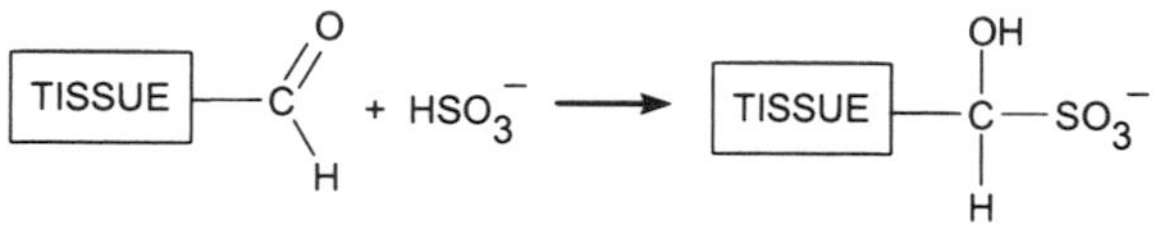

$$\boxed{\text{TISSUE}}-\overset{\overset{\displaystyle O}{\|}}{\underset{\underset{\displaystyle H}{|}}{C}} + HSO_3^- \longrightarrow \boxed{\text{TISSUE}}-\overset{\overset{\displaystyle OH}{|}}{\underset{\underset{\displaystyle H}{|}}{C}}-SO_3^-$$

The addition compound is a sulphonic acid, so it will bind cationic dyes such as toluidine blue (Rommanyi *et al.*, 1975) or alcian blue (Klessen, 1974) from solutions at pH 1.0 or lower (Section 6.1.1). This reaction is exploited in a method for staining *Helicobacter pylori*, a spirochaete implicated in peptic ulceration, in biopsies of gastric mucosa. Hydroxy groups in the neutral carbohydrates of the mucus are oxidized by periodic acid to give aldehydes (see Chapter 11), which are then converted to sulphonic acids and stained with a yellow cationic dye. The yellow mucus provides a contrasting background for the organisms, which are stained with a subsequently applied blue cationic dye (Leung *et al.*, 1996).

10.10.5.1. Leung and Gibbon method for *Helicobacter pylori*
This method is applied to paraffin sections of formaldehyde-fixed biopsies of gastric mucosa.

Solutions required
A. 1% Periodic acid

Periodic acid ($HIO_4.2H_2O$):	2.0 g
Water:	200 ml

Keeps for several weeks and may be used repeatedly. Discard the solution when it is no longer colourless.

B. Acidified bisulphite solution

Sodium metabisulphite ($Na_2S_2O_5$):	5.0 g
Water:	100 ml
1.0 M hydrochloric acid:	1.0 ml

This is made on the day it is to be used.

C. 1% Alcian yellow

Alcian yellow (C.I. 12840):	1.0 g
50% ethanol:	100 ml
Glacial acetic acid:	3.0 ml

Filter before using. Alcian yellow solutions decompose with formation of insoluble products.

D. Toluidine blue

Toluidine blue (C.I. 52040) (1 ml of a stock 1% aqueous solution of the dye):	10 mg

Water: 100 ml
3% aqueous sodium hydroxide: 4 drops

This solution is made up before using.

Procedure
(1) De-wax and hydrate paraffin sections.
(2) Immerse slides in 1% periodic acid (Solution A) for 10 min.
(3) Wash in 3 changes of water.
(4) Immerse slides in acidified metabisulphite solution (B) for 5 min.
(5) Wash in water for 2 min.
(6) Stain in alcian yellow (Solution C) for 5 min.
(7) Wash in 3 changes of water.
(8) Stain in toluidine blue (Solution D) for 3 min.
(9) Wash in 3 changes of water.
(10) Blot the sections with filter paper.
(11) Dehydrate in 3 changes of 100% alcohol, clear in xylene and apply cover-slips, using a resinous mounting medium.
(12) Examine, using an oil-immersion objective.

Result
Mucus on surface of gastric mucosa yellow. Nuclei and cytoplasm blue. *Helicobacter* organisms appear as dark blue curved and spiral forms within the mucus. Other organisms that cause gastrointestinal disturbances, notably *Giardia* and *Cryptosporidium*, can also be recognized by this method (Vartanian *et al.*, 1998).

**10.10.6.
Blocking
procedures**

Three blocking procedures for the carbonyl group are histochemically valuable. Most of the other available methods are unduly time-consuming, are damaging to the sections, or are too easily reversible. The three useful blocking agents are:

(a) **Phenylhydrazine:**

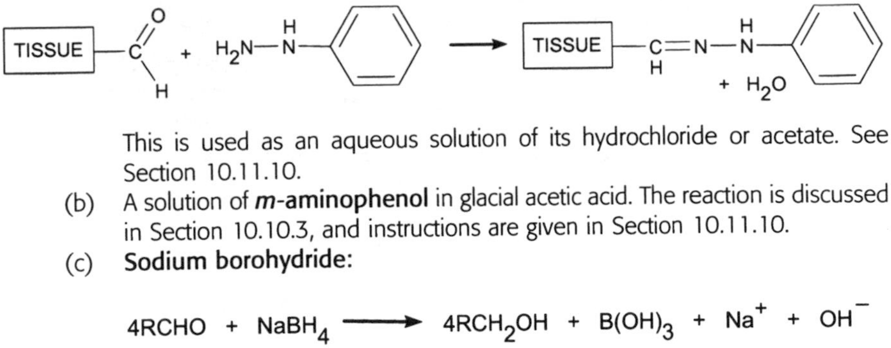

This is used as an aqueous solution of its hydrochloride or acetate. See Section 10.11.10.

(b) A solution of **m-aminophenol** in glacial acetic acid. The reaction is discussed in Section 10.10.3, and instructions are given in Section 10.11.10.

(c) **Sodium borohydride:**

$$4RCHO + NaBH_4 \longrightarrow 4RCH_2OH + B(OH)_3 + Na^+ + OH^-$$

This reducing agent is used as a mildly alkaline aqueous solution. It reduces aldehydes to primary alcohols and ketones to secondary alcohols. No other organic functional groups likely to be present in tissues are reduced, but it is worth noting that the −C=N− linkages of imines and hydrazones are reduced to −C−N− by this reagent (Billman and Diesing, 1957). Sodium borohydride is the reagent of first choice for irreversible histochemical blocking of the carbonyl group. It is important that the pH of the solution be greater than 8.2. Neutral or less alkaline solutions will not reduce all the aldehyde groups present in a section (Bayliss and Adams, 1979).

10.10.6.1 Borohydride reduction procedure

Take sections to water and transfer to a freshly prepared solution:

Sodium phosphate, dibasic (Na_2HPO_4):	0.5 g
Water:	50 ml

Dissolve, then add:

Sodium borohydride ($NaBH_4$):	25 mg

Leave slides in this for 10 min, with occasional agitation to release bubbles of hydrogen from surfaces of slides. Wash in four changes of water.

Caution. Sodium borohydride releases hydrogen on contact with acids. Do not use this reagent near any naked flame. Do not acidify its solutions. Discard the alkaline solution by flushing down the drain with several litres of tap water.

After reduction, aldehyde groups such as those formed by Feulgen hydrolysis (Chapter 9) or periodate oxidation (Chapter 11) can no longer be demonstrated with Schiff's reagent or by other methods.

10.11. Chemical blocking procedures

The reactions described in this section bring about modifications of the organic functional groups of macromolecules. They are used as control procedures in protein and carbohydrate histochemistry.

Table 10. 2. Some blocking and unblocking reactions

Functional group	Blocking reaction	Product of blockade	Unblocking reaction
Hydroxy	Acetylation (3 h)	Acetyl ester	Saponification
	Benzoylation	Benzoyl ester	Saponification
	Sulphation	Half-sulphate ester	Methylation (2 h)
Carboxyl	Methylation (2 h)	Methyl ester	Saponification
Phosphate	Methylation (24 h)	Obstruction of phosphate by nearby methylated amines	Saponification
Sulphate (of carbohydrate)	Methylation (24 h)	Hydroxyl	Irreversible
Amino	Acetylation (48 h)	Acetyl amide	Saponification
	Benzoylation	Benzoyl amide	Saponification
	Sulphation	Sulphoamino	Methylation (2 h)
	Deamination	Hydroxy etc.	Irreversible

10.11.1. Sulphation

Solutions required

A. Sulphation reagent

Pack ice around a 100 ml conical flask containing 25 ml of diethyl ether. Slowly add 25 ml of concentrated sulphuric acid (which should have been pre-cooled by leaving at 4°C for 30–60 min). The mixture becomes hot. Use it when it has cooled to room temperature. After use, pour the mixture carefully into about 500 ml of tap water and neutralize with sodium hydroxide (about 50 ml of 10N NaOH is needed).

B. A cationic dye

A dilute solution of a thiazine dye (Chapter 6) at pH 1.0 is suitable. Alcian blue at pH 1.0 (Chapter 11) may also be used.

Procedure
(1) Take sections to absolute ethanol and then into diethyl ether.
(2) Place the slides in the sulphation reagent (A) for 5–10 min.
(3) Rinse in 95% alcohol and then immerse in water, two changes, each 30 s.
(4) Stain with a suitable cationic dye (Solution B).
(5) Wash in water, dehydrate appropriately for the dye used, clear in xylene, and mount in a resinous medium.

Notes
(1) A control section that has not been sulphated is necessary to demonstrate the distribution of sulphated mucosubstances.
(2) Sulphation-induced basophilia is most prominent in carbohydrate-containing structures. Comparison with a section stained by the PAS method (Chapter 11) is useful for distinguishing between carbohydrates and proteins.
(3) Sites of sulphate esters are stained. When thiazine dyes are used, metachromatic effects are often seen. If the staining (Step 4) is omitted, sulphation is a blocking reaction of low specificity for hydroxy groups. Some amino groups are N-sulphated, and become basophilic instead of acidophilic.

10.11.2.
Acetylation and benzoylation

Acetylation reagent
Pyridine (anhydrous):   24 ml
Acetic anhydride: 16 ml

Make as needed and use only once. Make the mixture in a fume cupboard.

Benzoylation reagent
Benzoyl chloride: 2 ml
Pyridine (anhydrous):   38 ml

Make as needed and use only once. Make the mixture in a fume cupboard.

Procedure
De-wax paraffin sections and take into absolute ethanol, and then into pyridine. Transfer to either the acetylation or the benzoylation reagent in a tightly capped container. Conditions are as follows:

Mild acetylation: 3 h at 37°C
Complete acetylation: 48 h at 37°C
Benzoylation: 24 h at room temperature

After treatment, wash the slides in absolute ethanol, and take to water.

Effects
Mild acetylation blocks hydroxy groups. Complete acetylation blocks hydroxy and amino groups. Benzoylation has the same effect as complete acetylation. These blockades are largely reversed by saponification (Section 10.11.5).

10.11.3.
Sulphation-acetylation

This is the fastest way to block amino groups (Lillie, 1964). Sulphation of hydroxy groups also occurs.

Reagent
Acetic anhydride: 10 ml
Glacial acetic acid: 30 ml
Concentrated sulphuric acid: 0.1 ml

Make as needed and use only once.

Procedure
De-wax paraffin sections and take to absolute ethanol and then into glacial acetic acid. Transfer to the reagent for 10 min at room temperature. Wash in running tap water for 5 min.

Effects

Amino and hydroxy groups are blocked, mainly by sulphation. This effect is reversed by treatment for 3 h at 60°C with the reagent used for methylation (Section 10.11.4, below). Some acetylation may also occur. Histochemical reactions of arginine are unimpaired. It is possible however that N-sulphation of guanidino groups occurs (preventing the attachment of anionic dyes and inducing basophilia) but is reversed by hydrolysis in the strongly alkaline reagents used in specific methods for arginine.

10.11.4.
Methylation and desulphation

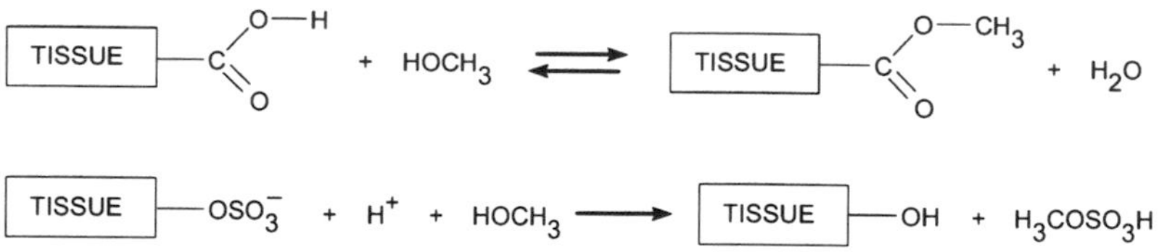

$$\boxed{\text{TISSUE}} - C \underset{O}{\overset{O-H}{<}} \ + \ HOCH_3 \ \rightleftharpoons \ \boxed{\text{TISSUE}} - C \underset{O}{\overset{O-CH_3}{<}} \ + \ H_2O$$

$$\boxed{\text{TISSUE}} - OSO_3^- \ + \ H^+ \ + \ HOCH_3 \ \longrightarrow \ \boxed{\text{TISSUE}} - OH \ + \ H_3COSO_3H$$

Methylating reagent

Methanol (absolute):	60 ml
Concentrated hydrochloric acid:	0.5 ml

Make as needed. Use immediately, and only once.

Procedure

De-wax paraffin sections, take into absolute ethanol, and then into absolute methanol. Transfer to the reagent in a tightly screw-capped Coplin jar, which should be no more than two-thirds full, at 60°C for the required time (see below). Rinse in 95% ethanol and bring to water.

Effects

The chemical changes produced depend on the length of time for which the reaction is allowed to proceed:

2 h: Carboxyl groups are esterified. Sulphate groups introduced experimentally are released with re-establishment of original $-NH_2$ or $-OH$. There is partial hydrolysis of naturally occurring sulphate esters (of carbohydrates) and partial blockade of phosphate–ester groups (of nucleic acids).

24 h: Carboxyl groups are esterified and phosphate groups of nucleic acids are blocked. All sulphate esters are hydrolysed. Primary amines are largely converted to tertiary amines. (This increases their acidophilia but prevents chemical reactions characteristic of the $-NH_2$ group.)

The effects of methylation, except for removal of sulphate groups, are reversible by saponification. Methylation blocks the basophilia of nucleic acids by different mechanisms (Prento, 1980 and see Section 11.7.2).

10.11.5.
Saponification

This procedure is used for reversal of effects of acylation or methylation. The reagent is alkaline and may remove sections from slides. Coating with a film of nitrocellulose (Chapter 4) is sometimes helpful in preventing losses of sections.

Reagent

Water:	25 ml
Potassium hydroxide (KOH):	1 g
Absolute alcohol:	75 ml

Make as needed and use only once.

Procedure

Take sections to 70% ethanol, then immerse in the reagent for 30 min at room temperature. Rinse with minimum agitation in 70% ethanol, blot to flatten sections if necessary. Rinse in water. Allow the sections to dry in air if they look as if they are only loosely adherent to the slides. Proceed with the staining method.

10.11.6.
Deamination with nitrous acid

Reagent

Sodium nitrite (NaNO$_2$):	7.0 g
Water:	94 ml

Dissolve, then add

Glacial acetic acid:	6.0 ml

Make as needed; use immediately, and only once.

Procedure
De-wax and hydrate paraffin sections. Immerse in the reagent for 4, 12, 24 or 48 h. Wash in gently running tap water for 5 min.

Effects
Primary amine groups are removed. The guanidino group of arginine is only slightly affected. Most of the deamination occurs in the first 4 h, but it is occasionally necessary to apply the reagent for 48 h.

10.11.7.
Blockade of arginine

For both methods the reagent solutions are made as needed and used only once.

Benzil method (Lillie *et al.*, 1971)
Reagent

Benzil:	1.6 g
Ethanol (absolute):	32 ml
Water:	8 ml
Sodium hydroxide (NaOH):	0.8 g

This is a saturated solution. Some benzil may remain undissolved.

Diacetyl method (Segura *et al.*, 1994)
Reagent

Barium hydroxide [Ba(OH)$_2$.8H$_2$O]:	1.5 g
Water:	40 ml
Diacetyl:	1.0 ml

Add in the order stated. Check the pH, which should be 12.4.

Procedure
De-wax paraffin sections and take to 95% ethanol. Transfer to the reagent and leave for 1 h at room temperature (25°C). Rinse in 70% ethanol and then in three changes of water.

Effects
Histochemical reactions of arginine are prevented. Acidophilia generally is depressed, indicating that there may also be partial blockage of amino groups.

Note
Montero *et al.* (1991) used 100 mg benzil in 40 ml of 50% ethanol (dissolve in hot 100% ethanol before adding water), containing 0.7 g Ba(OH)$_2$ (saturated solution). Sections were immersed for 1 h at room temperature, then rinsed in 1% aqueous sodium acetate.

10.11.8.
Sulphydryl blocking procedures

Either of the following will block sulphydryl groups effectively. Sections are hydrated and then treated as described below. Both reagents should be freshly dissolved.

N-ethylmaleimide
Dissolve 625 mg of this compound in 50 ml of phosphate buffer, pH 7.4. Treat sections for 4 h at 37°C, rinse in 1% acetic acid, wash thoroughly in water.

Iodoacetate

Dissolve 0.9 g of iodoacetic acid in 40 ml of water. Add 1.0 M (4%) NaOH until the pH is 8.0. Make up to 50 ml with water. Treat sections for 18–24 h at 37°C. Wash thorouhly in water.

10.11.9.
Reduction of cystine to cysteine

Many reagents are available for the conversion of –S–S– to –SH. Two are given below. The first of these, sodium thioglycollate, is the most widely used. The second, dithiothreitol, is just as effective and can be used in a less strongly alkaline solution. It is more expensive, but less malodorous than thioglycollate. The solutions are prepared immediately before using, and used only once, in full screw-capped containers (to minimize atmospheric oxidation).

Thioglycollate reduction

Take sections to water and immerse for 15 min in a freshly made solution containing:

Thioglycollic acid ($HSCH_2COOH$):	5.0 ml
Water:	80 ml
4% (1.0 M) sodium hydroxide (NaOH):	Add dropwise until the pH is 9.5
Water:	to make 100 ml

Wash carefully in five changes of water before staining.

Dithiothreitol reduction

Take sections to water and immerse for 30 min in:

Dithiothreitol (Cleland's reagent):	1.5 g
0.03 M phosphate buffer, pH 8.0:	50 ml

Wash carefully in five changes of water before staining.

Effects

Disulphides are reduced to thiols, for which histochemical tests become positive.

10.11.10.
Blocking aldehydes and ketones

Borohydride reduction, explained with practical instructions in Section 10.10.6, removes the carbonyl group of aldehydes and ketones. The following two procedures add aromatic substituents to the carbonyl group. **Phenylhydrazine** blocks aldehydes and ketones, but *m*-**aminophenol** probably combines only with aldehydes (Section 10.10.3).

Phenylhydrazine

Take sections to water and transfer to the following solution in a screw-capped coplin jar:

Phenylhydrazine:	5 ml
Glacial acetic acid:	10 ml
Water:	to make 50 ml

Prepare when needed and use only once. **Caution.** Poisonous. Avoid contact with skin.

Leave the slides in this reagent at about 60°C for 3 h. Rinse in three changes of 70% alcohol and then in water. *Alternatively*, use a fresh 0.5% (w/v) aqueous solution of phenylhydrazine hydrochloride, for 2 h at room temperature, and then wash in water.

In some circumstances, blockade by phenylhydrazine is reversible by acids (including the H_2SO_3 of Schiff's reagent), and this is exploited in carbohydrate histochemistry (Chapter 11).

Amine-aldehyde condensation

Take sections to absolute ethanol and then into glacial acetic acid. Transfer to the following solution:

m-Aminophenol:	5.5 g
Glacial acetic acid:	50 ml

This keeps for about 2 weeks and may be used three or four times.

Take sections to absolute alcohol, transfer to the *m*-aminophenol reagent, and leave there, at room temperature, for 1 h. Rinse the slides in 95% alcohol and take to water.

This procedure can be extended to provide a staining method for aldehydes. After reaction with *m*-aminophenol and washing as described above, the slides are immersed for 2 min at 0–4°C in a freshly prepared solution containing 150 mg fast black K salt (Chapter 5) in 50 ml of 0.1 M barbitone–HCl buffer, pH 8.0 (Chapter 20). Other buffers are probably suitable, but I have not tested them. The slides are then washed in three changes of 0.1 M hydrochloric acid (each 5 min) to remove excess diazonium salt (and perhaps also to decompose triazenes), rinsed in water, dehydrated, cleared, and mounted in a resinous medium. Sites of aldehydes are stained black to deep purple. Background staining due to azo-coupling with proteins also occurs in various shades of pink and brown. The theory and practice of this technique are discussed in great detail by Lillie (1962).

11 | Carbohydrate histochemistry

Although 'carbohydrate' applies to all the sugars and their derivatives, the only such substances available in sections of fixed tissue are those in which the sugars form parts of lipids, nucleic acids and mucosubstances. The glycolipids are considered in Chapter 12 and the nucleic acids in Chapter 9. **Mucosubstance** is a collective term that includes **polysaccharides**, **glycoproteins** and **proteoglycans**, which form the subject of this chapter.

11.1. Constituent sugars of mucosubstances

Mucosubstances are identified histochemically by virtue of the properties of their constituent sugars. The monosaccharide units most commonly encountered in polysaccharides, glycoproteins, and proteoglycans will now be described. The chemistry is explained at greater length in textbooks of biochemistry. For an intro- ductory review of terminology, intended for histochemists, see Barrett (1971). Some specialized chemical terminology is used in this chapter, and in *Table 11.1*. Consult the Glossary for definitions. Varki *et al.* (1999) provide comprehensive cov- erage of carbohydrate biochemistry.

The structural formulae of monosaccharides are shown here as Haworth formulae: rings that lie in a plane perpendicular to the paper (*Fig. 11.1*). The thickened lines represent bonds in the side of the ring that is nearer to the reader. All the sugars illustrated exist as six-membered pyranose rings. The numbering system is shown for α-D-glucose. In the β-anomers of sugars of the D-series, the hydroxyl group at position C1 is directed downwards. The formulae for the L-enantiomers are obtained by envisaging the images in a mirror held *in the plane of the ring*. In α-L- sugars, therefore, the hydroxyl at position C1 is directed upwards and C6 lies below rather than above C5. **Anomers** differ only in the configuration at position C1. **Epimers** differ in the direction of the hydroxyl group at one carbon atom other than C1. Thus, α-D-glucose and β-D-glucose are anomers. Galactose and mannose are epimers of glucose, but not of one another. Haworth structures give a false impression that the rings are planar, but they simplify the recognition of monosaccharide

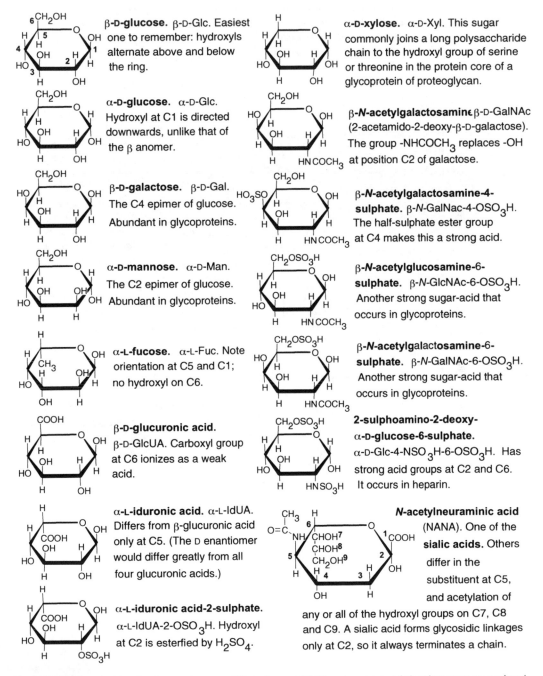

β-D-glucose. β-D-Glc. Easiest one to remember: hydroxyls alternate above and below the ring.

α-D-glucose. α-D-Glc. Hydroxyl at C1 is directed downwards, unlike that of the β anomer.

β-D-galactose. β-D-Gal. The C4 epimer of glucose. Abundant in glycoproteins.

α-D-mannose. α-D-Man. The C2 epimer of glucose. Abundant in glycoproteins.

α-L-fucose. α-L-Fuc. Note orientation at C5 and C1; no hydroxyl on C6.

β-D-glucuronic acid. β-D-GlcUA. Carboxyl group at C6 ionizes as a weak acid.

α-L-iduronic acid. α-L-IdUA. Differs from β-glucuronic acid only at C5. (The D enantiomer would differ greatly from all four glucuronic acids.)

α-L-iduronic acid-2-sulphate. α-L-IdUA-2-OSO$_3$H. Hydroxyl at C2 is esterfied by H$_2$SO$_4$.

α-D-xylose. α-D-Xyl. This sugar commonly joins a long polysaccharide chain to the hydroxyl group of serine or threonine in the protein core of a glycoprotein of proteoglycan.

β-N-acetylgalactosamine β-D-GalNAc (2-acetamido-2-deoxy-β-D-galactose). The group -NHCOCH$_3$ replaces -OH at position C2 of galactose.

β-N-acetylgalactosamine-4-sulphate. β-N-GalNac-4-OSO$_3$H. The half-sulphate ester group at C4 makes this a strong acid.

β-N-acetylglucosamine-6-sulphate. β-N-GlcNAc-6-OSO$_3$H. Another strong sugar-acid that occurs in glycoproteins.

β-N-acetylgalactosamine-6-sulphate. β-N-GalNAc-6-OSO$_3$H. Another strong sugar-acid that occurs in glycoproteins.

2-sulphoamino-2-deoxy-α-D-glucose-6-sulphate. α-D-Glc-4-NSO$_3$H-6-OSO$_3$H. Has strong acid groups at C2 and C6. It occurs in heparin.

N-acetylneuraminic acid (NANA). One of the **sialic acids.** Others differ in the substituent at C5, and acetylation of any or all of the hydroxyl groups on C7, C8 and C9. A sialic acid forms glycosidic linkages only at C2, so it always terminates a chain.

Figure 11.1. Monosaccharide units of mucosubstances. All but xylose and NANA are hexoses, and their carbon atoms are numbered as shown for β-D-glucose.

units and their α- or β- linkages, and the presence of L-series sugars (fucose and iduronic acid) in some biologically important mucosubstances.

In the complex carbohydrates, monosaccharide units are joined together by **glycosidic** linkages. Each unit or residue may be called a glycosyl group. Carbon atom C1 of one sugar is connected via an oxygen atom to one of the carbons (most commonly C3, C4, or C6) of another sugar. In the names of glycosides, the linkage is indicated in an abbreviated form such as α-1→4, which shows which carbon atoms are joined and what the configuration is at C1. In a free monosaccharide or one at the end of a chain with C1 not involved in a glycosidic linkage, the ring (hemiacetal) structure is in equilibrium with an open-chain (aldehyde) isomer, as shown for α-D-glucose.

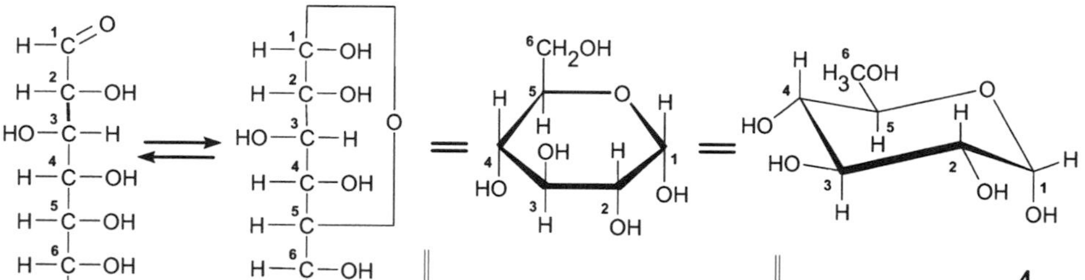

aldehyde   cyclic hemiacetal

Fischer projection formulae.

Haworth plane ring structure. Downwardly directed bonds correspond to bonds that project to the right in the Fischer projection formulae.

α-Glucose in the $^4C_1$ chair conformation, which more realistically shows the shape of the molecule.

Only a small proportion is present as an aldehyde, but this functional group is responsible for some of the chemical properties of glucose and other carbohydrates, including reduction of Fehling's solution and ammoniacal silver nitrate, but not of Schiff's reagent.

11.2. Classification and composition of mucosubstances

The macromolecular carbohydrates may be classified on the basis of their chemistry, their behaviour in selected histochemical tests, or their distribution in nature. Pearse (1985) presented a system of classification in which an attempt was made to correlate chemical compositions with histochemically discernible properties, but with the advent of techniques for the demonstration of individual monosaccharides residues (Section 11.5) this scheme is now somewhat outdated. Classifications based solely on staining properties, such as those of Cook (1974) and Culling *et al.* (1985), are used in diagnostic pathology, but they lead to identifications that do not correspond very closely with known chemical entities. Indeed, the mucosubstances known to biochemists cannot all be distinguished by means of histochemical procedures. The differing approaches of the two disciplines have also led to a wealth of confusing terminology. In this account, the recommendations of Reid and Clamp (1978) are followed as far as possible. Ambiguous terms such as mucin, mucoid, mucopolysaccharide, mucoprotein, sialomucin sulphomucin, and several others that abound in the literature are avoided.

The following scheme is not so much a classification as a descriptive list. It includes the major mucosubstances of vertebrate animals and a few others. For each mucosubstance the major constituent sugars and the forms of glycosidic linkage are stated; other organic functional groups are identified, and histochemically relevant physical properties are mentioned.

POLYSACCHARIDES
Composed entirely of carbohydrate
(polyglycosides)

PROTEOGLYCANS
Long polysaccharide side-chains
(glycosaminoglycans) that have repeating
disaccharide units, attached to a
relatively small protein core

MUCOSUBSTANCES
Macromolecular compounds
composed in whole or in
part of carbohydrate

GLYCOPROTEINS
Proteins bearing numerous covalently
bound oligosaccharide chains

11.2.1
Polysaccharides

A polysaccharide consists of many monosaccharide units, joined by glycosidic link-ages. The macromolecular carbohydrate is not covalently linked to a protein.

The following polysaccharides are all **homopolysaccharides**, composed of many identical monosaccharide units. The chains may be unbranched, typically when the same glycosidic linkage occurs throughout the molecule, or branched when some of the units are connected through more than one hydroxyl group.

Glycogen: $-D-Glc(\alpha-1\rightarrow4)D-Glc(\alpha-1\rightarrow4)-$. The chain is branched because there are some $-D-Glc(\alpha-1\rightarrow6)D-Glc-$ linkages in each molecule of glycogen. This poly-saccharide is fairly soluble in water, and is best preserved by alcoholic fixatives.

The only important functional group in glycogen is $-OH$. Adjacent hydroxy groups occur at C2 and C3 in every monosaccharide unit (see structure of α-glucose in *Fig. 11.1*). This is known as the **glycol** formation (also called vicinal diol, *vic*-glycol or 1,2-diol) and it is present in many other mucosubstances.

Starch. This plant polysaccharide has the same general chemical structure as glyco-gen, differing only in the size, branching and conformation of its molecules. The unbranched form is **amylose**, and the branched type, which is similar to glycogen, is **amylopectin**. (Pectin, the principal polysaccharide of the middle lamellae of plant cell walls, consists largely of galacturonic acid units.)

Cellulose: $-D-Glc(\beta-1\rightarrow4)D-Glc(\beta-1\rightarrow4)-$. This, the principal component of plant cell walls, is absent from animal tissues, with the exception of the exoskeleton in tunicates. It differs from starch and glycogen in being a β- rather than an α-polyglu-coside. Cellulose is insoluble in all the reagents commonly used in microtechnique.

Chitin: $-D-GlcNAc(\beta-1\rightarrow4)D-GlcNAc(\beta-1\rightarrow4)-$. This is the principal component of the exoskeleton in insects, crustacea, and various other invertebrates. It also occurs in some fungi and algae. The polysaccharide constitutes about half the dry weight of exoskeletal material, with the balance consisting largely of proteins and insoluble salts of calcium.

11.2.2.
Proteoglycans

The carbohydrate components of proteoglycans are **heteropolysaccharides**, each long chain being composed of repeating units of two or more different monosac-charide units. The polysaccharide chains of proteoglycans, considered in isolation, are often called glycosaminoglycuronans or **glycosaminoglycans** (GAGs). The term 'mucopolysaccharide' was formerly used as synonym for either 'proteoglycan' or the heteropolysaccharide component. The repeating units always include a nitro-gen-containing sugar and an acid sugar. The latter, which may be a uronic acid or a sulphate–ester of a hexose, confers affinity for cationic dyes. The repeating units given below for some individual GAGs are not completely constant: smaller quantities of other monosaccharides are also present in the molecule, and the distribution of sulphate–ester groups is somewhat variable. For a longer account of these compounds, see Varki *et al.*, 1999.

Hyaluronan (hyaluronic acid). The repeating unit is: −D-GlcUA(β-1→3)D-GlcNAc(β-1→4)−. This GAG exists in a variable state of polymerization. The polymers of low molecular weight are soluble in water and have low viscosity. The high polymers are more viscous and are less easily extracted by water. Glycol and carboxyl groups are present in the β-D-glucuronic acid component of each repeating unit.

Chondroitin-4-sulphate (synonym: chondroitin sulphate A). The repeating unit is −D-GlcUA(β-1→3)D-GalNAc-4-OSO₃H(β-1→4)−. Insoluble in all commonly used histological reagents and has glycol, carboxyl, and sulphate–ester groups.

Chondroitin-6-sulphate (synonym: chondroitin sulphate C). The repeating unit is −D-GlcUA(β-1→3)D-GalNAc-6-OSO₃H(β-1→4)−. Chemically and physically this is closely similar to chondroitin-4-sulphate, differing only in the position of the sulphate–ester group.

Dermatan sulphate (formerly 'chondroitin sulphate B'). The repeating unit is −L-IdUA(α-1→3)D-GalNAc-4-OSO₃(β-→>4)−. This is another sulphated proteoglycan, differing from chondroitin-4-sulphate only in the configuration at position C5 in the uronic acid (see *Fig. 11.1*).

Keratan sulphates. The repeating unit is −D-Gal(β-1→4)D-GlcNAc-6-OSO₃H(β-1→3)−. Type I is joined by an *N*-glycoside linkage from asparagine in the associated core protein of the proteoglycan to GalNAc. Type II is O-linked from serine to GalNAc, and the protein core molecule is larger than in Type I. Keratan sulphates also contain small quantities of mannose, fucose and sialic acids.

These closely related proteoglycans are insoluble in all commonly used histological reagents. Sulphate–ester groups are present but glycol formations are absent because position C3 of the galactose is involved in the glycosidic linkage.

Heparin. The protein core of the molecule bears several long heteropolysaccharide chains, the principal repeating unit of which is

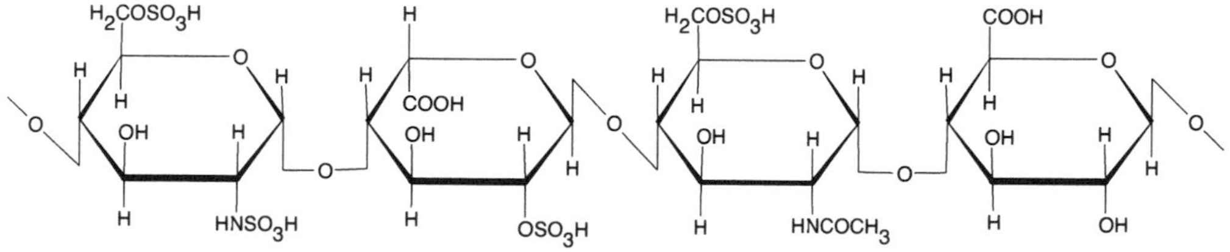

All the glycosidic linkages are α-1→4. The monosaccharide units are variously sulphated derivatives of L-iduronic and D-glucuronic acids and *N*-acetyl-D-glucosamine. Small amounts of D-galactose and D-xylose are also present (see Jeanloz, 1975; Jansson *et al.*, 1975). All the organic functional groups that occur in mucosubstances are present in heparin, but sulphate–ester groups predominate.

Heparin occurs principally in the cytoplasmic granules of mast cells, but it is possible that lower concentrations are also present in other cells and in connective tissues (Jaques *et al.*, 1977). Heparin is used clinically as an anticoagulant.

Heparan sulphate. This is a group of substances that occur within and on the surfaces of animal cells. Heparan sulphate has been studied mainly by chemical and pharmacological methods. It is a by-product of the manufacture of heparin from animal tissues. At least four different GAGs are embraced by the name. They are similar to heparin but contain fewer sulphate and more *N*-acetyl groups. Heparan sulphate, which has also been called heparitin sulphate and heparin monosulphuric acid, is produced in almost all animal cells and is not now considered a metabolic precursor of heparin (Silbert *et al.*, 1975; Backstrom *et al.*, 1975; Varki *et al.*, 1999); it has less than 1% of the anticoagulant power of heparin.

A **proteoglycan molecule** consists of chondroitin, dermatan, keratan or heparan sulphate molecules, which are typically 50–200 nm long, joined to a core protein that is some 300 nm long. Oligosaccharide chains similar to those of glycoproteins (5–15 sugar units) are also attached to the core protein. In an extracellular matrix, the proteoglycan molecules are joined, through smaller linking protein molecules, to strands of hyaluronan of indefinite (>2 µm) length (*Fig. 11.2*). Most of the protein-carbohydrate linkages are *O*-glycosidic bonds to the side chain of serine, but there are also some *N*-glycoside linkages to basic amino acids. Proteoglycans and hyaluronan form a three-dimensional macromolecular mesh that occupies the spaces between collagen fibrils.

The extracellular matrices of tissues vary in their proportions of collagen, proteoglycan and hyaluronan, and in the relative abundances of the different glycosaminoglycans.

Proteoglycans are preserved chemically intact by all non-oxidizing fixatives, though there may be extraction of some heteropolysaccharide material, such as the lower polymers of hyaluronan. It is advisable, when investigating a previously unstudied tissue, to try more than one fixative mixture. A proteoglycan in the rat's brain, for example, has been shown to be histochemically detectable after fixation in formalin–acetic acid or Bouin, but not after fixation in pure formaldehyde solutions (Lai *et al.*, 1975). Cetylpyridinium chloride (Williams and Jackson, 1956) has been proposed as a special fixative for the precipitation of proteoglycans, though it can depress staining by competition with cationic dyes. Cyanuric chloride (Goland *et al.*, 1967), which combines covalently with hydroxyl groups, has also been used as a fixative for mucosubstances, though it would be expected to prevent many histochemical reactions.

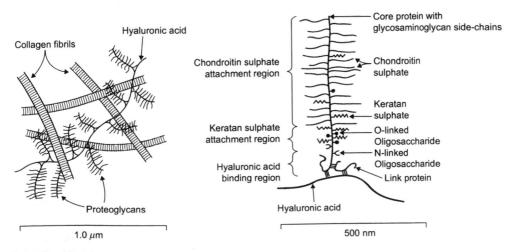

Figure 11.2. Structural relations of collagen, hyaluronan (hyaluronic acid) and proteoglycans in a tissue such as cartilage matrix (After Hascall and Hascall, 1981; reproduced with permission.)

11.2.3.
Glycoproteins

These mucosubstances are more varied than the polysaccharides and proteogly-cans. The oligosaccharide chains consist of 2–12 monosaccharide units. The commonest sugars in glycoproteins are β-D-galactose, α-D-mannose, α- and β-N-acetylglucosamine, α- and β-N-acetylgalactosamine, α-L-fucose and sialic acids. The two last-named always occupy terminal positions (farthest from the protein). In a branched side-chain, however, these terminal sugars can be nearer to the polypeptide core than some of the residues in the interior of the chain (see Podolsky, 1985). Examples of glycoproteins are:

Serum proteins
These include immunoglobulins.

Blood-group specific substances
These occur on the surfaces of erythrocytes.

Secretory products
Both exocrine and endocrine glands secrete glycoproteins. Some of these, especially in the alimentary canal, contain sulphated sugars and sialic acids. Histochemical methods cannot determine whether such substances are single glycoproteins or mixtures.

Constituents of the glycocalyx
Glycoproteins form the 'cell coat' on the outside surface of the plasmalemma of every cell. The glycocalyx is an integral part of the cell membrane (see Cook, 1995).

Collagen
This is unusual in that α-D-glucosyl units form a major part of the carbohydrate component (see also Chapter 8).

The traditional histochemical demonstration of glycoproteins is based on the presence of carboxyl, hydroxyl and sulphate–ester groups. They are preserved by most fixatives, but mixtures containing oxidizing agents (which would attack the glycol formation) should not be used. The carbohydrate components of glycolipids are similar to those of glycoproteins, and the two groups of substances can be confused with one another when frozen sections are used. In many sites, especially in mucus that lubricates epithelial surfaces, several different glycoproteins are present. The histochemist can identify and localize various functional groups and some individual monosaccharide residues, but cannot determine whether these occur in the same or different molecules.

11.2.4.
Amyloid

Amyloid is named from its resemblance to starch; both substances give a blue colour reaction with iodine. It is considered in this chapter for convenience, even though it is predominantly composed of proteins. Deposits of amyloid accumulate in various organs as a consequence of chronic inflammatory diseases and in the brain in Alzheimer's disease. A rare condition known as primary amyloidosis is also encountered occasionally by pathologists.

The deposits consist of fibrillary and other proteins, including basement membrane components such as Type IV collagen and perlecan, a heparan sulphate proteoglycan. The proteins are in β-pleated sheet conformation and are organized as fibrils 7–13 nm in diameter, which occur in interlacing bundles (see Glenner *et al.*, 1980; Kisilevsky, 2008). One major protein, the amyloid P component, is different for each of the more than 20 types of amyloidosis.

The techniques of carbohydrate histochemistry fall into three categories: those in which **dyes** and related reagents are used, **chemical methods**, and methods involving use of **lectins**. All types of method can also be used in conjunction with chemical blocking procedures for reactive groups and with enzymatic degradation of specific mucosubstances. Several techniques exist other than the ones described in this chapter. It is also possible to demonstrate many mucosubstances by immunohistochemical methods, which can detect individual proteoglycans and glycoproteins with high specificity. Most of the methods discussed in this chapter show only major groups of mucosubstances.

11.3. Histochemical methods using dyes

Four techniques will be discussed: the uses of the alcian blue, the observation of metachromasia, staining with a cationic dye in conjunction with a metal salt, and the use of anionic dyes with large molecules.

11.3.1. Alcian blue

This dye (Chapter 5) binds to carboxyl and sulphate–ester groups at pH 2.5, but only to the latter at pH 1.0. With the more strongly acid solution, carboxyl groups are not ionized and therefore cannot electrostatically attract the cations of the dye. It is therefore possible to identify with some degree of certainty mucosubstances that owe their acidity wholly to carboxyl groups, but it is not possible to tell whether a substance stained at both pH levels owes its acidity only to sulphate groups or to both sulphate and carboxyl groups. If, however, a section is subjected before staining to an adequate treatment with hot, acidified methanol (Chapter 10; also this chapter, Section 11.7.2), the sulphate–ester groups and probably also most of the sialic acids will be removed, and the carboxyl groups will be esterified. Nothing will be stained by alcian blue. The section can next be subjected to a 'saponification' procedure (Section 11.7.2), which will cause hydrolysis of the methyl esters and restore the carboxyl groups. These will regain their stainability by alcian blue at pH 2.5. The sulphate esters, however, will have been irreversibly removed and will no longer be detectable. Thus, provided that at least six sections of the same tissue are available, it is possible to determine whether affinity for alcian blue at pH 1.0 and 2.5 is due solely to sulphate esters or to both sulphate ester and carboxyl groups coexisting at the same site.

It is quite feasible to study acid mucosubstances by staining with cationic dyes other than alcian blue. Some effects of pH on the affinities of thiazine dyes for different anions were reviewed in Chapter 6. The main reason for using alcian blue in carbohydrate histochemistry is the fact that this dye does not usually stain nuclei or cytoplasmic deposits of RNA in sections, though it is known to be able to bind to nucleic acids in solution (Scott et al., 1964).

Studies with molecular models (Scott, 1972b) have revealed that the four tetramethylisothiouronium groups attached to the phthalocyanine ring of alcian blue 8G (Section 5.9.14) make the dye molecule too big to fit between the coils of the DNA helix. Electrostatic attraction between the phosphate groups and the auxochromes is weakened by distance and there can be no close-range interaction (van der Waals forces, etc., see Section 5.5) between the aromatic rings of the dye and the purine and pyrimidine rings of the DNA. The access of the large cations of alcian blue to the phosphate groups of nucleic acids in a fixed tissue is hindered also by the presence of the associated nucleoproteins (Chapter 9). Steric hindrance may also explain the failure of alcian blue to stain RNA. Sometimes, especially in the tissues of very young animals, nuclei are stained by alcian blue at pH 2.5. Such staining may be due at least in part to acid mucosubstances present in the chromosomes of dividing cells (Ohnishi et al., 1973). Another advantage of alcian blue over most other cationic dyes is that its solubilizing tetramethylisothiouronium groups are lost, as a result of base-catalyzed hydrolysis, when the stained sections are washed in water. The resulting pigment (copper phthalocyanine) is not extracted by water, alcohols, acids, or solutions of other dyes used for counterstaining. The PAS procedure (Section 11.4) is frequently applied to tissues already stained with alcian blue.

Solutions required
Some batches of alcian blue are unsatisfactory when new. The use of a BSC-certified dye is strongly recommended. Some initially satisfactory batches deteriorate with storage, even as dry powders.

A. Alcian blue, pH 1.0
Alcian blue 8G (C.I. 74240):	1.0 g
0.1 M hydrochloric acid:	100 ml

See Chapter 20 for instructions for making 0.1 M HCl. The stability of this dye solution is variable. Sometimes all the coloured material precipitates after 2 or 3 weeks. Other batches are stable for more than 1 year. Filter before using.

B. Alcian blue, pH 2.5
Alcian blue 8G (C.I. 74240):	1.0 g
Water:	97 ml
Glacial acetic acid:	3.0 ml

Takes about 1 h to dissolve (magnetic stirrer). Filter into a clean bottle. Keeps for several years but eventually decomposes and precipitates. If the stored solution needs filtering, it has probably deteriorated enough to need replacing.

Procedure
(1) De-wax and hydrate paraffin sections.
(2) Stain in *either* solution A *or* solution B for 30 min.
(3) Rinse in 0.1 M HCl or 3% acetic acid (the solvent for the dye), then wash in running tap water for three min.
(4) (Optional.) Apply a pink or red counterstain if desired.
(5) Dehydrate in graded alcohols. Alcian blue is not removed by alcohol, but the counterstain may be differentiated.
(6) Clear in xylene and mount in a resinous medium.

Result
All acid mucosubstances are stained at pH 2.5. Only sulphated mucosubstances are stained at pH 1.0.

Notes
(1) A dye marketed as **alcian blue pyridine variant** is as efective as alcian blue 8G in this method (Henwood, 2002).
(2) Mucosubstances with carboxyl or sulphate–ester groups may be distinguished from one another if control sections are methylated and saponified (See Section 11.7.1). Neuraminidase (Section 11.6.3) and mild acid hydrolysis (Section 11.7.4) may be used to identify glycoproteins that owe their acidity to sialic acids.
(3) Ordinary red cationic dyes, especially safranine (Spicer, 1960), may be used in conjunction with alcian blue. Differential staining effects have been described in carbohydrate-containing structures such as mast cell granules (Jasmin and Bois, 1961; Combs *et al.*, 1965), but the tinctorial variations have been shown by Tas (1977) to have no histochemical significance. For further information concerning the histochemical properties of alcian blue, see Scott *et al.* (1964) and Quintarelli *et al.* (1964a,b).
(4) Alcian blue has also been used mixed with an inorganic salt (usually magnesium chloride) at various ionic strengths. The cations of the salt compete with those of the dye for binding sites in the tissue. The dye is used at a high pH

(5–6) so that the results will not be complicated by incomplete ionization of carboxyl groups. The highly dissociated acids ($-OSO_3^-$ in this case) can bind the dye in the presence of high concentrations of the salt, whereas the weaker acids ($-COO^-$) cannot. This assertion forms the basis of the **critical electrolyte concentration** (CEC) method of Scott (1970), with which each acidic mucosubstance can be assigned a concentration of $MgCl_2$ above which it is not stainable by alcian blue. This chemical interpretation of CEC effects has been questioned (Horobin and Goldstein, 1974). Horobin (1982,1988) suggests that dyes in solutions of increasing ionic strength are bound by substrates of increasing porosity rather than increasing acidity. Solutions of alcian blue 8G with $MgCl_2$ at pH 5–6 are stable for only a few hours. Alcian blue pyridine variant (see *Note 1* above) is more stable and works well in CEC methods (Churukian *et al.*, 2000).

11.3.2. Metachromasia

When a cationic dye imparts its own colour to an object, the staining is said to be **orthochromatic**. In some circumstances the bound dye ions have an altered wavelength of absorption, so that the observed colour of the stained object is different from that of the dye. This phenomenon is known as **metachromasia** and substrates that stain metachromatically are said to be **chromotropic**. In most cases the metachromatic colour of the dye is of a longer wavelength than the orthochromatic colour. Blue dyes, such as thionine and toluidine blue, stain chromotropic materials in shades of red and purple. The red and purple colours produced by such dyes have been called γ- and β- metachromasia, respectively, but this distinction is probably of little importance. Only γ-metachromasia is of interest in the histochemistry of mucosubstances. The change in colour is due to a shift to shorter wavelengths (a hypsochromic shift) in the absorption spectrum of the dye and to an associated reduction in the intensity of the colour.

Metachromatic effects are produced when the coloured ions of a dye are brought in close proximity to one another. This occurs when anionic radicals of the substrate are close together, as in some proteoglycans. The dye-substrate complex of a metachromatically stained object has the form shown in *Fig. 11.3*.

The water molecules interposed between the stacked dye ions are believed to be necessary for modifying the distribution of electrons in the chromophoric system in such a way as to reduce the wavelength at which light is maximally absorbed (Bergeron and Singer, 1958). The dyes with which metachromatic effects can be obtained are thiazines, oxazines, azines, and xanthenes (Chapter 5). These have planar molecules that are able to stack closely (*Fig. 11.3*) and they can be formulated with positively charged auxochromic groups on either side of the systems of fused rings. When the auxochromes are more bulky than the $-N(CH_3)_3$ group,

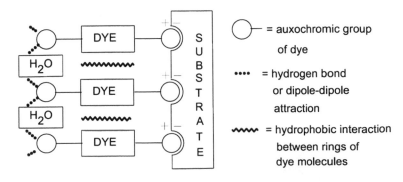

Figure 11.3. Arrangement of stacked dye molecules in a metachromatically stained substrate.

metachromatic staining does not occur (Taylor, 1961), probably because there is not room for the interposition of water molecules. The bound water is thought to resist extraction by dehydrating agents: indeed, it is generally agreed that metachromasia must persist in dehydrated, cleared preparations if it is to have any significance in relation to macromolecular carbohydrates (Kramer and Windrum, 1955).

Another cause of metachromasia may be the formation of dimers of dye molecules in the staining solution and the subsequent attachment of these dimers to anionic sites in the tissue (see Schubert and Hamerman, 1956; Wollin and Jaques, 1973 for discussion). This does not seem a very probable mechanism, however, because dye solutions display metachromasia only when they are concentrated, but metachromatic histological staining is easily obtained from very dilute solutions.

Acid mucosubstances are not the only sources of metachromasia found in animal tissues. Nucleic acids are also chromotropic in some circumstances, though their metachromasia usually reverts to orthochromasia after dehydration. Despite the low histochemical specificity of metachromatic staining with cationic dyes, the method is useful for the morphological study of structures known to contain sulphated glycoproteins (some types of mucus), heparin (mast-cell granules) and proteoglycans in the intercellular matrices of cartilage and some other connective tissues.

Solution required

A 0.05–0.25% (w/v) solution of toluidine blue (C.I. 52040), azure A (C.I. 52005), or thionine (C.I. 52000) in 1% (v/v) aqueous acetic acid. These solutions can be kept for several years, but they lose potency with repeated use. Filter before each use.

Procedure

(1) De-wax and hydrate paraffin sections.
(2) Stain for 1–5 min (see *Note 1*).
(3) Wash in water.
(4) Dehydrate in 70%, 95%, and two changes of absolute ethanol (see *Note 2*).
(5) Clear in xylene and mount in a resinous medium.

Result

Orthochromatic colour (nuclei, cytoplasm of some cells, Nissl substance of neurons) blue. Metachromatic colour red.

Notes

(1) If staining is excessive, add more acetic acid to the toluidine blue. (Older dye solutions lose acidity with storage.) The pH of the solution should be approximately 4.0. A lower pH will give weaker orthochromatic staining.
(2) The dye is differentiated mainly by the 70% ethanol. The sections should be pale blue before being cleared. If the staining is initially weak, take the slides directly from water into the first of three changes of 100% alcohol. Alternatively, blot the sections after washing and dehydrate in two changes (each 3–5 min) of *n*-butanol.
(3) For microspectrophotometric studies of glycosaminoglycans in cartilage, Kiraly *et al.* (1996b) found that thionine and safranine O gave measurements that correlated with chemical estimations more closely than the results obtained with other basic dyes.

11.3.3.
Heath's
aluminium–
basic dye method

A dilute (approximately 10^{-3} M) solution of a cationic dye in 0.1–0.5 M aluminium sulphate gives selective staining of structures that contain sulphated mucosubstances. Heath (1962) investigated this phenomenon thoroughly. The most effective dyes were found to be *N*-methyl azines and thiazines, including neutral red and toluidine blue. Cationic dyes with larger molecules, including some triarylmethanes, gave specific staining of sulphated mucosubstances but the colour was easily lost in washing and dehydration. Heath also found that the same result could be obtained by treating sections with the aluminium salt before the dye, and that aluminium could be replaced by other metals that readily formed coordination compounds. Specificity for sulphate esters was confirmed by ascertaining that the stainability was prevented by methylation of the tissue, and not restored by saponification (see also Chapter 10 and later in this chapter). Strong acid groups artificially introduced into tissues (by sulphation of hydroxyls or oxidation of cystine; see Chapter 10) were also stained by aluminium–basic dye combinations.

Aluminium ions bind, by coordination or ionic attraction, to all parts of a section immersed in a solution of $Al_2(SO_4)_3$. It seems probable that the metal forms complexes with carboxyl groups of proteins and carbohydrates, and perhaps also with the phosphate groups of nucleic acids, leaving sulphates as the only anionic groups free to combine with a cationic dye.

Solutions required

A. Aluminium-dye solution

Neutral red (C.I. 50040) or Toluidine blue (C.I. 52040): 0.1 g
Water: 100 ml
Aluminium sulphate ($Al_2(SO_4)_3.18H_2O$): 5.0 g

Boil, allow to cool, and filter to remove insoluble material; then add 5% (w/v) aqueous $Al_2(SO_4)_3.18H_2O$: to make 300 ml.

B. 70% ethanol, for differentiation of stained sections.

Procedure

(1) De-wax and hydrate sections. Remember to remove mercury deposits, if necessary.
(2) Stain for 5–30 min.
(3) Rinse in water.
(4) Differentiate in 70% ethanol for 20–30 s, or until the background (nuclei, cytoplasm, collagen) is colourless.
(5) If desired, apply a suitably contrasting counterstain, such as eosin or fast green FCF (Chapter 6).
(6) Complete the dehydration, in 95% and 2 changes of 100% alcohol, clear in xylene and cover, using a resinous mounting medium.

Result

Sites of sulphated mucosubstances (mast cells, cartilage matrix, some goblet cells, etc.) red with neutral red, or red to purple (metachromatic) with toluidine blue.

Note

Heath (1962) tested 57 dyes for this method and strongly recommended one that he called 'nuclear fast red'. Probably this dye was really neutral red (see Frank *et al.*, 2007). The anthraquinone dye usually known as nuclear fast red (C.I. 60760), is not suitable, however, because it is not a cationic dye and its aluminium complex stains nuclei. Confusion about the identity of a suitable dye may account for the lack of popularity of Heath's simple and reliable method, which uses inexpensive reagents and deserves to be used more widely.

11.3.4.
Dye methods for glycogen and amyloid

Anionic dyes that exist in solution as large molecules or aggregates of molecules are used for staining collagen, as explained in Chapters 5 and 7. Some of these dyes can also be used for the demonstration of polysaccharides. Neutral polysaccharides like **glycogen** have no charged groups, so the binding and retention of a dye necessarily occur by non-ionic mechanisms. The classical stain of this kind for glycogen is Best's carmine technique, in which the dye is dissolved in a mixture of water and alcohol. The structural formula of carmine (Chapter 5) shows a large molecule with numerous hydrophilic substituents (carboxyl, phenolic hydroxyl, and the hydroxyls of the sugar moieties). Glycogen, a macromolecule, also bears great numbers of hydroxyl groups. Horobin (1982) has suggested that this may be one of the few instances in which hydrogen bonding plays an important part in a staining mechanism. Evidence in support of this idea comes from the observation that the intensity of staining of glycogen by carmine is reduced if the proportion of water in the solvent of the dye is increased. Water competes for hydrogen bonding sites on the molecules of dyes and substrates, as explained in Chapter 5.

The staining of **amyloid** by Congo red and other direct cotton dyes at high pH is non-ionic, and has been attributed to hydrogen bonding to the carbohydrate component of the substrate (Puchtler et al., 1964). The staining of amyloid by solutions of these dyes is retarded, however, by addition of alcohol (which should enhance hydrogen bonding), and under certain conditions of application Congo red simultaneously stains amyloid and hydrophobic objects such as elastic fibres (Mera and Davies, 1984). Hydrophobic and van der Waals forces are therefore probably the most important factors involved in the binding of the dye (see also Section 5.5). Carbohydrates are not hydrophobic, so the substrate of the dye is presumably proteinaceous. Amyloid stained by Congo red acquires a conspicuous dichroism: the deposits show as bright green areas on a black background when viewed in a polarizing microscope with crossed polarizer and analyser. (For information on polarizing microscopy, see Robinson and Bradbury, 1992.) The dichroism indicates alignment of dye molecules in a highly ordered structure, in this case the parallel filaments of protein molecules with β-pleated sheet structure (Wolman and Bubis, 1965; see also Glenner et al., 1980; Pearse, 1985).

Different proteins are present in the amyloids associated with different diseases. These can be distinguished on the basis of the preservation or destruction of their Congo red dichroism after such treatments as autoclaving or immersion in alkaline guanidine. Immunohistochemical methods specific for the proteins are preferred, however, for identifying different types of amyloid (Elghetany and Saleem, 1988).

Amyloid can also be stained with cationic dyes, which are attracted to the sulphate ester anions of perlecan. Cationic dyes often give unusual metachromatic colours, presumably due to aligned glycosaminoglycan chains within the proteinaceous matrix of the amyloid fibrils. Thioflavine S and thioflavine T (Section 5.9.12.2) are used for fluorescent staining of amyloid; these methods have high sensitivity but low specificity (McKinney and Grubb, 1965; Sun et al., 2002).

11.3.4.1. Best's carmine for glycogen
An alcoholic fixative should be used to preserve glycogen (Chapter 5). If an aqueous fixative must be used, it should be perfused through the animal's vascular system. A classical diffusion artifact is seen in specimens of liver fixed by immersion in aqueous liquids. In every hepatocyte the stained glycogen is present only in the cytoplasm of the side of the cell that faces away from the surface of the specimen. This gives a curious striated pattern when the section is examined with a low-power objective. The artifact is caused by dissolving of glygogen in water and diffusion along a concentration gradient until the cell mambrane, impermeable to large molecules, is encountered. After their migration, the glycogen molecules become immobilized in a sponge of fixed protein. Aqueous formaldehyde, because it diffuses quickly but cross-links proteins slowly, is the fixative with which this artifact is most pronounced. With correct fixation, glycogen staining is uniformly distributed in the cytoplasm of hepatocytes.

Solutions required

A. Nuclear counterstain
An iron–haematoxylin or a haemalum (Chapter 6 for several suitable mixtures).

B. Stock solution of carmine
Water:	60 ml
Carmine:	2.0 g
Potassium carbonate (K_2CO_3):	1.0 g
Potassium chloride (KCl):	5.0 g

Boil for 5 min, in a 500 ml flask (large volume because of effervescence). Cool, filter, and add the filtrate to 20 ml of strong ammonium hydroxide (SG 0.880). Store in a dark place. The solution keeps for 2–3 months.

C. Working staining solution
Stock solution (above):	15 ml
Ammonium hydroxide (SG 0.880):	12.5 ml
Methyl alcohol:	12.5 ml

Make up as required. Keeps for about one week, and can be re-used, but its potency declines with time.

D. Best's differentiator
Absolute methyl alcohol:	40 ml
Absolute ethyl alcohol:	80 ml
Water:	100 ml

Stable, but usually mixed before using.

Procedure
(1) De-wax the slides and coat with nitrocellulose (celloidin) as described in Chapter 4 (Section 4.2.2). The coating is not an essential part of the staining method, but without it some sections will be lost. Take to water.
(2) Stain the nuclei with solution A. Follow the instructions in Chapter 6 for the method you have chosen. Wash in water.
(3) Stain in the working solution of carmine (C) for about 15 min (more or less, according to intensity obtained).
(4) Transfer (without rinsing) directly to Best's differentiator (solution D). Agitate gently for about 10 s.
(5) Wash in 2 changes of 95% alcohol and examine. If necessary, repeat the differentiation (step 4 above).
(6) Complete the dehydration in 2 changes of 100% alcohol, clear in xylene and cover, using a resinous mounting medium.

Result
Glycogen bright crimson. Fibrin, mast cell granules and some mucus pink. Nuclei black or blue, according to counterstain.

Notes
(1) Control sections may be incubated, before staining, in **amylase**, which removes glycogen (Section 11.6.1 for instructions).
(2) The periodic acid–Schiff method (Section 11.4) also stains glycogen; it is frequently used for the purpose, and has the advantage of being a thoroughly understood histochemical method.
(3) A section of liver provides a positive control. The artifactual striated appearance in formalin-fixed material is unmistakable.

11.3.4.2. Congo red method for amyloid

This method (Highman, 1946) is suitable for paraffin sections of formaldehyde-fixed material. The differentiation in alkali removes most of the dye that binds initially to collagen and cytoplasm.

Solutions required

A. Congo red solution

Congo red:	1.0 g
50% (v/v) ethanol:	200 ml

Keeps for at least 3 years.

B. Differentiating solution

Ethanol:	160 ml
Water:	40 ml
Potassium hydroxide:	0.4 g

Dissolve, then add water if necessary to bring the final volume to 200 ml. (Keeps indefinitely if not contaminated; replace if it goes brown.)

C. Nuclear stain

An iron–haematoxylin or an alum–haematoxylin (Chapter 6).

Procedure

(1) De-wax and hydrate the sections.
(2) Stain with Congo red (Solution A) for 1–5 min, until sections are deep red.
(3) Differentiate in Solution B, 2–10 s, then rinse in copious distilled water and examine. The only red colour remaining in the section should be in elastic fibres and laminae and in strongly acidophilic structures such as the cytoplasmic granules of eosinophils and Paneth cells. Amyloid deposits are also stained, but may be quite inconspicuous in the wet section. The differentiation may be repeated if necessary, and the staining may be repeated if differentiation has been excessive.
(4) Counterstain nuclei with an iron–haematoxylin or haemalum (Chapter 6).
(5) Wash in water, dehydrate in acetone, clear in xylene and cover, using a resinous mounting medium.

Result

Amyloid deposits red. With polarizing microscopy, green dichroism in amyloid. This may reveal deposits that are hardly visible with ordinary illumination. Nuclei blue or black, according to counterstain.

11.4. The periodic acid–Schiff method

The chemical technique most extensively used in carbohydrate histochemistry is the periodic acid–Schiff (PAS) reaction which, as will be seen below, is positive with structures containing neutral hexose sugars and/or sialic acids. Other chemical methods are available for sulphate–ester groups, for sialic acids, and for some amino sugars; such methods (see Pearse, 1968b; Pearse and Stoward, 1985) are little used and will not be discussed here.

In the PAS method sections are treated with periodic acid, which oxidizes glycols to aldehydes. The aldehydes are then rendered visible by reaction with Schiff's reagent.

The term 'neutral sugar' though not strictly accurate in the chemical sense, is used by histochemists for monosaccharide residues that do not have sulphate–ester, carboxylic acid, or nitrogen-containing functional groups. Glucose, galactose, mannose, and fucose (*Fig. 5.1*) are the principal neutral sugars present in mucosubstances.

11.4.1.
Periodate
oxidation

Periodic acid, $HIO_4 \cdot 2H_2O$, is used in histochemistry as a 1% aqueous solution (0.044 M) and is normally allowed to act upon sections of tissue for 5–10 min at room temperature, though oxidation for 30 min is necessary for some specimens (Culling and Reid, 1977). The sodium salt of the acid may also be used. The effect of this treatment is a selective oxidation by the periodate ion of hydroxyl groups attached to adjacent carbon atoms (i.e. glycols), with fission of the intervening carbon-to-carbon bond and production of two aldehydes:

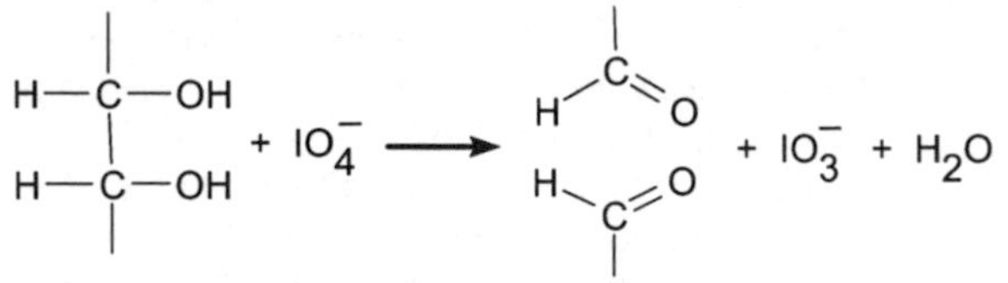

$$
\begin{array}{l}
H-C-OH \\
H-C-OH
\end{array}
+ IO_4^- \longrightarrow
\begin{array}{l}
H-C=O \\
H-C=O
\end{array}
+ IO_3^- + H_2O
$$

Where there are three neighbouring carbon atoms bearing hydroxyl groups a similar reaction occurs but with the elimination of a molecule of formic acid:

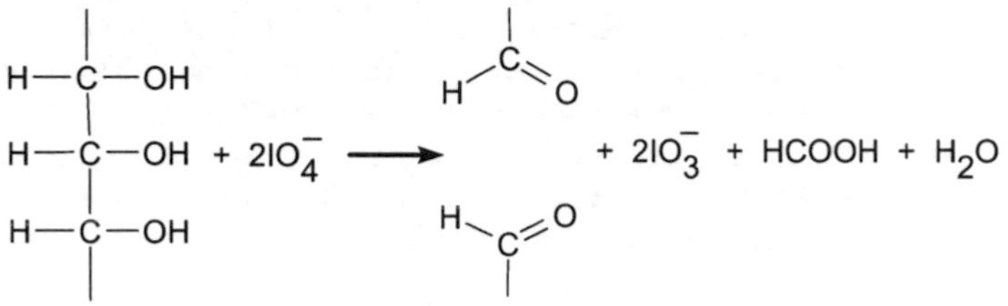

$$
\begin{array}{l}
H-C-OH \\
H-C-OH \\
H-C-OH
\end{array}
+ 2IO_4^- \longrightarrow
\begin{array}{l}
H-C=O \\
 \\
H-C=O
\end{array}
+ 2IO_3^- + HCOOH + H_2O
$$

Glycol groupings are present in the neutral sugars and in the uronic and sialic acids and some of the *N*-acetylamino sugars (see *Fig. 11.1*).

Periodic acid can also oxidize the α-amino alcohol formation:

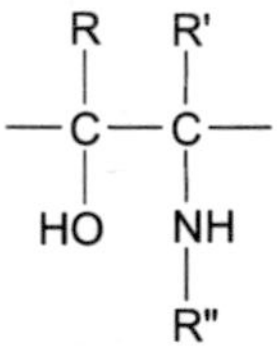

$$
\begin{array}{cc}
R & R' \\
-C-C- \\
HO & NH \\
& | \\
& R''
\end{array}
$$

where R, R' and R'' may be hydrogen or alkyl radicals (Nicolet and Shinn, 1939). This configuration occurs in the amino acids serine and threonine (but not when these are incorporated into peptide linkages), in the side-chain of hydroxylsine, and also in sphingosine, an amino alcohol present in certain lipids. The only common sugars that are α-amino alcohols are glucosamine and galactosamine, but these do not occur in significant quantities in tissues. The nitrogen-containing sugars of proteoglycans and glycoproteins, *N*-acetylglucosamine and *N*-acetylgalactosamine, contain the structural arrangement:

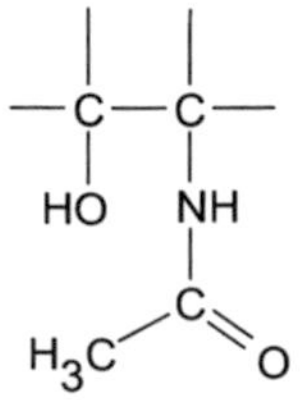

$$
\begin{array}{cc}
-C-C- \\
HO & NH \\
& | \\
& C=O \\
H_3C &
\end{array}
$$

They are α-N-acetylamino alcohols and, as such, are almost completely resistant to oxidation by periodate (Nicolet and Shinn, 1939; Carter et al., 1947). (In principle, the N-acetyl hexosamines could be oxidized by periodate if they formed glycosidic linkages at position C6, leaving C3 and C4 with free hydroxyl groups; see *Fig. 11.1*. In mucosubstances these sugars are connected to others through glycosidic linkages involving position C3 or C4, so they are never responsible for stainability by the PAS method.)

Lead tetraacetate (Glegg et al., 1952) and sodium bismuthate (Lhotka, 1952) have been used for the same purpose as periodic acid. They act in the same way, but as histochemical reagents they have not been investigated as thoroughly as periodic acid. Oxidizing agents that are less selective in their actions include potassium permanganate and chromium trioxide. These can generate aldehydes from sugars, and are used for this purpose in silver methods for reticulin and for fungi (Chapter 18); they are not appropriate for histochemical work because they can bring about further oxidation of aldehydes to carboxyl groups.

If the histochemical situation were as simple as the foregoing account might lead one to believe, all carbohydrate-containing structures would be expected to yield aldehydes with periodic acid. This is not the case, however. It has been shown that the GAGs of proteoglycans (consisting of uronic acids and acetylhexosamines, sulphated or not) are not PAS-positive (Hooghwinkel and Smits, 1957). In sections of fixed tissue, periodic acid produces aldehydes from glucosyl, galactosyl, mannosyl, and fucosyl residues (Leblond et al., 1957) and sialic acids. These are components of glycogen and of glycoproteins.

Proteoglycans are PAS-negative because the usual treatment with periodic acid fails to oxidize the glycol formations at C2-C3 in glucuronic and iduronic acids. Scott and Harbinson (1969) have shown that uronic acids in GAGs are not attacked by periodic acid on account of repulsion of the periodate ion by the carboxylate anions and perhaps also by the nearby sulphate–ester anions, when these are present. This electrostatic effect can be overcome by using periodate for a longer time and at a higher temperature than usual. Although the uronic acid components of GAGs yield aldehydes under these more rigorous conditions, the N-acetyl hexosamines are still unaffected. Scott and Dorling (1969) have developed a modified PAS technique, based on the principle outlined above, for the selective demonstration of uronic acid-containing mucosubstances (i.e. proteoglycans). A preliminary treatment with periodate is followed by reduction with sodium borohydride:

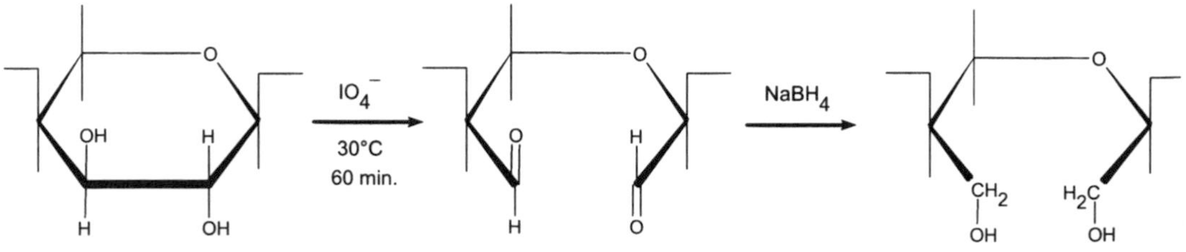

This procedure changes all neutral hexoses into compounds that can no longer yield aldehydes by reaction with periodate. In the next stage of the technique, the sections are again exposed to periodate, but for a time sufficient to oxidize the glycol groups of uronic acids:

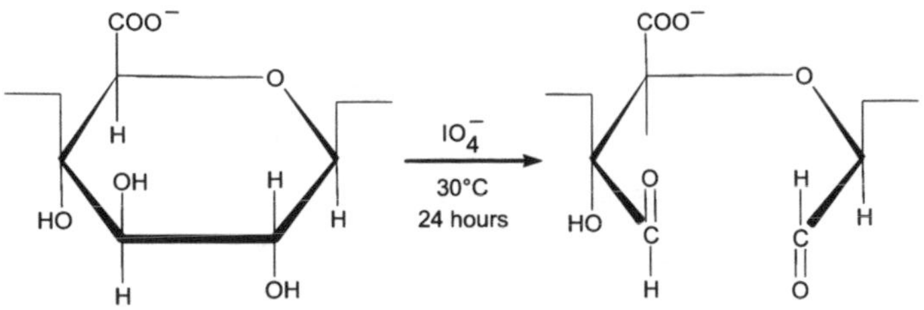

The aldehyde groups produced by the second oxidation are demonstrated with Schiff's reagent. Scott and Dorling's modified PAS method therefore demonstrates mucosubstances whose uronic acid residues have free hydroxyl groups at positions C2 and C3. From Section 11.2.2 of this chapter it can be seen that these are hyaluronan, chondroitin-4-sulphate, chondroitin-6-sulphate, dermatan sulphate, heparan sulphate and heparin. The polysaccharides, the glycoproteins, and the keratan sulphates will not be stained.

The versatility of periodic acid as a histochemical reagent is further exemplified in its ability, under appropriate conditions, to produce aldehydes selectively from sialic acid residues. Sialic acids are glycosidically linked at position C2 (see *Fig. 11.1*). The only potentially periodate-reactive part of a sialic acid molecule is therefore the side-chain (C7, C8, and C9) attached at C6, which bears three adjacent hydroxyl groups. The side-chain reacts with periodate much more rapidly than do the glycols of hexoses (see Hughes, 1976). By using dilute periodic acid for a short time it is possible to oxidize the sialic acid residues but not the hexoses of glycoproteins:

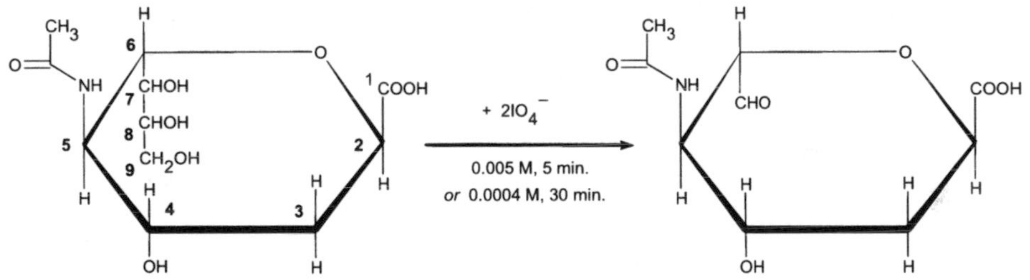

The resultant aldehyde can be demonstrated either with Schiff's reagent (Roberts, 1977) or with a fluorescent hydrazine (Weber *et al.*, 1975). Volz *et al.* (1986, 1987) have determined that a strongly acidified very dilute solution of periodic acid used at 40°C provides optimum selective oxidation of sialic acid side-chains.

In some intestinal glycoproteins, *O*-acetyl groups replace the hydroxyls at position C7, C8, or C9 of NANA. These acetylated sialic acids can be recognized histochemically by means of a sequence of treatments.

(1) Oxidation by periodic acid (glycol → aldehyde). It is important to convert all available glycol groups to aldehydes; thus, sections are oxidized for 30–120 min in 0.044 M periodic acid.
(2) Reduction by borohydride (aldehyde → primary alcohol). (PAS staining carried out after this reduction should give a negative result if the initial oxidation has been adequate.)
(3) Saponification with alcoholic potassium hydroxide (acetyl ester → hydroxyl).
(4) Second oxidation with periodate (glycol → aldehyde).

The production of aldehydes is sought, with Schiff's reagent, after stages 1 and 4. The side-chains of the sialic acids react as shown in *Fig. 11.4*.

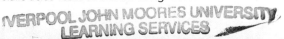

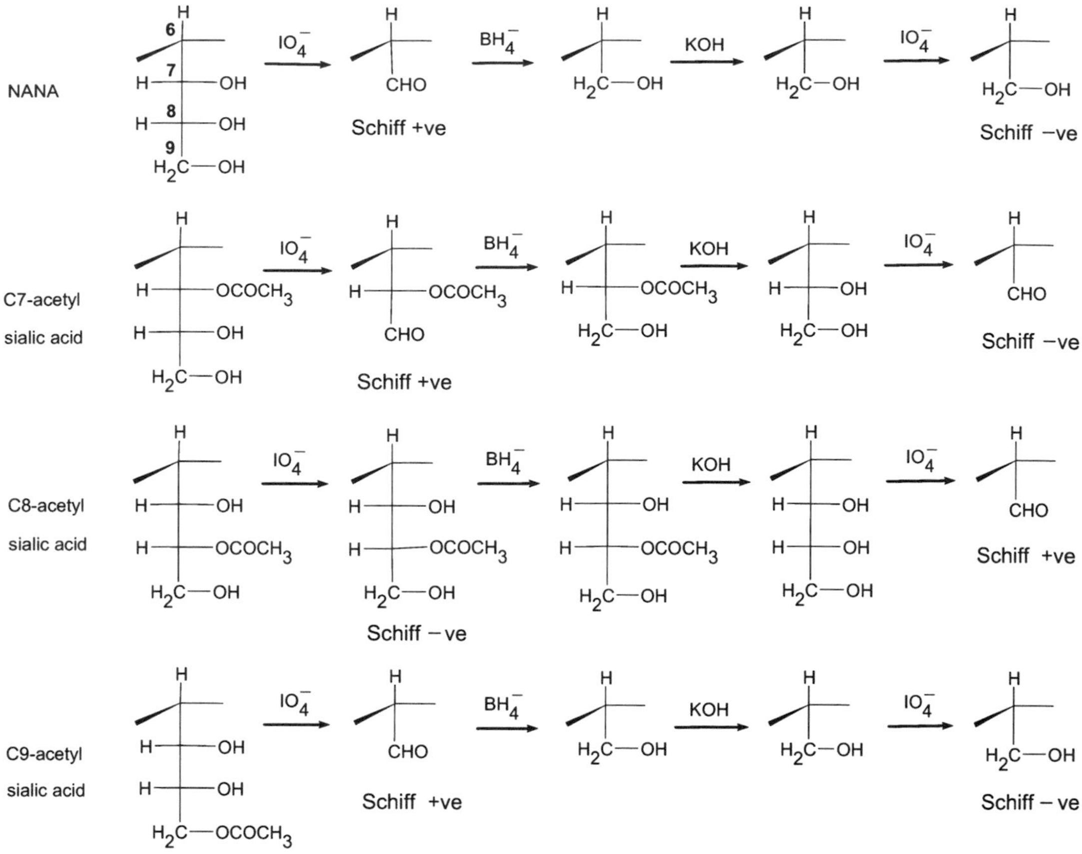

Figure 11.4. Reactions of sialic acid side-chains in the periodic acid-borohydride-saponification-periodic acid–Schiff staining method.

Unsubstituted and C9-acetylated sialic acids are Schiff-positive only after the first periodate oxidation and cannot be distinguished from one another. The C7-acetylated sialic acid is Schiff positive after both oxidations and the C8-acetylated compound is Schiff-positive only after the second oxidation. If acetyl groups are present on any two or all three of the positions C7, C8, and C9, positive Schiff reactions will be obtained only after the second oxidation with periodate. It must be emphasized that this histochemical analysis (Reid *et al.*, 1978, 1984a) involves oxidation of sialic acids and neutral hexoses, so it is applicable only when it has already been proved that the sialic acids are the sole substances responsible for stainability by the PAS method at the sites being investigated.

Another method, related to the procedure described above, is that of Culling *et al.* (1976). In this, the first oxidation with periodic acid is followed by staining with a 'pseudo-Schiff' reagent (Section 10.10.1) made from thionine. The sections are then saponified, oxidized for a second time with periodic acid, and stained with conventional Schiff's reagent. Sialic acids that bear no *O*-acetyl groups or are acetylated only at C9 are stained blue. Those acetylated at C8 are red and those acetylated at C7 or at more than one of the positions C7 C8 and C9 are purple.

Two strategies are available to enhance the selectivity for sialic acids of these modified PAS procedures. The simpler is the use of selective (mild) oxidation, which leaves the neutral hexoses unchanged. The other procedure makes use of the fact that the products of periodate oxidation of sialic acids and neutral hexoses react differently with phenylhydrazine. The single aldehyde group resulting from oxidation of a sialic acid side-chain gives an ordinary phenylhydrazone (Section 10.11.10), which is unstable in an aqueous acidic medium such as Schiff's reagent. The aldehyde is regenerated, and promptly reacts to give a coloured product. In contrast, the two nearby aldehydes produced by oxidation of a hexose react with one molecule of phenylhydrazine to form a cyclic compound. The latter is not affected by Schiff's reagent. Consequently, treatment of a section of an animal tissue with periodic acid, followed by phenylhydrazine, and then by Schiff's reagent, gives selective staining at the sites of sialic acids (except for the unoxidizable C8-acylated ones). If a Schiff-like reagent made from thionine is used to colour the sites of sialic acids blue, it is then possible to stain the section again by the ordinary PAS method, to show the distribution of neutral hexoses in red. If neutral hexoses are absent, or if selective (mild) periodate oxidation is used, a saponification can be interposed between the treatment with thionine–Schiff and the second periodate oxidation. A second PAS routine will then stain the C8-acylated sialic acids (Park *et al.*, 1987; Reid *et al.*, 1987, 1988).

11.4.2.
PAS procedures

These methods are commonly applied to paraffin sections of specimens that have been fixed in neutral buffered formaldehyde. Other fixatives that do not contain oxidizing agents are also suitable. If glutaraldehyde has been used, the aldehyde groups formed in the tissue must be blocked or removed (Section 10.10) before treating the sections with periodic acid.

11.4.2.1. Standard PAS method

Solutions required
A. Periodic acid solution

Periodic acid ($HIO_4.2H_2O$):	2.0 g
Water:	200 ml

Keeps for several weeks and may be used repeatedly, but should be discarded if it goes brown.

B. Schiffs reagent
See under the Feulgen technique (Section 9.3.2).

C. Solutions for counterstaining
A suitable sequence is: alum–haematoxylin or iron-chromoxane cyanine R for blue nuclei, with fast green FCF as a counterstain for cytoplasm and collagen. Methods are given in Chapter 6. For critical evaluation of the PAS reaction it is preferable to use no counterstain.

Procedure
(1) Allow the Schiff's reagent to warm to room temperature.
(2) De-wax and hydrate paraffin sections. (See *Note 1*).
(3) Oxidize for 10–30 min in periodic acid (Solution A).
(4) Wash in running tap water for 3 min.
(5) Immerse in Schiff's reagent (Solution B) for 20 min.
(6) Transfer to copiously running tap water and leave to wash for 10 min (see *Note 2*).
(7) Apply counterstains, as desired.
(8) Dehydrate in alcohols, clear in xylene, and cover, using a resinous mounting medium.

Result

Hexose-containing and sialic acid-containing mucosubstances pink to bright purplish red. In an adequately stained preparation reticulin, basement membranes and mucous glands should stand out sharply against the background of faintly coloured or unstained components of the tissue.

Notes

(1) Remove mercurial deposits if introduced by the fixative. A control slide should be treated with Schiff's reagent **without** prior oxidation by HIO_4. This will indicate whether any reactive aldehyde groups (from the fixative, for example) were previously present in the tissue. If found, such aldehydes must be chemically blocked **before** the treatment with HIO_4. If pink staining occurs in the absence of aldehydes, the Schiff's reagent has deteriorated.

(2) A bisulphite rinse is often recommended between stages 5 and 6, but Demalsy and Callebaut (1967) found that this caused some fading of the stain and was not necessary provided that the Schiff's reagent was washed away rapidly.

(3) Glycogen can be identified if the PAS reaction is applied in conjunction with amylase-digested control sections (Section 11.6.1). Neuraminidase and/or mild acid hydrolysis will assist in the identification of sialic acids. The PAS reaction is blocked by acetylation, though this procedure has little analytical value.

(4) If frozen sections are used, some glycolipids are stained. A pseudoplasmal reaction is also usually obtained with frozen sections (Chapter 12), which are therefore unsuitable for the study of glycoproteins unless lipids are extracted before staining.

11.4.2.2. Specialized PAS methods

The theoretical basis of these procedures, which should be used in conjunction with appropriate enzymatic digestions and other controls, was explained and discussed in Section 11.4.1 of this chapter. The methods for sialic acids are useful for distinguishing different types of mucus in tumours of the colon (see Roe *et al.*, 1989).

(a) For sialic acids

To generate aldehydes from sialic acids (NANA and possibly others), oxidize in a freshly prepared solution of *either* 4×10^{-4} M sodium metaperiodate ($NaIO_4$; 0.0086% aqueous, for 30 min) *or* 5×10^{-3} M periodic acid (0.11% aqueous H_3IO_5, for 5 min). Transfer the slides directly into 0.1 M sodium sulphite (1.3% Na_2SO_3) for 5 min to arrest the oxidation. Wash in running tap water for 5 min and then proceed with Step 5 of the standard technique.

(b) For O-acetylated sialic acids

Treat hydrated sections as follows:

(1) Oxidize in 1% periodic acid ($HIO_4.2H_2O$), 2 h.
(2) Wash in running tap water for 10 min.
(3) Stain some of the slides with Schiff's reagent (Step 5 of standard technique).
(4) Immerse the remaining slides in 0.05% sodium borohydride ($NaBH_4$) in 1% Na_2HPO_4 for 10 min. Use this solution within 30 min of dissolving the $NaBH_4$. (**Caution.** See Section 10.10.6.1.)
(5) Wash in four changes of tap water.
(6) Immerse in 0.5% potassium hydroxide (KOH) in 70% ethanol for 15 min.
(7) Wash gently in four changes of tap water.
(8) Oxidize for a second time with 1% periodic acid for 10 min.
(9) Stain with Schiff's reagent (Step 5 of standard technique).

If **positive reactions due to hexoses have been excluded**, staining at Step 3 above is due to NANA or to sialic acids acylated at position C7. Staining obtained at Step 9 but not at Step 3 is due to sialic acids acylated at C8 or at more than one of the positions C7, C8, and C9. A positive result at Steps 3 **and** 9 indicates a sialic acid acylated at C7. The results may be difficult to interpret if mucosubstances containing different sialic acids occur at the same site. From the scheme in *Fig. 11.4*, C9-acylated sialic acids should also stain, but in practice it is found that acyl substitution at C9 prevents oxidation of the C7-8 glycol formation (P.E. Reid, personal communication 1988).

(c) For uronic acids

Treat hydrated paraffin sections as follows:

(1) Oxidize for 1 h at 30°C in 2% aqueous sodium metaperiodate ($NaIO_4$).
(2) Wash in running tap water for 10 min.
(3) Treat with freshly dissolved 0.1% sodium borohydride in 1% Na_2HPO_4 for 10 min. (**Caution.** See Section 10.10.6.1.)
(4) Wash in running tap water for 10 min.
(5) Oxidize for a second time in 2% $NaIO_4$ for 24 h at 30°C.
(6) Wash in running tap water for 10 min.
(7) Stain with Schiff's reagent (Step 5 of the standard technique).

A positive result is seen at the sites of proteoglycans with free hydroxyl groups at positions C2 and C3 of their uronic acid residues. Hexoses and sialic acids are unstained.

11.4.3.
Artifacts associated with the PAS method

A structure coloured pink or purple by the PAS technique cannot be assumed to contain periodate-reactive sugars unless the following causes of false-positive staining have been excluded.

(1) Aldehydes may be initially present in the tissue. These will be stained by Schiff's reagent without prior oxidation by periodic acid and may be derived from the fixative (especially glutaraldehyde) or from atmospheric oxidation of olefinic linkages in unsaturated lipids (the **pseudoplasmal** reaction). Fixatives containing mercuric chloride may produce aldehydes from plasmalogen phospholipids (the **plasmal** reaction). Lipids (Chapter 12) rarely interfere with the interpretation of PAS staining in paraffin sections. Blocking procedures for pre-existing aldehyde groups have been described in Chapter 10. Sodium borohydride is the aldehyde-blocking agent of first choice for use in carbohydrate histochemistry.
(2) Periodic acid can produce aldehydes from olefinic bonds of lipids as well as from glycols. Consequently, a genuinely positive PAS reaction in a frozen section may not be due to glycoprotein or glycogen, or even to glycolipid, especially if an aqueous mounting medium is used. Adams (1965) describes a modified PAS method in which the reactivity of unsaturated linkages is chemically suppressed before the oxidation of carbohydrates by periodic acid. Sphingosine, an amino alcohol present in several lipids, is also oxidized by periodic acid (Chapter 12). Glycolipids (which are commonly PAS-positive on account of their content of galactose and sialic acids) are distinguished from mucosubstances by virtue of the solubility of the former in a hot mixture of methanol and chloroform. Some glycolipids are largely extracted by water.
(3) Hydroxylysine, an amino acid that occurs only in collagen (Chapter 8), might be expected to be PAS-positive, but Bangle and Alford (1954) showed that the stainability of collagen by the PAS method was due almost entirely to its carbohydrate content. The hydroxylysine may not be present in sufficient

quantity to be histochemically detectable, or its amino groups may be involved in an amide linkage with another part of the collagen fibril.

(4)   Some batches of Schiff's reagent prove unsatisfactory and may give either false positive or false negative results. An untried sample of the reagent should be tested on sections in which the correct localizations of PAS-positive structures are already known. An aldehyde-blocking reaction applied after oxidation with periodate will serve as a control for false positive coloration by an unsatisfactory sample of Schiff's reagent.

11.5. Lectins as histochemical reagents

The word 'lectin' was originally applied to proteins that were extracted from plants and that had the property of agglutinating mammalian erythrocytes (see Boyd, 1970). Such proteins were also called **agglutinins**. An agglutinin molecule can bind to two or more glycoprotein molecules on the outside surfaces of cells, and thereby join the cells together. The term lectin has come into widespread use, and its meaning has been etended to all proteins that have non-catalytic carbohydrate-binding sites. Proteins with only one such site per molecule cannot agglutinate cells. Enzymes such as glycosidases with only catalytic carbohydrate-binding sites are not lectins (Van Damme et al., 1998; Kilpatrick, 2000; Sharon and Lis, 2003).

11.5.1.
Properties of
lectins

It has been known for many years that whereas some lectins agglutinate all types of human red blood cells, others are selective for particular blood groups in much the same ways as circulating antibodies. The blood group determinant substances are glycoproteins located on the surfaces of the erythrocytes, and lectins bind to specific carbohydrate moieties of these glycoproteins.

The lectins can bind to appropriate carbohydrates whether these be located on the surfaces of erythrocytes or elsewhere. Makela (1957) showed that the specific agglutination of red cells of particular blood groups was due to affinity of the lectins for the terminal monosaccharide residues of the determinant glycoproteins. The blood group O glycoprotein, for example, has terminal α-L-fucosyl residues, and the lectins that agglutinate group O erythrocytes bind to L-fucose and its α-glycosides. Lectins that agglutinate erythrocytes of all blood groups are those that bind to sugars such as mannose and N-acetylglucosamine, which are universally distributed on the surfaces of cells. Irrespective of specificity for human blood groups, all the lectins are remarkably selective with respect to the types of sugar to which they bind. Lectins are classified into 5 groups according to their affinities for different sugars (see Table 11.1). Binding is principally to the terminal sugar of a polysaccharide or oligosaccharide, and can be competitively inhibited by adding the free sugar or an appropriate glycoside to a solution of the lectin. The affinity of a lectin is usually influenced, however, by the next one to three units in the chain (see Goldstein and Poretz, 1986). Consequently a particular cell-type or glycoprotein may be able to bind different amounts of different lectins of the same group.

Many lectin molecules exist as a dimers or tetramers, and the subunits, which are not always identical, can be separated and recombined. Different subunits or combinations are called **isolectins**; they may vary in their sugar-binding properties.

The binding of a lectin molecule to a carbohydrate does not involve the formation of covalent bonds. It is similar in nature to the attachment of an antigen to its specific antibody (Chapter 19). The molecules of some lectins incorporate ions of calcium and a transition metal (usually manganese), and the presence of these metal ions is essential for the carbohydrate-binding activity.

Table 11.1. Some lectins used as histochemical reagents

Source of lectin (Name, where available)	Common abbreviation[a]	Specific affinity[b]
Group 1. Affinity for glucose and mannose		
Canavalia ensiformis (concanavalin A)	Con A	α-Man > α-Glc > α-GlcNAc
Galanthus nivalis (snowdrop lectin)	GNL	α-1→3-Man
Lens culinaris (lentil lectin)	LCA	α-Man > α-Glc > α-GlcNAc
Narcissus pseudonarcissus (daffodil agglutinin)	NPA	α-1→6-Man-α-1→6-Man-α-1→6-Man
Pisum sativum (pea lectin)	PSA	α-Man > α-Glc > α-GlcNAc
Group 2. Affinity for *N*-acetylglucosamine		
Griffonia simplicifolia (= *Bandeiraea simplicifolia*; Griffonia lectin II)	GSL-II *or* BSL-II	α-GlcNAc and β-GlcNAc
Lycopersicon esculentum (tomato lectin)	LEL *or* TL	GlcNAc oligomers
Phytolacca americana (pokeweed mitogen)	PAA *or* PWM	GlcNAc-β-1→4-GlcNAc = Gal-β-1→4-GlcNAc
Solanum tuberosum (potato lectin)	STA	GlcNAc-β-1→4-GlcNAc
Triticum vulgare (wheat germ agglutinin)	WGA	GlcNAc-β-1→4-GlcNAc > β-GlcNAc > Sialic acids
Group 3. Affinity for galactose and *N*-acetylgalactosamine		
Arachis hypogaea (peanut agglutinin)	PNA	Gal-β-1→3-GalNAc > α- and β-Gal
Artocarpus integrifolia (jacalin, jackfruit lectin)	Jac	Gal-β-1→3-GalNAc
Bauhinia purpurea (Bauhinia lectin)	BPL	Gal-β-1→3-GalNAc > α-GalNAc
Dolichos biflorus (horse gram lectin)	DBA	GalNAc-α-1→3-GalNAc >> α-GalNAc
Glycine max (soybean agglutinin)	SBA	α- and β-GalNAc > α- and β-Gal
Griffonia simplicifolia (= *Bandeiraea simplicifolia*; Griffonia lectin I)	GSL-I	α-GalNAc (isolectin A) and α-Gal (isolectin B)
Maclura pomifera (osage orange lectin)	MPA	α-GalNAc > α-Gal
Phaseolus vulgaris (kidney bean lectin)	PHA-E & PHA-L	Gal-β-1→4-GlcNAc-β-1→2-Man (isolectins E and L agglutinate erythrocytes and leukocytes respectively)
Ricinus communis (castor bean agglutinin I)	RCA-I or RCA$_{120}$	β-Gal > α-Gal >> GalNAc
Vicia villosa (hairy vetch lectin)	VVA	(Protein)-α-GalNAc > Gal-α-1→3-GalNAc > β-GalNAc
Group 4. Affinity for L-fucose		
Anguilla anguilla (eel lectin)	AAA	α-L-Fuc
Lotus tetragonobolus (*Tetragonobolus purpureus*; asparagus pea lectin)	LTA	α-L-Fuc
Ulex europaeus (gorse lectin I)	UEA-I	α-L-Fuc

continued

Table 11.1. Some lectins used as histochemical reagents (continued)

Source of lectin (Name, where available)	Common abbreviation[a]	Specific affinity[b]
Group 5. Affinity for sialic and uronic acids		
Aplysia depilans (Aplysia gonad lectin)	AGL	Galacturonic acid >> D-Gal
Bovine or porcine lung, pancreas salivary glands (aprotinin; bovine trypsin inhibitor)		Uronic and sialic acids[c]
Limax flavus (slug lectin)	LFA	N-acetylneuraminic acid > N-glycolylneuraminic acid
Limulus polyphemus (limulin or horseshoe crab lectin)	LPA	N-acetyl (*or* N-glycolyl) neuraminic acid-α-2→ 6-GalNAc
Sambucus nigra (elder bark lectin)	SNA	N-acetylneuraminic acid-α-2→6(-Gal *or* GalNAc)
Tritrichomonas mobilensis	TML	Some sialic acids (Babal and Gardner, 1996)

[a]The terminal A in abbreviations stands for 'agglutinin;' L is for 'lectin.' A subscript number indicates the MW × 10^{-3} of one of a number of lectins extracted from the same source (e.g. RCA_{120}, whose MW is 120 000).

[b]See Section 11.1.2 for the structures of the sugars corresponding to the abbreviations in this column of the table. The information on specificity is derived largely from Toms and Western (1971), Cook and Stoddart (1973), Nicolson (1974), Goldstein and Poretz (1986), Benhamou *et al.* (1988) and Taatjes *et al.* (1988). For lectins that bind to more than one terminal sugar, ligands are listed in order of decreasing affinity (>> indicates much greater affinity; > greater, and = equal affinity for the lectin.)

[c]Aprotinin is not a lectin, but the fluorescently labelled polypeptide can be used to stain glycoproteins and gycosaminoglycans that owe their acidity to carboxyl rather than to sulphate groups (Kiernan and Stoddart, 1973; Stoddart and Kiernan, 1973a). Fluorescent aprotinin also binds to the proteolytic enzymes it inhibits, but this latter affinity does not permit the use of the reagent for histochemical demonstration of the enzymes in sectioned tissues.

Lectins are proteins with large molecules (MW 20 000–300 000), so it is possible to attach dye molecules or other labels covalently to some of their free amino groups without interfering with the carbohydrate-binding properties. The most frequently used labels are fluorochromes (especially fluorescein and rhodamine derivatives), [³H]acetyl groups (for subsequent autoradiography) and biotin (for detection with avidin–biotin systems, see Chapter 19). Histochemically demonstrable enzymes (horseradish peroxidase, alkaline phosphatase) and ferritin (an electron dense protein) are also used, but these large labelling molecules can interfere with binding to specific sites in tissues (Brooks *et al.*, 1997; Van Damme *et al.*, 1998). Bound lectins can also be detected by immunohistochemical methods, using anti-lectin antisera.

11.5.2
Techniques for use of lectins

Histochemical methods involving the use of lectins have much in common with immunohistochemical techniques (Chapter 19). Only the simplest type of procedure is described here: a solution of the fluorescently labelled lectin, usually at a concentration of 1–100 µg/ml in water or saline, usually buffered to pH 7.0–7.6, is applied to the sections of tissue for 15–60 min. Excess reagent is washed off and the preparation is either mounted in an aqueous medium or dehydrated, cleared, and mounted in a non-fluorescent resinous medium. Fluorescence is observed at sites of binding of the lectin. For reviews of other techniques and their uses, see Spicer and Schulte (1992) and Brooks *et al.* (1997). The latter gives detailed practical instructions for many techniques.

Lectin histochemistry is useful for the demonstration of cells that are not easily distinguished by ordinary dye-based staining. For example, lectin affinities allow the recognition of microglial cells in nervous tissue (Streit, 1990; Hauke *et al.*, 1993; Glenn *et al.*, 1993; Acarin *et al.*, 1994), nerve fibres in the peripheral nervous system (Spicer et al., 1996), age-related changes in the brain (Sato et al., 2001), muscle fibre types in paraffin sections (Bardosi et al., 1989), capillary blood vessels in various organs (Tyler and Burns, 1991; Qu et al., 1997) and different parts of renal tubules (Engel et al., 1997).

Materials needed
Fluorescent conjugates of lectins can be prepared in the laboratory (Smith and Hollers, 1970; Roth et al., 1978b; Brooks et al., 1997). The procedure is not as easy as the labelling of most other types of protein, because it is necessary to protect the sugar-binding sites, and lectin molecules are prone to aggregation, leading to insoluble labelled products. Most histochemists now use labelled lectins from commercial suppliers, and these are entirely satisfactory. **It is important to buy the correct lectin**, especially when more than one is available from the same plant (e.g. *Ulex europaeus* or *Ricinus communis*). A few lectins are toxic; warnings are given in catalogues and on the outsides of containers. The supplier should also provide information about the purity and specificity of each product.

It is usual to buy 0.5 or 1 mg of a fluorescently labelled lectin. The almost invisible amount of freeze-dried powder will be in a vial that can hold 1–10 ml. The most frequently encountered labels are fluorescein and rhodamine derivatives. There is little to choose between the two fluorochromes. I prefer rhodamine because its orange–red fluorescence is not easily confused with autofluorescence. To make a stock solution of the fluorescently labelled lectin, add 0.5–1.0 ml of the following buffered saline solution to the vial.

TRIS base:	60.57 g
Trace metal solution:	10 ml
Sodium azide (NaN$_3$):	0.65 g
Water:	900 ml

Add drops of concentrated hydrochloric acid, with stirring, until the pH is 7.2–7.6, then make the volume up to 1000 ml with water. The 'trace metal solution' contains calcium, magnesium and manganese chlorides, each at 0.01 M concentration. Phosphate buffer is avoided because the trace metals have insoluble phosphates.

The Ca^{2+}, Mg^{2+} and Mn^{2+} satisfy the requirements of lectins for these metals. The NaN$_3$ is to inhibit growth of microorganisms in the solution. The same solution is used for further dilutions of the lectin, and for washing sections before and after staining.

The initial stock solution of the fluorescently labelled lectin usually should contain 1 mg of protein per ml. A tiny drop of this should be diluted 10 times and tested by staining a section (see below). Probably the fluorescence will be too intense, with non-specific background staining. Other sections should then be stained with further dilutions until the observed fluorescence is confined to structures that are known or expected to contain stainable material. Such structures commonly include collagen fibres, basement membranes and mucus-secreting cells. When the optimum concentration has been found, an appropriate volume of the buffer is added to the initially dissolved lectin in its container, to give a working solution. This solution should be kept at 4°C, **not frozen**. It is stable for several weeks. For many fluorescently labelled lectins, the optimal concentration is 10 µg/ml.

Staining procedure
Fixation is not critical, but ethanol and mercuric chloride were found by Allison (1987) to be somewhat superior to Carnoy, Bouin, neutral buffered formal–saline and calcium acetate–formaldehyde. Hoyer and Kirkeby (1996) favoured Carnoy or Zenker. Glutaraldehyde should be avoided because it causes non-specific binding

of proteins to tissues (Rittman and Mackenzie, 1983). Carbodiimides are unsuitable for the same reason (Hoyer and Kirkeby, 1996). Paraffin or cryostat sections may be used.

(1) Bring sections to water, rinse in buffer containing trace metals (see above) and blot dry.
(2) Place the slides, sections up, on a piece of wet filter paper on a flat bench top.
(3) Carefully apply the smallest possible drop of fluorescent lectin solution to cover the sections to be stained.
(4) Cover the slides with a suitable airtight lid, such as a petri dish. The air inside must be saturated with water vapour, to prevent drying of the sections.
(5) Wait for 30 min. (Sometimes 10 min will be enough; rarely 2 h may be needed.)
(6) Rinse the slide in 3 changes of buffer containing trace metals.
(7) Dehydrate in 95% and 2 changes of absolute alcohol, clear in xylene and cover, using a non-fluorescent resinous mounting medium. *Alternatively*, mount from water into buffered glycerol (Section 4.3.2.2). The latter method is useful if the same section is to be stained again by some other technique.

Result
Lectin binding sites are fluorescent.

Notes
(1) Lectins can also be bought labelled with horseradish peroxidase. When these are used, the working solution can be more dilute than that of a fluorescent lectin. After Stage 5 above, the sections are subjected to a histochemical method for peroxidase, usually with DAB as the chromogen (Chapter 16).
(2) For whole suspended cells, wash by suspending in in buffered saline and centrifuging. Repeat the procedure two more times before making smears or cytocentrifuge preparations (Chapter 7). It is important to remove serum or tissue culture medium, which contain sugars and glycoproteins.
(3) Controls are important in lectin histochemistry. They are discussed in the next section of this chapter.

11.5.3. Interpretation of results

Two considerations are important in assessing the significance of observed binding of a lectin to a component of a tissue.

(1) The specificity of the binding must be established by means of suitable controls. **Competitive inhibition** with appropriate sugars or glycosides is the most important control procedure. This is done by staining control slides in the presence of high (0.2–1.0 M) concentrations of sugars or glycosides that will occupy binding sites on the lectin molecules before the latter can attach to the tissue. For example, staining with concanavalin A should not occur from a solution containing α-methyl-D-glucoside but should occur normally in the presence of β-methyl-D-glucoside (Stoddart and Kiernan, 1973). **Chemical blocking methods** destroy or modify the glycosyl residues to which the lectin is expected to bind. Acetylation, for example, prevents the binding of concanavalin A, but not of aprotinin, and methylation prevents staining by fluorescently labelled aprotinin or limulin but not by concanavalin A and most other lectins. The reasons for these effects can be determined by consulting *Table 11.1* and Section 11.7. Oxidation by periodic acid prevents the binding of concanavalin A at most sites in tissues, but some structures paradoxically acquire the ability to bind this lectin, even though all glucosyl and mannosyl residues would be expected to be destroyed. It has been suggested that certain mannosyl units of glycoproteins, previously inaccessible to the large molecules of

concanavalin A, are 'unmasked' but not oxidized as a result of the treatment with periodic acid (Katsuyama and Spicer, 1978).

(2) It may not be assumed that the amount of lectin bound at any site (as judged by intensity of staining) is proportional to the local concentration of the appropriate monosaccharide in the tissue. The binding of any lectin is profoundly affected by neighbouring sugar residues in the oligosaccharide chains of glycoproteins, even though these may not be ones that attach themselves directly to the lectin (see *Table 11.1*). The histochemical recognition of individual monosaccharide units forms only a small part of the study of the interactions between lectins and glycoproteins (see Nicolson, 1974). In their excellent *Lectin Histochemistry*, Brooks *et al.* (1997) emphasized this point: 'Do not make the mistake of thinking that, for example, all gal-binding lectins will give the same results – they certainly won't'.

11.6. Enzymes as reagents in carbohydrate histochemistry

Three enzymes are commonly used in the histochemical study of mucosubstances. These are amylase, hyaluronidase, and neuraminidase. The precautions discussed in Chapter 9 (Section 9.4.1) apply equally to the use of these enzymes.

11.6.1. Amylase

Amylase is a collective name for α-1,4-glucan hydrolases (E.C. 3.2.1.1, 3.2.1.2 and 3.2.1.3) These enzymes catalyze the hydrolysis of the glycoside linkages of starch and glycogen. The enzyme usually used in histochemistry is α-amylase (E.C. 3.2.1.2), the action of which yields the soluble disaccharide maltose. Glycogen or starch can therefore be identified as a substance whose stainability by any method is prevented by digestion of the sections with amylase.

Procedure

Use a solution containing 1.0 mg of enzyme per ml of water. Ideally a pure preparation of α-amylase should be used. An effective alternative is human saliva, though this also contains various proteolytic enzymes and a ribonuclease. An adequate supply of saliva may be obtained by thinking of lemons and drooling into a small beaker. Bubbles should be removed by stroking the surface of the collected liquid with filter paper before applying it to the sections.

Incubate for 30 min at 37°C. The treatment is somewhat destructive to the sections, which may need to be covered with a film of celloidin after applying the enzyme but before staining. A control section should be incubated with water.

11.6.2. Hyaluronidase and chondroitinases

Hyaluronidase (hyaluronate lyase, E.C. 4.2.99.1.) attacks the glycosidic linkages of some GAGs, including hyaluronan, causing depolymerization of these substances. Hyaluronidases of different types are available, the one most often used by histochemists being that extracted from ovine testes. The specificities of the enzymes were reviewed by Pearse (1985), who concluded that the testicular enzyme would remove hyaluronan, chondroitin-4-sulphate, and chondroitin-6-sulphate from fixed tissues. Streptococcal hyaluronidase is specific for hyaluronan.

Chondroitinase AC and **chondroitinase ABC** are enzymes of bacterial origin that degrade chondroitin sulphates. They are occasionally used histochemically, in the same way as the hyaluronidases. The formal names of these enzymes are chondroitin AC lyase (E.C. 4.2.2.5) and chondroitin ABC lyase (E.C. 4.2.2.4).

Most samples of hyaluronidases and of chondroitinases are contaminated with proteolytic enzymes, but these probably do not affect the specific degradation of glycosaminoglycans (Harrison, Van Hoof and Vanroelen, 1986).

Procedure

Testicular and streptococcal hyaluronidases are used as solutions containing 1.0 mg of enzyme per ml of 0.9% aqueous NaCl.

Incubate overnight at 37°C.

11.6.3.
Neuraminidase

Neuraminidase is *N*-acetylneuraminate glycohydrolase (E.C. 3.2.1.18). The enzyme from *Vibrio cholerae* is usually used. It removes the terminal NANA residues of glycoproteins, enabling the histochemist to determine whether staining is due to the presence of these sugars. Unfortunately, not all sialic acid groups are removed, so no significance can be attached to a failure to prevent staining by pre-treating the sections with the enzyme. Prior saponification (see below) makes some previously neuraminidase-resistant sialic acid residues susceptible to the action of neuraminidase, probably by converting *O*-acylated sialic acids to NANA. The type of fixative does not usually affect digestibility by neuraminidase, but cyanuric chloride, which cross-links hydroxyl and amino groups, is exceptional in that it prevents the subsequent action of the enzyme (Sorvari and Lauren, 1973). The identity of the sugar to which NANA is glycosidically bound can affect the susceptibility of the linkage to attack by neuraminidases from different sources. The *Vibrio* enzyme catalyzes the hydrolysis of all the types of linkage studied by Drzeniek (1973). Acid hydrolysis (Section 11.7.4) will detach all sialic acid residues from glycoproteins.

Procedure

The sections may be saponified (Section 10.11.5) before exposure to neuraminidase. This will make some otherwise resistant sialic acid residues susceptible to removal by treatment with the enzyme.

Make up the enzyme solution immediately before using.

0.1 M acetate buffer, pH5.5:	1.0 ml
Calcium chloride (CaCl$_2$)	
(or 0.1ml of a 1% aqueous solution)	1.0 mg
Neuraminidase:	0.025 IU
(IU = international units)	

Incubate overnight at 37°C.

11.6.4.
Other
glycosidases

There are many enzymes that split glycosidic linkages, in addition to those mentioned in the preceding paragraphs (see Hughes, 1976). Some of these are histochemically useful, especially in conjunction with lectins (Whyte *et al.*, 1978). Enzymatic removal of the terminal residue of an oligosaccharide makes the next sugar in the chain accessible to lectin molecules. For example, removal of terminal fucose by an α-L-fucosidase will abolish the affinity of the tissue for UEA (see *Table 11.1*), and may unmask binding sites for other lectins. Sequential degradation with glycosidases is extensively used in the biochemical study of glycoproteins. Caution in the interpretation of results is necessary, however. Glycoside linkages other than those to the terminal sugar unit may be attacked, and commercially available preparations of glycosidases often contain more than one enzyme (Stoddart, 1984).

11.7. Chemical blocking procedures

The reactive groups of carbohydrates are hydroxy, carboxy, and half-sulphate esters. These can be chemically changed (blocked) to prevent their subsequent histochemical demonstration. The significance of a negative result produced in this way depends on the selectivity of the blocking procedure. Blocking reactions are discussed more fully in Chapter 10 and the following notes apply only to the histochemical study of carbohydrates.

**11.7.1.
Acetylation of
hydroxyl groups**

Sections are treated with acetic anhydride in dry pyridine. Hydroxyl groups are converted to acetyl esters:

$$H-\overset{|}{\underset{|}{C}}-OH \ + \ \overset{\displaystyle O}{\underset{\displaystyle O}{O}}\overset{\displaystyle C-CH_3}{\underset{\displaystyle C-CH_3}{}} \longrightarrow H-\overset{|}{\underset{|}{C}}-O-\overset{\displaystyle O}{\overset{\|}{C}}-CH_3 \ + \ CH_3COOH$$

Histochemical reactions due to the hydroxyl groups of carbohydrates are prevented. Acetic anhydride also causes *N*-acetylation of amines and can react with carboxyl groups (of proteins, but probably not of carbohydrates) to form carbonyl compounds, though the optimum conditions for these reactions are different from those used for acetylating sugars. The acetyl esters of carbohydrates are hydrolysed by treatment with alkali (saponification), which restores the reactivity of the hydroxyl groups.

Procedure
(1) Take sections to absolute alcohol.
(2) Immerse overnight at room temperature in a mixture of acetic anhydride (2 volumes) and pyridine (3 volumes) in a closed glass container. Exercise care in handling acetic anhydride, which reacts with water to form acetic acid.
(3) Wash in two changes of absolute alcohol and then pass through 70% alcohol to water.

It is often said that the pyridine must be anhydrous, but ordinary reagent-grade pyridine, which may contain up to 0.025% water, is perfectly satisfactory. This is not surprising because the traces of water in it will react rapidly with acetic anhydride to form acetic acid, though not in quantities sufficient to interfere with the function of the pyridine as a basic catalyst.

**11.7.2.
Methylation and
desulphation**

When sections are treated with a solution of either HCl or thionyl chloride in methanol (or by any of several other procedures), methyl esters are formed with carboxyl groups:

$$H-\overset{|}{\underset{|}{C}}-\overset{\displaystyle O}{\underset{\displaystyle OH}{C}} \ + \ HOCH_3 \longrightarrow H-\overset{|}{\underset{|}{C}}-\overset{\displaystyle O}{\overset{\|}{C}}-O-CH_3 \ + \ H_2O$$

(In the case of the uronic acids it is likely that other reactions also occur; see Sorvari and Stoward, 1970.)

The same reagent, if applied for sufficient time, also **removes** *O*-sulphate and *N*-sulphate groups and methylates amino groups. Methylation prevents the staining of nucleic acids with cationic dyes, but this effect is not due to esterification of their phosphate anions. Prento (1980) attributes the abolition of basophilia to (a) depolymerization and extraction of RNA, and (b) the induction of a high concentration of positively charged groups in the chromatin in which the DNA is located. This positive charge is due to the excess of amino groups following methylation of the carboxyl groups of the nucleoproteins. Another effect of the methylating agent is that it causes acid hydrolysis of most of the glycosidic linkages of sialic acid residues. The loss of basophilia of sialic acid-containing glycoproteins therefore cannot, for the most part, be restored by saponification. This last effect is rather unpredictable, so methylation is more useful for the study of uronic acids in proteoglycans than for the investigation of glycoproteins.

As with acetylation, the esters can be saponified with restoration of carboxyl groups, but this treatment does not, of course, restore any tinctorial properties that were due to the presence of sulphate esters. Hydroxyl groups are not blocked by methanolic HCl under the conditions in which the reagent is normally used. Free hydroxyls at position C1 of a monosaccharide unit would be converted to methyl glycosides, but in mucosubstances almost all the sugars are already linked at this position. The formation of methyl ethers with the alcoholic hydroxyl groups of carbohydrates requires methyl iodide or dimethyl sulphate with a basic rather than an acid catalyst, and does not occur in histochemical methylations.

Procedure
(1)   Take sections to absolute methanol.
(2)   Immerse in methanol containing 1% by volume of concentrated hydrochloric acid in a tightly closed container at 58–60°C for 48 h.
(3)   Rinse in absolute methanol and pass through 70% alcohol to water.

Methylation for only 4 h is usually adequate for blocking carboxyl groups and removing sulphate ester groups. The completeness of the desired consequences of methylation is easily determined by staining with alcian blue at pH 1.0 and 2.5.

11.7.3.
Saponification

This unblocking procedure can be used after acetylation or methylation.

(1)   Take sections to absolute ethanol.
(2)   Cover with a film of celloidin (optional; instructions in Chapter 4), drain, dry, and harden the film in 70% ethanol.
(3)   Immerse for 20 min in a freshly prepared 0.5% solution of potassium hydroxide (KOH) in 70% ethanol.
(4)   Rinse gently in three changes of 70% ethanol.

11.7.4.
Mild acid hydrolysis

Sialic acids are attached by an α-2-glycosidic linkage to the subjacent sugars of the oligosaccharide chains of glycoproteins. This link is easily broken by acid-catalyzed hydrolysis. Sections are treated with an aqueous acid (pH 2.5 or lower) for 1 or 2 h at 70–80°C. All sialic acid residues are removed, including those that resist digestion by neuraminidase. Most other glycosidic linkages remain intact.

Procedure
(1)   Take sections to water.
(2)   Make some 0.05 M sulphuric acid:
Concentrated sulphuric acid (SG 1.84, 96% H_2SO_4):   2.8 ml
Water: 800 ml
Mix thoroughly and add water to obtain: 1000 ml. Heat 50–100 ml to 80°C.
(3)   Place the slides in the hot, dilute acid and keep at 80°C for 1 h.
(4)   Wash in running tap water for 2 min, rinse in distilled or de-ionized water, and proceed with the histochemical testing. (Sections often come off their slides and are lost in this procedure.)

11.8. Combinations of techniques

It is often informative and convenient to apply two or more different methods for carbohydrates to the same section. A counterstain for nuclei is often added, to provide general morphological information. Notes on two such procedures follow. Many other combinations are possible.

11.8.1.
Alcian blue and PAS procedure

Sections may be stained with alcian blue before or after the PAS method. The results are not the same (see *Note* below).

(1)   Take sections to water.

(2)   Stain with alcian blue, either at pH 1.0 or at pH 2.5.
(3)   Wash in running tap water, then rinse in distilled water.
(4)   Stain by the PAS method. The periodate oxidation may be the standard one (Section 14.4.2.1) or the mild oxidation that is selective for sialic acids (Section 14.4.2.2).
(5)   Wash thoroughly in rapidly running tap water.
(6)   Counterstain nuclei blue with an alum–haematoxylin or with an iron–eriochrome cyanine R mixture (Chapter 6).
(7)   Wash in water, dehydrate, clear, and mount in a resinous medium.

Result

Alcian blue-positive materials turquoise-blue. (With the dye at pH 1.0, only sulphated glycoproteins and glycosaminoglycans are stained.) PAS-positive material magenta. With the mild oxidation, sialic acids are the only PAS-positive substances. A purple colour is seen in material stained by both alcian blue and PAS. Nuclei are a clear blue colour, quite different from alcian blue.

Note

Usually the alcian blue is applied before the PAS staining. If the sequence is reversed, staining by alcian blue is stronger, especially in mucus that is also PAS-positive. The additional blue staining has been attributed by Johannes and Klessen (1984) to the formation of aldehyde bisulphite addition compounds, by reaction of the periodate-engendered aldehyde groups with the bisulphite in Schiff's reagent. Aldehyde bisulphite compounds are sulphonic acids, and can therefore bind alcian blue even at pH 1.0 (Chapter 10). The purple and blue colours produced in sialoglycoproteins by the PAS-alcian blue sequence are not uniformly distributed. Yamabayashi (1987) has suggested that the variations may be due to differences in the positions of the sialic acid groups. Steric hindrance by parts of other macromolecules might keep the alcian blue cations away from some anionic sites. Alcian blue also binds to the coloured tissue–Schiff compound (Reid and Owen, 1988), which contains a sulphonic acid group (Chapter 10). For microspectrophotometric studies, it is necessary to apply alcian blue and PAS procedures to separate sections (Roe et al., 1989).

11.8.2.
A two colour periodate method for sialoglycoproteins

This method (Reid et al., 1984b) is based on principles explained in Section 11.4.1 of this chapter. Aldehydes formed from neutral hexoses are irreversibly blocked by phenylhydrazine, and those derived from oxidizable sialic acids are stained with a blue Schiff-like reagent (thionine–Schiff). Saponification then releases more hydroxyl groups by removing O-acyl groups from esterified sialic acid residues. The newly formed glycols are then demonstrated by the ordinary PAS reaction. The borohydride reduction (Step 11) blocks any aldehyde groups that failed to combine with the thionine–Schiff reagent, and also changes the colour imparted by the thionine–Schiff from purple to blue.

Solutions required

Thionine–Schiff reagent (van Duijn, 1956)
Add 0.5 g thionine (C.I. 52000) to 250 ml of water. Boil for 5 min. Leave to cool, then add water to restore the volume to 250 ml. Add 250 ml t-butanol (freezes at 26°C; may need to be warmed). Do not filter at this stage, even though some of the dye is undissolved. Add 37.5 ml of 1.0 M hydrochloric acid, followed by 5.0 g of sodium metabisulphite ($Na_2S_2O_5$), shake, and leave in a stoppered bottle for 24 h at room temperature, then transfer to a refrigerator for storage. The reagent may be used after 48 h at 4°C. Filter what is needed into a coplin jar, and use it only once.

Phenylhydrazine

Phenylhydrazine hydrochloride:	0.25 g
Water:	50 ml

Prepare as needed, and use only once. **Caution.** Phenylhydrazine is poisonous.

Other solutions needed are described with the other components of the method (see section references below).

Procedure

(1)   Take sections to water.
(2)   Oxidize with 1% periodic acid for 2 h at room temperature.
(3)   Wash in running tap water, 10 min.
(4)   Transfer to 0.5% phenylhydrazine hydrochloride, 2 h.
(5)   Wash in running tap water for 10 min, then leave overnight in distilled water.
(6)   Immerse in thionine–Schiff for 4 h.
(7)   Wash in running tap water, 10 min.
(8)   Transfer to 70% alcohol.
(9)   Saponify in alcoholic KOH (Section 11.7.3)
(10) Wash in running tap water, 10 min.
(11) Immerse in a freshly prepared sodium borohydride solution (Section 10.10.6.1.) for 20 min.
(12) Wash in running tap water, 10 min.
(13) Oxidize with 1% periodic acid for 30–60 min at room temperature.
(14) Wash in running tap water for 10 min, then rinse in distilled water.
(15) Immerse in ordinary Schiff's reagent for 1 h.
(16) Wash in running tap water, 10 min.
(17) Apply a counterstain if desired (see *Note* below).
(18) Dehydrate, clear and cover, using a resinous mounting medium.

Results

Sialic acids with free hydroxyls at C7, C8 and C9: blue. Sialic acids acylated at C7: blue. Sialic acids acylated at C8 or C9: magenta. Sialic acids acylated at two or three of positions C7, C8, C9: magenta. Mixtures are stained purple. Mucosubstances that do not contain sialic acids are unstained.

Note

The counterstain should be one that contrasts well with the blue, magenta and purple colours imparted to glycoproteins. The usual blue and red nuclear stains are obviously not ideal for this purpose. See Chapter 6 for some other possibilities.

12 | Lipids

The term 'lipid' is applied to a chemically heterogeneous group of substances that are extracted from tissues by non-polar organic solvents such as chloroform and ether. These substances vary greatly in structural complexity but are built from a limited number of simpler molecules joined together in different ways. These component substances do not occur in large amounts in the free state in living tissue but are present as metabolic precursors of the lipids themselves. Accounts of lipid chemistry and metabolism are found in textbooks of biochemistry (e.g. Voet *et al.*, 2006) and there are detailed accounts of individual lipids in Gunstone *et al.* (1986).

12.1. Components of lipids

In the following brief account the symbols R, R' and R'' indicate alkyl radicals, mostly of 16–20 carbon atoms. Simplified structural formulae are used for whole lipids: most carbon atoms are represented only as junctions of bonds, hydrogen atoms attached to carbon are omitted, and usually no attempt is made to show the real shape of the molecule.

(a) Aliphatic alcohols
ROH. Present in waxes as their esters. An example is cetyl alcohol, $CH_3(CH_2)_{14}CH_2OH$. Long-chain alkyl groups are also present as glyceryl ethers in the ether phosphatides.

(b) Fatty acids
RCOOH. Present as acyl groups in all those lipids that are esters or amides. Most have unbranched chains of even numbers of carbon atoms. Olefinic (unsaturated; CH=CH) linkages may or may not be present. In the following list of the common fatty acids of animals, the length of chain is shown as C16, C18, etc., and the number of double bonds is indicated by the symbol Δ.

Saturated:	Myristic acid	C14	
	Palmitic acid	C16	
	Stearic acid	C18	
	Lignoceric acid	C24	
Unsaturated:	Palmitoleic acid	C16,	$\Delta1$
	Oleic acid	C18,	$\Delta1$
	Linoleic acid	C18,	$\Delta2$
	Linolenic acid	C18,	$\Delta3$
	Arachidonic acid	C20,	$\Delta4$
	Clupanodonic acid	C22,	$\Delta5$

In normal animals, all lipids (with the exception of some cholesterol esters and sulphatides) contain at least one unsaturated acyl group per molecule.

(c) Glycerol

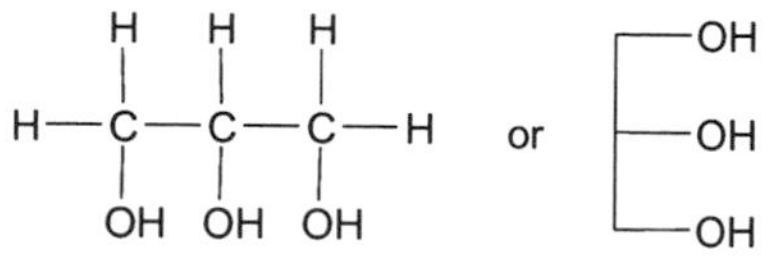

This trihydric alcohol is present as its esters in most lipids.

(d) Phosphoric acid

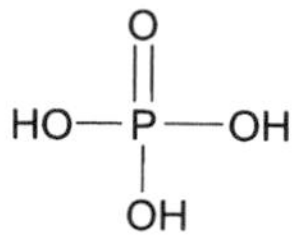

This formulation, though not strictly in accord with modern chemical notation, is the one usually used by biochemists. In phospholipids the H_3PO_4 is esterified through one or two of its hydroxyl groups. The unesterified hydroxyls ionize as acids.

(e) Choline, ethanolamine and serine

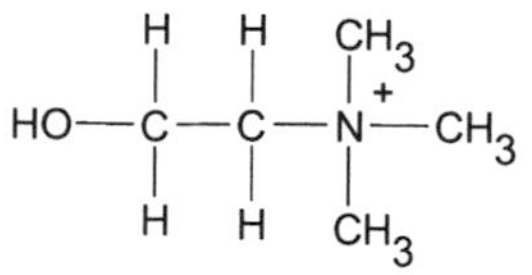

or $HOCH_2CH_2\overset{+}{N}(CH_3)_3$

CHOLINE (as cholinium cation; a quaternary ammonium compound)

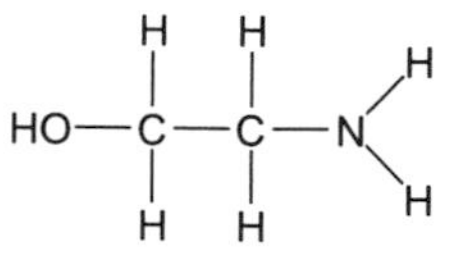

or $HOCH_2CH_2NH_2$

ETHANOLAMINE

(an amino alcohol)

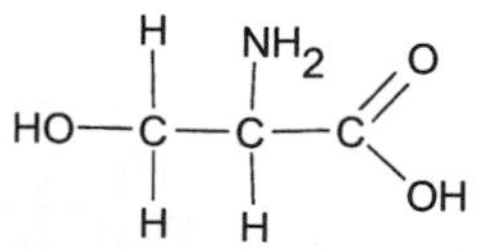

or $HOCH_2CH(NH_2)COOH$

SERINE (an amino acid, also present in proteins)

These three bases are esterified through their hydroxyl groups with phosphoric acid in phosphoglycerides and sphingomyelins.

(f) myo-Inositol

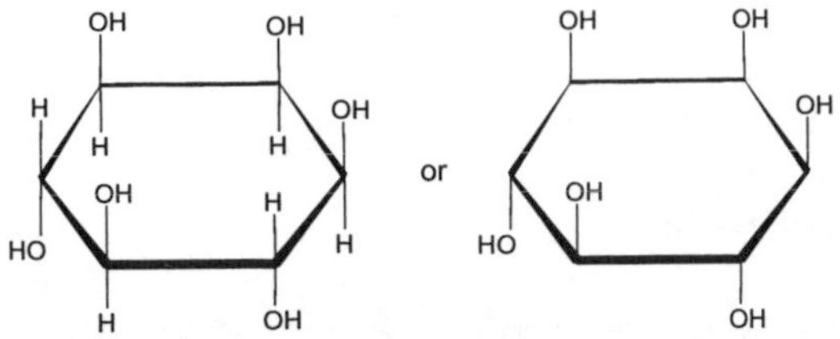

This cyclic alcohol is esterified through phosphoric acid to glycerol in the phosphoinositides, in which some other hydroxyl groups of the inositol are also phosphorylated.

(g) Sugars
Galactose, N-acetylgalactosamine, N-acetylglucosamine, glucose, N-acetylneuraminic acid, and other monosaccharides, sometimes carrying sulphate–ester groups, are present in the glycosphingolipids. See Chapter 11 for structures and abbreviated formulae.

(h) Sphingosine

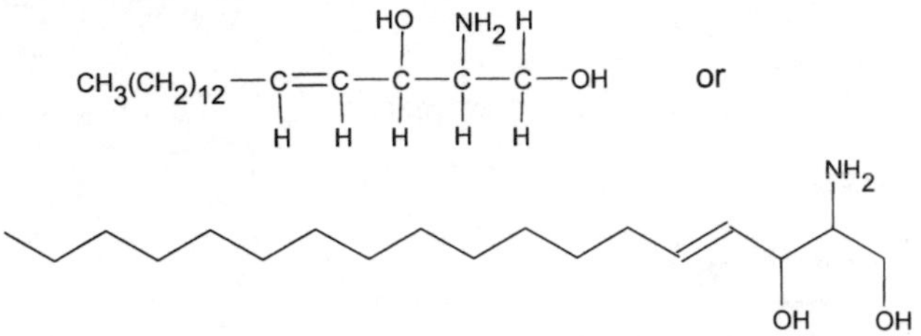

This long-chain (C18) unsaturated amino alcohol is joined in amide linkage to fatty acids and is esterified with phosphoric acid through the hydroxyl group shown at the right-hand side of the formula. In the related compound **dihydrosphingosine** the bond between C4 and C5 is saturated. In the **dehydrosphingosines**, more than one unsaturated linkage is present in the hydrocarbon chain.

(i) Cholesterol

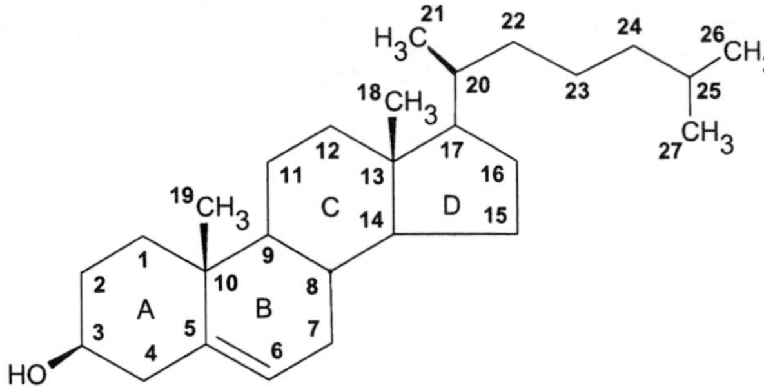

The numbering system and the letters identifying the fused aliphatic rings are applicable to all **steroids**. Cholesterol is a **sterol** (a steroid alcohol). It is insoluble in water or cold ethanol, but freely soluble in ether or acetone, so it is a hydrophobic lipid (see *Table 12.1*).

(j) Isoprene

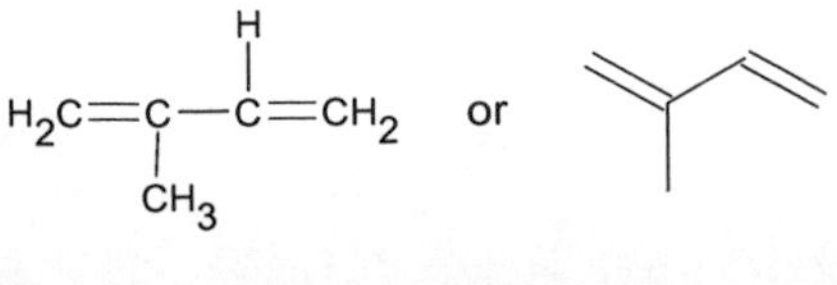

This unsaturated hydrocarbon is the monomer from which the carbon skeletons of cholesterol and the terpenes are constructed.

(k) Proteins

These are frequently conjugated with phospholipids, in proteolipids and lipoproteins.

12.2. Classification of lipids

The following scheme applies principally to the lipids of vertebrate animals. Substances with similar histochemical properties are, as far as possible, grouped together. For a modern classification that includes all types of lipid, see Fahy *et al.* (2005). The classification is summarized in *Table 12.1*. Brief descriptions of the main groups of lipids follow.

Table 12.1. A classification of the major groups of lipids

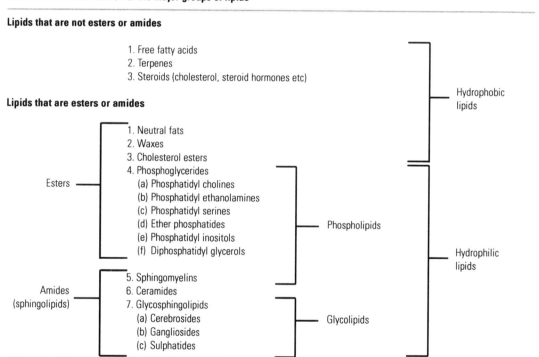

Note: phospholipids and sphingolipids are often covalently bound to proteins in proteolipids and lipoproteins.

12.2.1. **Free fatty acids**	These occur only in traces in normal tissues, but the amounts are increased in some pathological states. Crystal-like deposits of free fatty acids may also form in lipid-rich tissues that have stood for long periods of time in formaldehyde solutions. The salts of fatty acids are called **soaps**. Sodium and potassium soaps are water-soluble, but the soaps of calcium and many other metal cations are insoluble.

The prostaglandins are cyclic unsaturated fatty acids (C20, Δ2-3) of great physiological and pharmacological interest. They are produced by all animal cells, but in minute quantities that are not histochemically detectable.

12.2.2. **Terpenes**	Numerous terpenes occur in plants. The only important one in higher animals is squalene:

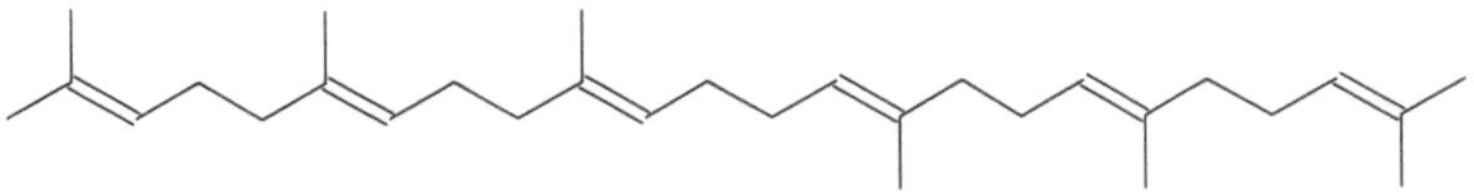

This hydrocarbon occurs in the sebum of mammals and birds, and in the oils of marine vertebrates. It is also a metabolic precursor of cholesterol.

12.2.3.
Steroids

Cholesterol is a waxy solid with a much higher melting point (150°C) than most other lipids. Inspection of its structural formula, in Section 12.1 (i), shows that it is an unsaturated secondary alcohol. It dissolves easily in most organic solvents but is insoluble in water. Cholesterol occurs in cell membranes and (together with its esters) in atheromatous lesions of arteries. Cholesterol forms needle-like crystals, which can be seen by polarizing microscopy in frozen sections (Doinikow, 1913).

The steroid hormones (corticosteroids, androgens, oestrogens and progestogens) are numerous but it is doubtful whether they can be identified histochemically. They are stored in minute quantities in the glands that secrete them, though metabolic precursors with similar chemical structure exist in detectable concentrations in steroid-secreting endocrine cells. Many steroid hormones are ketones.

12.2.4.
Fats (neutral fats)

These may be mono-, di-, or triglycerides:

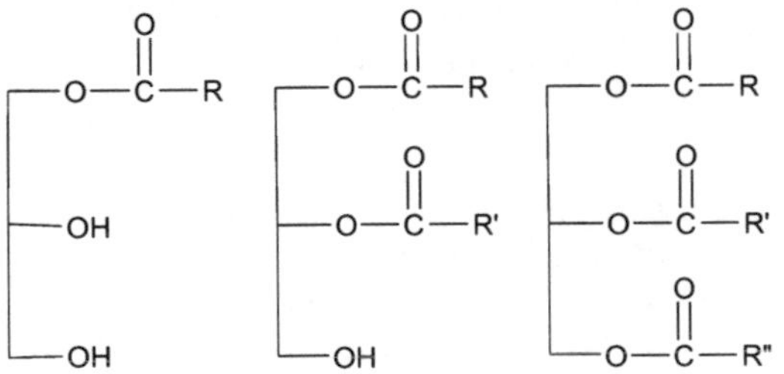

mono-   di-   tri-

The last-named type is the most abundant. Neutral fats occur principally in adipose connective tissue.

12.2.5.
Waxes

Natural waxes are esters of long-chain aliphatic alcohols with fatty acids:

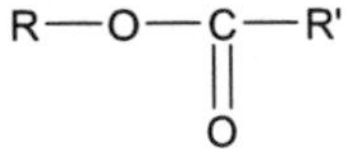

Waxes occur in a wide variety of organisms (spermaceti and beeswax are well-known examples) but are unlikely to be encountered in the tissues of laboratory animals or of man. The waxy substances of plants, **cutin** and **suberin**, are linear polymeric esters of ω-hydroxy fatty acids.

12.2.6.
Cholesterol esters

These compounds resemble waxes, but the alcohol half of the ester is derived from the hydroxyl group at position 3 of cholesterol. Cholesterol esters occur in regions of axonal degeneration in the nervous system (Miklossy and van der Loos, 1987), in intracellular lipid droplets (Pelletier and Vitale, 1994), and in atheromatous lesions of arteries.

12.2.7.
Phosphoglycerides

These lipids are hydrophilic on account of their content of polar groups such as phosphate ester, hydroxyl, and primary or quaternary amino. They fall into six groups:

(a) **Phosphatidylcholines**
These phospholipids are commonly known as **lecithins**. They are soluble in all lipid solvents, including ethanol, with the notable exception of acetone.

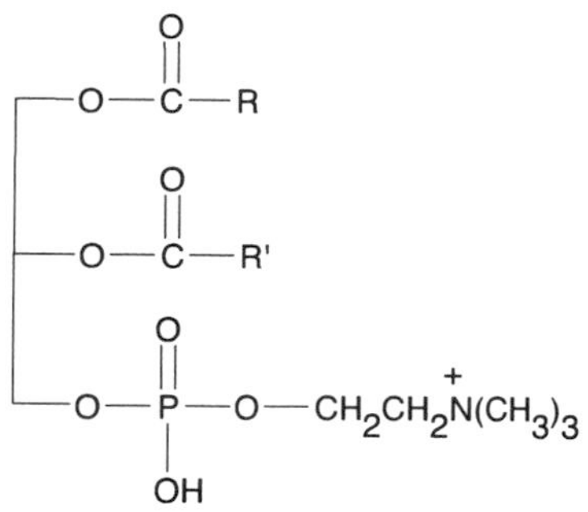

$$
\begin{array}{l}
\text{—O—C(=O)—R} \\[4pt]
\text{—O—C(=O)—R'} \\[4pt]
\text{—O—P(OH)—O—CH}_2\text{CH}_2\overset{+}{\text{N}}\text{(CH}_3)_3
\end{array}
$$

(b) **Phosphatidyl ethanolamines**

$$
\begin{array}{l}
\text{—O—C(=O)—R} \\[4pt]
\text{—O—C(=O)—R'} \\[4pt]
\text{—O—P(OH)—O—CH}_2\text{CH}_2\text{NH}_2
\end{array}
$$

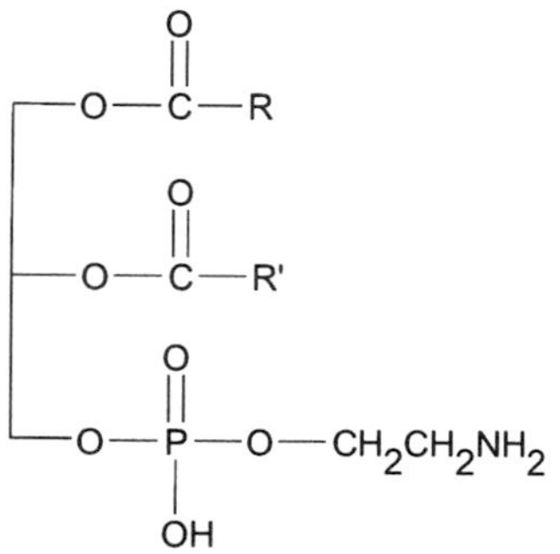

An old synonym is 'cephalins'. The ethanolamine has sometimes been called 'cholamine' or 'colamine'. In the pure state, phosphatidyl ethanolamines are, like the lecithins, soluble in ethanol but insoluble in acetone. However, the crude mixture of cephalins isolated from tissues, which is a mixture of phosphatidyl ethanolamines, serines, and inositols, is insoluble in ethanol. Extractions with solvents are of little value when attempting to distinguish histochemically between different phosphoglycerides in sections of tissues.

(c) **Phosphatidyl serines**

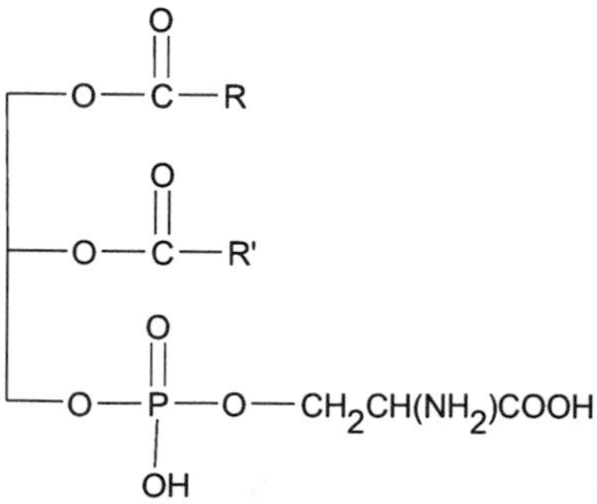

$$
\begin{array}{l}
\text{—O—C(=O)—R} \\[4pt]
\text{—O—C(=O)—R'} \\[4pt]
\text{—O—P(OH)—O—CH}_2\text{CH(NH}_2)\text{COOH}
\end{array}
$$

These phospholipids normally are part of the inner surface of the cell membrane. They are translocated to the outside surface early in the course of programmed cell death (apoptosis, see Chapter 9).

(d) **Ether phosphatides**
In these phospholipids one of the oxygen atoms of glycerol is joined to a long-chain alkyl group to give an ether. The most important ether phosphatides to the histochemist are those in which there is an unsaturated linkage adjacent to the ether oxygen. These are the **plasmalogens**:

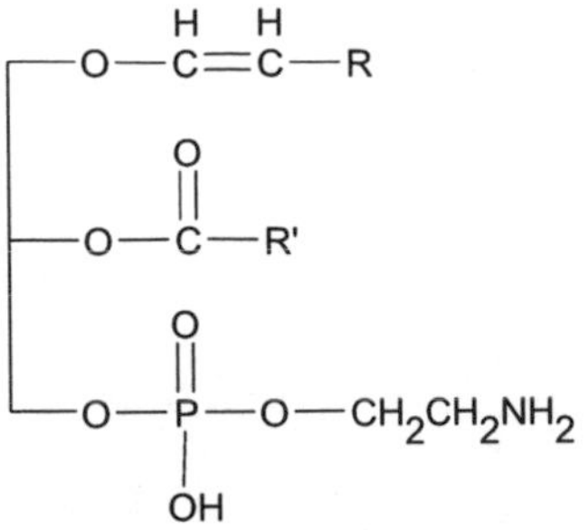

$$
\begin{array}{l}
-\text{O}-\overset{\text{H}}{\text{C}}=\overset{\text{H}}{\text{C}}-\text{R} \\[2mm]
-\text{O}-\overset{\text{O}}{\overset{\|}{\text{C}}}-\text{R}' \\[2mm]
-\text{O}-\overset{\text{O}}{\underset{\underset{\text{OH}}{|}}{\overset{\|}{\text{P}}}}-\text{O}-\text{CH}_2\text{CH}_2\text{NH}_2
\end{array}
$$

It was once thought that plasmalogens were acetals rather than ethers, hence the old name 'acetal lipids'. The basic component is most commonly ethanolamine (as shown) but sometimes choline. Plasmalogens are extracted rapidly from sections of tissue by 80% ethanol but only slowly by 60% ethanol.

(e) **Phosphatidyl inositols**
The simplest lipids of this type, which are also known as 'inositol cephalins', have the structure:

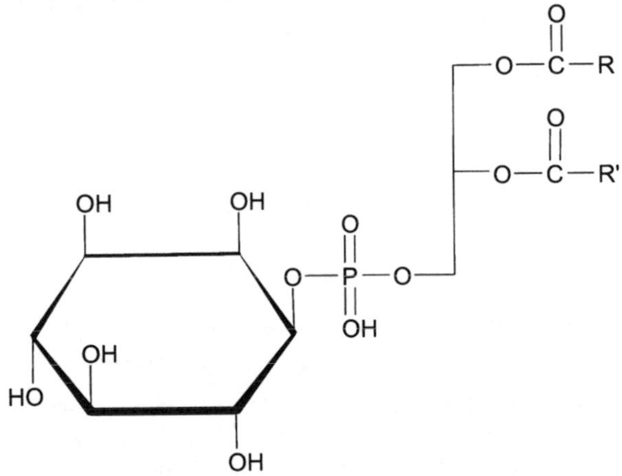

$$
\begin{array}{l}
-\text{O}-\overset{\text{O}}{\overset{\|}{\text{C}}}-\text{R} \\[2mm]
-\text{O}-\overset{\text{O}}{\overset{\|}{\text{C}}}-\text{R}'
\end{array}
$$

(myo-inositol ring) $\;\;\text{O}-\overset{\text{O}}{\underset{\underset{\text{OH}}{|}}{\overset{\|}{\text{P}}}}-\text{O}-$

Commonly one or two of the hydroxyl groups shown in the *myo*-inositol ring are esterified by phosphoric acid.

(f) **Diphosphatidyl glycerols**

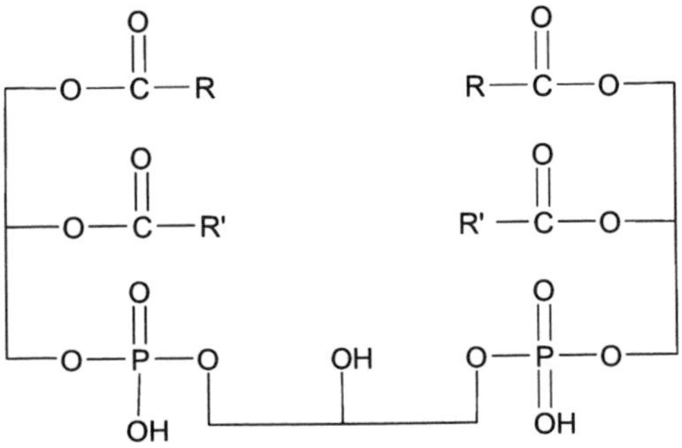

$$
\begin{array}{ll}
-\text{O}-\overset{\text{O}}{\overset{\|}{\text{C}}}-\text{R} & \quad \text{R}-\overset{\text{O}}{\overset{\|}{\text{C}}}-\text{O}- \\[2mm]
-\text{O}-\overset{\text{O}}{\overset{\|}{\text{C}}}-\text{R}' & \quad \text{R}'-\overset{\text{O}}{\overset{\|}{\text{C}}}-\text{O}- \\[2mm]
-\text{O}-\overset{\text{O}}{\underset{\underset{\text{OH}}{|}}{\overset{\|}{\text{P}}}}-\text{O}\quad\text{OH}\quad \text{O}-\overset{\text{O}}{\underset{\underset{\text{OH}}{|}}{\overset{\|}{\text{P}}}}-\text{O}-
\end{array}
$$

The most important lipid of this type is **cardiolipin**, a component of the inner mitochondrial membrane. Cardiolipin is unusual among lipids in that it can serve as an antigen.

12.2.8.
Sphingomyelins

These choline-containing phospholids are derived from sphingosine, choline and fatty acids, the last named being connected by an amide linkage:

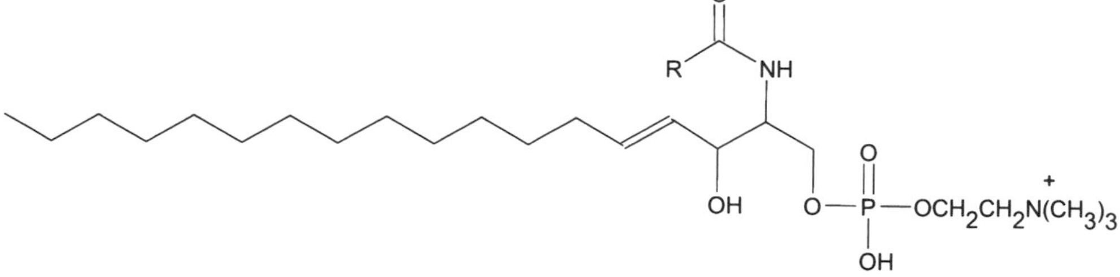

The sphingosine may be replaced by dihydrosphingosine or dehydrosphingosine. The amide linkage of sphingomyelins is more resistant to alkali-catalysed hydrolysis than are the ester linkages of other phospholipids.

Sphingomyelins, which dissolve in hot ethanol but not in ether or acetone, have more hydrophilic character than do the phosphoglycerides, which are all soluble in ether.

12.2.9.
Ceramides

These lipids, which are simple amides of sphingosine containing no phosphorus, are widely distributed but are never present in high concentration in tissues.

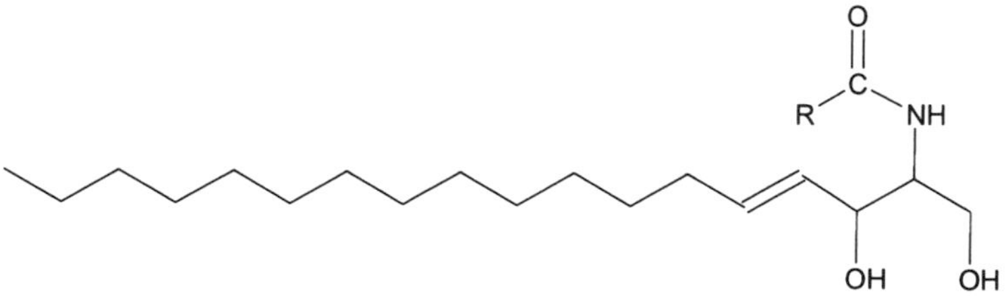

12.2.10.
Glycosphingosides (glycolipids)

Because of their carbohydrate content, these lipids are strongly hydrophilic and are easily lost from tissues owing to their solubility in water. There are three types:

(a) **Cerebrosides**. These are ceramides in which the terminal hydroxyl group of sphingosine is joined by a glycosidic linkage to a hexose sugar, which is most commonly a β-D-galactosyl residue:

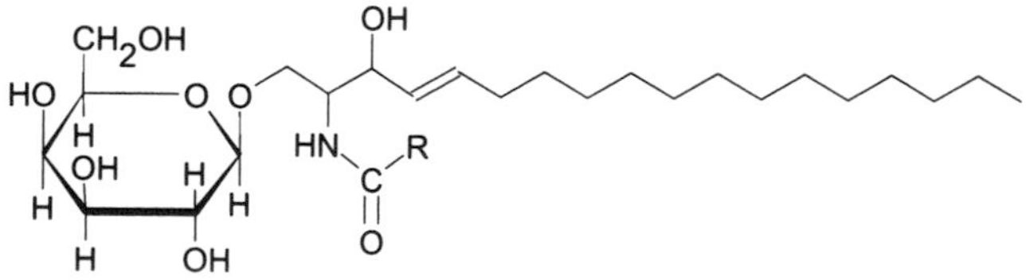

(b) **Gangliosides** resemble the cerebrosides, but have an oligosaccharide chain in place of the single hexose residue. Sialic acids and N-acetyl hexoses are always present. They have structures such as: NANA(α-2→4)D-GalNAc(β-1→4)D-Gal(β-1→Ceramide).

(c) **Sulphatides** are cerebrosides in which one of the hydroxyl groups of the hexose is esterified by sulphuric acid. In the commonest sulphatides of mammalian nervous tissue a β-galactosyl residue is sulphated at position C3.

12.2.11.
Lipids conjugated to protein

Proteolipids are compounds in which each protein molecule is combined with several of lipids, so that the complete molecule is soluble in nonpolar solvents.

Lipoproteins are large protein molecules with some bound lipid. They are insoluble in nonpolar solvents and are also insoluble in most polar solvents, so they are not extracted from tissues by the process of embedding in paraffin wax. A typical lipoprotein molecule is globular, with fatty acid chains and hydrophobic amino acid side-chains in the centre, and the hydrophilic parts of the protein on the outside (see Voet *et al.*, 2006). The lipid moieties of lipoproteins, which include phospholipids and cholesterol, can be dissolved out of sections only if the bonds to protein are broken. The cleavage can be brought about by adding a strong acid to a suitable solvent (Section 12.4).

12.3. Histochemical methodology

The many techniques of lipid histochemistry have been thoroughly reviewed by Adams (1965) and Bayliss High (1984). Some older methods, valuable especially for revealing structural features of invertebrate tissues, are reviewed by Wigglesworth (1988). Only a few of the available procedures selectively demonstrate any of the classes of lipid described above. It is possible, however, to obtain information about several physical properties and chemical constituents of these substances. Methods are available that will detect with reasonable certainty the presence of:

(1) Any lipids.
(2) The hydrophobic or hydrophilic nature of a lipid.
(3) Unsaturation.
(4) Carbohydrates.
(5) Free fatty acids.
(6) The 1,2-unsaturated ether groups of plasmalogens.
(7) Cholesterol and its esters.
(8) Choline in phospholipids.
(9) Amide rather than ester linkages.

Both physical and chemical properties have to be taken into consideration when attempting to identify and localize lipids in tissues. The specificities of techniques for the demonstration of lipids have been determined mainly by experiments using pure lipids incorporated into thin paper, which is then treated as if it were a section being stained. Kaufmann and Lehmann (1926), Baker (1946) and Adams (1965) have carried out thorough studies of this kind.

Most lipids are unaffected by chemical fixation of tissue (Heslinga and Deierkauf, 1961; Deierkauf and Heslinga, 1962), but the presence of calcium ions in the fixative (as in Baker's formal–calcium) increases the preservation of the hydrophilic phospholipids, possibly by forming insoluble calcium-phosphate–lipid complexes.

Bayliss High and Lake (1996) state that fixation in formal–calcium should not exceed 2 or 3 days' duration for blocks of tissue or 1 h for cryostat sections of fresh tissue. Longer fixation impairs the staining of phosphoglycerides. Calcium ions derived from the fixative form salts (calcium soaps), insoluble in non-polar solvents, with free fatty acids. Treatment with a strong acid (e.g., 1.0 M HCl for 60 min) will regenerate the fatty acids.

Frozen sections are used for the histochemical examination of lipids, but appreciable quantities of phospholipids persist in sections of paraffin-embedded tissue. They occur mainly in myelin sheaths of nerve fibres and in erythrocytes. These lipids are stained in some of the histological techniques for the demonstration of myelin (Chapter 6). They can be extracted from paraffin sections by suitable mixtures of solvents. Aldehyde fixation does not enhance the preservation of lipids through the process of embedding in epoxy resin; freeze-substitution of unfixed tissue is preferred (Maneta-Peyret *et al.*, 1999).

Phospholipids are rendered completely insoluble in organic solvents by prolonged treatment with potassium dichromate. This technique, known as **chromation**, has been known for over a century (Elftman, 1954), but the chemical mechanism is still unknown. Lillie (1969) showed that the chromating reagent reacted with double bonds in lipids, though other functional groups such as –OH may also have been involved in the binding of chromium, especially if chromation was carried out at 60°C rather than at 3°C or 24°C. He suggested that a cyclic ester was produced:

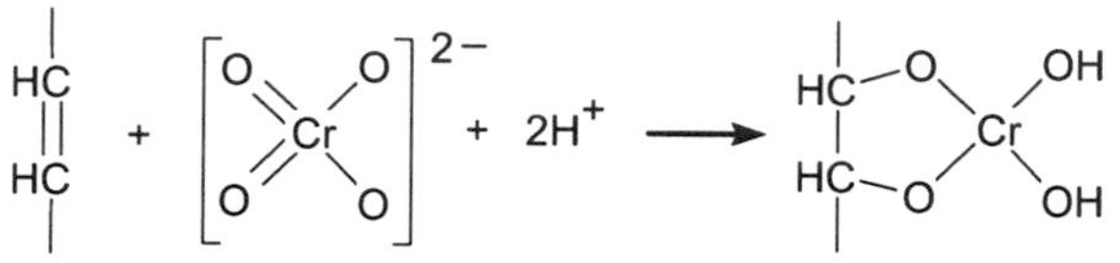

The oxidation number of the chromium in Lillie's proposed product is +4. Compounds of Cr(IV) are rare, though some stable organometallic complexes are known. The free hydroxyl groups of such a complex would be expected to participate in the formation of dye–metal complexes (e.g. with haematein) if the coordination number of the chromium atom were 6. Coordination numbers 4 and 6 exist in known Cr(IV) complexes. Lillie's speculations did not take into account the fact that the chromating reagent, between pH 2 and pH 6, exists as an equilibrium mixture of hydrogen chromate and dichromate ions:

$$2HCrO_4^- \rightleftharpoons Cr_2O_7^{2-} + H_2O$$

The chromate ion $[CrO_4]^{2-}$ required by Lillie's equation is formed when the pH of the solution is above 6 (see Cainelli and Cardillo, 1984 for chemistry of chromium). A dichromate ion might be able to combine with the two unsaturated sites to give a Cr(IV) *bis*-ester. Such cross-linking could account for the insolubilization of chromated lipids.

12.4. Extraction and chemical degradation

The pre-treatments described in this section can be applied to sections before carrying out any staining or other histochemical method for lipids. Chemical reactions of narrower specificity are discussed in their context, elsewhere in the chapter.

**12.4.1.
Rationale**

The hydrophobic lipids, of which the neutral fats of adipose tissue are the most abundant, are extracted by **cold acetone**. It is important that the acetone be anhydrous. If traces of water are present, partial extraction of hydrophilic lipids occurs (Elleder and Lojda, 1971). Ordinary laboratory acetone contains about 0.5% water.

Either **pyridine** or a mixture of **chloroform and methanol** will extract all lipids except those that are firmly bound to protein. Proteolipids are soluble in methanol–chloroform but lipoproteins are not. In order to extract the firmly bound lipids of lipoproteins it is necessary to use an **acidified solvent**, which will hydrolyse the protein-lipid linkages and then dissolve the lipids (Adams and Bayliss, 1962).

Extractive methods may be used in conjunction with any staining method in order to confirm the specificity for the demonstration of lipids.

With some lipoproteins it is necessary to employ acid hydrolysis in an aqueous medium to release the lipid components for staining with solvent dyes (see below). Without such treatment, the hydrophilic protein prevents access of hydrophobic dye molecules to the lipids.

The ester linkages between fatty acids and glycerol in fats and phosphoglycerides can be broken by **alkaline hydrolysis (saponification)**. The fatty acids are liberated as their soluble sodium soaps. Amide linkages (with sphingosine) are not hydrolysed under the same conditions of time, temperature, and concentration of alkali. Consequently the fatty acid moieties of ceramides and sphingomyelins remain insoluble in water after saponification of the other lipids in the tissue. Glycosphingolipids may also be presumed to resist saponification, but they are largely extracted from tissues by aqueous reagents.

12.4.2. **Solvent extraction procedures**	Times given are for frozen sections of formaldehyde-fixed tissue. Sections are mounted onto slides and allowed to dry before extraction. Use solvents in tightly screw-capped containers to avoid evaporative losses and risk of fire. For extraction with heated solvents a water bath in a fume cupboard is safer than a 60°C oven.

Cold acetone. Acetone (4°C, 1 h, but sometimes may need to be left overnight) extracts hydrophobic lipids only. It is important that no water be present in the acetone. Ordinary acetone is dehydrated by adding anhydrous calcium chloride, one-fifth of the total volume of $CaCl_2$ + acetone, and allowing to stand for 2 days. Use a bottle of at least 500 ml capacity, because much acetone is lost by absorption into the desiccant. Glassware must be dry and the sections must be allowed to dry in air before and after immersion of the slides in the anhydrous acetone (Elleder and Lojda, 1971).

Hot methanol–chloroform. A mixture of methanol (2 volumes) and chloroform (1 volume), at 58–60°C for 18 h (2 h is sometimes sufficient) removes all lipids except those firmly bound to protein.

Methanol–chloroform–HCl. Methanol, 66 ml; chloroform, 33 ml; concentrated hydrochloric acid, 1.0 ml. Extract sections for *either* 18 h at room temperature (25°C) *or* 2 h at 58°C. This removes all lipids, including the phospholipid moieties of lipoproteins (Adams and Bayliss, 1962).

12.4.3. **Hydrolysis of esters (saponification)**	Esters (but not amides) are hydrolysed by treating free-floating sections for 1 h at 37°C with 2 M (8%) sodium hydroxide (NaOH). The sodium soaps of the liberated fatty acids are dissolved out. After hydrolysis the sections are fragile and should be gently washed in water, followed by 1% aqueous acetic acid (to neutralize residual alkali), and then returned to water.
12.4.4. **Unmasking masked lipids**	Lipids firmly bound to protein (Section 12.2.11) are released by acid hydrolysis prior to staining with a solvent dye. Sections are treated with 25% (v/v) aqueous acetic acid for 2 min and then washed in five changes of water. After this treatment the released ('unmasked') lipids are amenable to staining with dyes and to extraction by solvents.

12.5. Solvent dyes

12.5.1. **Solvent dyes (lysochromes)**	Coloured, non-polar substances dissolve in lipids and render them visible under the microscope. These substances belong to the Colour Index class of solvent dyes (Section 5.7). Baker (1958) called these dyes **lysochromes**. They stain lipid material because they are more soluble in it than in the solvents from which they are applied. The first solvent dyes to be used for staining fat were Sudan III and Sudan IV. Later, oil red O, which is more hydrophobic, was introduced. (See Chapter 5 for

the chemistry of these and related solvent dyes.) Solvent dyes dissolve in those hydrophobic lipids that are liquid at the temperature used for staining: neutral fats and those esters of cholesterol whose acyl groups are unsaturated (Section 12.6). They give only weak colour to the hydrophilic phospholipids, in which they are less soluble.

A solvent dye that can colour all types of lipid is Sudan black B. This is a mixture of two main components and 8–11 coloured contaminants (Marshall, 1977). Several other unwanted dyes form in solutions that are more than one month old. Some of these products of deterioration stain proteins and nucleic acids (Frederiks, 1977). Even in fresh solutions, contaminating anionic dyes can give rise to false positive identification of lipids (Malinin, 1977).

Lysochromes can dissolve in lipids only at temperatures above the melting points of the latter. This is a point of some importance, because lipids in which all the fatty acid chains are saturated melt above 60°C. Unsaturated lipids are mostly liquid at room temperature for a reason given in Section 12.6. Cholesterol melts at 150°C and its esters with saturated fatty acids also have high melting points. However, it is possible to stain these lipids with Sudan black B if the sections have first been treated with bromine water. This reagent reacts with unsaturated linkages in fatty acids (Section 12.6.3). Bromine also reacts with cholesterol to form an oily derivative that is liquid at room temperature (Bayliss and Adams, 1972). This derivative is not 5,6-dibromocholesterol (which has a higher melting point), and its chemical structure is unknown. The bromine–Sudan black method stains virtually all lipids. (The only lipid materials not stained would be those consisting entirely of fully saturated triglycerides, fully saturated waxes, or saturated free fatty acids.)

The staining of lipids is affected by the solvent (Adams, 1965). Thus, phospholipids are more likely to be stained from a solution of Sudan black B in 70% than from one in 100% alcohol. Phosphoglycerides and free fatty acids are generally supposed to be more prone to extraction by the solvent than are lipids of other types. Some lipoproteins cannot be stained by solvent dyes without prior acid hydrolysis (Sections 12.2.11 and 12.4.4). In such substances the lipid is said to be 'masked' by the protein.

**12.5.2.
Sudan IV
method**

Sudan III (C.I. 26100) may be substituted for Sudan IV in this method, but its colour is less intense. Oil red O, which is similar to Sudan IV, is commonly applied from a different solvent (Section 12.5.3).

Preparation of stain
Prepare a saturated solution of Sudan IV (C.I. 26105) by adding an excess of dye powder (about 0.5 g per 100 ml) to 70% ethanol in a tightly capped or stoppered bottle. Shake well and then allow to stand for 2 or 3 days before using the supernatant solution. Keeps for at least 10 years and can be used repeatedly. Replace when the colour weakens.

Procedure
(1)   Cut frozen sections and rinse them in 70% ethanol.
(2)   Stain in Sudan IV solution for 1 min.
(3)   Transfer to 50% ethanol for a few seconds, until no more clouds of dye leave the section.
(4)   Wash in two changes of water.
(5)   (Optional.) Counterstain nuclei progressively with alum–haematoxylin.
(6)   Wash in water.
(7)   Mount in an aqueous medium.

Result

Lipids (especially neutral fats) orange-red. Small intracellular droplets cannot be resolved and hydrophilic lipids, such as those of myelin, are only weakly stained. This simple method is adequate for adipose tissue and for the detection of isolated fat cells. Nuclei are blue if counterstained with haemalum.

12.5.3.
Oil red O from a supersaturated solution

In this method a supersaturated solution is made by adding water to a saturated stock solution of the solvent dye in isopropanol. The difference of dye solubility (in the solvent and in lipids) is consequently greater than it is when the stain is a stable solution in an alcohol–water mixture. Other solvent dyes, including Sudan III, Sudan IV and Sudan black B can be substituted for oil red O in this technique. Both the stability and dye content of the working solution of oil red O are increased by the presence of dextrin.

Solutions required

A. Oil red O in isopropanol (stock solution)
Prepare a saturated solution of oil red O (C.I. 26125) by adding excess dye powder (about 1 g per 100 ml) to 99% isopropyl alcohol in a tightly capped or stoppered bottle. Shake well and then allow to stand for 2 or 3 days before using the supernatant solution. Keeps for at least 10 years. Replace when the colour of the working solution weakens.

B. 1% dextrin
In water.

C. Working solution (make as required)
Add 2 volumes of 1% dextrin (Solution B) to 3 volumes of the stock solution (A) of oil red O in isopropanol. Leave for at least 2 days, then filter through slow (Whatman no. 4) filter paper. This working solution can be kept and reused for two years (Churukian, 1999).

Alternatively (Lillie and Ashburn, 1943), add 2 volumes of water to 3 volumes of stock oil red O (Solution A), wait 30 min and filter into the staining jar. This working solution is stable for only 4–6 h. It may be used more than once if it remains transparent.

D. Counterstain
A counterstain, if used, must be one that is not red and is stable in an aqueous mounting medium. Any alum–haematoxylin is suitable (Chapter 6 for technical details and discussion of other possible counterstains).

Procedure
(1) Cut frozen sections and rinse them in 60% ethanol.
(2) Stain in the working solution of oil red O (C) for 10–20 min.
(3) Rinse in 60% ethanol, then in four changes of water.
(4) (Optional.) Counterstain with Solution D.
(5) Wash in water.
(6) Mount in an aqueous medium.

Result
Hydrophobic lipids (especially neutral fats) red. Small intracellular droplets should be clearly visible. Hydrophilic lipids are weakly stained. Other features in the tissue are appropriately coloured by the counterstain.

12.5.4. Sudan black B methods

The complete procedure presented here is is the bromine–Sudan black B method of Bayliss and Adams (1972), for the demonstration of all types of lipid. If the bromination is omitted (the usual practice), free cholesterol is not stained and phospholipids are less strongly coloured. (See *Note 1* below.)

Solutions required

A. Bromine water

Bromine:	about 5.0 ml
Water:	about 200 ml

Bromine is caustic, and its brown, pungent vapour is injurious to the respiratory system. Keep it in a fume cupboard and don't even think of pipetting it by mouth! The aqueous solution is no more hazardous than most other laboratory chemicals. Bromine water is stable for about 3 months at room temperature in a glass-stoppered bottle and may be used repeatedly. It should be replaced when there are no drops of dark brown bromine in the bottom of the bottle.

B. Sodium metabisulphite

Approximately 0.5% aqueous $Na_2S_2O_5$. Dissolve on the day it is to be used.

C. Sudan black B

Add 600 mg of Sudan black B (C.I. 26150) to 200 ml of 70% ethanol. Place on a magnetic stirrer for 2 h, then pour into a screw-capped bottle. Leave to stand overnight. To use the solution, filter it into a coplin jar and try not to disturb the sediment of undissolved dye in the bottom of the bottle.

The solution of Sudan black B may be kept (and used repeatedly) for only 4 weeks. With older solutions there is grey non-lipid background staining and weaker coloration of lipids.

D. A counterstain

Alum–brazilin and Mayers carmalum (Chapter 6) are suitable red nuclear counterstains because they act progressively and are stable in aqueous media.

Procedure

(1)   Cut frozen sections, mount them onto slides and allow them to dry.
(2)   Immerse slides in bromine water (Solution A) for 1 h.
(3)   Rinse in water.
(4)   Immerse in sodium metabisulphite (Solution B) for about 1 min until the yellow colour of bromine has been removed from the sections. (See *Note 2* below.)
(5)   Wash in four changes of water.
(6)   Rinse in 70% ethanol.
(7)   Stain in Sudan black B (Solution C) for 10 min, with occasional agitation of the slides.
(8)   Rinse in 70% ethanol, 5–10 s (see *Note 3* below), with agitation, then wash in water.
(9)   Apply counterstain if desired.
(10) Wash in water and mount in an aqueous medium.

Result

Lipids appear in shades of deep grey, very dark blue, and black.

Notes

(1)   Steps 2–5 are commonly omitted. Cholesterol is then unstained.
(2)   In the original account of this method, 'sodium bisulphate' was specified as the reagent for decolorizing the brominated sections: obviously an error. Dilute aqueous solutions of sodium or potassium sulphite, bisulphite, or thiosulphate may be used instead of sodium metabisulphite.
(3)   This differentiation is the only critical step in the method. Ideally a lipid-extracted control section should be included with those being stained. When the lipid-free section is completely decolorized the end-point of the differentiation has been reached.

12.6. Tests for unsaturation

Olefinic linkages occur in isoprene, cholesterol, and sphingosine, and in the very widely distributed unsaturated fatty acids. Consequently, the histochemical demonstration of the carbon-carbon double bond is tantamount to the staining of all lipids. Double bonds in fatty acids can be of the *cis* or *trans* type. The *cis* configuration is the more abundant in fatty acids of animal tissues.

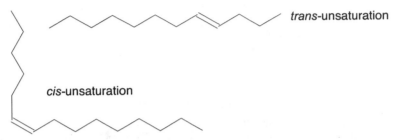

trans-unsaturation

cis-unsaturation

It can be seen that a *cis* double bond produces a bend in the chain of carbon atoms. This impairs the packing of the molecules in the solid state and in consequence *cis*-unsaturated lipids have lower melting points than do saturated or *trans*-unsaturated ones. Thus, glyceryl tripalmitate melts at 65.1°C whereas glyceryl trioleate melts at −4°C. Lysochromes dissolve only in lipids that are in the liquid phase, so these dyes impart their colours only to structures containing unsaturated lipids. The ordinary lysochromes, such as Sudan III, Sudan IV, and oil red O, stain only those unsaturated lipids that are hydrophobic. Sudan black B (Section 12.5.2) is different and can also enter hydrophilic domains. The methods based on the use of oil-soluble dyes demonstrate lipids by virtue of their physical properties and may reasonably be called 'histophysical' techniques (Adams, 1965; Bayliss High and Lake, 1996). There are, however, several genuinely histochemical reactions for the demonstration of unsaturation. Some of these will now be discussed.

12.6.1.
Osmium
tetroxide

The reactions of osmium tetroxide with various substances present in tissues were discussed in some detail in Chapter 2. There it was shown that this compound oxidizes the −CH=CH− bond and is reduced to a black substance, probably osmium dioxide. Osmium tetroxide is soluble in both polar and non-polar solvents; consequently it serves as a stain for both hydrophilic and hydrophobic lipids. It is possible, however, to distinguish between the two types by mixing the osmium tetroxide with an oxidizing agent that dissolves only in polar liquids. Potassium chlorate is a suitable oxidizing agent for this purpose. When frozen sections are treated with such a mixture, the osmium tetroxide forms cyclic esters (Section 2.4.6) at both hydrophilic and hydrophobic sites. The other product of the reaction, the unstable osmium trioxide, then disproportionates to give osmium tetroxide (soluble) and dioxide (insoluble and black). However, at hydrophilic sites in the tissue, the newly formed osmium dioxide is immediately be oxidized by chlorate ions:

$$3OsO_2 \ + \ 2ClO_3^- \ \longrightarrow \ 3OsO_4 \ + \ 2Cl^-$$

Hydrophilic unsaturated lipids therefore remain converted to cyclic osmium esters, which may be colourless or brown and are barely visible in the sections. At hydrophobic sites, the precipitation of osmium dioxide is unimpeded, so that intense black staining will be observed. The cyclic esters of the unsaturated hydrophilic lipids can be stained subsequently by treating the sections with α-naphthylamine, which forms a red or orange complex with the bound osmium. These reactions form the basis of the OTAN (osmium tetroxide-α-naphthylamine) method for differential staining of hydrophobic and hydrophilic lipids. The Marchi method for degenerating myelin (Chapter 18) is similar. The chemical reactions described above follow Adams *et al.* (1967) and Adams and Bayliss (1968), but have been slightly modified from the original accounts in the light of the work of Korn (1967).

In practice, osmium tetroxide seems to be a sensitive and specific reagent for the demonstration of unsaturation, though the OTAN reaction may sometimes fail to distinguish correctly between hydrophilic and hydrophobic lipids (see Bayliss High and Lake, 1996). The reactions of osmium tetroxide with phenolic compounds and with proteins (Nielson and Griffith, 1978,1979; see also Chapter 2) should not be ignored, however. The specificity can be checked by staining control sections in which unsaturated linkages have been blocked by bromination (Section 12.6.3) and others from which the lipids have been extracted by solvents.

Solutions required

Osmium tetroxide stock solution

The following instructions are for preparing 2% aqueous osmium tetroxide, which can be used in lipid histochemistry and also for preparing fixative mixtures (Chapter 2) and reagents for other osmium-based staining methods (Chapter 18).

Water:	50 ml
Osmium tetroxide:	1.0 g

To prepare this solution, carefully clean the outside of the sealed glass ampoule in which the OsO_4 is supplied, removing all traces of the label and any gum with which it was attached. Score the glass with a file or a diamond scriber, clean off sebum (from your skin) by dipping the ampoule in acetone, and allowing it to dry. Drop the scored, cleaned ampoule into a very clean bottle containing 50 ml of the purest available water. Insert the glass or black rubber stopper (no grease may be used) and shake the bottle until the ampoule breaks. If necessary, the ampoule may be broken by striking it with a clean, degreased glass rod. The OsO_4 often takes several hours to dissolve completely.

In a clean, tightly stoppered bottle, this solution keeps for a few months at 4°C. The solution may be used several times provided that all glassware is very clean. Debris derived from sections may be removed by filtration (in fume cupboard) when the solution is poured back into its bottle. The used filter paper should be soaked overnight in 10% alcohol to reduce OsO_4 to $OsO_2.2H_2O$, before throwing it away.

Caution. Osmium tetroxide should always be used in a fume cupboard. Its vapour attacks the respiratory system and the eyes. It can cause corneal opacity.

Deterioration is indicated by the presence of a blue–grey colour in the solution, due to colloidal osmium dioxide. Old solutions should be pooled in a screw-capped container that contains some alcohol, and kept for recycling (see Kiernan, 1978).

Osmium tetroxide working solution

The concentration of OsO_4 for this technique is not critical. It is usual to use a 1% solution, which is made by diluting the 2% stock solution with an equal volume of water. The 1% solution can be kept for a few months (see above), and used repeatedly if it remains transparent.

Procedure

(1) Cut frozen sections of formaldehyde– or formal–calcium-fixed specimens and collect them in water. They may be mounted onto slides, preferably without any adhesive.

(2) Transfer to the working OsO_4 solution and leave in a closed container for 1 h, in a fume cupboard.

(3) Wash free-floating sections in five changes of water (at least 10 ml per section), 2 min in each change. Mounted sections may be washed in running tap water (for at least 30 min) if they are still firmly adherent to their slides.
(4) Dry free-floating sections onto slides *or* blot mounted sections with filter paper.
(5) Mount in an aqueous medium. Alternatively, dehydrate in dioxane (two changes, each 4 min with occasional agitation), clear in carbon tetrachloride (two changes, each 1 min), and mount in a resinous medium. (See *Note 3* below.)

Result
Unsaturated lipids black.

Notes
(1) The hydrophobic lipids can be extracted with acetone (Section 2.4.2). This may reveal hydrophilic lipids in the same sites.
(2) Thorough washing is necessary to remove excess OsO_4.
(3) Alcohols are avoided for dehydration because they would reduce any OsO_4 not removed by aqueous washing. The clearing agent recommended is one in which OsO_4 is extremely soluble. **Caution.** Toxic vapours from dioxane and carbon tetrachloride.

12.6.2.
Palladium
chloride

Unsaturated hydrophilic lipids can be demonstrated by virtue of their ability to reduce the chloropalladite ion $[PdCl_4]^{2-}$ to metallic palladium. The chloropalladite ion is formed when palladious chloride is dissolved in aqueous hydrochloric acid:

$$PdCl_2 + 2HCl \longrightarrow [PdCl_4]^{2-} + 2H^+$$

$$(H_2PdCl_4 = \text{chloropalladious acid})$$

An unstable complex is formed with olefinic compounds and the complex is reduced to the metal, which is visible as a black deposit. Because the reagent is used in aqueous solution, it is reduced only by hydrophilic unsaturated lipids. The chloropalladite ion also behaves as an anionic dye, imparting a yellow background colour to non-lipid substances. This non-specific staining can be largely removed by treating the sections with pyridine, with which are formed complexes of the type $[Pd(pyr)_2Cl_2]$. The chemistry of the technique is discussed in greater detail by Kiernan (1977).

Palladium chloride has been used in empirical staining procedures for the nervous system (Paladino, 1890) and in electron microscopy to impart electron density to elastin (Morris *et al.*, 1978). The reaction with elastin has not been studied chemically, but it does not result in the formation of black products, so there is no possibility of confusion with hydrophilic lipids in light microscopy.

In addition to its use as a histochemical test, this method (Kiernan, 1977) is suitable for the histological demonstration of myelinated nerve fibres in the peripheral nervous system. In the central nervous system, myelin is also coloured, but stained lipids in the grey matter reduce the contrast (see Kiernan, 2007b).

Solutions required

Chloropalladious acid solution
Stock solution

Palladium chloride ($PdCl_2$):	1.0 g
Concentrated hydrochloric acid:	1.0 ml
Water:	5.0 ml

Mix thoroughly to disperse the $PdCl_2$, then add:

Water:	to make 50 ml

Keeps for several months.

Working solution

Stock solution:	1.0 ml
Water:	9.0 ml

This diluted solution can be used repeatedly until it becomes cloudy.

20% aqueous pyridine

Pyridine:	20 ml
Water:	80 ml

This could be kept indefinitely, but it is convenient to make it up when required. Use a fume cupboard because pyridine has a strong smell that many people find unpleasant.

Procedure

(1) Wash frozen sections in water. (See *Note 1* below.)
(2) Transfer to the working solution of chloropalladious acid for 2 h at 37°C. (See *Note 2* below.)
(3) Rinse in two changes of water, 1 min in each.
(4) Immerse sections in 20% aqueous pyridine for 1 min.
(5) Rinse in water.
(6) Dehydrate through graded alcohols, clear in xylene, and mount in a resinous medium.

Result

Unsaturated hydrophilic lipids dark brown or black. Background pale yellow. (See *Note 3* below.)

Notes

(1) Either free-floating sections or sections dried onto slides may be used.
(2) Alternatively, leave the sections in chloropalladious acid overnight at room temperature, or for 30 min at 58°C.
(3) Bromination or extraction of hydrophilic lipids prevents the reaction but the yellow background coloration is unaffected.

12.6.3.
Bromination

Unsaturated linkages are **blocked** by bromination, either by exposure to bromine vapour or by treatment with bromine water or an aqueous solution of bromine in potassium bromide ($KBr + Br_2 = KBr_3$).

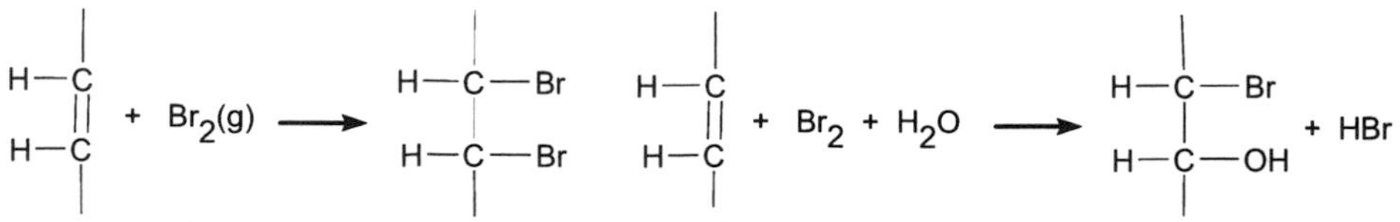

This test, though not entirely specific, may be used to confirm the unsaturated nature of substances stained by the methods discussed above.

The bromo derivatives of unsaturated lipids are decomposed with liberation of bromide ions when treated with a dilute mineral acid. The bromide ions can be precipitated as silver bromide, which can then be reduced to black metallic silver. These reactions constitute the bromine-silver method for the histochemical detection of unsaturation (Norton *et al.*, 1962):

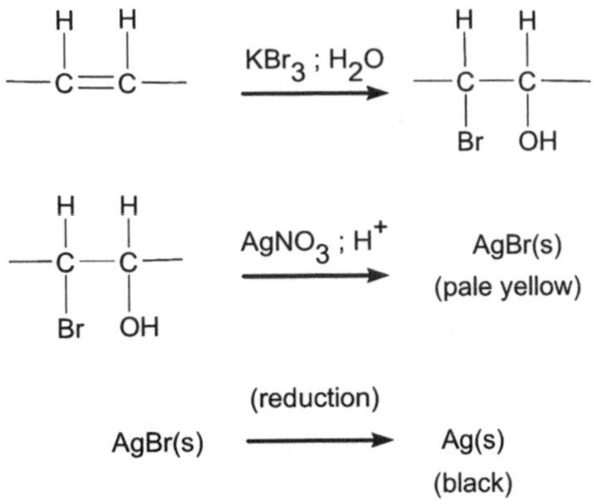

$$
\underset{\substack{H \quad H \\ | \quad | \\ -C=C-}}{} \xrightarrow{\text{KBr}_3 \; ; \text{H}_2\text{O}} \underset{\substack{H \quad H \\ | \quad | \\ -C-C- \\ | \quad | \\ \text{Br} \quad \text{OH}}}{}
$$

$$
\underset{\substack{H \quad H \\ | \quad | \\ -C-C- \\ | \quad | \\ \text{Br} \quad \text{OH}}}{} \xrightarrow{\text{AgNO}_3 \; ; \text{H}^+} \quad \begin{array}{l} \text{AgBr(s)} \\ \text{(pale yellow)} \end{array}
$$

$$
\text{AgBr(s)} \xrightarrow{\text{(reduction)}} \begin{array}{l} \text{Ag(s)} \\ \text{(black)} \end{array}
$$

The specificity of this technique is marred, however, by the occasional non-specific deposition of silver at sites in the tissue that do not contain lipids.

Procedure for bromination

Potassium bromide, 6 g; water, 300 ml; bromine, 1.0 ml. (**Caution.** Use fume cupboard; see also Section 12.5.4.) Keeps for a few months. Replace when the colour has faded.

Treat sections with this solution for 5 min at room temperature. Rinse in a bisulphite or thiosulphate solution to remove yellow stain of bromine and wash thoroughly with water.

This treatment prevents reactions due to unsaturated (–CH=CH–) linkages.

12.7. Glycolipids

Carbohydrates in glycosidic combination with lipids are demonstrated by the techniques of carbohydrate histochemistry. It should be remembered that inositol, though not a sugar, has an arrangement of hydroxyl groups similar to that found in some hexoses. Phosphatidyl inositols contain the glycol configuration unless three or more of their hydroxyl groups are phosphorylated. Distinction between glycolipids and mucosubstances is made by using extractive procedures for the lipids. It is not possible to draw satisfactory conclusions when the two types of substance are present in the same place.

When the PAS reaction is used with frozen sections, allowance must be made for the possible presence of aldehydes generated by atmospheric oxidation of unsaturated fatty acids. Direct positive staining with Schiff's reagent from this cause is known as the **pseudoplasmal** reaction. A related phenomenon is **DAB-induced fluorescence**, which is seen in frozen sections of nervous tissue examined for peroxidase activity using 3,3'-diaminobenzidine (DAB) as the chromogen (Chapter 16). This is the most commonly used technique for localizing peroxidase-labelled antibodies in immunohistochemical procedures (Chapter 19). Even in the absence of H_2O_2, the substrate of peroxidase, exposure to DAB results in the formation of a stable fluorescent product. Histochemical tests (Section 12.4 and Chapter 10) indicate that this fluorescence results from combination of DAB with aldehyde groups derived from oxidized lipids (von Bohlen und Halbach and Kiernan, 1999; see also Chapter 10).

In addition to its well known action on adjacent hydroxyl groups of carbohydrates, the periodate ion oxidizes a proportion of the double bonds of lipids to pairs of aldehyde groups. This results in a truly positive PAS reaction that is not due to carbohydrate. Performic acid oxidizes double bonds even more effectively.

A modified PAS method, devised to circumvent the unwanted reactions of olefinic bonds, is described by Bayliss High (1984). Primary amine groups are oxidatively deaminated (producing aldehydes), and double bonds are oxidized to aldehydes, with performic acid. All the free aldehyde groups are blocked with 2,4-dinitro-phenylhydrazine, and a conventional PAS staining is then carried out. The aqueous reagents used in this procedure extract gangliosides, so that the only lipids stained by this method are cerebrosides (and possibly phosphatidyl inositols).

Lipids containing acid sugars (i.e. gangliosides and sulphatides) are conspicuous only in the tissues of patients with certain lipid-storage diseases. They may be stained with techniques of carbohydrate histochemistry (Chapter 11), to show the sialic acid of gangliosides or the sulphate ester groups of sulphatides. The results are negative in lipid-extracted control sections (see Jones, 2002).

12.8. Free fatty acids

The soaps formed from fatty acids and heavy metals are insoluble in water. The cationic component of such a soap can be demonstrated by any suitable chromogenic reaction.

In **Holczinger's method**, sections are treated with a dilute solution of cupric acetate. Loosely bound copper is then removed by a brief treatment with a chelating agent, EDTA. The residual metal, which has been shown by Adams (1965) to be associated only with fatty acids, is made visible by forming an insoluble dark-green compound with dithiooxamide (Chapter 13).

Elleder and Lojda (1972) were less impressed with the specificity of this technique than was Adams (1965). They found that free fatty acids were sometimes weakly stained when known to be present in considerable quantities in some tissues and that there was false-positive coloration of some phospholipids and of calcified tissue, as well as background staining of proteinaceous and carbohydrate-containing material. They showed that pre-treatment with 1.0 M hydrochloric acid enhanced the staining of free fatty acids, probably by causing hydrolysis of the calcium soaps formed during fixation in formal–calcium. This pre-treatment also dissolved calcium phosphates and carbonate. The differentiation in EDTA could usefully be extended beyond the time suggested in the original method, to minimize the staining of copper bound to 'background' structures, but extraction of control sections with cold acetone was necessary in order to ensure that positive results were due to free fatty acids and not to phospholipids. The modifications recommended by Elleder and Lojda (1972) are incorporated into the practical instructions for Holczinger's method given here.

Use unfixed cryostat sections or frozen sections of tissue fixed in formal–calcium. Acetone-extracted control sections must also be examined.

Solutions required
A. 1.0 M hydrochloric acid

Concentrated hydrochloric acid (SG 1.19):	40 ml
Water:	to 500 ml

Keeps indefinitely.

B. Copper acetate

Cupric acetate $(CH_3COO)_2Cu.H_2O$:	5.0 mg
Water:	100 ml

Prepare before using.

C. 0.1% EDTA

Disodium ethylenediamine tetraacetate (Na$_2$(EDTA).2H$_2$O): 100 mg
Water: 80 ml

Adjust to pH 7.1 with drops of 1.0 M (=4%) NaOH, then add:

Water: to make 100 ml

Prepare on the day it is to be used.

D. Dithiooxamide solution

Dithiooxamide: 100 mg
Ethanol: 70 ml

Dissolve and then add:

Water: 30 ml

Prepare on the day it is to be used.

Procedure

(1)   Affix frozen sections to slides.
(2)   Immerse in 1.0 M HCl (Solution A) for 1 h.
(3)   Rinse in three changes of water, drain, and allow sections to dry. Carry out acetone extraction of control sections at this stage (Section 12.4.2).
(4)   Immerse sections in copper acetate (Solution B) for 3–4 h.
(5)   Transfer to two changes of 0.1% EDTA (Solution C), 30 s in the first, 60 s in the second.
(6)   Wash in two changes of water.
(7)   Immerse in dithiooxamide solution (D) for 30 min. A shorter time (e.g. 10 min) will usually suffice. The time need not be extended after the sections have stopped darkening.
(8)   Rinse in 70% ethanol, two changes, 1 min in each.
(9)   Wash in water and apply a coverslip, using an aqueous mounting medium.

Result

Free fatty acids dark green to black. Any staining seen in acetone-extracted control sections is not due to free fatty acids.

12.9. The plasmal reaction

In frozen sections, plasmalogens yield aldehydes following a brief treatment with a 1% aqueous solution of mercuric chloride. The aldehydes are then demonstrated by means of Schiff's reagent (Chapter 10). The chemistry of the plasmal reaction was worked out by Terner and Hayes (1961), whose paper should be consulted for the experimental evidence upon which the following account is based.

In most publications dealing with plasmalogens, the double bond of the vinyl ether is said to be between the α and β-carbon atoms. This is an incorrect usage of the Greek letters (see 'Conventions and Abbreviations' at the beginning of this book). These two carbons should be designated as 1 and 2, as in the present account. The letters α and β, used correctly, would refer to carbon atoms 2 and 3.

Mercuric chloride adds to the double bond of the vinyl (1,2-unsaturated) ether linkage of plasmalogens:

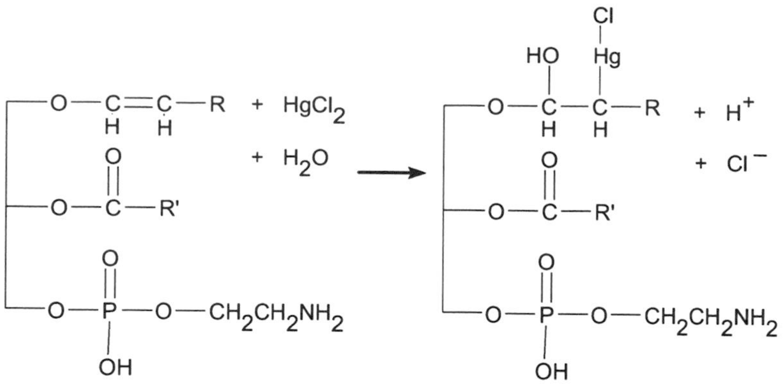

The initial product, a hemiacetal, is unstable. It immediately dissociates into an alcohol and an aldehyde:

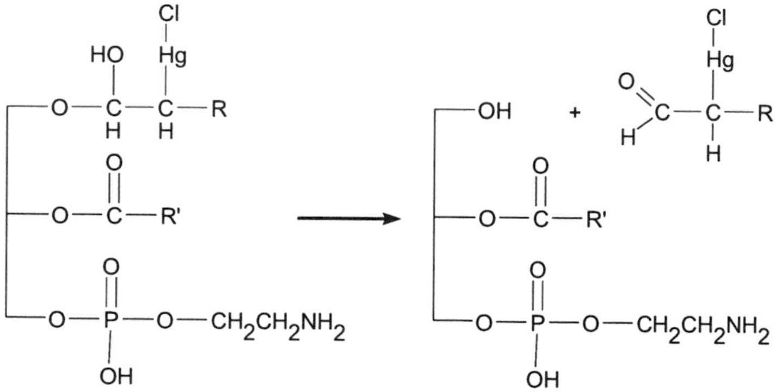

The mercury atom remains attached to carbon 2 of the aldehyde; its presence there can be demonstrated histochemically.

Vinyl ethers are more easily hydrolysed in the presence of acids than are ordinary ethers, but the pH of the mercuric chloride solution used in the plasmal reaction (3.5) is not low enough to catalyse the hydrolysis. However, 6 M hydrochloric acid is just as effective as 1% mercuric chloride in generating aldehydes from plasmalogens:

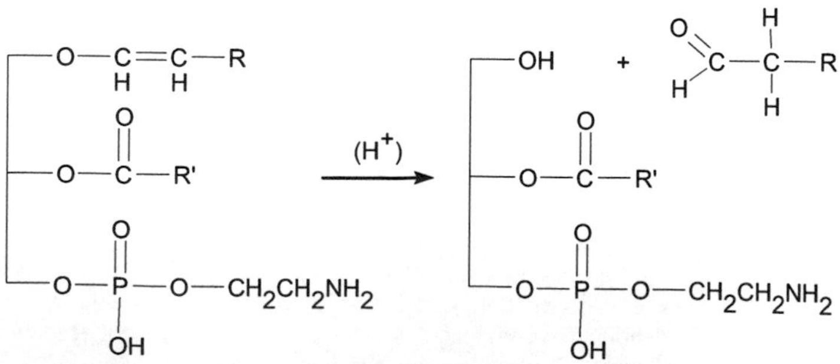

(The obvious product of hydrolysis of this ether would be an enolic "vinyl alcohol," RCH=CHOH. These compounds do not exist as such, but as the tautomeric aldehydes.)

In practice, 6 M HCl is not used because it is more injurious to the sections than aqueous mercuric chloride. However, acid-catalysed hydrolysis of plasmalogens can occur in Schiff's reagent (pH 2.5), especially if the sections are immersed in it for more than 20 min (Elleder and Lojda, 1970). Consequently, omission of the treatment with mercuric chloride is not always an adequate control procedure for the plasmal reaction. Staining with Schiff's reagent alone could be due to plasmalogens as well as to a pseudoplasmal reaction (Section 12.7). However, if there is no staining with Schiff's reagent alone, a positive reaction after treatment with mercuric chloride certainly indicates the presence of plasmalogens.

It is important to control for aldehydes already present in the tissue. If found, these must be chemically blocked with sodium borohydride (Chapter 10). If any staining occurs when there are no aldehyde groups in the tissue, the Schiff's reagent is not working properly and must be replaced.

For the plasmal reaction, use either cryostat sections of unfixed tissue or frozen sections of small specimens that have been fixed in formaldehyde for no more than 6 h. The sections should be used within 1 h of being cut.

Solutions required
A. 1% mercuric chloride

Mercuric chloride ($HgCl_2$):	1.0 g
Water:	100 ml

Keeps indefinitely.

B. Schiff s reagent
See under the Feulgen reaction (Section 9.3.2). Allow the Schiff's reagent to warm to room temperature before use.

C. Bisulphite water

Potassium metabisulphite ($K_2S_2O_5$):	5.0 g
Water:	1000 ml
Concentrated hydrochloric acid:	5.0 ml

Prepare before using and use only once.

D. Counterstain
A progressive haemalum (see Section 6.1.3.2) is suitable. Alternatively, use any other blue, green or yellow stain that is stable in an aqueous mounting medium.

Procedure
(1) Wash sections (mounted on slides or coverslips) in three changes of water. This step is omitted for sections of unfixed tissue.
(2) Immerse in 1% $HgCl_2$ (Solution A), 1 min.
(3) Transfer slides directly to Schiff's reagent (Solution B) for 5 min.
(4) Transfer to bisulphite water (Solution C), three changes, 2 min in each.
(5) Wash in three changes of water.
(6) (Optional) Apply a counterstain. Wash in running tap water after counterstaining.
(7) Mount in an aqueous medium.

Result
Plasmalogens pink to purple, provided that a positive reaction in the absence of treatment with $HgCl_2$ is not obtained. Nuclei blue if counterstained with haemalum.

12.10. Cholesterol and its esters

Needle-like birefringent crystals are likely to be of cholesterol (See Section 12.2.3) but frozen sections commonly contain other, unidentifiable birefringent material, so more specific tests are needed. Various chromogenic chemical reactions have been devised for steroids; the one with the most certain specificity for cholesterol is the perchloric acid-α-naphthoquinone (PAN) reaction. There is also a simpler affinity-based technique that makes use of a fluorescent antibiotic, filipin,

Free cholesterol may be distinguished from its esters by treating sections with a solution of **digitonin** before staining. Digitonin is a glycoside of a plant sterol and it forms with cholesterol an adduct that is insoluble in cold acetone. Esters of cholesterol remain soluble in cold acetone, along with other hydrophobic lipids. Digitonin has also been incorporated into fixatives for the purpose of making cholesterol insoluble and also osmiophilic for histochemical studies with the electron microscope. However, Vermeer *et al.* (1978) have found that digitonin added to aqueous fixatives fails to immobilize cholesterol on filter paper and that it accelerates the diffusion of cholesterol esters. The specificity of histochemical tests involving the use of digitonin to insolubilize cholesterol is therefore doubtful.

12.10.1.
The PAN method

Adams (1965) showed that this method gave a positive result with no lipids other than cholesterol, its esters, and a few other closely related sterols. The sections are heated in a solution containing perchloric acid, 1,2-naphthoquinone-4-sulphonic acid, formaldehyde and ethanol.

Perchloric acid is thought to convert cholesterol to a conjugated diene:

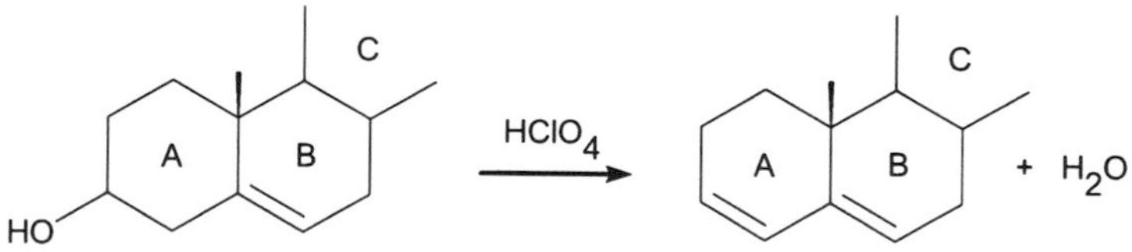

(Only the A and B rings of the cholesterol molecule are shown.

The remainder of the structure does not take part in the reaction.)

This reaction is analogous to the well-known preparative technique whereby ethylene is formed by elimination of water from ethanol in the presence of concentrated sulphuric acid. Esters of cholesterol may be hydrolysed in the strongly acid reagent and the resultant cholesterol then converted to the diene. In the next phase of the method, the diene reacts with 1,2-naphthoquinone-4-sulphonic acid (see also Chapter 10, Section 10.5) to form a blue compound. The chemistry of the second reaction and the nature of the end-product are not understood. Neither are the roles of the ethanol and the formaldehyde contained in the reagent. The method does not work with pure cholesterol. Prior oxidation either by air or by ferric chloride is necessary (Bayliss High, 1984).

Fixation in formal–calcium is recommended for this method. Nicholson and Monkhouse (1985) have shown that much cholesterol is retained in tissue that has been fixed in glutaraldehyde and embedded (without alcoholic dehydration) in glycol methacrylate.

Preparation of reagents
A. Perchloric acid-naphthoquinone (PAN) solution
Ethanol:	60 ml
60% aqueous perchloric acid (SG 1.54) (Handle with care):	10 ml

Formalin (40% HCHO):	1.0 ml
Water:	9.0 ml
1,2-naphthoquinone-4-sulphonic acid:	40 mg

This is made as needed and used only once.

B. 60% aqueous perchloric acid (S.G. 1.54) (Handle with care)

Procedure

(1) Cut frozen sections and leave them (unmounted) in 4% aqueous formaldehyde (from formalin) for 1 week. Alternatively, leave the sections in a freshly
prepared 1% (w/v) aqueous solution of ferric chloride ($FeCl_3.6H_2O$) for 4 h.
Before starting the staining procedure, preheat a hotplate to approximately
65°C.
(2) Wash the sections in water and dry them onto slides.
(3) Paint the sections with a thin layer of the PAN reagent (A) and place on the
hotplate for 10 min. Use a brush to apply more PAN solution at intervals to
prevent drying. The colour changes from red to blue.
(4) Place a drop of 60% $HClO_4$ (Reagent B) on the section and apply a coverslip. Carefully remove excess perchloric acid from the edges of the coverslip,
with filter paper.

Result

Cholesterol, its esters and a few closely related steroids are stained dark blue. (See
Note below.) Pink background colours are not due to lipids. The colour is not stable in water or in ordinary mounting media.

Note

To demonstrate free cholesterol alone, proceed as follows:

(a) Carry out stages 1 and 2 of the above method.
(b) Place slides in a 0.5% solution of digitonin in 40% ethanol for 3 h.
(c) Immerse slides in acetone for 1 h at room temperature.
(d) Rinse in water.
(e) Proceed with steps 3 and 4 of the above method. Esters of cholesterol are
extracted by the acetone, but free cholesterol is rendered insoluble by combination with digitonin.

The PAN method is damaging to sections, so the stained preparations show poor
structural preservation. There are other histochemical tests for steroids, but most
are just as destructive and have less chemical specificity. Cholesterol can be stained
by the bromine–Sudan black method (Section 12.5.3) and by the fluorescent Nile
red method described in Section 12.11.2 of this chapter. These techniques are not
injurious to the tissue, but they have little specificity for cholesterol, even when
used in conjunction with solvent extractions and digitonin.

**12.10.2.
Filipin affinity
method**

Filipin is a mixture of three similar antifungal antibiotics produced by *Streptomyces
filipini*, a soil-dwelling bacterium first found in in the Philippines. As antibiotics, the
filipins are classified as macrolide polyenes (large rings with numerous double
bonds). The major component is **filipin III**:

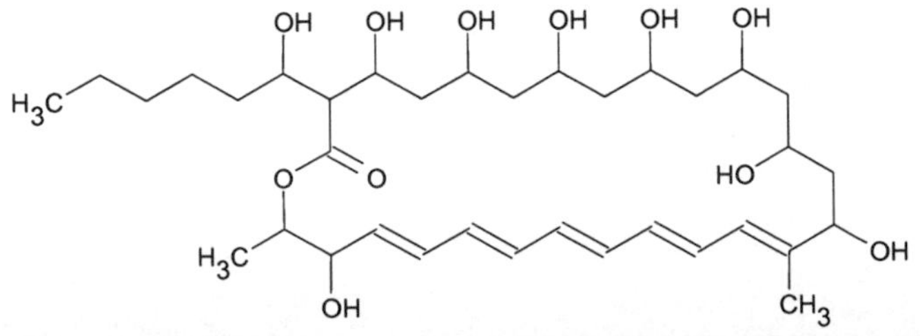

Filipin is yellow and fluorescent. It is almost insoluble in water but soluble in most organic solvents. Filipin binds specifically to 3β-hydroxysterols, notably cholesterol. This affinity forms the basis of histochemical methods for localizing free cholesterol by fluorescence microscopy (Bornig and Geyer, 1974) and electron microscopy (see Pelletier and Vitale, 1994). The affinity is attributed to similar shapes of the cholesterol and filipin molecules; hydrophobic interactions between the hydrocarbon parts of the molecules are reinforced by hydrogen bonding of cholesterol's only –OH to an –OH at one end of the filipin molecule (Volpon and Lancelin, 2000).

A cholesterol ester cannot bind filipin because it does not have a free –OH group.

The filipin affinity method is applicable to frozen sections of formaldehyde- or glutaraldehyde-fixed tissues (Volpon and Lancelin, 1974) or to unfixed cell cultures (Kruth and Vaughan, 1980). Jones (2002) considers this the method of first choice for histochemical demonstration of cholesterol.

Solutions required
Filipin stock solution
Filipin complex:	5 mg
Either N,N′-dimethylformamide or dimethylsulphoxide:	2 ml

Store at 4°C. Protect from light. Pure filipin III is commercially available, at 25 times the price of filipin complex, but offers no advantage.

Filipin working solution
Stock solution:	0.1 ml
Phosphate-buffered saline (PBS):	to make 5.0 ml

Procedure
This is applicable to frozen sections mounted on slides or coverslips, or to cell cultures on coverslips or in petri dishes.

(1) Rinse with PBS.
(2) Cover the preparation with filipin working solution, under a lid to prevent evaporation, for 1 h. (See also *Note 1* below.)
(3) Wash in 3 changes of PBS, total time 5 min.
(4) Apply a coverslip, with PBS as the mounting medium and examine by fluorescence microscopy, with near UV excitation (340–380 nm) and a 500–530 nm barrier filter.

Result
Sites of free cholesterol show blue fluorescence, which should be photographed immediately because of rapid photobleaching.

Notes
(1) Thick (40 μm) sections require incubation with filipin for 3 h (Distl *et al.*, 2001).
(2) For a negative control, pre-incubate a preparation in a solution of cholesterol oxidase, 0.04 mg/ml in 0.1 M phosphate buffer, for 2 h at 37°C. This converts cholesterol to a ketone that does not combine with filipin.
(3) To release cholesterol from its esters, preincubate in a solution of cholesterol esterase, 0.4 mg/ml in 0.1 M phosphate buffer, for 2 h at 37°C
(4) Klinkner *et al.* (1997) combined filipin with Nile red in a study of the distribution of cholesterol and other lipids in early atheroma lesions. Their paper includes coloured micrographs.

12.11. Miscellaneous techniques

Two useful methods for lipids remain to be considered. Baker's acid–haematein test is a valuable staining method for mitochondria, myelin and other structures rich in phospholipids. Nile blue and Nile red have been in occasional use for many years, but have recently enjoyed a resurgence of popularity with the rediscovery and further investigation of the fluorescence of Nile red.

12.11.1.
Acid-hematein
for choline
containing lipids

Various techniques are available for the selective demonstration of phosphatidyl cholines and sphingomyelins. Some of them (e.g. Bottcher and Boelsma-van Houte, 1964; Hadler and Silveira, 1978) are derived from analytical chemical methods for choline and its derivatives. They will not be discussed here because they are not very frequently used. A more popular technique is Baker's (1946) acid–haematein test. Model experiments with lipids and other substances on paper have revealed that it is specific for choline-containing phospholipids (Adams, 1965) if the instructions are followed faithfully. Baker's (1946) investigation indicated a lower degree of specificity, but it is likely that his specimens of phosphatidyl ethanolamines ('cephalin') and cerebrosides ('brain galactolipine') were less pure than those available to Adams (1965).

In the first stage of the acid–haematein procedure, sections fixed in either formal–calcium or a mixture similar to Bouin's fluid are exposed to a solution containing potassium dichromate. As explained earlier (Section 12.3), this reagent probably combines covalently with unsaturated linkages and also with nearby hydroxyl groups. The chromated sections are then stained with an acidic solution of haematein (Chapter 5), which forms a dark blue dye–metal complex with the bound chromium. Destaining in an alkaline solution of potassium ferricyanide leaves the strong colour only in structures such as mitochondria and myelin sheaths, which contain phosphatidyl cholines and sphingomyelin. The chemical mechanism of the differentiation is unknown. Baker (1958) suggested that the ferricyanide ion might oxidize haematein to more faintly coloured compounds (Chapter 5). The blue product of the acid–haematein test is insoluble in alcohols and xylene, so the preparations can be mounted permanently in resinous media. A yellow background coloration is probably due to haematein acting as a simple anionic dye in the absence of a metal with which to form a strongly coloured complex. Aside from its histochemical value, the acid–haematein method is one of the best techniques for staining **mitochondria**. Other methods for the demonstration of these organelles by light microscopy of fixed tissues are purely empirical (see Gabe, 1976, for detailed descriptions).

Baker (1946) prescribed an extraction with pyridine as a control procedure to confirm that stained structures were lipids. Nowadays other solvents are preferred, and it is also possible to employ a saponification procedure (Section 12.4.3) that removes phosphatidyl cholines and makes the method selective for sphingomyelins.

In the original method of Baker (1946) the chromation was carried out before sectioning, and the procedure took 4 days to complete. The current practice is to treat sections with dichromate, and to use much shorter times for staining and differentiation.

Solutions required
A. Dichromate-calcium

Potassium dichromate ($K_2Cr_2O_7$):	15 g
Calcium chloride ($CaCl_2$):	3.0 g
Water:	300 ml

This solution keeps indefinitely, but is used only once.

B. Acid–haematein

Haematoxylin (C.I. 75290):	50 mg
Water:	300 ml
1% aqueous sodium iodate ($NaIO_3$):	1.0 ml

Heat until it just boils, then allow to cool to room temperature and add:

Glacial acetic acid:	1.0 ml

This reagent is used on the day it is prepared.

C. Borax-ferricyanide differentiator

Potassium ferricyanide, $K_3Fe(CN)_6$:	15 g
Borax (sodium tetraborate, $Na_2B_4O_7.10H_2O$):	0.75 g
Water:	300 ml

Stable indefinitely at 4°C. Use only once.

Procedure

(1) Cut frozen (or cryostat) sections of tissue that has been fixed in formal–calcium, and mount on slides.
(2) Transfer the slides to the dichromate-calcium solution (A), and leave overnight at about 60°C. (4 h is usually enough.)
(3) Wash in 5 changes of water, 1 min in each.
(4) Stain for 2 h in acid–haematein (Solution B), at about 37°C.
(5) Wash in water until excess dye is removed.
(6) Differentiate in borax ferricyanide (Solution C) for 2 h at 37°C.
(7) Wash in water (3 or 4 changes, taking care to avoid detachment of the sections after treatment with the alkaline differentiator).
(8) Either mount in an aqueous medium or dehydrate through graded alcohols, clear in xylene, and mount in a resinous medium.

Result

Certain phospholipids (phosphatidyl cholines and sphingomyelins) are coloured blue, blue-black, or grey. Background yellow. Blue-stained objects may only be assumed to contain phospholipid if they are unstained after appropriate solvent extraction. (See *Note 1* below.) Mitochondria and myelin sheaths are shown well by the acid–haematein method.

Notes

(1) All lipids are extracted from frozen sections by methanol–chloroform or acidified methanol–chloroform (Section 12.4.2) prior to chromation.
(2) Sections may be subjected to alkaline hydrolysis (Section 12.4.3) before chromation. Sphingomyelins will then be the only lipids stained by acid–haematein.

12.11.2
Nile blue and Nile red

The chemistry of Nile blue and its oxidation product Nile red has been reviewed in Chapter 5 (Section 5.9.9). The staining solution used in lipid histochemistry is a mixture of the two dyes, made in the laboratory by boiling an acidified aqueous solution of Nile blue. Although Nile red is insoluble in pure water, it dissolves easily in mixtures of alcohol or acetone with water, or in an aqueous solution of Nile blue. Presumably the hydrophobic molecules of the red dye are held by van der Waals forces to the similarly shaped Nile blue cations. Nile red can be extracted from the mixture of dyes by shaking with a non-polar solvent. The purified dye is used alone as a fluorochrome.

The fluorescence of Nile red is quenched in the presence of water, so the dye is a probe of hydrophobic environments. The wavelengths of maximum excitation and emission are affected by the polarity of the solvent. Thus, in a strongly hydrophobic medium Nile red is excited by blue (450–500 nm) light and emits yellow-orange (maximum at 528 nm). In an organic solvent miscible with water, the excitation maximum is around 550 nm (green), with an emission maximum at 628 nm (Greenspan and Fowler, 1985). Equivalent differences in fluorescence are seen in hydrophobic and hydrophilic lipids stained with Nile red.

When a frozen section of a tissue is treated with a solution of Nile red, this dye behaves like any other lysochrome and dissolves in hydrophobic lipids: principally the neutral fats. These are coloured red. If a very dilute solution of Nile red is used (Greenspan et al., 1985), there is fluorescence at the sites in which the dye is present. Unlike the red colour seen by ordinary microscopy, this fluorescence is visible even in inclusions composed of cholesterol, which is solid at the temperature of staining. The visibility of fluorescence in cholesterol is due to the fact that fluorescence microscopy is more sensitive than bright-field microscopy. Even minute amounts of a fluorochrome stand out conspicuously against a dark background.

In frozen sections stained with an aqueous solution of Nile blue and Nile red, the cations of the former dye stain some of the hydrophilic lipids. These are the ones that are acidic due to the presence of ionized phosphate (or sulphate) ester groups. Free fatty acids, if present, are stained blue or purple, because they are somewhat hydrophilic on account of their carboxyl groups.

The staining of phospholipids and fatty acids by Nile blue cannot be explained simply by attraction of oppositely charged ions. The pH of the reagent is approximately 2, so most of the non-lipid macromolecular cations, such as nucleic acids, acquire little of the blue colour (Chapters 6 and 9 for reasons). Sulphated carbohydrates, which can bind cationic dyes even at pH 1 (Chapter 11), are stained by Nile blue, and the resulting colour is metachromatic (i.e. red), so it must not be confused with that of Nile red. When using Nile blue and Nile red, it is necessary to stain suitable control sections from which lipids have been extracted.

Nile blue and red staining solution

Nile blue sulphate (C.I. 51180):	1.0 g
Water:	200 ml
Sulphuric acid (10% v/v aqueous):	10 ml

Boil for 4 h (use a reflux condenser to prevent loss of water, or make up the volume manually from time to time). Cool and filter. Keeps for several months.

Nile red stock solution

Shake 100 ml of the Nile blue and red solution (above) in a separating funnel with three changes of 100 ml of xylene. Collect the xylene (with extracted Nile red) and evaporate to dryness in a rotary evaporator, to obtain about 0.4 g of solid dye. The powder is probably stable indefinitely. A stock solution is made by dissolving it in acetone to a concentration of 0.5 mg/ml. The solution in acetone can be kept for several months in a tightly capped container in darkness (e.g. in a refrigerator).

Nile red working solution (for fluorescence)

Nile red stock solution (above):	0.05 ml
Glycerol–water (75:25 by volume) mixture:	50 ml

Stir vigorously. Removal of bubbles is facilitated by exposing the mixture to reduced atmospheric pressure for a few minutes. This is the highest concentration of Nile red likely to be needed for fluorescence microscopy. Dilution (fivefold) is necessary if over-staining occurs.

(Greenspan and Fowler, 1985, started with Nile blue chloride, rather than the sulphate. The chloride is less soluble in water, and is not used in staining methods for ordinary light microscopy.)

Nile blue sulphate method
This is the method developed by Cain (1947).

(1)   Cut frozen sections and attach to slides.
(2)   Stain in the Nile blue and red solution at 37°C, for 30 min.
(3)   Differentiate in 1% acetic acid, 2 min.
(4)   Wash in water, and mount in an aqueous medium.

Result
Unsaturated hydrophobic lipids pink to red. Free fatty acids and phospholipids blue to purple. There is sometimes some blue staining of nuclei. Mast cell granules and other glycosaminoglycan-containing structures are red to purple (metachromasia). Free fatty acids can be extracted (cold acetone), leaving phospholipids as the only stainable substances; they then stain blue (see Bayliss High, 1984).

Nile red fluorescence method
This procedure (Fowler and Greenspan, 1985) is applicable to frozen or cryostat sections or to monolayers or suspensions of cultured cells. They may be unfixed or fixed in a mixture suitable for lipid histochemistry.

(1)   Place a drop of the Nile red working solution (see above) on the preparation, apply a coverslip, and wait for 5 min.
(2)   Examine in a fluorescence microscope. Two filter sets are needed: one for blue excitation (as used for fluorescein) and one for green excitation (as used for rhodamine derivatives).

Result
With blue exciting light, hydrophobic lipids (neutral fat or cholesterol) show orange-yellow fluorescence. This can be prevented by prior extraction with acetone or alcohol. With green excitation, phospholipids show red fluorescence.

Notes
(1)   Nile blue sulphate (presumably containing Nile red) has been used as a fluorochrome for the examination of muscle biopsies (Bonilla and Prelle, 1987).
(2)   Malinin (1980) found that different types of intracellular lipid inclusions could be distinguished from one another by staining with Nile red at various temperatures from 19–65°C. (See also Section 12.5.1).
(3)   Anilinonaphthalene sulphonic acid (ANSA) was used by Cowden and Curtis (1974) as a supravital fluorochrome for hydrophobic cytoplasmic inclusions in the cells of invertebrates. ANSA can also impart fluorescence to hydrophobic proteins such as elastin (Vidal, 1978).

13.1. General considerations

Inorganic ions are present in all parts of all tissues, but owing to their solubility they are not generally amenable to detection by histochemical methods. It has been possible to demonstrate some soluble ions, such as potassium and chloride, by making use of freeze-dried material or by including in the fixative a reagent that forms an insoluble salt with the ion concerned. It is, however, difficult to determine the extent to which a soluble ion has diffused during the course of the procedure from its location *in vivo* to the site at which the end-product of the histochemical reaction is seen.

When inorganic substances are present in tissues as insoluble compounds, be these salts such as calcium carbonate or complexes with protein, such as haemosiderin, they remain *in situ* while the specimens are being processed and can therefore be localized accurately by histochemical methods. Some metals, such as calcium, iron, and zinc, are present in animal tissues in sufficient quantity to allow their demonstration in normal material. Others are normally present but can be detected histochemically only when large amounts accumulate as the result of disease or experimental manipulation. There are other metals that are not involved in normal mammalian metabolism but may be found in the tissues following intoxication or excessive environmental exposure. Of the inorganic anions, phosphate and carbonate of mineralized tissue are the only ones normally present in an insoluble form.

Histochemical techniques for inorganic ions fall into two categories: those in which the visible products are black or coloured inorganic substances, and those in which coloured compounds are formed by chelation of metals by organic ligands. The chemistry of chelation was introduced in connection with dyeing (Chapter 5). It is important to realize that the methods described in this chapter will only detect metals present as ions in the tissue. Metals already bound by strong coordinate bonds to organic ligands cannot react with the reagents used to demonstrate their ions. For example, the iron in erythrocytes is so firmly combined with the haem group of haemoglobin that it will not give a positive reaction in histochemical tests for iron.

Comprehensive accounts of inorganic histochemistry are given by Lillie and Fullmer (1976, Chapter 12) and Pearse (1985, Chapter 20). It should be remembered that histochemistry is only one approach to the examination of metals and other elements in tissues. There are valuable physical methods too, including electron probe microanalysis, cathodoluminescence, mass spectrometry and laser microprobe emission spectroscopy. (For reviews, see Moreton, 1981; Schmidt and Moenke-Blankenburg, 1986.)

As examples of histochemical techniques for inorganic substances, we will consider some of the methods for calcium, phosphate (and carbonate), iron, zinc, copper, and lead.

13.2. Calcium

This metal is demonstrated by virtue of its ability to form coloured chelates with dyes and other organic compounds. Dyes are chosen that do not form complexes of similar colour with other naturally occurring metals such as magnesium and iron. Acidic fixatives, which can dissolve calcium phosphate and carbonate, should not be used. Soluble calcium salts are present at low concentrations in extracellular and intracellular fluids. They can be immobilized by snap freezing and freeze-drying the tissue, or precipitated by including in the fixative an ion that forms an insoluble salt with calcium. Phosphate, fluoride, dichromate, oxalate and pyroantimonate ions are all suitable precipitants (see Vohringer *et al.*, 1995 for technical details and comparisons).

13.2.1.
Alizarin red S
method

Alizarin red S, is a synthetic anthraquinone dye (Chapter 5). Like other hydroxyanthraquinones, it forms chelates in which a quinone oxygen and a phenolic oxygen serve as electron donors to the metal atom, so that a stable six-membered ring is formed. Calcium, with coordination number 4, combines with two molecules of the dye:

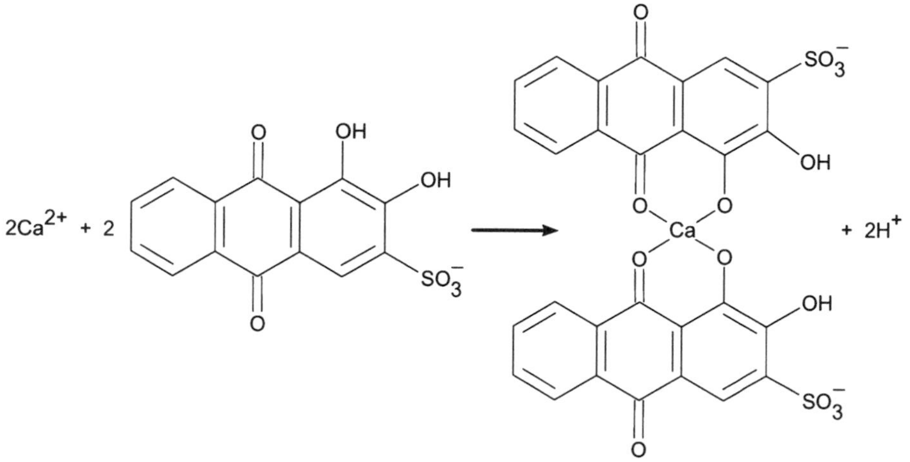

The structure shown is widely accepted but has been challenged by Lievremont *et al.* (1982), who found that when the complex was precipitated *in vitro*, the ratio of metal:dye was close to 1.0. They suggested chelation by the ionized phenol and sulphonic acid groups.

Alizarin red S is also an anionic dye in its own right and, as such, imparts non-specific pink 'background' coloration to the tissue.

The calcium ions must be released from the insoluble deposits in which they occur before they can combine with the dye to form an insoluble chelate. Consequently, some diffusion from the original site of deposition of calcium is inevitable. The histological picture is greatly influenced by the pH of the stain. An acid solution will extract much calcium and produce a conspicuous coloured deposit, but this will be diffusely localized. An alkaline solution will liberate fewer calcium ions, so that although the accuracy of localization will be greater the sensitivity of the method will be less. Different authors have recommended pH values ranging from 4–9 for solutions of alizarin red S.

An alcoholic or a neutral aqueous fixative should be used. Maximum preservation of calcium is probably achieved by fixation in 80% ethanol, though this is a poor fixative for histological purposes. Neutral, buffered formaldehyde is satisfactory.

Solutions required
A. Alizarin red

Alizarin red S (C.I. 58005):	1.0 g
Water:	90 ml

Add dilute NH_4OH (28% ammonia diluted 100 times with water) in small aliquots until the pH is approximately 6.1. Keeps for 4 weeks.

B. Differentiating fluid

Ethanol (95%):	500 ml
Concentrated hydrochloric acid:	0.05 ml

Mix before using, and use only once.

Procedure
(1) De-wax and hydrate paraffin sections.
(2) Stain in solution A for 2 min.
(3) Wash in water for 5–10 s.
(4) Differentiate in solution B for 15 s.
(5) Complete the dehydration in two changes of absolute ethanol, clear in xylene, and mount in a resinous medium.

Result
Calcium, orange to red. Background, dull pink.

13.2.2.
GBHA method

A more sensitive histochemical method for calcium involves a chelating agent that is not a dye. This is glyoxal-bis-(2-hydroxyanil), also known as GBHA:

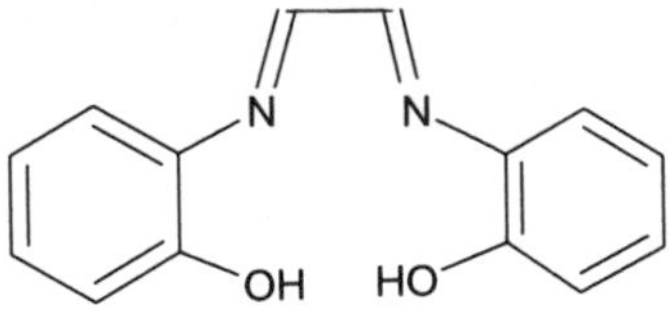

In the presence of a strong base such as sodium hydroxide, the phenolic hydroxyl groups ionize. The anion of GBHA forms insoluble chelates with several metals, including calcium:

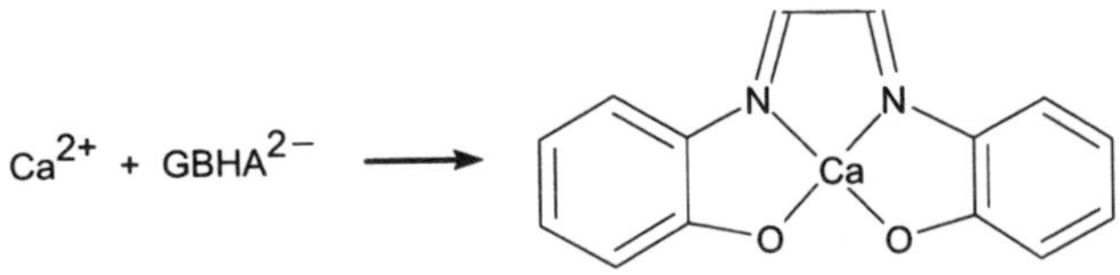

$$Ca^{2+} + GBHA^{2-} \longrightarrow$$

Metal chelates are also formed with strontium, barium, cadmium, cobalt, and nickel. If any of these metals are likely to be present in the tissue their chelates can be decomposed by treating the stained sections with an alkaline solution containing cyanide ions.

The GBHA method is very sensitive and can be used to detect calcium ions other than those of insoluble salts of the metal, provided that the tissue has been freeze-dried or freeze-substituted. After fixation in an aqueous reagent, the soluble calcium diffuses and some of it can be detected in nuclei of cells by the GBHA method. This artifact is presumably due to electrostatic attraction of calcium ions by the phosphate groups of nucleic acids. As with alizarin red S, the solution of GBHA used for staining deposits of insoluble calcium salts must contain some water and must not be too strongly alkaline. 'soluble' calcium salts, however, are best stained with a solution of GBHA in absolute ethanol containing some sodium hydroxide.

For this technique (Kashiwa and Atkinson, 1963; Kashiwa and House, 1964) it is essential to prepare the tissues as described and to avoid the use of any reagents (including water) that might contain traces of calcium.

Solutions required

A. GBHA stock solution

Glyoxal *bis*-(2-hydroxy-anil):	200 mg
Absolute ethanol:	50 ml

Keeps for several weeks at 4°C.

B. 10% NaOH solution

Sodium hydroxide(NaOH):	10 g
Water:	to make 100 ml

Keeps for several weeks.

C. GBHA working solution I

GBHA stock solution (A):	2.0 ml
10% NaOH (solution B):	0.15 ml
Water:	0.15 ml

Mix just before using.

D. GBHA working solution II

GBHA stock solution (A):	2.0 ml
10% NaOH (solution B):	0.6 ml

Mix just before using.

E. Alkaline cyanide solution

Absolute ethanol:	45 ml
Water:	5.0 ml
Sodium carbonate (Na_2CO_3):	to saturation (approx. 1.0 g)
Potassium cyanide (KCN):	to saturation (approx. 1.0 g)

Stable for a few weeks at room temperature.

Caution. Potassium cyanide is poisonous. Do not allow it to come into contact with acids. Before throwing it away add an excess of sodium hypochlorite solution and wait for 10 min. Then flush down sink with plenty of water.

F. Fast green FCF counterstain

Fast green FCF (C.I. 42053):	0.24 g
95% ethanol:	300 ml

Keeps for at least 5 years and may be used repeatedly.

Preparation of specimens

Freeze small blocks, no more than 2.0 mm³, in isopentane cooled in liquid nitrogen. *Either* freeze dry and embed in paraffin wax *or* freeze substitute in acetone at −80°C, clear in xylene, and embed in paraffin wax. Wolters *et al.* (1979) state that superior results are obtained by freeze substitution for 10 days at −80°C in acetone containing 1% oxalic acid (presumably as $H_2C_2O_4.2H_2O$). Cut sections at 7 μm and mount them onto slides without using water or any adhesive. Dry the slides at 40°C or less, so that the wax ribbons will not soften or melt. The sections are not dewaxed before staining. (See also *Note 2* below.)

Staining procedure

(1) Place the slides bearing the sections on a horizontal staining rack. **Do not remove wax.**
(2) *Either:* flood with GBHA working solution I (C) for 3 min,
     or: apply one or two drops of GBHA working solution II (D) per section and allow to evaporate to dryness.
(3) Rinse in 70% ethanol, then in 95% ethanol.
(4) (Optional, see *Note 1* below.) Immerse for 15 min in alkaline cyanide solution (E).
(5) Rinse in three changes of 95% ethanol.
(6) Apply a counterstain, if desired: rinse in absolute ethanol; de-wax in xylene; rinse in absolute, followed by 95% ethanol. Stain in alcoholic fast green FCF (solution F) for 3 min. Rinse in three changes of 95% ethanol, then proceed to Step 7 below.
(7) Dehydrate in four changes of absolute ethanol, clear in xylene, and mount in a resinous medium.

Results

When GBHA working solution I is used, a red colour is seen at sites of soluble calcium salts, but insoluble calcified material is largely unstained. With GBHA working solution II, the red colour is seen predominantly at sites of insoluble calcium salts. If the fast green FCF counterstain is used, the background is bluish green. The red colour fades after 2 or 3 days, so the sections should be photographed to obtain a permanent record.

Notes

(1) The alkaline cyanide reagent decolorizes the chelates of metals other than calcium (Sr^{2+}, Ba^{2+}, Cd^{2+}, Co^{2+}, Ni^{2+}). Step 4 may be omitted if the presence of other metals is unlikely.
(2) It is necessary to use freeze-dried or freeze substituted tissue in order to minimize the diffusion of the calcium ions dissolved in the cytoplasm and extracellular fluid. If the method is applied to sections of conventionally fixed tissue, calcified material is stained but there is also red staining of nuclei, cytoplasmic RNA, and sites of proteoglycans (Chapter 11). These artifacts are due to electrostatic attraction of diffused calcium ions to macromolecular anions.
(3) A green filter in the illuminating system of the microscope enhances the contrast of the red stained calcium deposits and is recommended for black and white photomicrography.

13.3. Phosphate and carbonate

The **von Kossa technique** is often designated as a histochemical method for calcium, but it is really a method for phosphate and carbonate, the anions with which the metal is associated in normal and pathological calcified tissues.

The sections are treated with silver nitrate. The calcium cations are replaced by silver:

$$CaCO_3(s) + 2Ag^{2+} \longrightarrow Ag_2CO_3(s) + Ca^{2+}$$

$$Ca_3(PO_4)_2(s) + 6Ag^+ \longrightarrow 2Ag_3PO_4(s) + 3Ca^{2+}$$

(The phosphates are really more complicated compounds than those indicated in this simple equation.)

The reaction is carried out in bright light, which promotes the reduction to metal of silver ions in the crystals of the insoluble silver phosphate and carbonate. Alternatively, the silver nitrate may be applied in darkness or subdued light and the reduction accomplished chemically with a solution of hydroquinone, metol or another photographic developing agent. Finely divided metallic silver is black. Any unreduced ionized silver is finally removed by treatment with sodium thiosulphate, which dissolves otherwise insoluble salts by forming complex anions such as $[Ag(S_2O_3)_3]^{5-}$.

The von Kossa procedure provides sharp and accurate localizations of calcified material in tissues, but it is less sensitive than the alizarin red S or the GBHA methods for calcium. Acid fixatives are best avoided for this method. Neutral formaldehyde is satisfactory.

Solutions required
Solution A must be made up in the purest available water. All these solutions can be used repeatedly until precipitates form in them.

A. 1% aqueous silver nitrate ($AgNO_3$)

B. 5% aqueous sodium thiosulphate ($Na_2S_2O_3.5H_2O$)

C. A counterstain
0.5% safranine or neutral red is suitable. See Chapter 6 for other possibilities.

Procedure
(1)   De-wax and hydrate paraffin sections. Wash in water.
(2)   Immerse in silver nitrate (Solution A) in bright sunlight or directly underneath a 100 W electric light bulb for 15 min.
(3)   Rinse in two changes of water.
(4)   Immerse in sodium thiosulphate (Solution B) for 2 min.
(5)   Wash in three changes of water.
(6)   Counterstain nuclei (Solution C), about 1 min.
(7)   Rinse briefly in water.
(8)   Dehydrate (and differentiate the counterstain) in 95% and two changes of absolute alcohol.
(9)   Clear in xylene and mount in a resinous medium.

Result
Sites of insoluble phosphates and carbonates black, brown or yellow. Nuclei pink or red.

Note
Instead of silver nitrate, Rungby et al. (1993) used 0.05% silver lactate, for 40 min without bright light, in Step 2 of the method. They then immersed the sections in freshly prepared 0.5% aqueous hydroquinone, followed by a wash in water, between steps 3 and 4. The use of silver lactate increased the sensitivity of the method and resulted in largely black deposits.

13.4. Iron

The major deposits of iron in mammals are in the red blood cells as haemoglobin, and in phagocytic cells (macrophages, microglia, etc.) as ferritin and haemosiderin. In these compounds, the metal is present in the ferric (oxidation state +3) form, but, being complexed to protein, it is not available as ions to participate in simple chemical reactions.

The iron of ferritin and haemosiderin is readily released as Fe^{3+} ions by treatment with a dilute mineral acid. In the presence of ferrocyanide ions, Prussian blue is immediately precipitated:

$$4Fe^{3+} + 3[Fe(CN)_6]^{4-} \longrightarrow Fe_4[Fe(CN)_6]_3(s)$$

Prussian blue is a more complicated compound than the simple ferric ferrocyanide implied above (Section 10.8.2). This is the simplest histochemical test for iron; it is known as the Prussian blue reaction of Perls.

An alternative strategy is to reduce all the ferric ions in the section to ferrous by treatment with a dilute aqueous solution of ammonium sulphide:

$$2Fe^{3+} + 3S^{2-} \longrightarrow 2FeS(s) + S$$

The sulphur dissolves in the excess of aqueous ammonium sulphide. Ferrous sulphide is soluble in dilute mineral acids, so when the sections are treated with an acidified potassium ferricyanide solution:

$$FeS(s) + 2H^+ \longrightarrow Fe^{2+} + H_2S(g)$$

$$3Fe^{2+} + 2[Fe(CN)_6]^{3-} \longrightarrow Fe_3[Fe(CN)_6]_2(s)$$

As explained in Chapter 10 (Section 10.8.2), the precipitate of 'Turnbull's blue' is not really ferrous ferricyanide, but is identical to Prussian blue. This method would, of course, also detect any ferrous ions that were initially present in a tissue.

The simple Perls method is adequate for the detection of iron in higher vertebrates, but according to Gabe (1976) the Turnbull blue technique is more sensitive and is preferred for the demonstration of iron in the tissues of cold blooded vertebrates and invertebrates. The Perls reaction is also suitable for the identification of exogenous ferritin introduced into animals as an experimental tracer protein (Parmley *et al.*, 1978).

It should be noted that the iron of haemoglobin cannot be released as ions by any method that does not totally destroy the section.

Stainable iron can be **removed** from sections by treatment with acid in the absence of a precipitant anion. Aqueous solutions of oxalic acid or sodium dithionite are also suitable for this purpose (Morton, 1978) and act more rapidly than dilute mineral acids.

13.4.1.
Perls' Prussian blue method

The fixative should not be acidic and should not contain dichromate. Hadler *et al.* (1969) compared several fixatives and found that the largest amounts of histochemically detectable iron were preserved by immersion of tissues for 24 h in 6% aqueous formaldehyde containing 0.27 M calcium chloride, with the pH adjusted to 4.0 by addition of 0.1 M NaOH or 0.1 M HCl. Alcoholic fixatives or buffered aqueous formaldehyde solutions were somewhat less satisfactory. Decalcification of a bone-containing specimen extracts stainable iron from cells in the marrow (DePalma, 1996).

Solutions required

A. Acid ferrocyanide reagent

Potassium ferrocyanide:	2.0 g
Water:	100 ml

Dissolve, and add:

Concentrated hydrochloric acid:	2.0 ml

Use reagent-grade HCl that does not contain iron. Prepare just before using.

B. Counterstain for nuclei

0.5% aqueous safranine or neutral red is suitable (Chapter 6 for other possibilities; nuclear fast red is commonly used).

Procedure

(1) De-wax and hydrate paraffin sections.
(2) Immerse in acid ferrocyanide reagent (Solution A) for 30 min.
(3) Wash in four changes of water.
(4) Counterstain nuclei (Solution B), about 1 min.
(5) Rinse briefly in water.
(6) Dehydrate (and differentiate the counterstain) in 95% and two changes of absolute alcohol.
(7) Clear in xylene and mount in a resinous medium.

Result

Blue precipitate with Fe^{3+} liberated from ferritin and haemosiderin. Nuclei pink or red. Haemoglobin is not stained. See *Note 1* below for a control procedure.

Notes

(1) Iron can be removed, before staining, by treatment of the hydrated sections with 5% aqueous oxalic acid ($H_2C_2O_4.2H_2O$) for 6 h or with freshly prepared 1% sodium dithionite (sodium hydrosulphite, $Na_2S_2O_4$) in acetate buffer, pH 4.5, for 5 min. Perls' method is also applicable to sections of plastic-embedded tissue, but the times required for extraction of iron are longer: 12 h for oxalic acid or 15 min for sodium dithionite (Morton, 1978). A negative result after this extraction shows that the sections were not coloured artifactually as a consequence of the presence of unwanted traces of iron in the acid ferrocyanide reagent.

(2) The stained slides fade after a year or two of storage. One way to avoid fading is based on the ability of Prussian blue to catalyse the oxidation of 3,3'-diaminobenzidine (DAB) by hydrogen peroxide (Nguyen-Legros et al., 1980). The product of the catalysed reaction is an insoluble brown polymer that does not fade. To make preparations permanent in this way, carry out the DAB reaction for peroxidase (Section 16.5.4) between Steps 3 and 4 of Perls' method. The DAB procedure increases the sensitivity of the Perls reaction, allowing the detection of intracellular iron deposits in the brain that are not otherwise visible (Morris et al., 1992; Connor et al., 1995). The sensitivity of the DAB-enhanced method can be further increased by treating the sections sequentially with methenamine-silver, gold chloride and uranyl nitrate; for details see Moos and Mollgard (1993).

13.5. Zinc

Zinc is associated with insulin in the B cells of the pancreatic islets, with various enzymes (notably carbonic anhydrase in exocrine glands), in the cytoplasmic granules of leukocytes and of the Paneth cells of the small intestine, and in synapses in certain regions of the brain. The proteins that bind zinc are easily denatured, with loss of the metal ions, so for histochemical demonstration it is desirable to use freeze-dried material, cryostat sections of unfixed tissue or air-dried smears. If a liquid fixative must be used, cold absolute ethanol is probably the least objectionable one. Alternatively, the zinc may be precipitated by sulphide ions and then demonstrated by the sensitive but non-specific sulphide-silver technique (Section 13.8.2). Histochemical methods certainly do not detect all the zinc that can be shown by chemical analysis to be present in animal tissues (Elmes and Jones, 1981).

A useful reagent for the detection of zinc is **dithizone** (diphenylthiocarbazone; 3-mercapto-1,5-diphenylformazan):

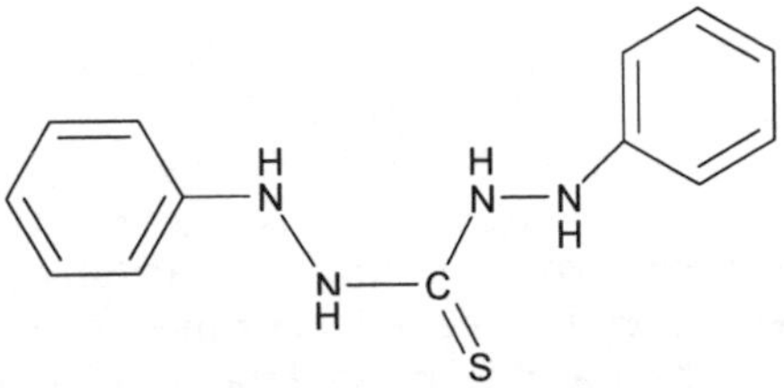

This compound forms a red chelate with zinc. Many other metal ions form differently coloured chelates with dithizone. The reagent has also been used for the histochemical detection of **mercury**, which forms a reddish-purple complex with the structure:

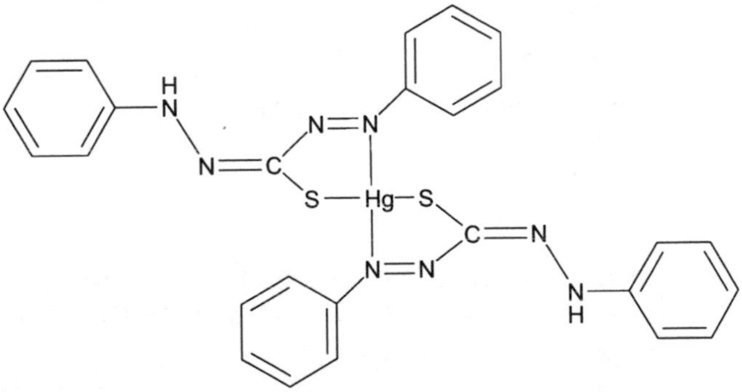

(See Harris and Livingstone, 1964). The zinc chelate probably has a similar structure (De *et al.*, 1970). Dithizone and metal–dithizone complexes are much more soluble in non-polar solvents than in water, so it is necessary to use an aqueous mounting medium for the stained preparations. However, it is necessary to use a non-polar solvent to wash off the excess of dithizone (which is itself coloured). The unusual procedure in the last three steps of the method described below is an attempt to reconcile the removal of the reagent with retention of the desired product.

**13.5.1.
Dithizone
method**

This method should be used with paraffin sections of freeze-dried tissue or with cryostat sections of unfixed tissue. Cryostat sections may be fixed for 10 min in absolute ethanol at 4°C to improve morphological preservation. If a liquid fixative is unavoidable, fix small pieces for 1 h at 4°C in absolute methanol or ethanol, clear in benzene or xylene, and prepare paraffin sections. Extraction of zinc may be reduced if sections are not flattened on water when mounting onto slides. Dinsdale (1984) fixed in absolute ethanol, cleared in propylene oxide, embedded in an epoxy resin, and used dithizone successfully on 1 µm sections that were collected directly into the staining solution.

Solutions required

A. Dithizone stock solution

Dithizone:	100 mg
Anhydrous acetone (Chapter 12, Section 12.4.2):	100 ml

Keeps for 1 or 2 months in darkness at 4°C

B. Complexing solution

Sodium thiosulphate ($Na_2S_2O_3.5H_2O$):	55 g
Sodium acetate (anhydrous):	5.4 g
Potassium cyanide (KCN) (**Caution.** Poisonous. See Section 13.2.2):	1.0 g
Water:	100 ml

Dissolve the salts in the water. Dissolve a little dithizone in 200 ml of carbon tetra-chloride. Shake the aqueous complexing solution in a separatory funnel with successive 50 ml aliquots of the solution of dithizone in CCl_4 until the CCl_4 layer is a clear green colour. This manipulation extracts traces of zinc from the reagents. The carbon tetrachloride fractions are discarded. (**Be careful.** The vapour of CCl_4 is toxic. Ideally, this solvent should be collected into a metal drum or canister designated for the disposal of 'chlorinated solvents', not a drum for ordinary 'waste solvents' such as alcohol and acetone.) The purified aqueous complexing solution is stable for a few months.

C. 1.0 M acetic acid

Glacial acetic acid:	60 ml
Water:	to make 1000 ml

Keeps indefinitely.

D. Sodium potassium tartrate solution

$NaKC_4H_4O_6.4H_2O$:	2 g
Water:	to make 100 ml

Keeps indefinitely.

E. Working dithizone solution (see also *Note 1* below)
This is mixed when needed and used immediately.

Solution A:	24 ml
Water:	18 ml

Add 1.0 M acetic acid (Solution C) in 0.1 ml aliquots until the pH is 3.7 (about 2 ml required).

Solution B:	5.8 ml
Solution D:	0.2 ml

F. Chloroform (required for rinsing)

Procedure

(1) *Cryostat sections:* Allow to dry on coverslips or slides.
   Paraffin sections: De-wax in xylene (three changes) and allow to dry by evaporation.
(2) Immerse the slides or coverslips bearing the sections in freshly mixed working dithizone solution (E) for 10 min.
(3) Rinse the slides or coverslips in two changes of chloroform (F), with agitation, for 30 s.
(4) Pour off the chloroform and allow the slides or coverslips to drain but do not let the solvent evaporate completely (to avoid cracking of the sections).

(5) Rinse in water, allow most of the water to drain off onto filter paper, and put a drop of an aqueous mounting medium onto each section. Apply slides or coverslips according to the type of preparation.

Result
A red to purple colour is formed where zinc is present in the tissue. See *Notes 1* and *2* below.

Notes
(1) The complexing solution is mixed with the dithizone to prevent the formation of coloured chelates with metals other than zinc. 24 ml of Solution A may be diluted with 16 ml of water instead of with Solutions B, C, and D as described above. This simple dithizone solution will form coloured complexes with Ag, Au, Bi, Cd, Co, Cu, Fe, Hg, In, Mn, Ni, Pb, Pd, Pt, Sn, and Tl, as well as with Zn.
(2) Zinc is removed by treating control sections for 5 min with 1% aqueous acetic acid before staining.
(3) The sulphide-silver method (Section 13.8.2) will detect concentrations of zinc that are too low to give a visible colour with dithizone.

13.6. Copper

Normal adult mammalian tissues do not contain enough copper to allow histochemical detection of the metal, but in Wilson's disease (hepato-lenticular degeneration) large quantities of the metal accumulate in phagocytic cells in the brain, liver, and cornea. The fetal liver has stainable copper in the hepatocytes. It is also possible, of course, to demonstrate copper that has been artificially introduced into an animal. In some arthropods and molluscs the haemocyanins, respiratory pigments equivalent to the haemoglobin of vertebrate animals, are copper-containing proteins dissolved in the plasma. Copper ions can be released from combination with protein by exposing sections to the fumes of concentrated hydrochloric acid.

The most satisfactory histochemical method for the detection of copper (as the cupric ion, oxidation state +2) makes use of a chelating agent, **dithiooxamide** (also called **rubeanic acid**):

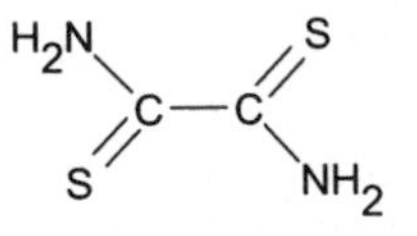

This reagent forms an insoluble dark-green chelate with copper in the presence of ethanol and acetate in alkaline solution. Other metals, such as nickel, cobalt, and silver, also form coloured complexes with dithiooxamide, but under these conditions they are unreactive or give soluble complexes. The copper chelate is believed to be a polymer with the structure:

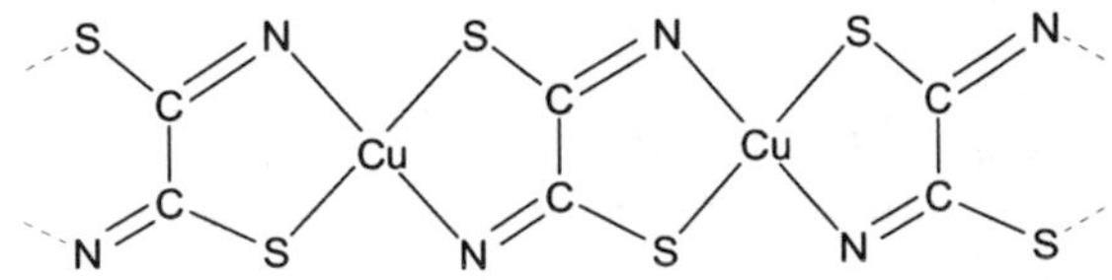

(Harris and Livingstone, 1964). Dithiooxamide combines only with cupric ions. A reagent that forms a coloured complex with cuprous ions is *p*-dimethylaminobenzylidenerhodanine:

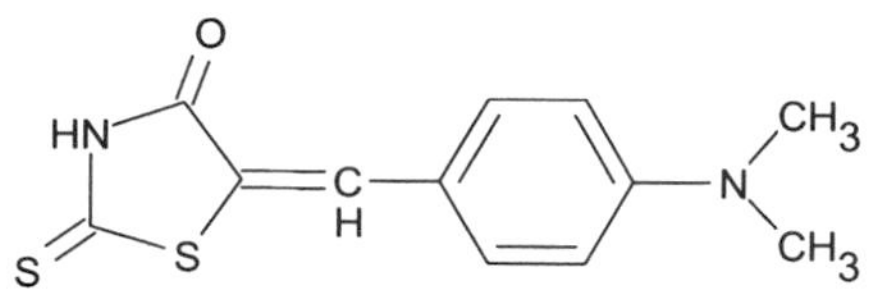

Copper probably replaces the hydrogen attached to the nitrogen atom in the five-membered ring to form a red product. Brown, red, and purple compounds are formed with several other metals. Irons *et al.* (1977) found that whereas dithiooxamide and *p*-dimethylaminobenzylidenerhodanine were equally sensitive reagents for the histochemical detection of copper, only the latter gave an intensity of staining proportional to the concentration of the metal in the tissue.

Little attention has been paid by histochemists to the oxidation states of copper in tissues. The invertebrate haemocyanins contain Cu(I), whereas coeruloplasmin, the copper-binding globulin of mammalian blood plasma, contains both Cu(I) and Cu(II). The copper-containing deposits in the tissues of patients with Wilson's disease are stainable with dithiooxamide, so they must consist partly or entirely of a compound capable of releasing cupric ions. Further study of the interconversion of Cu(I) and Cu(II) in tissues, which is readily brought about by treatment with oxidizing and reducing agents, might lead to broadening of the applicability of histochemical techniques for the demonstration of copper.

13.6.1.
Dithiooxamide method

This technique is applicable to frozen or paraffin sections of specimens fixed in phosphate-buffered formaldehyde, to cryostat sections of unfixed tissue, and to de-waxed paraffin sections of freeze-dried material. Fixatives other than formaldehyde are probably acceptable but have not been investigated. It is probably desirable for the fixative to contain anions such as phosphate, hydroxide, or carbonate that form insoluble copper salts.

Solution required

Dithiooxamide (rubeanic acid):	0.2 g
70% aqueous ethanol:	200 ml
Sodium acetate (CH_3COONa):	0.4 g

Keeps for several months.

Procedure

(1) Take frozen or paraffin sections to water. (See *Note 1*.)
(2) Immerse in the dithiooxamide reagent for 30 min.
(3) Rinse in two changes of 70% ethanol. (See *Note 2*.)
(4) Dehydrate, clear, and mount in a resinous medium.

Result

Sites of copper deposits dark green to black.

Notes

(1) According to Pearse (1985), protein-bound copper can be released by placing the slides (after de-waxing) face downwards over a beaker of concentrated hydrochloric acid for 15 min followed by immersion for 15 min in 100% ethanol.
(2) A counterstain may be applied after stage 3.

13.6.2.
p-Dimethyl-
aminobenzyl-
idenerhodanine
method

The following method is for paraffin sections of material that has been fixed in neu-tral fuffered formalin (Churukian, 1997).

Solutions required
A. 0.4% p-dimethylaminobenzylidenerhodanine

p-Dimethylaminobenzylidenerhodanine:	24 mg
100% alcohol:	6.0 ml

Prepare on the day it is to be used.

B. 65 mM sodium acetate

Sodium acetate: *Either* $CH_3COONa.3H_2O$:	2 g
or CH_3COONa:	1.6 g
Water:	100 ml

This is stable indefinitely, but should not be used if it shows signs of mould or bac-terial growth.

C. Working p-dimethylaminobenzylidenerhodanine solution
Immediately before using, filter Solution A (Whatman No. 4 paper) into 45 ml of Solution B.

D. A counterstain
A haemalum is suitable; see Chapter 6 for methods.

Procedure
(1) De-wax and hydrate paraffin sections.
(2) Place slides in the working p-dimethylaminobenzylidenerhodanine solution (C) in a closed coplin jar, overnight at 37°C. (See also *Note 1* below.)
(3) Wash in 6 changes of water.
(4) Counterstain nuclei (but not strongly) with haemalum.
(5) Wash in 4 changes of water.
(6) Apply coverslips, using an aqueous mounting medium such as Apathy's (see *Note 3* below).

Result
Sites of copper brownish-red, as granular deposits within cells. Nuclei (if counter-stained as suggested) are blue.

Notes
(1) Churukian (2000) reduced the staining time to 11 mins by increasing the temperature to 80°C, in a microwave oven. He stated the the result was sometimes less satisfactory than with the overnight method.
(2) See also *Note 1* following the preceding method.
(3) Instructions for making aqueous mounting media are given in Chapter 4 (Section 4.3.2).

13.7. Lead

Lead has no known physiological function. It can be demonstrated histochemically in the tissues of animals or people poisoned by its salts. The element accumulates in intranuclear inclusion bodies, especially in the kidney (Goyer and Cherian, 1977).

The simplest histochemical method for lead is based on the formation of the insol-uble chromate, $PbCrO_4$, which is yellow. In order to ensure precipitation of lead ions, it is prudent to include sulphate ions in the fixative. Lead sulphate is insoluble in water (solubility product $= 1.6 \times 10^{-8}$), but the chromate is even less soluble (solubility product $= 2.8 \times 10^{-13}$), so the reaction:

$$PbSO_4(s) \ + \ CrO_4{}^{2-} \longrightarrow PbCrO_4(s) \ + \ SO_4{}^{2-}$$

can proceed, though slowly, in the direction indicated.

This is a fairly specific test for lead. (The other metals that have insoluble yellow chromates are Ba, Sm, Sr, Tl, and Zn.) The product, however, is not conspicuous in thin sections. A brighter coloration is obtained by using a chelating agent, sodium or potassium rhodizonate:

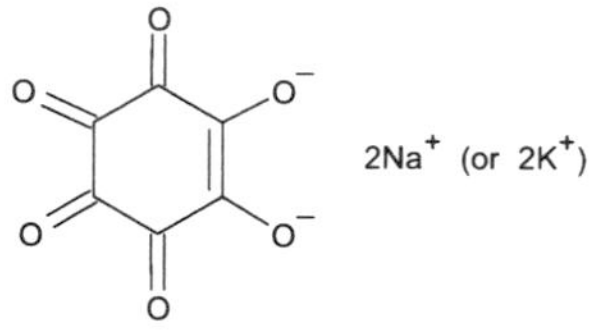

13.7.1.
Rhodizonate method

Under mildly acid conditions this forms a pink to red chelate with lead. Neutral solutions of the reagent give a brown product (Molnar, 1952). Barium, strontium, and mercury can also form red compounds with rhodizonate, and a blue-black product is formed with iron (Pearse, 1985).

This method is applicable to frozen or paraffin sections of formaldehyde-fixed specimens. An anion such as sulphate or phosphate should be present in the fixative to ensure precipitation of salts of lead. If the technique is to be applied to bone, sodium sulphate ($Na_2SO_4.10H_2O$; 5–10% w/v) should be added to the decalcifying fluid.

Solution required

Sodium (or potassium) rhodizonate:	0.2 g
Water:	99 ml
Glacial acetic acid:	1.0 ml

This should be prepared just before using and protected from light.

Procedure
(1) Take sections to water.
(2) Immerse in rhodizonate solution for 30 min, in darkness.
(3) Wash in water.
(4) Mount in a water-soluble medium.

Result
Sites of salts of lead are pink to red, or brown.

Notes
(1) Several other metals form coloured rhodizonate complexes, notably Ag, Ba, Bi, Ca, Cd, $Hg_2{}^{2+}$, Sn, Sr, Tl and $UO_2{}^{2+}$. Confusion with Pb is unlikely in tissues from experimental animals. See Feigl and Anger (1972) and Lillie and Fullmer (1976) for suggested methods for increasing the specificity of the method if you suspect the presence of one of these other metals.
(2) Normal keratinizing structures can be coloured by rhodizonate (Shelley, 1970). Sections of tissue known not to contain lead should be stained as negative controls.

13.8. Methods of high sensitivity but low specificity

Some histochemical techniques for metal ions have greater sensitivity than those described in the preceding sections of this chapter. Such methods, however, do not identify the detected element with any certainty. The specificity can sometimes be improved by the use of control procedures, or the investigator may already know what the metal is, and be interested only in its localization in the tissue. Two of these methods will now be discussed.

13.8.1.
Detection of metals with haematoxylin

The chemistry of haematoxylin and haematein was reviewed in Chapter 5. The ability of haematein to form darkly coloured complexes with many metals makes the dye useful in the histochemistry of inorganic ions. For greatest sensitivity, the solution should be freshly made from haematoxylin. According to Lillie and Fullmer (1976) haematoxylin itself is the reagent in this histochemical test. It seems likely, however, that haematein (formed by atmospheric oxidation) is the substance that forms coloured metal complexes.

Procedure
This method may be applied to frozen or paraffin sections. The fixative should contain an appropriate precipitating ion (a phosphate buffer, pH 7–8 is generally suitable), and the purest available water and other chemicals must be used in the fixative and all other solutions used.

(1) Take the sections to water (which must not be contaminated with traces of metal salts).
(2) Dissolve 50 mg haematoxylin (C.I. 75290) in 1 ml of absolute ethanol. Add the solution to 99 ml of the purest available water. The solution is almost colourless at first and becomes pink on standing.
(3) Stain the sections in the freshly prepared haematoxylin solution. Examine after 2 h. If nothing is seen, leave overnight.
(4) Do not wash in water. Transfer from the staining solution to 95%, then 2 changes of 100% ethanol.
(5) Clear in xylene and mount in a synthetic resinous mounting medium.

Results
Colours are obtained with the following metals (cited from Lillie and Fullmer, 1976):

Al	Blue-black	Nd	Blue
Be	Blue	Ni	Blue
Bi	Purple	Os	Blue or greenish-brown
Cr	Blue-black	Pb	Blue
Cu	Greenish-blue	Pt	Blue
Dy	Blue	Rh	Blue
Fe	Blue-black	Sn	Purplish-red
Ga	Blue-black	Ta	Brownish-red
Hf	Blue-black	Tb	Blue
Ho	Blue	Ti	Brown
In	Blue-black	Tl	Purplish-red
Ir	Blue	U	Blue
Mn	Blue	Yb	Blue
Mo	Blue	Zn	Blue
Nb	Brown	Zr	Blue-black

Notes
(1) All the above metals react with unbuffered haematoxylin (pH 5–6). Optimum pH levels for staining a few metals are given by Lillie and Fullmer (1976), who also recommend a mounting medium with a low refractive index, so that the architecture of the unstained parts of the section can be seen.
(2) The sensitivity of the method can be increased by prolonging the staining time, which may be as long as 48 h.
(3) Another chromogenic chelating agent of low specificity is bromopyridylazo-diethylaminophenol (bromo-PADAP):

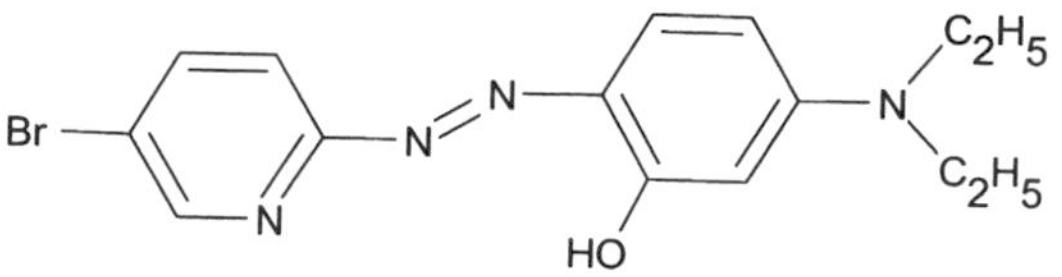

This has been used by Sumi *et al.* (1983a, 1999) as an extremely sensitive histochemical reagent for several metals. By treating the sections with suitable mixtures of colourless complexing agents, it is possible to 'mask' the colour reactions of some metals with bromo-PADAP while preserving those of others. Masking is derived from a comparable practice widely used in analytical chemistry, but chelating agents for histochemical use cannot be selected only on the basis of their chemical properties. The reactivities of chelating agents with metal salts in tissues often differ significantly from the reactions with the same salts in a test tube (Sumi *et al.*, 1983b).

13.8.2.
Timm's sulphide-silver method

In this technique, the fresh specimen is fixed in a liquid containing sulphide ions, either as hydrogen sulphide (bubbled through the fluid before use) or as sodium sulphide (more convenient and less smelly, but usable only with aqueous fixatives). Metals are precipitated:

$$M^{2+} + S^{2-} \longrightarrow MS(s)$$

In the above equation, M^{2+} is a cation of any metal that has an insoluble sulphide. The method has been used histochemically to detect Ag, Au, Ca, Co, Cu, Fe, Hg, Ni, Pb, Pt and Zn. Of these, copper, lead, mercury and zinc have been most often studied.

The next stage of Timm's method is the preparation of sections of the fixed and sulphide-treated specimen. The sections are treated with a **physical developer**, which is a solution containing silver ions, a reducing ('developing') agent, and a stabilizing agent that retards the reduction of silver ions to metal. Deposition of silver occurs first at sites where there are deposits of metal sulphide, because these have a catalytic action. Deposited silver also acts as a catalyst, so the black deposits of silver continue to accumulate, thus increasing the sizes and optical densities of the original sulphide precipitates. The slides must be removed from the physical developer and washed in water before there is appreciable reduction of Ag^+ to Ag at non-catalytic sites. For more information about physical developers, see Chapter 18.

The method now described is based on the modification of Timm's original method by Danscher and Zimmer (1978).

Solutions required
A. Aqueous fixative (for perfusion)

Sodium sulphide (Na_2S):	11.7 g
Sodium phosphate, monobasic ($NaH_2PO_4.H_2O$):	11.9 g
Water:	1000 ml

Mix in fume cupboard, immediately before use. Sodium sulphide is deliquescent, and cannot be weighed accurately unless it is new and dry.

About 1 l of a phosphate-buffered 3% glutaraldehyde solution (Chapter 2) will also be needed.

B. Alcoholic fixative (for immersion)

Bubble hydrogen sulphide (from a Kipp's apparatus or similar generator) through 200 ml of *either* 70% ethanol *or* Carnoy's fluid (Chapter 2), for 5 min in a fume cupboard.

Caution. Hydrogen sulphide is malodorous and poisonous.

C. Physical developer
This is made from four stable stock solutions.

The first three ingredients of the developer may be mixed several hours in advance, but the last ($AgNO_3$) is added immediately before using.

50% (w/v) aqueous gum arabic (see *Note 1* below):	60 ml
Citrate buffer (see *Note 2*):	10 ml
Hydroquinone (5.67% w/v, aqueous):	30 ml
Silver nitrate (17% w/v, aqueous):	0.5 ml

Procedure
(1) Arrange to fix an anaesthetized rat by vascular perfusion (Chapter 2). Inject 5 ml of the sodium sulphide solution (A) into the tubing, then perfuse the buffered glutaraldehyde for 3 min. Next, perfuse sodium sulphide (Solution A) for about 10 min. This uses up some 250 ml of the solution. Remove the organs of interest, and continue their fixation by immersion of small pieces (no more than 2 mm thick) in buffered glutaraldehyde for 1 h.
Alternatively, fix pieces of tissue by immersion in an alcoholic fixative that is saturated with hydrogen sulphide (Solution B), overnight at room temperature.
(2) Dehydrate in graded alcohols.
(3) Either embed in plastic (after the aqueous fixative) or dehydrate, clear (48 h in toluene recommended) and embed in paraffin wax (after either fixative). Cut sections and mount them on slides.
(4) Bring the sections to water. (Wax must be removed, but plastic need not be removed.)
(5) Add the last ingredient to the physical developer (Solution C) and immerse the slides in it for 30–90 min. *Remove a slide from time to time, rinse in water, and check with a microscope.* With excessive time in the developer there will be non-catalytic reduction of silver, with generalized non-specific brown staining of the sections.
(6) Rinse slides in water, then wash for 5 min in running tap water.
(7) Counterstain, if desired. Any method that does not give dark colours is suitable.
(8) Wash, dehydrate, clear, and cover, using a resinous mounting medium.

Result
Sites of heavy metals black. Background according to counterstain. If no counterstain is used, a faint yellow-brown background colour may be discernible.

Notes
(1) Gum arabic is slow to dissolve. The viscous solution should be filtered through cloth, and stored frozen in 60 ml aliquots.
(2) Preparation of stock citrate buffer:

Citric acid ($H_3C_6H_5O_7.H_2O$):	25.5 g
Sodium citrate ($Na_3C_6H_5O_7.2H_2O$):	23.5 g
Dissolve in water and make up to:	100 ml

The pH is 3.7. Keeps for several months.
(3) Timm's sulphide-silver method can also be used for electron microscopy. Practical instructions are given by Danscher and Zimmer (1978) and Danscher and Norgaard (1985). Zinc can be detected in synaptic vesicles of certain neurons in the brain (Danscher, 1996).
(4) Sodium selenide can be used, with advantage, instead of sulphide, to precipitate endogenous zinc in the central nervous system. The technique is described and discussed in detail by Danscher and Stoltenberg (2005).

14 Enzyme histochemistry: general considerations

This chapter introduces the large subject of enzyme histochemistry. A short account of the general properties of enzymes is followed by a discussion of the physical and chemical principles underlying the methods used for their localization in tissues. These techniques are exemplified by more detailed treatments of the histochemistry of some hydrolytic enzymes (Chapter 15) and some oxidative enzymes (Chapter 16).

14.1. Some properties of enzymes

An enzyme is a protein that serves as a catalyst. The catalysis is brought about by combination of a molecule of the enzyme with a molecule of one of the reactants, known as the **substrate**. The substrate, which is nearly always an organic compound or ion, is thereby made more chemically active than it otherwise would be towards another reactant. The products of the reaction are released from the enzyme molecule, which will then be free to bind another molecule of the substrate. It is an important feature of enzymatic catalysis that reactions are enabled to occur at ambient or body temperature, usually in a medium whose pH is near to neutrality. In the absence of enzymes, the same chemical reactions might never proceed, or would take place only at unphysiologically high temperatures, in strongly acid or alkaline solutions, or in non-aqueous solvents.

Individual enzymes are highly specific for their substrates and for the types of reaction they catalyse. The substrate specificity is not always absolute, however, and this is fortunate for the biochemist or histochemist. By providing an artificial substrate, similar to the natural one, it is often possible to study the enzymatic catalysis of a reaction that yields products more easily detectable than those generated from the physiological substrate. Insoluble coloured end-products are desirable in enzyme histochemistry.

For more information about enzymes and their physiological functions the reader should consult a textbook of biochemistry or enzymology. A comprehensive work of reference is that of Dixon and Webb (1979). The histochemistry of enzymes is treated in great detail by Burstone (1962), Lojda et al. (1979) and Stoward and Pearse (1991). Useful shorter books on the subject include Chayen and Bitensky

(1991) and Van Noorden and Frederiks (1992). For plant enzymes, see Vaughn (1987). For enzyme histochemistry with the electron microscope, see Hayat (1973–1977) or (in German) Wöhlrab and Gossrau (1991).

14.2. Names of enzymes

Knowledge of enzymes and their properties has, like all other scientific information, been acquired gradually. The recognition of more and more enzymes has led to a bewildering profusion of names for these substances. The International Union of Biochemistry has introduced a scheme of nomenclature in which each enzyme is named according to the reaction it catalyses. The system also embraces a classification of enzymes and allows the use of approved trivial names when the full systematic names are cumbersome. Each enzyme is given a number (the Enzyme Commission, **E.C. number**), which establishes its place in the classification. For example, E.C.3.1.1.3 is one of the major group (Group 3) of hydrolases. It acts on ester bonds (3.1) of carboxylic acids (3.1.1) and is the third member (3.1.1.3) of the list of carboxylic ester hydrolases. Its systematic name is triacylglycerol ester hydrolase, and its recommended trivial name is triacylglycerol lipase. It catalyses the reaction:

$$\text{A triglyceride} \;+\; H_2O \xrightarrow{\text{(lipase)}} \text{A diglyceride} \;+\; \text{a fatty acid}$$

The approved trivial names of enzymes are used in this and the following two chapters. The E.C. numbers and systematic names are given at the first mention in the text. Some non-approved names must also be used and discussed. This is an unfortunate consequence of the fact that the histochemical study of enzymes is a less precise science than biochemical enzymology.

14.3. Scope and limitations of enzyme histochemistry

The accurate identification of the cellular and subcellular locations of many enzymes has been one of the most conspicuous achievements of modern histochemistry. When using a method for the detection of a particular enzyme, a histochemist seeks answers to two questions.

(1) *Is the activity detected in the tissue the same as the activity of the purified enzyme identified by biochemical methods?* This is a re-statement of the requirement for chemical specificity associated with every histochemical technique. It is important to remember that the biochemist purifies enzymes from homogenized tissue and usually studies their properties in solution. In a section of tissue, many enzymes are present, and all of them may be available to act upon the histochemical reagents chosen for the purpose of demonstrating just one of their number.

    The sequestration of an enzyme in an organelle can impede the access of histochemical reagents and apparently suppress the activity of that enzyme in a section. Histochemical techniques are usually devised in such a way as to detect as much enzymatic action as possible, but an enzyme is not necessarily fully active, all the time, in all parts of all the cells in which it is present.

(2) *Where in the tissue is the enzyme located in vivo?* This is usually the more difficult question to answer. The problems associated with accuracy of localization are different for the three principal types of method used for the histochemical demonstration of enzymes. These will now be discussed.

14.4. Methods not based on enzymatic activity

Enzymes are proteins and are antigenic. It is therefore possible to prepare antibodies to purified enzymes and to use these antibodies in immunofluorescent and other **immunohistochemical techniques**. For accurate localization it is necessary that the antigenic (though not necessarily the catalytic) properties of the enzyme be unaffected by fixation or other pretreatment of the tissue, and that the enzyme does not diffuse away from its normal position before forming an insoluble complex with its antibody. Antigenicity is more resistant than catalytic activity to fixation and other preparative procedures. Large numbers of enzymes, including many for which there are no activity-based histochemical methods, are localized immunohistochemically, often with commercially available antibodies. The method is immunological, however, so it will not be further discussed in this chapter. Immunohistochemical techniques are dealt with in Chapter 19.

Another technique is that of **affinity labelling with specific inhibitors** of enzymes. The first method of this type to be described involved the binding of radioactively labelled DFP (Chapter 15) to sections. The bound inhibitor was then detected by autoradiography. Unfortunately this inhibitor attaches to and inhibits many enzymes that have serine residues at or near their substrate binding sites, so the specificity of the technique is low. Sodium, potassium-adenosine triphosphatase (**Na, K-ATPase**; a variant of E.C. 3.6.1.3, ATP phosphohydrolase), which is the sodium-potassium pump in cell mambranes, has been detected by virtue of its binding of ouabain, a specific inhibitor of the enzyme. The ouabain was covalently coupled to a peptide with peroxidase activity. The peptide could then be identified by a histochemical method for peroxidase (Chapter 16). This gave an osmiophilic product, visible with the electron microscope (Mazurkiewicz *et al.*, 1978).

Carbonic anhydrase (E.C. 4.2.2.1) was demonstrated by means of a fluorescent inhibitor, dimethylaminonaphthalene-5-sulphonamide, by Pochhammer *et al.* (1979). This inhibitor was given orally to animals, which were killed 7–12 h later. Cryostat sections of unfixed tissue were examined and it was possible, with appropriate filters, to distinguish the fluorescence of the enzyme-bound from that of the unbound inhibitor. Dermietzel *et al.* (1985) applied the same fluorescent inhibitor directly to unfixed cryostat sections. Controls for specificity included mixing the fluorescent compound with competitive non-fluorescent inhibitors.

Some irreversible enzyme inhibitors can be covalently tagged with a fluorochrome or other label, without impairment of the specificity. Thus, α-difluoromethylornithine is firmly and specifically bound by **ornithine decarboxylase** (L-ornithine carboxylyase; E.C. 4.1.1.17) after labelling with rhodamine or with biotin (Gilad and Gilad, 1981). Rhodamine is fluorescent. Labelling with biotin is discussed in Chapter 19.

A related application of enzyme-substrate affinity is the use of **polymers of an enzyme to detect its substrate** in sections of tissue. Thus, each molecule of glucose oxidase has two substrate-binding sites. Aggregates (made by mixing the enzyme with glutaraldehyde) will attach to α-D-glucosyl groups in sections of fixed tissue. The free active sites of the enzyme aggregates are then demonstrated histochemically (Dermietzel *et al.*, 1985).

14.5. Methods based on enzymatic activity

14.5.1.
Substrate-film methods

In this type of technique, the enzyme acts upon a substrate carried in a film of some suitable material which is closely applied to the section of tissue. After incubation for an appropriate time, the change in the substrate is detected by any expedient means. The sites of change in the film can then be seen to correspond to sites in the underlying (or overlying) section.

Substrate-film techniques are potentially very versatile, but they have two important limitations. Firstly, **the enzyme must diffuse** from its original locus to the film. Diffusion takes place in all directions, not just straight up or down, so changes in the film occur at some distance from the place in which the enzyme was located in the section. The inaccuracy from this cause is minimized if the contact between section and film is uniformly very close, and if the film is as thin as is compatible with seeing the changes in it. Secondly, **the change produced in the substrate must be immediate** and irreversible, otherwise lateral diffusion of products of enzymatic action within the film would render the method useless. Probably the highest resolution that can be expected with a substrate-film technique is the identification of the cells in which an enzyme is contained.

A method related to the substrate-film procedure is the **enzyme transfer technique**, developed by Schulz-Harder and Graf Von Keyserlingk (1988) for the localization of ribonuclease activity. The enzyme is transferred electrophoretically from a cryostat section to a polyacrylamide gel containing RNA. The gel is incubated for a suitable time, and the remaining RNA is then fluorescently stained with ethidium bromide (Chapter 9). The original section is stained, and its microscopic appearance is compared with that of the gel. This approach may be suitable for other enzymes too.

Soluble substrates and other reagents are often included in a gelatinous film applied to the section, but in this case the substrate diffuses into the section, and the enzyme (ideally) does not move. This approach reduces diffusion of the enzyme and of intermediate reaction products. It is technically similar to the substrate film methods, but is really a dissolved substrate procedure, because the visible end-product is formed in the section, not in the film.

14.5.2.
Dissolved substrate methods

In these methods all reagents are used in solution and the end-products of enzymatic action are deposited within the sectioned tissue. The great majority of histochemical methods for enzymes fall into this category. In all such techniques, the enzyme in the section acts upon a substrate (often not the natural substrate of the enzyme), which is provided in an **incubation medium**. Depending upon the enzyme, the substrate may be hydrolysed, or it may be oxidized or reduced by another substance provided in the incubation medium or already present in the section. Other chemical reactions are also possible. The enzymatic reaction results in the formation of **products** (of hydrolysis, oxidation, etc.), one of which must be immobilized at its site of production and eventually made visible under the microscope. This immobilization of the product is accomplished by means of a **trapping agent**, usually a compound that reacts rapidly with the product to form an insoluble, coloured **final deposit**. Sometimes the precipitate produced by the trapping agent is colourless and must be made visible by a third chemical reaction. At least two chemical processes occur in every histochemical method in which a dissolved substrate is used: the enzyme-catalysed reaction and the trapping of a product. Techniques of this type are subject to five possible sources of artifact.

(1) The enzyme may diffuse, either during preparation of the tissue or during incubation with the substrate and trapping agent. The diffusion of many soluble enzymes can be greatly reduced by incorporating an inert synthetic polymer, such as polyvinyl alcohol, in the incubation medium. Fixation of the tissue will also immobilize enzymes, but most fixatives also cause sufficient denaturation to destroy the catalytic properties. If it is possible the tissue should always be fixed: many histochemical methods will work even when only a small fraction of the original enzymatic activity survives.

(2) The product of the enzymatic reaction may diffuse away from its site of production before it is precipitated by the trapping agent. The diffused product may then attach itself to nearby structures that are different from the sites in which the enzyme is located. For example, if the product is a positively charged ion, it may be bound to anionic sites in the nucleus of the cell in whose cytoplasm it was formed. In order to minimize diffusion of the primary product of the enzyme-catalysed reaction, it is important that: (a) the trapping reaction occurs very rapidly, and (b) the final deposit has a very low solubility in the incubation medium. The latter condition depends, in some cases, on the solubility product of the final deposit. For example, if phosphate ions, released by a phosphate ester hydrolase, are to be trapped by precipitation of calcium phosphate, the incubation medium must contain as high a concentration of calcium ions as possible. In this way, the product $[Ca^{2+}]^3[PO_4^{3-}]^2$ is likely to exceed the low solubility product of $Ca_3(PO_4)_2$ in the presence of only minute traces of phosphate.

(3) The final deposit is necessarily precipitated somewhere in the section. If the deposit is insoluble in water but somewhat soluble in lipids, there may be erroneous localization of the enzyme in the latter. Protein is ubiquitous in cells, so it is preferable for the final deposit to be bound to protein once it has been precipitated. The term **substantivity** is used to denote the affinities of different types of final deposit for lipid or protein. High substantivity for protein is clearly a desirable property.

(4) If a third reaction is necessary to make the trapped product visible, diffusion can occur at this stage. This is not often a cause of artifact in light microscopy, but may assume greater significance in enzyme histochemistry at the higher level of resolution of the electron microscope.

(5) At any stage of the procedure, coloured deposits may be formed that do not result from activity of the enzyme being studied. False-positive reactions of this type may be due to (a) other enzymes acting upon constituents of the incubation medium, (b) other enzymes acting on a product of the primary enzyme-catalysed reaction, (c) spontaneous occurrence of the reaction catalysed by the enzyme, or (d) unwanted non-enzymatic reactions of other kinds. As controls to exclude some of these types of artifact it is necessary to try out the method in the absence of the substrate, and also on sections in which specific enzymatic activity is prevented (e.g. by heating or, preferably, by a specific inhibitor of the enzyme). Large numbers of compounds that inhibit enzymes are classified, reviewed and indexed by Jain (1982). The occurrence of artifacts of false localization, due to diffusion of products and unwanted reactions, must always be considered in the development of new histochemical methods for enzyme activities. The principles of accurate enzyme localization were critically evaluated by Holt and O'Sullivan (1958), a publication that should be read by anyone intending to develop a new histochemical method.

14.6. Types of enzymes

Biochemists classify enzymes according to the types of chemical reaction they catalyse. The systematic classification of enzymes is too thorough for the histochemist, whose repertoire of techniques is much more limited than that of the enzymologist. Histochemically demonstrable enzymes fall into the following rather broad categories:

Hydrolytic enzymes (hydrolases)
These catalyse the reactions of their substrates with water. The substrate molecule is split into two parts, one of which can be trapped. Some examples of hydrolase histochemistry are discussed in Chapter 15.

(1) Phosphatases. Catalyse the hydrolysis of esters and amides of phosphoric acid.
(2) Sulphatases. Catalyse the hydrolysis of sulphate esters.
(3) Carboxylic esterases. Catalyse the hydrolysis of ester linkages between carboxylic acids and any of a variety of alcohols or phenols.
(4) Glycosidases. Catalyse the hydrolysis of glycosidic linkages.
(5) Proteolytic enzymes. Several types, which catalyse the splitting of peptide and amide bonds.

Oxidoreductases

These enzymes, which catalyse oxidation–reduction reactions, are discussed in Chapter 16. They include dehydrogenases, peroxidases and oxidases.

Transferases

A transferase is an enzyme that removes part of a molecule to form a new compound. A number of chemical reactions (degradation, synthesis, changes in coenzymes) are associated with the activities of transferases, and there is a varied assortment of histochemical methods for enzymes of this type.

Lyases

This group includes enzymes that catalyse the decomposition of larger into smaller molecules. Commonly one of the products is a small molecule such as water or ammonia.

14.7. Technical considerations

**14.7.1.
Preparation of
tissue**

The preservation of an enzyme in a tissue may be achieved in one of three ways.

(a) The tissue may be rapidly frozen and sectioned with a cryostat. The unfixed sections can then be incubated to detect enzymatic activity. This procedure is strongly recommended by Chayen and Bitensky (1991) for all histochemical methods for enzymes. However, most histochemists prefer to fix the tissue if possible.
(b) A chemical fixative that does not inhibit the enzyme may be used. This procedure is convenient for those enzymes that resist fixation. For example, most carboxylic ester hydrolases can be demonstrated in frozen sections of formaldehyde-fixed tissue, and some phosphatases survive fixation in acetone followed by paraffin embedding. Cryostat sections of unfixed tissue may be fixed for a few minutes (usually in cold formaldehyde or acetone) before incubation, and several enzymes will survive this treatment. Fixation limits diffusion of enzymes.
(c) The tissue may be freeze-dried and then embedded in glycol methacrylate. The resin must be kept cold during the exothermic polymerization. Many enzymes are demonstrable in sections of the embedded tissue. For details, see Litwin (1985), Murray, Burke and Ewen (1989) and Van Noorden and Frederiks (1992).

**14.7.2.
Conditions of
reaction**

Many incubations are carried out at 37°C, though room temperature or even 4°C is preferred in some methods. The enzymes of homoiothermic animals generally function optimally at 37°C; those of poikilotherms and plants at 25°C. There is less diffusion of the enzymes and of the products of reaction at lower temperatures. Sections mounted on slides or coverslips are most conveniently incubated in coplin jars. When only a small volume of medium is available (as when an expensive ingredient is used), a drop may be placed over an individual section. The slides are then enclosed in a humid container, such as a covered petri dish containing wet gauze, to prevent evaporation. Free-floating frozen sections are incubated in small petri dishes, glass cavity-blocks, or the wells of a haemagglutination tray or cell culture plate.

Clean glassware is essential, even more so when dealing with enzymes than in other branches of histochemistry, because contaminating substances may inhibit the enzymes or react with constituents of the incubation media.

Safety note. Some enzyme inhibitors (e.g. potassium cyanide, diethyl-*p*-nitrophenyl phosphate and many others) are toxic and must be handled with care. It should also be noted that some reagents (e.g. benzidine and related compounds) are carcinogenic and that the possible hazards associated with the use of many substances are unknown.

15 Hydrolytic enzymes

Methods for three groups of enzymes are discussed in this chapter. The techniques have been selected with a view to illustrating a wide variety of histochemical principles. It should be remembered that many other methods are available for these and related hydrolytic enzymes.

15.1. Phosphatases (Phosphoric monoester hydrolases; E.C. 3.1.3)

These enzymes catalyse the hydrolysis of esters of phosphoric acid. Acid and alkaline phosphatases are distinguished by their widely separated pH optima. The former are typical lysosomal constituents, whereas the latter group includes enzymes that hydrolyse specific substrates (e.g. adenosine triphosphate, thiamine pyrophosphate) as well as ones that can attack a variety of substrates.

15.1.1.
Acid phosphatase
(Orthophosphoric monoester phosphohydrolase – acid pH optimum; E.C. 3.1.3.2)

This name is applied to a family of lysosomal enzymes that catalyse the hydrolysis of phosphate esters optimally at around pH 5.0.

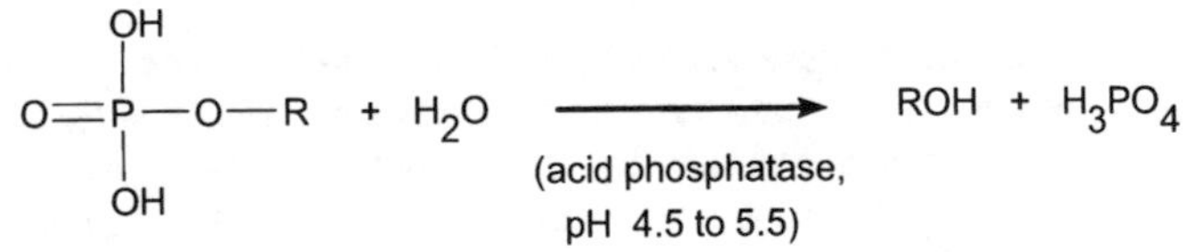

$$O = \overset{\displaystyle OH}{\underset{\displaystyle OH}{\overset{|}{\underset{|}{P}}}} - O - R \ + \ H_2O \ \longrightarrow \ ROH \ + \ H_3PO_4$$

(acid phosphatase,
pH 4.5 to 5.5)

R may be an alkyl or aryl radical. Only one hydroxyl group of phosphoric acid may be esterified in a substrate for this enzyme.

In the lysosomes acid phosphatase is associated with several other enzymes, all with acid pH optima, that catalyse the hydrolysis of a wide variety of esters, amides, and proteins. These enzymes occur in high concentrations in cells of the renal tubules and the prostate gland, in phagocytes, and in cells undergoing degeneration. Smaller numbers of lysosomes are found in most other types of cells.

In Gomori's lead phosphate method, which has been improved upon by many later investigators, the phosphate ions released by hydrolysis of the substrate (sodium β-glycerophosphate) are trapped by lead ions, with which they combine to form insoluble lead phosphate. This salt is white, but the colour can be changed to black by treatment with hydrogen sulphide or a solution of sodium or ammonium sulphide.

$$\text{β-glycerophosphate anion} \quad + \quad H_2O \quad \xrightarrow[\text{(pH 5)}]{\text{(acid phosphatase)}} \quad \text{glycerol} \quad + \quad HPO_4^{2-}$$

$$Pb^{2+} \quad + \quad HPO_4^{2-} \quad \longrightarrow \quad PbHPO_4(s)$$

(white, insoluble)

$$PbHPO_4(s) \quad + \quad S^{2-} \quad \longrightarrow \quad HPO_4^{2-} \quad + \quad PbS(s)$$

(black, insoluble)

Although lysosomal enzymes are enclosed in membranous organelles, the substrate can penetrate the membranes at the optimum pH of acid phosphatase.

The concentration of Pb^{2+} is critical and the incubation medium has to be mixed well in advance in order to allow any spontaneous precipitation of insoluble lead salts to occur before the sections are introduced. The effects of variations in concentration of Pb^{2+} and substrate, the pH, and the overall ionic strength of the incubation medium have all been examined (see Pearse, 1972, 1985; Chayen and Bitensky, 1991, for references to original literature). The mixture is formulated to minimize the binding of lead ions to nuclei and other structures, including the lysosomes that contain the enzyme.

Lead phosphate precipitates are electron dense, but are coarsely crystalline and adhere to membranes. A finely granular precipitate is obtained, within lysosomes, if aluminium ions are substituted for lead in the incubation medium (Berry *et al.*, 1982). The electron-opacity is surprising in view of the low atomic number of aluminium (see Lewis, 1987). Possibly there is deposition of osmium, from the post-fixation solution, upon the precipitated aluminium phosphate. Lanthanide metals, notably cerium, have also been used to precipitate phosphate ions in ultrastructural histochemical methods for phosphatases (Halbhuber *et al.*, 1988a,b).

Acid phosphatase in most sites is inhibited by fluoride ions (e.g. 10^{-3} to 10^{-2} M NaF in the incubation medium). Certain neurons in sensory ganglia, however, contain a fluoride-resistant acid phosphatase. These neurons also contain a peptide, substance P, and are believed to be involved in the perception of pain (see Jancso *et al.*, 1985). Other inhibitors include cupric ions (5×10^{-4} M) and tartrate ions (10^{-2} M) (Lojda *et al.*, 1979). The acid phosphatase of osteoclasts is notable for being resistant to tartrate. Phosphate ions are also inhibitory, but cannot, of course, be added to the lead-containing incubation medium. It is desirable to **avoid phosphate buffers in fixatives or washing solutions** for specimens in which phosphatases are to be histochemically demonstrated.

Fixation and processing
Acid phosphatase survives brief fixation in cold (4°C) acetone or aqueous formaldehyde. Decalcification in formic acid inhibits the enzyme in osteoclasts, but this can be reactivated by incubating the sections, before staining, for 1 h at 37°C in the buffer that will be used for the histochemical incubation (Liu *et al.*, 1987). Frozen or cryostat sections retain the greatest amounts of enzymatic activity, but the histochemical method will work with material embedded in glycol methacrylate, and even on paraffin sections if a wax with a low melting point has been used.

Solutions required
A. Incubation medium (Waters and Butcher, 1980)
Dissolve 132 mg of lead nitrate, $Pb(NO_3)_2$, in 25 ml of 0.2 M acetate–acetic acid buffer, pH 4.7. (Instructions for making the acetate buffer are in Chapter 20.) Dissolve 315 mg sodium β-glycerophosphate in 75 ml water. Combine the two solutions and warm to 37°C before use.

This medium is more stable than earlier formulations and it does not form a precipitate on standing. It may be used immediately or stored at room temperature for several days.

B. Sulphide solution
Add about 0.5 ml of yellow ammonium sulphide to about 100 ml of water immediately before use. Do not allow fumes from the ammonium sulphide bottle to come into contact with the incubation medium (Solution A). Ammonium sulphide is malodorous and toxic and should be used in a fume cupboard. Discard the used solution by washing it down the sink with plenty of running tap water.

Procedure
(1) Incubate sections in Solution A for 30 min at 37°C.
(2) Wash in four changes of water, 1 min in each.
(3) Immerse in dilute ammonium sulphide (Solution B) for about 30 s.
(4) Wash in three changes of water.
(5) Mount in a water-miscible medium. (See *Note 1* below.)

Result
Black deposits of lead sulphide indicate sites of acid phosphatase activity. (See also *Note 2* below.)

Notes
(1) An aqueous mountant is preferred because small amounts of PbS may be dissolved during dehydration and clearing. Saturation of the alcohols and xylene with PbS is sometimes recommended when it is desired to use a resinous mounting medium.
(2) Control sections should be incubated (a) without substrate, (b) in the full incubation medium containing, in addition, 0.01 M sodium fluoride, which inhibits the enzyme in most sites. For other inhibitors, see above.

15.1.2.
Alkaline
phosphatase
(Orthophosphoric
monoester
phosphohydrolase –
alkaline pH
optimum; E.C.
3.1.3.1)

The reaction catalysed by this group of enzymes (which excludes, in the present context, those phosphomonoesterases that have specific substrates) is the same as for acid phosphatase except that the pH optimum lies around 8.0. Alkaline phosphatase occurs in many types of cell, especially in regions specialized for endocytosis and pinocytosis.

Although it is possible to demonstrate alkaline phosphatases by a method similar to the one described above, which produces an eventual precipitate of a metal sulphide, we shall consider instead two other techniques. In the first, the released phosphate ions are precipitated by cerium ions; a second chemical reaction generates a visible product at sites of cerium phosphate deposition. In the second method, the organic product of hydrolysis is trapped by coupling to a diazonium salt, to form an insoluble azoic dye (see also Chapter 5). Cerium precipitation and azo coupling are versatile methods that are also used in histochemical techniques for other enzymes.

15.1.2.1. Cerium-DAB method for alkaline phosphatase
This technique resembles Gomori's lead phosphate method for acid phosphatase in that phosphate ions are precipitated as an insoluble but invisible salt. The way

the cerium phosphate is made visible is quite different. Compounds of cerium, one of the rare earth metals, may have oxidation numbers +3 or +4. (See Chapter 16 for more about oxidation numbers.) The ordinary salts (chloride, nitrate, sulphate) are cerous: those of cerium(III). They are soluble over a wider pH range than those of many other metals. Cerous phosphate is insoluble. It is therefore possible to prepare an incubation medium that has a pH appropriate for alkaline phosphatase while containing a concentration of Ce^{3+} high enough to precipitate $CePO_4$ in the presence of phosphate ions in low concentration, at sites of enzymatic activity. The substrate is the β-glycerophosphate ion.

$$\beta\text{-glycerol}-\text{phosphate} + H_2O \xrightarrow[\text{(pH 9 - 10)}]{\begin{array}{c}\text{(alkaline}\\\text{phosphatase)}\end{array}} \text{glycerol} + PO_4^{3-}$$

$$Ce^{3+} + PO_4^{3-} \longrightarrow CePO_4(s)$$

The white precipitate of cerous phosphate is electron-opaque (Hulstaert *et al.*, 1983; Robinson and Karnovsky, 1983) but optically inconspicuous. The generation of a visible product is possible because Ce(III) can be oxidized to Ce(IV) by treating with hydrogen peroxide. The product, cerium(IV) perhydroxide, is also insoluble. Ce(IV) compounds are strong oxidizing agents, and cerium(IV) perhydroxide can oxidize 3,3'-diaminobenzidine (DAB) to a brown polymer. In the presence of H_2O_2 this reaction occurs repeatedly, amplifying the original deposit. If nickel ions are added to the DAB solution, the final reaction product is blue–black rather than brown. (See Section 16.5.2.2 for DAB oxidation; Section 16.5.3.1 for more about cerium perhydroxide.)

The following method, based on Halbhuber *et al.* (1988a,b,1991), is for specimens fixed by vascular perfusion of cacodylate-buffered 2% glutaraldehyde for 5 min. The fixed pieces of tissue are stored at 4°C in a 15% solution of sucrose in water. Sections may be cut with a freezing microtome, vibrating microtome or cryostat. Other preparative methods are permissible, including cold acetone or formaldehyde fixation (see next method, Section 15.1.2.2), or quick freezing followed by fixation at −20°C in acetone and embedding (also at −20°C) in glycol methacrylate (van Goor *et al.*, 1989). Phosphate buffers should not be used because they could lead to non-specific precipitates.

Solutions required

A. Glycine–sodium hydroxide buffer, pH 9.2
(See Chapter 20). About 200 ml will be needed.

B. Incubation medium

Glycine–sodium hydroxide buffer (Solution A), pH 9.2:	50 ml
Cerium chloride ($CeCl_3.H_2O$):	185 mg (0.014 M)
Sodium citrate ($C_6H_5Na_3O_7.2H_2O$):	162 mg (0.011 M)
Magnesium chloride ($MgCl_2.6H_2O$):	41 mg (0.004 M)
(*or* 0.2 ml of a 0.1 M stock solution)	
Disodium β-glycerophosphate.$5H_2O$):	107 mg (0.007 M)

This is mixed shortly before using. You may have some reagents with waters of hydration different from those stated above. The molarities indicated are concentrations of the principal ion in the complete mixture.

Some incubation medium without the glycerophosphate substrate is also needed, for the pre-incubation (Step 1) and for control sections (see *Note 1* below).

C. 0.3% Hydrogen peroxide

A 0.3% aqueous solution, freshly diluted from stock 30% ('100 volumes') H_2O_2, is made alkaline by adding one drop (0.05 ml) of strong ammonia (ammonium hydroxide) to 30 ml. See also *Note 2* below.

D. DAB–nickel–H_2O_2 solution

While the sections are in the incubation medium, mix:

3,3'-diaminobenzidine dihydrochloride:	7.5 mg

Dissolve this in 1 ml of water, then add:

0.1 M acetate buffer (Chapter 20), pH 5.2:	41.5 ml
Methanol:	7.5 ml
Nickel ammonium sulphate $Ni(NH_4)_2(SO_4)_2.6H_2O$:	1.0 g

Immediateley before using, add 0.025 ml (a small drop) of 30% ('100 volumes') hydrogen peroxide. See also *Note 2* below.

Procedure

(1) Pre-incubate the sections for 60 min in medium without substrate. (This is to ensure thorough permeation by Ce^{3+}.)
(2) Incubate for 30 min in the complete incubation medium (Solution B). See also *Note 1* below.
(3) Wash in 3 changes of buffer (Solution A), each one for 1 min.
(4) Immerse in 0.3% Hydrogen peroxide (Solution C) for 10 min.
(5) Immerse in the DAB–nickel–H_2O_2 solution (D) for 45 min.
(6) Wash in 3 changes of water, apply a counterstain if desired, dehydrate, clear and cover, using a resinous mounting medium.

Result

Sites of alkaline phosphatase activity blue-black.

Notes

(1) Control sections should be incubated without the glycerophosphate substrate. For other controls, include 10^{-3} M levamisole or tetramisole in the pre-incubation (Step 1) and also in the complete incubation medium. (See next method for some other alkaline phosphatase inhibitors.)
(2) **Caution.** Be careful with 30% H_2O_2, which is a strong oxidizing agent and is corrosive to skin and clothing. An alternative is **urea hydrogen peroxide**, a solid compound that is treated as approximately 35% H_2O_2. It is more stable than the strong solution but also must be handled carefully. Simply dissolve it in water to obtain the desired dilution. DAB is chemically similar to known carcinogens. To destroy it, pour the solution into a jar containing some sodium hypochlorite (household bleach) and leave overnight.
(3) Many methods have been developed for ultrastructural visualization of alkaline phosphatase activity. Those based on precipitation of cerium phosphate are probably the most satisfactory (see Van Noorden and Frederiks, 1993).

15.1.2.2. An azo-coupling method for alkaline phosphatase

The substrate is the monobasic sodium salt of α-naphthyl phosphate, the monoester of α-naphthol and phosphoric acid. The α-naphthol freed by hydrolysis is a phenolic compound and can therefore couple with a diazonium salt, which is included in the incubation medium. Coupling occurs rapidly at an alkaline pH and an insoluble, coloured azoic dye is produced.

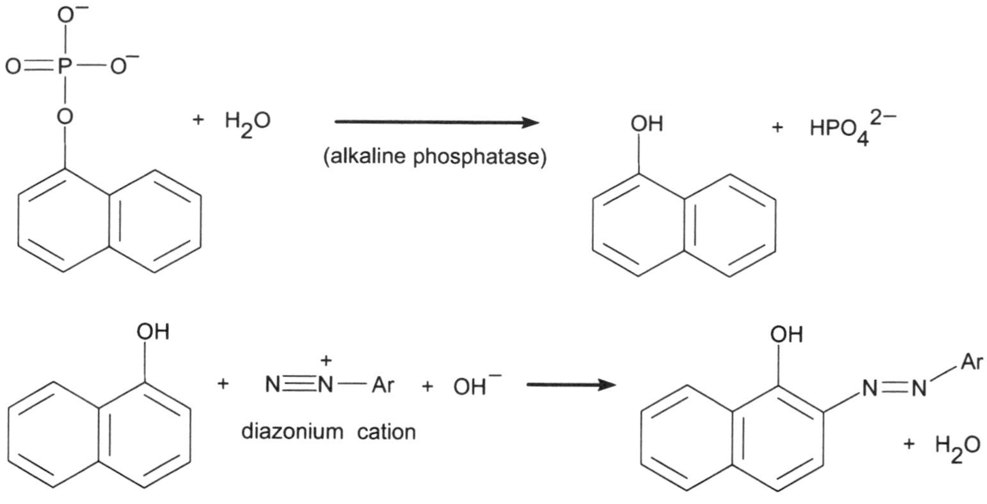

Notice that the azo compound is also phenolic and is therefore an acid dye, albeit one that is insoluble in water at pH 8. This property may confer some substantivity for protein. However, the azo dyes formed from naphthols are usually soluble in non-polar organic liquids. A phosphate ester of naphthol-AS (Chapter 5) can also be used as a substrate. Naphthol-AS forms more intensely coloured azoic dyes than α-naphthol, but its rate of coupling with diazonium salts is slower (Burstone, 1962). The diazonium salt used as a trapping agent should be as stable as possible and must not inhibit the enzyme. The dye formed as the end product of the histochemical reaction should precipitate as exceedingly small particles, with substantivity for protein. The perfect diazonium salt has not yet been found, but fast blue RR salt (Chapter 5) is one of the best available. The relative merits and faults of many stabilized diazonium salts used in enzyme histochemistry are discussed by Pearse (1972, 1985), Lillie (1977) and Horobin and Kiernan (2002).

There are no inhibitors of high specificity for alkaline phosphatase, but enzymatic activity is prevented by prior treatment of the sections with a solution of iodine in potassium iodide. Some alkaline phosphatases are inhibited when cysteine is added to the incubation medium. Mammalian alkaline phosphatases other than that of the intestinal epithelium are inhibited by including 10^{-3} M levamisole or tetramisole in the incubation medium. Levamisole is L[−]-2,3,5,tetrahydro-6-phenylimidazo[2,1-b]thiazole. Tetramisole is the slightly cheaper racemic ([±]) form of the same compound. The latter two compounds are useful for inhibiting endogenous alkaline phosphatase when antisera labelled with the intestinal enzyme are used as reagents in immunohistochemical techniques (Ponder and Wilkinson, 1981; Appenteng et al., 1986; see also Chapter 19).

Fixation and processing
Alkaline phosphatase can be detected after brief fixation in cold acetone or cold aqueous formalin followed by careful embedding in paraffin (see Bancroft and Cook, 1984), nitrocellulose or glycol methacrylate. Nitrocellulose embedding is valuable for demonstrating the enzyme in capillary blood vessels in thick sections of large organs (see Bell and Scarrow, 1984 for details of technique). Formaldehyde-fixed blocks may be stored for a few weeks at 4°C in gum-sucrose (Section 15.2.3). Frozen or cryostat sections are preferred for most purposes. The latter, if previously unfixed, are fixed on their slides or coverslips by immersion for 2 min in cold (4°C) acetone.

The following instructions apply to free-floating frozen sections, which must be handled carefully to minimize physical damage in the alkaline incubation medium.

Solutions required
A. Incubation medium

0.05 M TRIS buffer, pH 10.0 (Chapter 20):	10 ml
α-naphthyl acid phosphate (sodium salt):	10 mg
Magnesium chloride (MgCl$_2$.6H$_2$O):	10 mg
Fast blue RR salt (C.I. 37155):	10 mg

Mix in the order stated. Filter and use immediately.

B. 1% Aqueous acetic acid

Procedure
(1) Carry sections through two changes of water to remove fixative, then incubate them in Solution A for 20 min at room temperature.
(2) Transfer to water (in a large dish) for 1 min.
(3) Transfer to 1% acetic acid (Solution B) for 1 min.
(4) Rinse in water.
(5) Mount sections onto slides and cover, using a water-miscible mounting medium.

Result
Sites of alkaline phosphatase activity purple to black.

Notes
(1) Incubate sections in Solution A without the substrate as a control for non-specific staining by the diazonium salt.
(2) To control for spontaneous hydrolysis of the substrate, treat some sections with an iodine solution for 3 min followed by a rinse in Na$_2$S$_2$O$_3$ (as for removal of mercurial deposits, see Section 4.4.1) and four rinses in water, before incubating in the substrate-containing Solution A. The treatment with iodine inhibits the enzyme.
(3) The magnesium salt may enhance enzymatic activity, but it is often omitted. The rinse in dilute acetic acid neutralizes the alkaline buffer and renders the sections less fragile.
(4) Substrates and couplers are available that yield a fluorescent azo dye as the final reaction product (Ziomek et al., 1990). The substrate 2-(5'-chloro-2'-phosphoryloxyphenyl)-6-chloro-4-quinazolinone yields on hydrolysis a fluorescent compound that is insoluble in aqueous mounting media (Larison et al., 1995). A fluorescent product can also be obtained in methods based on calcium phosphate precipitation, by staining the calcium with a suitable fluorochrome (Murray and Ewen, 1992).

15.1.2.3. Indoxyl-tetrazolium method for alkaline phosphatase
Alkaline phosphatase is a commonly used label in immunohistochemical techniques. On account of its high sensitivity and the stability of the end product an indoxyl-tetrazolium method is currently in favour. The substrate is 5-bromo-4-chloroindoxyl phosphate (also called BCIP or X-phos). This can serve as a substrate for acid or alkaline phosphatases but for various reasons it is unsatisfactory the former group of enzymes (McGadey, 1970; see also Kiernan, 2007a). The organic product of hydrolysis of BCIP is 5-bromo-4-chloroindoxyl, a compound that is easily oxidized.

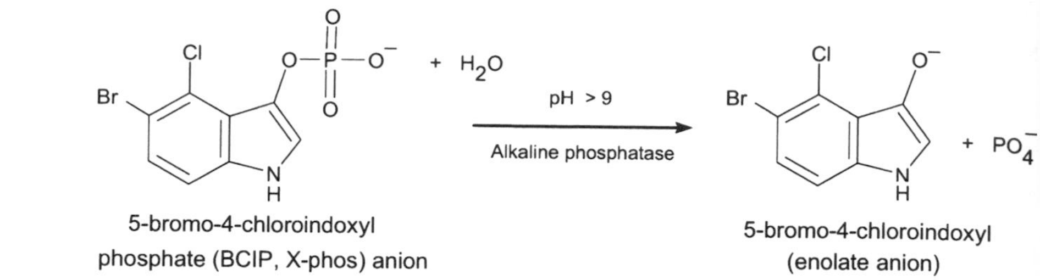

5-bromo-4-chloroindoxyl
phosphate (BCIP, X-phos) anion

5-bromo-4-chloroindoxyl
(enolate anion)

In some histochemical methods indoxyls are oxidized to insoluble indigoid dyes (Section 15.2.3). In the indoxyl-tetrazolium methods, however, the oxidizing agent is a tetrazolium salt such as nitro-BT, which is reduced to an insoluble blue formazan pigment. The reaction occurs only at high pH:

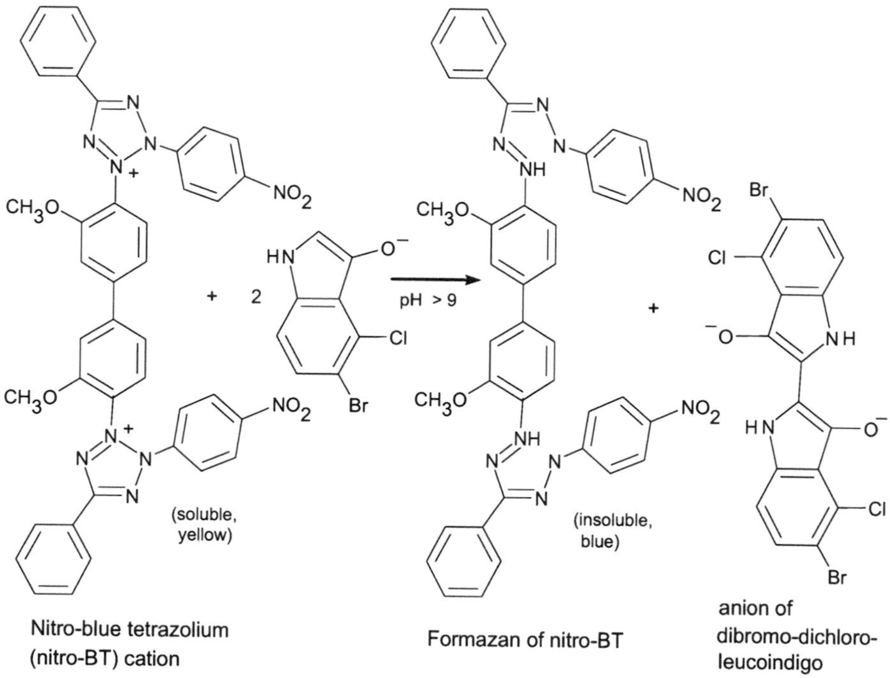

Nitro-blue tetrazolium
(nitro-BT) cation

Formazan of nitro-BT

anion of
dibromo-dichloro-
leucoindigo

The other product of the reaction is a leuco compound that can react with oxygen to form an insoluble blue indigoid pigment (Section 15.2.3). It is likely that the end-product contains both the formazan and the halogenated indigo (Kiernan, 2007a).

Solutions required
Incubation medium

5-bromo-4-chloroindoxyl phosphate: 2.5 mg

(This compound is also sold under the names 5-bromo-4-chloroindolyl phosphate, 5-bromo-4-chloro-3-indolyl phosphate, 5-bromo-4-chloroindol-3-yl phosphate, BCIP and X-phos.)

Dissolve in 0.5 ml *N,N'*-dimethylformamide, then add:

0.1 M TRIS-HCl buffer, pH 9.5:   10 ml
(See Chapter 20 for TRIS buffer)
Nitro blue tetrazolium chloride: 5 mg

4% Formaldehyde
Any formaldehyde fixative solution (Chapter 2).

Procedure (See also *Note 1* below)
(1) Incubate mounted cryostat sections for 10–20 min, either at room tempera-ture or 37°C. (This may be done either in a miniature Coplin jar or as lying drops in an airtight container with high humidity, such as a Petri dish.) See also *Note 2*.
(2) Pour off the incubation medium and carefully rinse the sections with water.
(3) Immerse in 4% formaldehyde (Solution B) for 30 min. (See *Note 3*.)
(4) Wash in water or 70% alcohol.
(5) Complete the dehydration, clear in xylene and apply coverslips using an aqueous mounting medium.

Notes
(1) This is the original simple method of McGadey (1970) for endogenous alka-line phosphatase of animal tissues, applicable to cryostat sections of unfixed tissue or tissue fixed in formal–calcium, or to paraffin sections of acetone-fixed intestine. It may also be applied to sections that have been used in *in situ* hybridization or immunohistochemical procedures that make use of reagents labelled with alkaline phosphatase.
(2) Examine the preparations with a microscope to determine the ideal time of incubation.
(3) The formaldehyde is to stop the enzymatic reaction and fix the tissue. For fixed tissues Step 3 may be replaced with a wash in water.
(4) **Controls.** (a) Omit the substrate (BCIP). This will control for non-enzymatic reduction of nitro-BT by –SH groups of proteins (Section 16.4.3.2). (b) Add inhibitors to the incubation medium (Section 15.1.2.2). Levamisole or tetramisole, 10^{-3} M is routinely added to the medium for detecting alkaline phosphatase-labelled immunoreagents, to inhibit endogenous enzyme in the tissue.

15.2. **Carboxylic esterases** (Carboxylic ester hydrolases; E.C. 3.1.1)

The carboxylic esterases catalyse the general reaction:

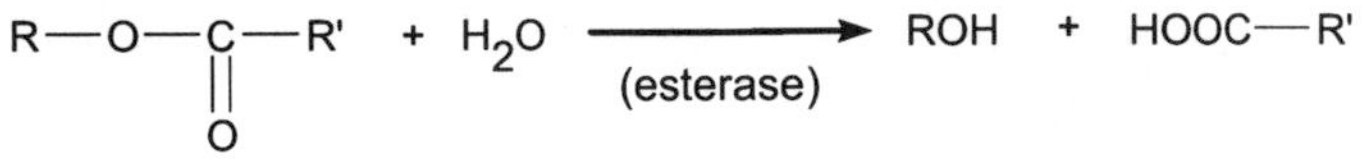

$$R\!-\!O\!-\!\underset{\underset{O}{\|}}{C}\!-\!R' \; + \; H_2O \xrightarrow[\text{(esterase)}]{} ROH \; + \; HOOC\!-\!R'$$

The alkyl or aryl radical R may be derived from one of many possible alcohols (including glycerol), or phenols, or from a hydroxylated base such as choline. The acyl group:

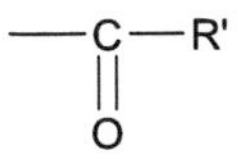

$$-\!\underset{\underset{O}{\|}}{C}\!-\!R'$$

may be derived from a simple carboxylic acid such as acetic or from one of the long-chain fatty acids.

15.2.1. Classification

Many names have been used for the histochemically demonstrable enzymes in this group. The synonymy is explained in *Table 15.1*. The substrates of the different enzymes and the products of their hydrolysis are listed in *Table 15.2*.

Table 15.1. Nomenclature of some carboxylic esterases

Recommended trivial name	E.C. number and systematic name	Synonyms which should no longer be used
Carboxylesterase	3.1.1.1. Carboxylic ester hydrolase	Ali-esterase B-esterase Organophosphate-sensitive esterase
Arylesterase	3.1.1.2. Aryl ester hydrolase	Arom-esterase A-esterase Organophosphate-resistant esterase E600-esterase DFP-ase
Acetylesterase	3.1.1.6. Acetic ester acetylhydrolase	C-esterase Organophosphate-resistant, sulphydryl inhibitor-resistant esterase
Acetylcholinesterase (AChE)	3.1.1.7. Acetylcholine acetylhydrolase	Specific cholinesterase True cholinesterase Cholinesterase (term still used by physiologists and pharmacologists)
Cholinesterase (ChE)	3.1.1.8. Acylcholine acylhydrolase	Pseudocholinesterase Butyrylcholinesterase Non-specific cholinesterase
Lipase	3.1.1.3. Glycerol ester hydrolase	
Phospholipase B	3.1.1.5. Lysolecithin acylhydrolase	

Table 15.2. Substrate and actions of some carboxylic esterases

Enzyme	Substrate whose hydrolysis is catalysed[a]	Products of reaction
Carboxylesterase	A carboxylic ester (may be of an aliphatic or aromatic alcohol or a phenol)	An alcohol or a phenol and a carboxylic acid
Arylesterase	An ester formed from acetic acid and a phenol	A phenol and acetic acid
Acetylesterase	An ester of acetic acid	An alcohol or a phenol and acetic acid
Acetylcholinesterase	Acetylcholine[b]	Choline and acetic acid
Cholinesterase	An acylcholine[b]	Choline and an acid
Lipase	A triglyceride[c]	A diglyceride and a fatty acid
Phospholipase B	A lysolecithin	Glycerolphosphocholine and a fatty acid

[a] These are the substrates that define the biochemical specificities of the enzymes, in conjunction with the effects of specific inhibitors. The enzymes also act upon other substrates, including those used in histochemistry. Some of these enzymes serve principally to catalyse the hydrolysis of exogenous substances (Satoh and Hosokawa, 1998).
[b] Histochemical substrates include phenolic esters and thioesters of choline.
[c] Histochemical substrates include esters of polyhydric alcohols other than glycerol and phenolic esters of higher fatty acids.

15.2.2. Substrates and inhibitors

In this text only the first five enzymes in *Table 15.2* will be considered. These are detected histochemically by providing them with synthetic substrates and trapping the products of hydrolysis. Unfortunately, no artificial substrate is available that is acted upon exclusively by any one of the individual enzymes. All five catalyse the hydrolysis of the substrates for carboxylesterase, arylesterase, and acetylesterase. The hydrolysis of some other substrates, which are not attacked by these three enzymes, is catalysed by both acetylcholinesterase and cholinesterase. Unlike the two phosphatases discussed earlier in this chapter, the carboxylic esterases cannot be distinguished from one another by taking advantage of their pH optima: they all function efficiently over the range of pH 5.0–8.0. It is therefore necessary to make use of toxic substances that specifically inhibit some of the enzymes.

The two choline esterases are inhibited by **eserine** (also known as physostigmine). This alkaloid competes with esters of choline for substrate binding sites on the enzyme molecules. Because it is a competitive inhibitor, eserine must be included in the incubation medium together with the substrate.

In the presence of eserine, a substrate for all five histochemically detectable carboxylic esterases will be hydrolysed only as a result of the activities of carboxylesterase, arylesterase, and acetylesterase. The first of these three is inhibited by low concentrations of **organophosphorus compounds** such as diisopropyl-fluorophosphate (DFP) or diethyl p-nitrophenyl phosphate (E600). These act by blocking serine residues at or near to the substrate binding sites of the enzyme molecules, thus preventing access of the substrate.

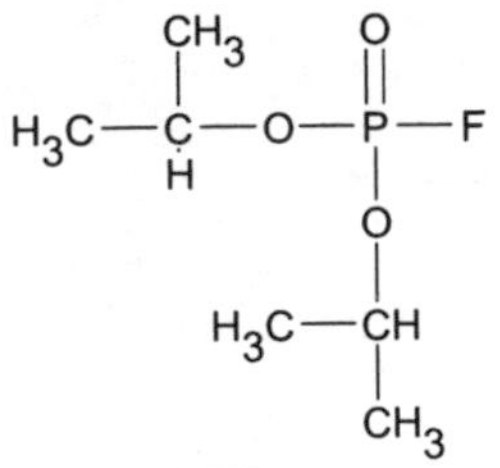

DFP 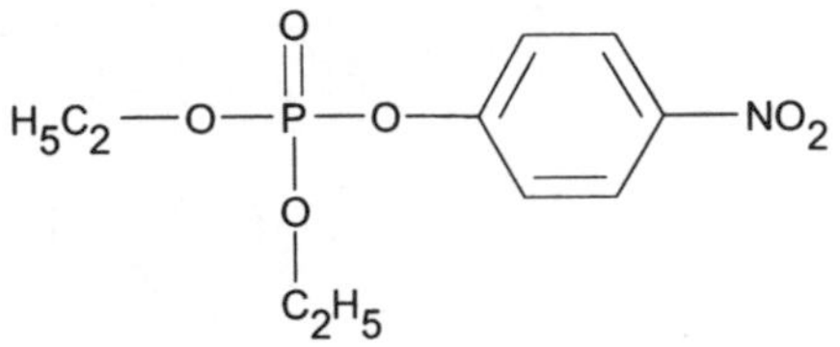   E600

The hydroxyl group of serine displaces the substituent shown on the right-hand side of the phosphorus atom in each of the above formulae. Organophosphorus compounds also inactivate the choline esterases and some proteinases. They are dangerously toxic, mainly because they inhibit acetylcholinesterase. Inhibition is irreversible, so when sections have been pre-incubated in DFP or E600 it is not necessary to add these inhibitors to the incubation medium.

Only arylesterase and acetylesterase are still active after exposure to an organophosphorus compound. The activity of arylesterase requires a free sulphydryl group at the substrate-binding site of the enzyme molecule. It can therefore be inhibited by blocking this sulphydryl group with an organic mercurial compound (Section 10.11.8). The inhibitor usually chosen is the p-chloromercuribenzoate ion (PCMB).

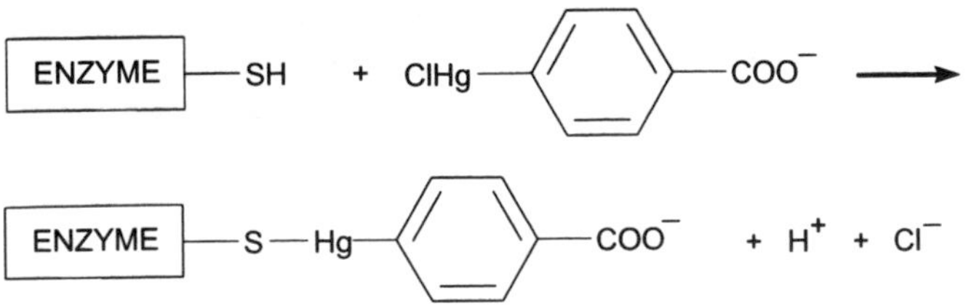

If the sections are first incubated in a dilute solution of E600, then in a solution of PCMB, and then in a substrate-containing medium with added PCMB, acetylesterase will be the only enzyme to give a positive histochemical reaction.

Selective inhibitors of acetylcholinesterase and cholinesterase will be mentioned later in connection with the histochemical methods for these enzymes. For reviews of the carboxylic esterases and their inhibitors, the reader is referred to Pearse (1972), Luppa and Andrä (1983), Oliver *et al.* (1991), Aldridge (1993) and Satoh and Hosokawa (1998).

Instructions for making solutions of esterase inhibitors are given in Section 15.2.6.

15.2.3.
Indigogenic method for carboxylic esterases

Acetyl esters of naphthols or of indoxyls are used as substrates in histochemical methods for these enzymes. The methods, with naphthyl esters, are similar in principle to the one for alkaline phosphatase discussed in Section 15.1.2. An example of such a technique, applied to blood films, is given in Chapter 7 (Section 7.4.2). The use of indoxyl esters will now be described.

The substrate may be one of a selection of halogenated derivatives of indoxyl acetate. 5-bromoindoxyl acetate is a typical example. The unsubstituted indoxyl ester (without Br) is not used because the end product of its hydrolysis forms unduly large crystals.

Hydrolysis yields the halogenated indoxyl:

5-bromoindoxyl acetate
(= 5-bromo-O-acetyl indoxyl)

5-bromoindoxyl

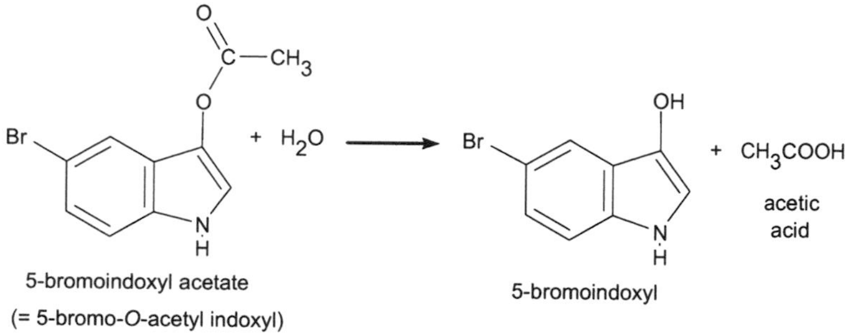

which exhibits keto-enol tautomerism. The indoxyl is light yellow, slightly soluble in water, and more soluble in lipids. The *enol* form is rapidly oxidized by atmospheric oxygen in the presence of a catalyst, which is a balanced mixture of ferrocyanide and ferricyanide ions present in the incubation medium. The desired product of oxidation of two molecules of the halogenated indoxyl is 5,5'-dibromoindigo (*Fig. 15.1*).

This compound is insoluble in water and also in histological dehydrating and clearing agents. It contains the indigoid chromophore (Chapter 5) and is blue. The oxidation catalyst is necessary because in its absence the lipophilic indoxyl is produced more slowly and diffuses into lipids and erythrocytes. There it is oxidized by hydrogen peroxide (a by-product of oxidation of indoxyls by oxygen), a reaction catalysed by the peroxidase-like activity of haemoglobin. In the presence of ferricyanide the oxidation proceeds rapidly, with the intermediate leuco compound binding to protein at the sites of esterase activity. Unfortunately, ferricyanide also facilitates oxidation of the leuco compound to substances other than the desired indigoid dye, perhaps reducing the potential sensitivity of the technique (Holt, 1956; Holt and Withers, 1958; Kiernan, 2007a).

All five of the carboxylic esterases under consideration are able to catalyse the hydrolysis of halogenated indoxyl acetates, so the individual enzymes must be identified by the judicious use of inhibitors, as outlined in the preceding section (15.2.2) of this chapter. No inhibitors are available that spare only the choline esterases. Consequently, the indigogenic method is used mainly for carboxylesterase, arylesterase, and acetylesterase. It is also useful, however, for the demonstration of acetylcholinesterase at motor endplates in skeletal striated muscle (McIsaac and Kiernan, 1974; Kiernan, 1996a), where other carboxylic esterases are absent.

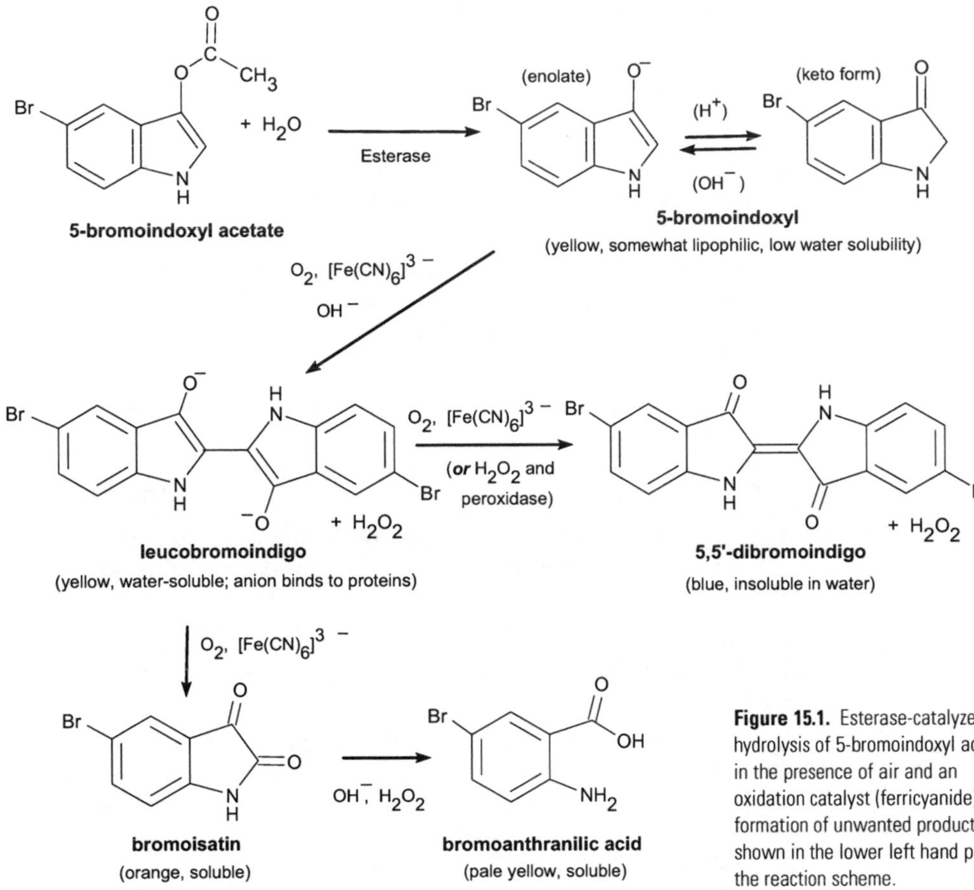

5-bromoindoxyl acetate

(enolate)

(keto form)

5-bromoindoxyl
(yellow, somewhat lipophilic, low water solubility)

O_2, $[Fe(CN)_6]^{3-}$
OH^-

leucobromoindigo
(yellow, water-soluble; anion binds to proteins)

O_2, $[Fe(CN)_6]^{3-}$
(or H_2O_2 and peroxidase)

5,5'-dibromoindigo
(blue, insoluble in water)

O_2, $[Fe(CN)_6]^{3-}$

bromoisatin
(orange, soluble)

OH^-, H_2O_2

bromoanthranilic acid
(pale yellow, soluble)

Figure 15.1. Esterase-catalyzed hydrolysis of 5-bromoindoxyl acetate in the presence of air and an oxidation catalyst (ferricyanide). The formation of unwanted products is shown in the lower left hand part of the reaction scheme.

Indigogenic methods for esterases have been in use for many years, and the original technique (Holt and Withers, 1952, 1958) is very reliable. It works well with frozen sections of tissues fixed in neutral, buffered formaldehyde for 12–24 h at 4°C. The fixed blocks may be stored for several months at 4°C if they are transferred directly from the fixative to gum-sucrose (Section 2.1.2). Several hydrolytic enzymes can be immobilized by soaking tissues in gum-sucrose. The large molecules of the gum, which is a polysaccharide, may hinder the diffusion of the enzyme molecules (Holt et al., 1960). The persistent gum can interfere with some counterstains, including reduced silver methods, and many workers prefer a simple sucrose solution (10–20% w/v in water). Sucrose also acts as a cryoprotectant. The following procedure (Holt and Withers, 1958) incorporates a minor improvement to the original method: the incorporation of 1.0 M NaCl, which limits diffusion of esterase during incubation.

Stock solutions
A. 0.05 M TRIS-HCl buffer
pH 8.5 (Chapter 20)

B. 0.2 M sodium chloride (NaCl; 11.7%)
Keeps for several months.

C. 0.05 M potassium ferricyanide (K₃Fe(CN)₆; 1.65%)
Keeps for several months.

D. 0.05 M potassium ferrocyanide ($K_4Fe(CN)_6.3H_2O$; 2.11%)

Keeps for about 4 weeks at 4°C. Replace when the colour becomes noticeably darker. (It is slowly oxidized by air to the ferricyanide, with consequent change of colour from almost colourless to yellow.)

E. A counterstain

Neutral red or safranine (Chapter 6) is suitable for nuclei (red). Van Gieson's stain (Chapter 8) shows cytoplasm (yellow) and collagen (red).

Incubation medium

Dissolve 1–5 mg of 5-bromoindoxyl acetate or 5-bromo-4-chloroindoxyl acetate (see *Note 1*) in about 0.2 ml of ethanol in a small beaker. (The amount of substrate is not critical. Use enough to cover about 1 mm^2 on the tip of a pointed scalpel blade or spatula.) To the solution, add:

Solution A (buffer):	8.0 ml
Solution B (NaCl):	10.0 ml
Solution C ($K_3Fe(CN)_6$):	1.0 ml
Solution D ($K_4Fe(CN)_6$):	1.0 ml

Mix just before using. This incubation medium is fairly stable if protected from bright light; it may be kept overnight and used the next day. See also *Notes 1* and *5* below.

Procedure

This is described for frozen sections, but the sections may be mounted on slides or coverslips.

(1) Cut frozen sections and transfer them to the incubation medium. Leave at room temperature for about 30 min. The time is variable; some tissues will show an adequate reaction in 5 min whereas others may require 2 h.
(2) Rinse sections in two changes of water.
(3) (Optional.) Apply a counterstain (see *Note 4* below).
(4) Rinse in water, mount onto slides, allow to dry, dehydrate, clear and mount in a resinous medium.

Result

Sites of carboxylic esterase activity, blue. The deposit is finely granular. See *Note 2* for comments on specificity and controls.

Notes

(1) 5-bromo-4-chloroindoxyl acetate generates an indigoid dye with a slightly less intense blue colour, but it is superior to 5-bromoindoxyl acetate in that the precipitate is more finely granular and therefore provides superior structural resolution.
(2) This method detects all carboxylic esterases. AChE and ChE are inhibited by eserine. (In skeletal muscle, the AChE of the postsynaptic component of the motor end-plate is the only enzyme detected by staining for bromoindoxyl esterase activity.) E600 and PCMB should be used to identify the other enzymes, but in critical histochemical studies it is necessary to determine the effects of other inhibitors as well, especially with species other than the rat. Instructions for making solutions of esterase inhibitors are given at the end of this chapter.
(3) Bromoindoxyl phosphate and various bromoindoxyl glycosides are available as substrates for phosphatases and glycosidases. In some of the methods, a diazonium salt is included in the incubation medium. This couples with the liberated indoxyl, and the final reaction product is therefore an azo dye, not a derivative of indigo. See Lojda *et al.* (1979) for more information.

(4) For many purposes a red nuclear counterstain (Chapter 6) is sufficient. A silver reduction method (Chapter 18) may be applied to display nerve fibres; the sequence is valuable for showing the motor innervation of skeletal muscle; the Winkelmann and Schmitt method (Chapter 18, Section 18.3.1.6) is recommended (see Kiernan, 1996a).

(5) Some esterases are inhibited by the oxidizing agent in the medium, and stronger staining is seen if the concentrations of $K_4Fe(CN)_6$ and $K_3Fe(CN)_6$ are reduced from 0.005 M to 0.0005 M (Kirkeby and Blecher, 1978). Reduce the volumes of Solutions C and D to 0.1 ml, and add water to make up the volume of the incubation medium to 20 ml

15.2.4.
Choline
esterases

Choline (Chapter 12) is a quaternary ammonium compound and a primary alcohol. Its hydroxyl group can combine with an acyl group (from a carboxylic acid) to form an ester. Mammalian tissues contain two enzymes that catalyse the hydrolysis of esters of choline. Both are inhibited by the alkaloid eserine.

15.2.4.1. Properties of the enzymes
Acetylcholinesterase (AChE; see *Table 15.1* for synonyms) is present in erythrocytes and in some neurons. This is the enzyme that terminates the action of acetylcholine at cholinergic synapses and neuromuscular junctions, though it must have other functions as well. An action on peptides has been detected (e.g. Chubb *et al.*, 1980). Highly purified AChE does not act on peptide bonds, however, though it does catalyze the hydrolysis of synthetic aryl acyl amides (Checler *et al.*, 1994).

Cholinesterase (ChE; also frequently called 'pseudocholinesterase', see *Table 15.1*) can also catalyse the hydrolysis of acetylcholine, but more slowly than AChE. The preferred substrates are esters of choline with acyl groups containing more carbon atoms than acetyl. ChE occurs in serum, in neuroglia, and in some neurons. It is also present in the endothelial cells of cerebral capillaries in some species, notably the rat.

Histochemical methods for AChE and ChE are valuable in the histological study of the nervous system, because they selectively demonstrate certain groups of neuronal somata, axons and certain regions of grey matter that are not distinctively coloured by dyes. The uses of the methods in neuroanatomy are reviewed by Kiernan and Berry (1975) and Butcher (1983).

15.2.4.2. Thiocholine ester hydrolysis
The substrate in the most widely employed technique (introduced by Koelle and Friedenwald, 1949) is **acetylthiocholine** (AThCh), the thioester analogous to acetylcholine:

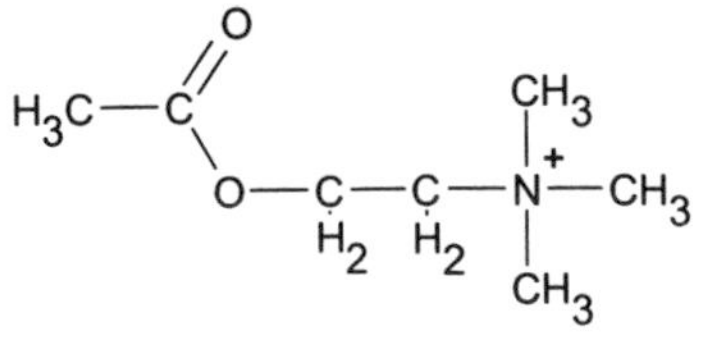

acetylcholine cation 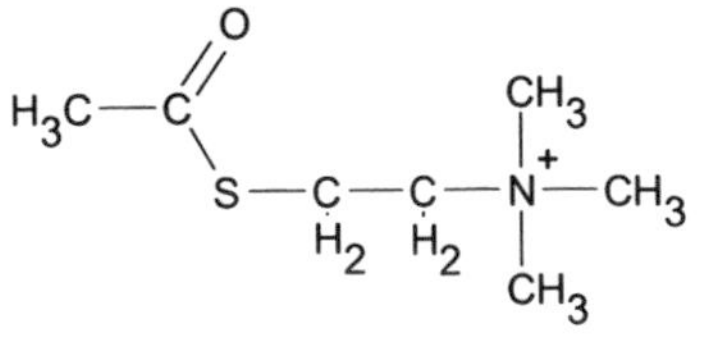   acetylthiocholine cation

Enzymatic cleavage of AThCh yields acetic acid and the thiocholine cation:

$$CH_3COS(CH_2)_2\overset{+}{N}(CH_3)_3 + H_2O \longrightarrow CH_3COOH + HS(CH_2)_2\overset{+}{N}(CH_3)_3$$

AThCh cation   Thiocholine cation

Thiocholine has a free sulphydryl group. The incubation medium also contains copper (complexed with glycine, so that the AChE is not inhibited by a high concentration of Cu^{2+}) and iodide ions. Thiocholine combines with copper and iodide ions to form an insoluble crystalline product, copper–thiocholine iodide, which is probably:

$$\left[Cu-S-\underset{H_2}{C}-\underset{H_2}{C}-\overset{\overset{\displaystyle CH_3}{|}}{\underset{\underset{\displaystyle CH_3}{|}}{N}}-CH_3 \right]^+ \quad I^-$$

(Tsuji, 1974). This product is usually made visible in the microscope by treatment with a soluble sulphide (H_2S, Na_2S or $(NH_4)_2S$), which results in the formation of brown cuprous sulphide. The crystals of copper–thiocholine sulphate are visible in light microscopy, but the deposits of cuprous sulphide are amorphous (Malmgren and Sylven, 1955) even under the electron microscope. This redistribution of the final product of the reaction must be remembered when the supposed localizations of AChE and ChE are studied at the ultrastructural level.

In another widely used technique (Karnovsky and Roots, 1964) the incubation medium contains a thiocholine ester, copper (as a citrate complex), and ferricyanide ions. The latter are reduced to ferrocyanide by the sulphydryl group of the thiocholine released by enzymatic hydrolysis. Brown copper ferrocyanide (Hatchett's brown) is formed and is immediately precipitated at the site of the enzymatic activity. This is known as a 'direct-colouring' technique to distinguish it from the procedures in which the product of the reaction has to be converted to cupric sulphide.

The efficiency of the direct-colouring method is reduced by simultaneous precipitation of copper-thiocholine iodide, which does not contribute colour to the final product (Tewari et al., 1982). In one modification of the technique (Tsuji and Larabi, 1983), the acetylthiocholine substrate is used as its chloride rather than iodide, so that Hatchett's brown is the only precipitated product of the reaction.

The deposits can be darkened by treatment with 3,3'-diaminobenzidine (DAB) and hydrogen peroxide. $Cu_2Fe(CN)_6$ resembles the enzyme peroxidase (Chapter 16) in that it catalyses the oxidation of aromatic amines by H_2O_2. The dark colour of oxidized DAB is made even darker if the reaction of formation occurs in the presence of nickel or cobalt ions.

15.2.4.3. Choline esterase substrates and inhibitors

AThCh is hydrolysed, though slowly, under the influence of catalysis by ChE, so it is necessary to include a selective inhibitor of this enzyme in the incubation medium if AChE is to be demonstrated in isolation. A more suitable substrate for the deliberate demonstration of ChE is **butyrylthiocholine** (BuThCh). This is, however, slowly attacked by AChE, so it is then necessary to inhibit the latter enzyme. The most generally useful selective inhibitor of AChE is a quaternary ammonium compound known as **B.W.284C51**, which is (1,5-*bis*(4-allyldimethylammoniumphenyl)pentan-3-one dibromide). **Ethopropazine** hydrochloride (a drug used to treat parkinsonism) is a convenient inhibitor of ChE, and this enzyme is also inhibited by concentrations of **DFP** that are too low to inhibit AChE. Another organophosphorus compound useful for selectively inhibiting ChE is tetraisopropylpyrophosphoramide (**isoOMPA**).

It should be remembered that there is considerable variation among different species of animals in the susceptibilities of choline esterases and other carboxylic esterases to different inhibitors. Except in well understood species (such as the rat), it is necessary to investigate the effects of several inhibitors before reaching a decision as to the identity of an enzyme. Interspecific variation is discussed by Kiernan (1964) and Pearse (1972). These references and a paper by Pepler and Pearse (1957) may be consulted for lists of substances that inhibit the different carboxylic esterases.

Instructions for making solutions of esterase inhibitors are given in Section 15.2.6.

15.2.5.
A method for acetylcholin-esterase and cholinesterase

This is the direct-colouring method of Karnovsky and Roots (1964), with modifications based on the work of Hanker *et al.* (1973) and Tago *et al.* (1986).

Frozen sections are cut from specimens fixed at 4°C for 12–24 h in formal–saline or neutral, buffered formaldehyde. Glutaraldehyde (1.0–3.0%, pH 7.2–7.6) is also a suitable fixative.

Two incubation media, **C.(1)** and **C.(2)**, are prescribed, each for a different purpose.

Reagents required
A. Substrate and inhibitors
(1)   Acetylthiocholine iodide (substrate for AChE)
(2)   Butyrylthiocholine iodide (substrate for ChE)
(3)   Inhibitors, according to the requirements of the investigation.

The solid substrates are stored desiccated at −20°C. Instructions for using inhibitors are given in Section 15.2.6.

B. Stock solution for incubating medium
0.1 M acetate buffer, pH 6.0 (Chapter 20):	65 ml
Sodium citrate (trisodium salt; dihydrate):	147 mg
Cupric sulphate (anhydrous):	48 mg
Water:	to make 100 ml

Dissolve, then add:

Potassium ferricyanide ($K_3Fe(CN)_6$):	17 mg

This pale green solution keeps for about 1 week at room temperature. It should not be used if it contains a brown precipitate.

C.(1). Incubation medium (working solution, full strength)
Dissolve 5.0 mg (approximately) of *either* acetylthiocholine iodide *or* butyrylthiocholine iodide in a drop of water and add 10 ml of solution B. This medium is stable for several hours and may be used repeatedly if not cloudy, but should be discarded at the end of the day. *This medium is used for tissues containing high enzymatic activity, including skeletal muscle (motor end-plates).*

C.(2). Incubation medium (working solution, 10-fold dilution)
Mix 10 ml of Solution C.(1) above with 90 ml of 0.1 M acetate buffer, pH 6.0 (Chapter 20). *This medium is used for tissues containing thin AChE-positive nerve fibres, or cell-bodies with low enzymatic activity.*

Inhibitors should be added to the medium C.(1) or C.(2) as needed. See Section 15.2.6 for instructions on use of inhibitors.

D. TRIS buffer, pH 7.2 (Chapter 20)

E. DAB solution
3,3′-diaminobenzidine tetrahydrochloride:	10 mg
Water:	1 ml

Dissolve, then add to

| TRIS buffer (Chapter 20; pH 7.6): | 20 ml |
| Nickel ammonium sulphate ($Ni(NH_4)_2(SO_4)_2.6H_2O$): | 150 mg |

Use within 1 h of dissolving the DAB.

F. Hydrogen peroxide (0.03%)

A stock solution of 30% H_2O_2 ('100 volumes available oxygen': handle carefully) is diluted to 0.03% with water, less than 15 min before it is needed (see *Procedure* below). 2 ml of the diluted solution will be needed.

Alternatively use urea hydrogen peroxide (UHP), which is a solid compound containing approximately 35% H_2O_2 by weight, which is released by dissolving in water. For 0.03% H_2O_2 dissolve 0.1 g of UHP in 115 ml of water.

Procedure

(1) Collect frozen sections into water in which they may remain for up to 1 h. Pre-incubate any control sections in appropriate inhibitors. Wash irreversibly inhibited sections in four changes of water. Do not wash after pre-incubation with competitive inhibitors.

(2) Transfer sections to the incubation medium, C.(1) *or* C.(2), for 10–30 min at room temperature. When regions of enzymatic activity go reddish brown, incubation is adequate. Check under a microscope for isolated sites of activity such as motor endplates.

(3) Wash in 3 changes of TRIS buffer, each about 2 min. The sections may be left in the last change, but total time in TRIS buffer should not exceed 30 min.

(4) Transfer sections to the 20 ml of DAB solution (E), and wait for 5 min.

(5) Add 2 ml freshly diluted 0.03% hydrogen peroxide (Solution F) to the DAB solution containing the sections. Mix well by stirring with a glass rod. Make sure the sections are not collapsed into little balls or knots.

(6) Wait for 10 min, then wash in 3 changes of water, each at least 1 min.

(7) Mount the sections onto slides and allow to dry.

(8) *Either* mount in an aqueous medium, *or* dehydrate through graded alcohols, clear in xylene, and mount in a resinous medium.

Result

Sites of enzymatic activity black (brown if Steps 4 and 5 are omitted).

Notes

(1) Steps 4 and 5 may be omitted when only sites of strong activity, such as AChE at motor end plates or ChE in cerebral capillaries and some central neurons, are of interest. Stages 4 and 5 are necessary when medium C.(2) is used.

(2) Although the substrates (especially butyrylthiocholine) show partial specificity, the use of inhibitors is imperative for certain identification of the two enzymes. A control with eserine should also be provided, though non-enzymatic precipitation of the end product is unusual with this technique. If the DAB–nickel–H_2O_2 intensification is carried out, there may be a non-specific grey background, and sites of endogenous peroxidase activity (erythrocytes, granular leukocytes, occasional groups of neurons in the brain) will be stained.

(3) Endogenous peroxidase activity can be blocked by treating the sections with 0.1% hydrogen peroxide for 30 min, before Step 1 of the method.

(4) A counterstain may be applied if desired between Steps 7 and 8. Most dye-based stains may be used. Silver reduction methods (Chapter 18) are unsatisfactory if Steps 4 and 4 are omitted, because the copper ferrocyanide deposit is slowly decolorized or removed when exposed to silver nitrate.

15.2.6.
Use of inhibitors

The carboxylic esterases are defined partly on the basis of their susceptibilities to different inhibitors. The following instructions relate to the practical uses of such compounds. *Remember: most substances that block the active sites of enzymes are poisonous, and the pure substances and stock solutions must be handled with great care.* Incubation media contain greatly diluted inhibitors, and do not pose any danger.

15.2.6.1. Preparation of inhibitor solutions

Eserine. Used as eserine (physostigmine) sulphate, MW 649; usually as a 10^{-5} M solution. Dissolve 6.5 mg of eserine sulphate in 10 ml of water. Add 0.1 ml of this to 9.9 ml of buffer (for pre-incubation) or incubation medium (for simultaneous incubation and inhibition). 10^{-5} M eserine inhibits AChE and ChE.

E600. Diethyl-*p*-nitrophenyl phosphate is sold as an oily liquid in an ampoule. It is poisonous and care must be taken to avoid ingestion, contact with the skin, or inhalation of vapour. Ampoules contain 1.0 ml (MW 275; SG 1.27). Drop an ampoule into 462 ml of propylene glycol in a stoppered reagent bottle under a fume hood. Break the ampoule with a glass rod and insert the stopper. This gives 10^{-2} M stock solution of E600, which keeps indefinitely at 4°C. The bottle should be stood in a container of absorbent material such as kieselguhr or vermiculite.

For use, dilute with buffer to obtain the desired concentration (usually 10^{-7} to 10^{-3} M). Dispose of old solution as described for DFP, below. 10^{-5} M E600 inhibits AChE, ChE, and carboxylesterase. Arylesterase and acetylesterase are inhibited only by higher concentrations (e.g. 10^{-2} M).

DFP. Diisopropylfluorophosphate is a liquid, supplied in a glass ampoule. On account of its volatility, it is more dangerous than E600. Ampoules contain 1.0 g of DFP (MW 208). In a fume hood, drop an ampoule into 480 ml of propylene glycol in a glass-stoppered reagent bottle. Break the ampoule with a glass rod and insert the stopper. This stock solution is 10^{-2} M DFP. Store at 4°C with the bottle standing in a container of absorbent material. Keeps indefinitely. Do not pipette by mouth! For use, dilute with buffer to obtain the desired concentration (usually 10^{-2} to 10^{-5} M). Solutions containing 10^{-2} M DFP should be discarded by pouring into an excess of 4% aqueous NaOH and leaving in the fume cupboard for 4 days before washing down the sink with plenty of water. More dilute solutions, in quantities less than 100 ml, may be discarded without special precautions.

AChE and ChE are inhibited by 10^{-5} to 10^{-4} M DFP. ChE is inhibited by 10^{-7} to 10^{-6} M DFP.

Ethopropazine. Available as its hydrochloride (MW 349), or as its methosulphate (MW 359), which is used clinically as a drug for relieving symptoms of Parkinson's disease. Ethopropazine is usually used as a 10^{-4} M solution. Dissolve 34.9 mg (hydrochloride) or 35.9 mg (methosulphate) in 10 ml of water. Add 0.1 ml of this to 9.9 ml of buffer (for pre-incubation) *and* to 9.9 ml of incubation medium (for simultaneous incubation and inhibition). ChE is inhibited selectively.

B.W.284C51 (1,5-bis-(4-allyldimethylammoniumphenyl)pentan-3-one dibromide) (MW 560). Dissolve 140 mg in 25 ml of water to give a stock solution which is 10^{-2} M. Keeps for a few months at 4°C. Dilute with buffer *and* with incubation medium to the desired concentration (10^{-5} to 10^{-4} M). B.W.284C51 inhibits AChE but not ChE.

p-**Chloromercuribenzoate** (PCMB). Available as *p*-chloromercuribenzoic acid (MW 357) or its sodium salt (MW 379). Dissolve 36 mg of the acid in the smallest possible volume (1–2 ml) of 2 M (8%) NaOH. Add 5 ml of buffer, then adjust to the desired pH by careful addition of 1.0 M HCl. Make up to 10 ml with buffer to obtain a 10^{-2} M solution of the inhibitor. The sodium salt (38 mg) can be dissolved directly in 10 ml of buffer. Dilute with buffer and with incubation medium to 10^{-4} to 10^{-6} M PCMB. Acetylesterase is *not* inhibited.

iso-**OMPA**. Tetraisopropylpyrophosphoramide (MW 342.4) is a somewhat sticky solid. Store in a metal can in a freezer. For use, weigh out approximately 10 mg, dissolve this in 5 ml of alcohol, and make up to 30 ml with water. The volume should be 3 ml for every 1.0 mg of *iso*-OMPA, giving a solution that is close to 10^{-3} M.

For use, dilute with buffer to obtain the desired final concentration. The principal use of *iso*-OMPA is in the histochemistry of choline esterases. A 10^{-7} to 10^{-6} M solution selectively inhibits cholinesterase but spares acetylcholinesterase. Higher concentrations (e.g. 10^{-4} M) inhibit AChE and carboxylesterase, in much the same way as E600 and DFP. Disposal of old solutions: as for DFP.

15.2.6.2. Methods of application

The **irreversible inhibitors** (i.e. the organophosphorus compounds E600, DFP and *iso*-OMPA) are used by **pre-incubation** in a solution with the same pH as the substrate-containing mixture. The sections are placed in a buffered solution containing the desired concentration of the inhibitor for 30 min at 37°C. The sections are rinsed in four changes of buffer before being transferred to the incubation medium. The rinsing is a particularly important part of the procedure when inhibited and uninhibited sections are to be incubated side by side in the same batch of medium.

Other inhibitors work by **competition** with the substrate for the active sites of the enzymes and must be **incorporated in the incubation medium**. Usually it is desirable also to pre-incubate the sections with a solution of the inhibitor, so that there will be no chance of enzymatic hydrolysis of the histochemical substrate during the earliest stages of incubation. Pre-incubation in a competitive inhibitor is *not* followed by washing; the sections are moved directly into the inhibitor-containing incubation medium.

In any attempt to identify carboxylic esterases it is necessary to use several inhibitors over a range of concentrations extending at least two orders of magnitude either side of that generally thought to be optimal for the inhibition of any particular enzyme. Inhibitors may not be necessary when a histochemical procedure is used only as a staining method for some structure that happens to contain one of the enzymes. Inhibitors additional to the ones described here are listed by Pearse (1972, pp 768, 770, 796 and 798) and Oliver *et al.* (1991).

15.3. Peptidases and proteinases

The proteolytic enzymes catalyse the hydrolysis of peptide bonds between amino acids in polypeptides and proteins:

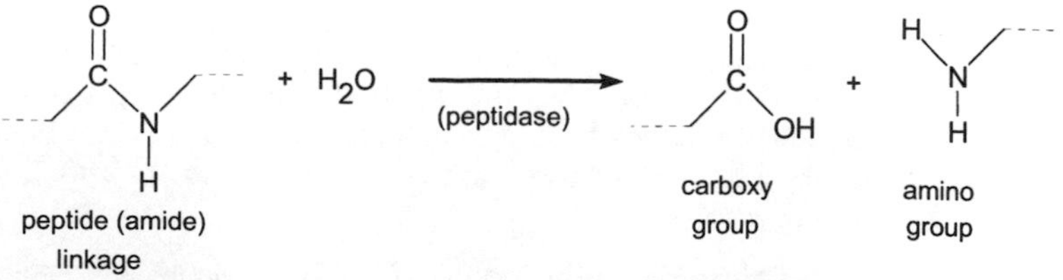

The different enzymes attack peptide linkages adjacent to particular amino acids or at one or other end (the C- or N-terminal amino acid) of a polypeptide chain.

| 15.3.1.
Classification of proteolytic enzymes | The scheme in *Table 15.3* is abstracted from Dixon and Webb (1979) and slightly modified to accommodate histochemically demonstrable enzymatic activities. Some peptidases catalyse the hydrolysis of synthetic substrates containing the pep- |

Table 15.3. Peptidases and proteinases

Peptidases (= exopeptidases) E.C. 3.4.11–3.4.17 (release single amino acids from peptide chain)

Aminopeptidases (= α-aminoacylpeptide hydrolases) E.C. 3.4.11 (release amino acids from N-terminus)
Many mammalian and bacterial enzymes. Some have little specificity; others are specific for the N-terminal amino acid. Most require metal ions (Zn^{2+}, Mg^{2+}, Mn^{2+}) for activity.

Dipeptidases E.C. 3.4.13 (act on dipeptide substrates)
Most of these are specific for one of the amino acids of the dipeptide. Related enzymes act at the penultimate peptide linkage, and liberate dipeptides from larger polypeptides.

Carboxypeptidases E.C. 3.4.16–3.4.17 (release amino acids from C-terminus)

Serine carboxypeptidases E.C. 3.4.16 (Acid pH optimum; inhibited by organophosphorus compounds that bind to serine residues).
Includes a group of enzymes of broad specificity, and enzymes that release C-terminal proline and tyrosine.

Metallocarboxypeptidases E.C. 3.4.17 (need a metal: Zn^{2+}, Co^{2+}, for activity)
Includes the pancreatic enzymes:
Carboxypeptidase A (E.C. 3.4.17.1; releases C-terminal amino acids other than arginine, lysine and proline).
Carboxypeptidase B (E.C. 3.4.17.2; releases lysine or arginine), and some enzymes that remove individual specific C-terminal amino acids.

Proteinases (= endopeptidases) E.C. 3.4.21–3.4.24 (attack non-terminal peptide linkage)

Serine proteinases E.C. 3.4.21 (have histidine and serine at active site; inhibited by organophosphorus compounds that bind to serine residues)
Includes **Chymotrypsin** (E.C. 3.4.21.1), which cleaves peptide linkages at the carboxyl end of phenylalanine, tyrosine, tryptophan or leucine; **Trypsin** (E.C. 3.4.21.4), which cleaves peptide linkages at the carboxyl end of lysine or arginine, and many enzymes with specialized metabolic functions.

Thiol proteinases E.C. 3.4.22 (have cysteine at active site; inhibited by compounds that react with -SH groups)
Include the plant proteinase **Papain** (E.C. 3.4.22.2), which cleaves peptide bonds at the carboxyl end of lysine or arginine or next-but-one to the carboxyl group of phenylalanine; **Cathepsin B** (E.C. 3.4.22.1) which has similar specificity and occurs in many vertebrate animal tissues.

Carboxyl (acid) proteinases E.C. 3.4.23 (acid pH optimum; unionized carboxyl group at active site)
Include **Pepsins A, B & C** (E.C. 3.4.23.1–3.4.23.3), which attack peptide linkages on the carboxyl side of leucine and phenylalanine; **Cathepsin D** (E.C. 3.4.23.5); and intracellular proteinases with similar specificity.

Metalloproteinases E.C. 3.4.24 (need a metal: Zn^{2+}, Ca^{2+}, Mg^{2+}, Fe^{2+}, for activity; inhibited by chelating agents)
Include various **Collagenases** (from bacteria and vertebrate animals), which peptide linkages joining glycine to proline, and numerous enzymes of invertebrates and microorganisms.

tide configuration, such as naphthyl amides. Histochemical methods are available in which the naphthyl amines liberated from substrates of this type are trapped by diazonium salts in a similar way to that in which α-naphthol is trapped in the method for alkaline phosphatase described in Section 15.1.2.2. Some proteinases are able to act upon esters, and this property has also been utilized histochemically. Unfortunately, uncertainty often exists as to the correspondence between histochemically demonstrated enzymes and those identified by biochemists.

| 15.3.2.
Method for enteropeptidase | Enteropeptidase (E.C. 3.4.21.9; also called enterokinase) is secreted in the duodenum. It catalyses the hydrolysis of a peptide bond between lysine and leucine in pancreatic trypsinogen, thus forming a hexapeptide and trypsin, which is a major enzyme of protein digestion: |

$$\text{TRYPSINOGEN} + H_2O \xrightarrow{\text{(enteropeptidase)}} \text{TRYPSIN} + \text{a hexapeptide}$$

The incubation medium for the histochemical detection of enteropeptidase (Lojda and Malis, 1972) contains trypsinogen, an artificial chromogenic substrate for trypsin, and a diazonium salt. Three reactions occur:

(1) Enteropeptidase catalyses the hydrolysis of its natural substrate, trypsinogen, releasing trypsin. At this stage, the newly formed trypsin is in the medium within and near to the cells that contain enteropeptidase.

(2) Trypsin catalyses the hydrolysis of N-benzoylarginine-2-naphthylamide (BANA):

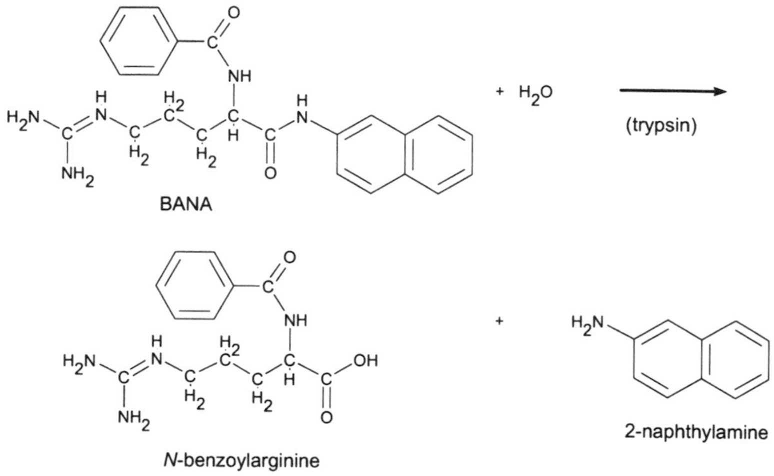

BANA

N-benzoylarginine

2-naphthylamine

(3) One of the products of the reaction is 2-naphthylamine (β-naphthylamine). This couples with the diazonium salt. Fast blue B salt has two $-N_2^+$ groups (Chapter 5), so it can combine with two molecules of the aromatic amine to form a disazo dye:

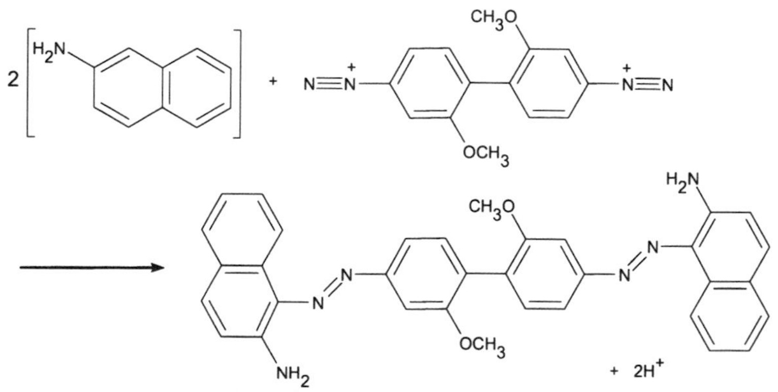

The dye can be rendered more stable by a treatment with aqueous copper sulphate. Probably an insoluble dye–metal complex is formed.

This is an example of a histochemical method in which two enzymatically catalysed reactions occur sequentially. The trypsin is formed in solution, and can be expected to diffuse away from the sites in which it is generated by the enteropeptidase-catalysed hydrolysis of trypsinogen. The accuracy of localization depends on rapid hydrolysis of BANA by the released trypsin and immediate production of the insoluble azo dye. The ingredients of the incubation medium are dissolved in a gel made from agar, and this is allowed to set in contact with the sections. The high viscosity of the gelled agar retards diffusion of trypsin and 2-naphthylamine, thereby improving the accuracy of localization of enteropeptidase.

Enteropeptidase is present at the luminal ends (brush borders) of the absorptive epithelial cells of the duodenum. Negative control specimens can be taken from the distal ileum. The tissue may be fixed for a few hours in neutral buffered formaldehyde at 4°C, but Lojda et al. (1979) preferred to use unfixed cryostat sections.

Solutions required

A. 0.1 M TRIS buffer, pH 6.5, with 0.01 M Ca²⁺
The TRIS buffer in Chapter 20 is 0.05 M. A 0.1 M buffer is prepared by making the final volume to only half that stated in the table. Adjustment of the pH may be necessary. Add 0.1 g calcium chloride ($CaCl_2$) to 100 ml of the buffer.

B. Agar solution
Dissolve 0.5 g of agar in 50 ml of water, by heating on a water-bath, almost to boiling. Allow to cool to about 60°C, and maintain at this temperature until ready to use. Make on the day it is to be used.

C. Copper sulphate solution (0.08 M)
2% (w/v) aqueous $CuSO_4.5H_2O$. Keeps indefinitely.

D. Incubation medium
This medium is made up immediately before it is to be used.

N-benzoyl-L-arginyl-2-naphthylamide:	8 mg
(If the pure L-isomer of BANA is not available, use the DL-form)	
N,N-dimethyl formamide (DMF):	0.5 ml

Dissolve the BANA in the DMF, then add to 5 ml of TRIS buffer with Ca^{2+} (Solution A). Mix well, then add:

Fast blue B salt (C.I. 37235):	5–10 mg

Filter the solution if it is not transparent, then add:

Trypsinogen:	2 mg

Swirl or stir to dissolve, then add 2 ml of the warm agar solution (B). Quickly check the pH, and adjust to 6.5 if necessary. Be careful to wash the pH meter electrode thoroughly after use. Proceed immediately to Step 2 of the procedure described below.

For a **control medium**, omit the trypsinogen.

Procedure
(1) Mount the sections on slides and allow to dry. Place on a horizontal staining rack.
(2) Pour the warm incubation medium (Solution D) onto the slides. It should spread to form a thin layer covering the sections, and set within about 1 min.
(3) Transfer the slides to an incubator with a moist atmosphere at 37°C, and inspect at 30 min intervals. Optimum staining is usually seen between 1 and 2 h.
(4) Immerse the slides in 0.08 M copper sulphate (Solution C) for 5 min at room temperature. Handle carefully to avoid damaging the agar layer and the sections.
(5) Transfer the slides to water, and leave for 5 min to remove copper sulphate and any other residual reagents.

(6)   Examine and photograph, then allow the slides to dry before storing. If they are to be examined later, a coverslip may be applied, using an aqueous mounting medium or a drop of immersion oil.

Result

The product of the reaction is purple; it is seen in the section, and in the overlying film of agar. There is also a brownish-yellow background, due to azo-coupling of the fast blue B salt with aromatic amino acid side-chains of proteins (Chapter 10, Section 10.9.2).

Enteropeptidase occurs at the luminal brush borders of the epithelial cells of the duodenum, and is absent from the distal ileum. Purple colour produced in the control medium (without trypsinogen) may be due to trypsin-like lysosomal enzymes, or to an enzyme present in the mast cells of some species, including man but not rats or mice (see Selye, 1965).

15.3.3.
Substrate film methods

We now consider a group of techniques that are based on principles quite different from those in which soluble substrates and trapping agents are used. In the first method of this kind to be described (Adams and Tuqan, 1961), unfixed cryostat sections were placed on the emulsion of an over-exposed, developed, fixed and washed photographic plate. The section and the film were kept slightly moist (but not wet) with a suitable buffer. The preparation was incubated for about an hour in a humid atmosphere and then dried and mounted for examination. A developed photographic emulsion contains tiny particles of metallic silver suspended in gelatin (which is a protein of high molecular weight made by boiling collagen in water). Proteolytic activity derived from the section changes the subjacent gelatin into soluble peptides of lower molecular weight, which diffuse into the surrounding regions of the emulsion, carrying the suspended silver particles with them. After a suitable time of incubation, the blackened emulsion has transparent holes in it that correspond to sites of proteinase activity in the tissue. The section itself is obscured by the black emulsion, so the positions of the digested holes have to be identified by comparison of the substrate-film preparation with an adjacent, stained section of the same specimen. Colour films have also been used as substrates, but most are unsuitable because their emulsions are made of gelatin that has been excessively cross-linked in the manufacturing process (Hasegawa and Hasegawa, 1977).

Finding that the emulsions on modern black and white photographic plates and films were not digestible by proteinases, Lee *et al.* (1999) used instead glass slides coated with Kodak NTB2, a liquid emulsion used for autoradiography. Their technique, described in detail in the cited publication, showed zones of proteolytic activity 25–30 μm wide in sections of growing bone. Studies with inhibitors and neutralizing antibodies, supplemented by immunohistochemistry and electron microscopy, identified the enzyme as gelatinase B, a matrix metalloproteinase (MMP). Another proteinase, collagenase-3 occurred at the same sites. These enzymes remove Type II collagen fibrils from cartilage in parts of bones that are remodeling during development (Lee *et al.*, 1999; Davoli *et al.*, 2001).

A gelatin substrate of more certain composition than a photographic emulsion may be prepared by covalently linking a dye to a layer of gelatin on a microscope slide (Cunningham, 1967; Kiernan, 1981). A dyed gelatin film is sufficiently transparent to allow examination of the section by phase-contrast microscopy, thereby permitting more accurate localization of the holes produced by the action of proteolytic enzymes. Pirila *et al.* (2001) used a conjugate of gelatin with a fluorescent dye, Oregon green 488 and was able to observe proteolysis for up to 4 days and, by using inhibitors, to identify the gelatinases as specific MMPs. An alternative approach is to use an undyed gelatin film and, after incubation, to stain both the film and the section by a general method for protein (Fried *et al.*, 1976). The colour is then strongest where both tissue and film are present, so that digested areas are easily seen only at the edges of the section. Another type of substrate film consists of colloidal silver particles suspended in gelatin. At sites of proteolytic digestion the particles clump together and the colour changes from yellow to red (Abiko *et al.*, 1999).

Substrate-film methods are not applicable only to proteolytic enzymes. It is possible to make gelatinous films containing other macromolecular substrates, such as nucleic acids or glycosaminoglycans, and to demonstrate local areas of degradation by appropriate staining (Section 14.5.1). In practice, none of these methods are much used, because of the imprecise localization of enzymatic activity.

Enzyme overlay membranes, which can be impregnated with a variety of fluorogenic substrates, are made commercially for application to gels that contain proteins separated by electrophoresis. The fluorescent product is released from combination with the substrate at sites where an enzyme diffuses into the membrane. The fluorochrome (typically 7-amino-4-trifluoromethylcoumarin, AFC) fluoresces more strongly in the free state than when it is joined by an amide or ester linkage to a peptide. Membranes containing AFC-peptide substrates for two proteolytic enzymes were applied to cryostat sections (fixed in cold methanol) by Day and Neufeld (1997), in conjunction with various inhibitors. This method is technically easier and more sensitive than earlier substrate film procedures, and is potentially applicable to a wide variety of enzymes. The resolution is, however, greatly inferior to that attainable with substrates that penetrate the tissue. Fluorescently labelled peptides can also be included in a thin layer of agarose that is layered over the preparation (Yi *et al.*, 2001). With enzyme overlay methods the fluorescent product must be photographed as it forms, and then compared with a phase-contrast image or a stained preparation of the same section.

16 Oxidoreductases

The following account is a simplified one, and several controversial issues are not taken into consideration. Stoward and Pearse (1991) and Wöhlrab, Seidler and Kunze (1979) discuss the subject in great detail, and shorter treatments are given by Lojda *et al.* (1979) and Chayen and Bitensky (1991). The metabolic functions of the oxidoreductases are explained in textbooks of biochemistry.

16.1. Oxidation and reduction

An atom or molecule is said to be oxidized when it loses one or more electrons and to be reduced when it gains one or more electrons. A simple example of a reaction of this type is a change in the oxidation state of a metal ion:

$$Fe^{2+} \underset{\text{reduction}}{\overset{\text{oxidation}}{\rightleftarrows}} Fe^{3+} + \varepsilon^-$$

The position of the equilibrium is determined by the presence of other substances which can accept or donate electrons (**oxidizing** and **reducing agents** respectively). For example, the ferric ion is reduced by hydroquinone in acid conditions:

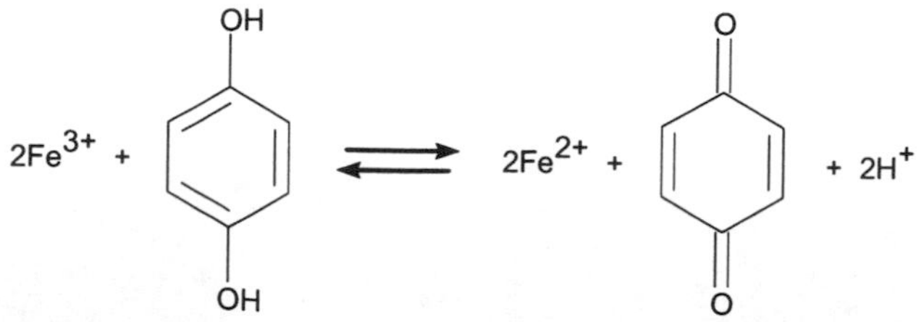

Here, the ferric ion is the oxidizing agent and it is reduced to the ferrous state. At the same time, hydroquinone is a reducing agent that acts upon the ferric ions and is itself oxidized (with loss of two hydrogen atoms) to *p*-quinone.

The reaction between ferric ions and hydroquinone is the algebraic sum of two half-reactions:

$$Fe^{3+} + \varepsilon^- \rightleftharpoons Fe^{2+} \qquad (16.1)$$

$$H_2Q \rightleftharpoons Q + 2H^+ + 2\varepsilon^- \qquad (16.2)$$

(H2Q = hydroquinone; Q = p-quinone)

Both sides of equation (16.1) are multiplied by 2 before adding, in order that the number of electrons (ε^-) participating in each half-reaction will be the same. Thus:

$$2Fe^{3+} + 2\varepsilon^- \rightleftharpoons 2Fe^{2+}$$

$$H_2Q \rightleftharpoons Q + 2H^+ + 2\varepsilon^-$$

$$\overline{}$$

$$2Fe^{3+} + H_2Q \rightleftharpoons 2Fe^{2+} + Q + 2H^+$$

It will be noticed that the electrons have been cancelled out and do not appear in the equation for the complete reaction. It will also be noticed that the reaction is reversible. The oxidation of hydroquinone in neutral and alkaline solutions is more complicated and leads to the formation of polymeric products.

The net effect of the oxidation of hydroquinone has been the loss of two atoms of hydrogen. The gain or loss of hydrogen is a feature of most oxidation–reduction reactions of biological importance. According to an earlier definition, a substance was said to be oxidized when it gained oxygen, lost hydrogen, or increased its positive charge and to be reduced when oxygen was lost, hydrogen gained, or negative charge increased. The modern definition, in terms of the transfer of electrons, simplifies the multiple requirements of the older one.

The number of electrons gained or lost by an organic molecule is not always as obvious as it is in the case of an inorganic ion. It may be determined (see Hendrickson et al., 1970, for more information) from the change in the **oxidation number** of the carbon atom at which oxidation or reduction takes place. The oxidation number of a carbon atom is found by adding the following values for each of its four bonds:

-1	for each bond to hydrogen
0	for each bond to another carbon
$+1$	for each bond to an atom other than hydrogen or carbon

Thus, for the carbon atom at the top of the p-quinone molecule there are two bonds to other carbon atoms ($2 \times 0 = 0$) and two to an oxygen atom ($2 \times +1 = +2$), so the oxidation number is +2. At the equivalent position in hydroquinone there are three bonds to carbon ($3 \times 0 = 0$) and one to oxygen ($1 \times +1 = +1$), giving the oxidation number +1. This carbon atom therefore gains one electron in the process of being reduced. The carbon on the opposite side of the ring behaves identically, so the reduction of the whole molecule of p-quinone involves the acquisition of two electrons. Conversely, the oxidation of hydroquinone is accomplished by its losing two electrons. Application of the rule given above will show that each of the other four carbon atoms has oxidation number -1 in both p-quinone and hydroquinone.

16.2. Oxidation–reduction potentials

It is possible to make an electrical cell in which one electrode is gaseous hydrogen and the other is an inert metal such as platinum, immersed in an electrolyte that is a solution of a substance capable of being oxidized or reduced. Completion of the external circuit by a wire will result in the passage of electrons from one electrode to the other as a consequence of the gain or loss of electrons by the electrolyte at the inert electrode. The potential difference between the electrodes can be measured, in volts, and its magnitude, under standardized conditions of temperature and concentration, is the **oxidation–reduction** potential (E_0) of the electrolyte. It is a measure of the ease with which the electrolyte is oxidized or reduced or, conversely, of the strength of the electrolyte as an oxidizing or reducing agent.

Hydrogen is arbitrarily assigned $E_0 = 0$. The oxidation–reduction potentials of other substances are, by the most widely used convention, applied to half-reactions in which electrons are gained. Thus, the half-reaction in which a strong oxidizing agent (which takes up electrons avidly) is reduced will have a high positive value of E_0. The half-reaction in which a weaker oxidizing agent than the hydrogen ion is reduced will have a negative E_0. These half reactions are reversible. If they are written the other way round, the negative or positive sign of E_0 is changed. Tables of half-reactions and their potentials are to be found in references books such as the *CRC Handbook of Chemistry and Physics* (Chemical Rubber Company, 2007) and *Lange's Handbook of Chemistry* (Dean, 1999).

Consider the following half-reactions, arranged in descending order of their oxidation–reduction potentials:

$$MnO_4^- + 8H^+ + 5\varepsilon^- \rightleftharpoons Mn^{2+} + 4H_2O \quad (E_0 = +1.51 \text{ V})$$

$$Fe^{3+} + \varepsilon^- \rightleftharpoons Fe^{2+} \quad (E_0 = +0.77 \text{ V})$$

$$2CO_2 + 2H^+ + 2\varepsilon^- \rightleftharpoons (COOH)_2 \quad (E_0 = -0.49 \text{ V})$$

$$Na^+ + \varepsilon^- \rightleftharpoons Na \quad (E_0 = -2.71 \text{ V})$$

Of the substances shown, permanganate ion is the strongest oxidizing agent, and sodium metal is the strongest reducing agent. A substance on the left-hand side of one of the above half-reactions can be expected to oxidize a substance on the right-hand side only if the latter has a more negative E_0 than the former. Permanganate ions in acid solution therefore react with oxalic acid (to give manganous ions and carbon dioxide), but sodium ions will not react with ferrous ions. The equation for the overall reaction is obtained by reversing the half-reaction that contains the reducing agent and adding it to the half-reaction containing the oxidizing agent. It may be necessary to multiply both sides of one or both of the equations by appropriate integers in order to obtain equal numbers of electrons on the two sides of the final equation. For the reaction between permanganate ion and oxalic acid, one reaction must be multiplied by 2 and the other by 5:

$$2MnO_4^- + 16H^+ + 10\bar{\varepsilon} \rightleftharpoons 2Mn^{2+} + 8H_2O$$

$$5(COOH)_2 \rightleftharpoons 10CO_2 + 10H^+ + 10\bar{\varepsilon}^-$$

$$\overline{2MnO_4^- + 6H^+ + 5(COOH)_2 \rightleftharpoons 2Mn^{2+} + 10CO_2 + 8H_2O}$$

Although this reaction is theoretically reversible, it proceeds from left to right, virtually to completion, because there is a large difference between the oxidation–reduction potentials of the two component half-reactions. (The continuous removal of carbon dioxide from the system, as gas or by combination with water to form carbonic acid, also helps to drive the reaction from left to right, in accordance with Le Chatelier's principle and the law of mass action.)

Tables of oxidation–reduction potentials are valuable for showing which oxidations are likely to occur and which are not, but they must be used with caution (see Latimer, 1952 and textbooks of inorganic and general chemistry). Other chemical properties of the reactants are not taken into account and may complicate the overall reaction. The mixing of ferric ions with oxalic acid, for example, will result in the formation not only of ferrous oxalate (a sparingly soluble salt) but also of soluble complexes in which one, two, or three oxalate ions are coordinately bound to iron ions in both oxidation states +2 and +3. These complications could only be predicted by taking into account the chemistry of complex formation as well as the oxidation–reduction potentials.

Of greater importance in biochemical oxidation–reduction reactions is the fact that the value of the potential for any system varies with temperature, with the pH of the solvent, and with the proportions of the oxidizing and reducing agents present. A constant more useful than E_0 is E_0', the oxidation–reduction potential of the half reduced system at specified temperature and pH. *Table 16.1* gives values of E_0' for some biochemically and histochemically important half-reactions at pH7 and 25°C.

16.3. Biological oxidations

The life of every cell depends upon the coordinated oxidation and reduction of many organic compounds. These chemical reactions, collectively known as **cellular respiration**, involve a great number of substrates and enzymes and a much smaller number of **electron carriers**. One electron carrier can function as coenzyme or prosthetic group to many different substrate-specific respiratory enzymes. A **coenzyme** is a soluble substance (itself enzymatically inert and not a protein) that can diffuse in the cytoplasm and attach itself, reversibly, to the proteinaceous **apoenzyme**. A **prosthetic group** is a non-protein organic compound that is covalently bound to the protein molecule constituting the enzyme.

When attached to the apoenzyme, the coenzyme accepts electrons from the substrate, and protons from either the substrate or the surrounding medium. Thus, the coenzyme is reduced and the substrate is oxidized. Effectively the coenzyme removes one or two atoms of hydrogen from the substrate, so it is equally valid to call the electron carrier a **hydrogen acceptor**.

The reduced form of the coenzyme acts as an electron donor for the enzymatic reduction of some other substrate. The original coenzyme is thus regenerated. Enzymes that catalyse the reoxidation of reduced coenzymes are often called **diaphorases**. They are more correctly named as the enzymes that catalyse the reduction of their specific substrates. The diaphorase activity (catalysis of the oxidation of reduced coenzyme) is incidental to the main function of such an enzyme. The histochemist, however, is often primarily interested in localizing the sites of reoxidation of reduced coenzymes. Because more than one enzyme may catalyse this reaction for a single reduced coenzyme, the conveniently vague term 'diaphorase' will continue to be used when the enzymes concerned cannot be accurately identified and named.

Before discussing some of the enzymes that catalyse oxidation and reduction and the histochemical methods for their identification, it is necessary to review the system that transfers electrons and protons from oxidized metabolites to the ultimate oxidizing agent, which is atmospheric oxygen. The transport takes place in several stages and involves the repetitive oxidation and reduction of various prosthetic groups, coenzymes, and cytochromes. The last-named substances are proteins with iron-containing haem groups. The oxidation number of the iron atom is +3 or

+2, when the molecule is in the oxidized or reduced state, respectively. Cytochromes are not, strictly speaking, enzymes, but one of them, cytochrome aa_3, is commonly known as **cytochrome oxidase**. It transfers electrons and protons to molecular oxygen. It is not itself consumed in this reaction. Thus, cytochrome aa_3 catalyses the reduction of molecular oxygen to water. The reactions of the electron-transport chain occur in an order dictated largely by the oxidation–reduction potentials of the various half-reactions that make up the system. These, together with the names of the more important coenzymes, prosthetic groups and cytochromes, are set out in *Table 16.1*. The data in the table are taken mainly from Loach (1976).

Table 16.1. Oxidation–reduction potentials in the electron-transport system

Half-reaction		E_0' (V) (at pH 7.0; 25°C)
$H_2O_2 + 2H^+ + 2\varepsilon^-$	$= 2H_2O$	+1.35
$O_2 + 4H^+ + 4\varepsilon^-$	$= 2H_2O$	+0.82
cyt. $aa_3^{3+} + \varepsilon^-$	$=$ cyt. aa_3^{2+}	+0.29
cyt. $a^{3+} + \varepsilon^-$	$=$ cyt. a^2+	+0.29
cyt. $c^{3+} + \varepsilon^-$	$=$ cyt. c^{2+}	+0.25
cyt. $c_1^{3+} + \varepsilon^-$	$=$ cyt. c_1^{2+}	+0.22
$UQ + 2H^+ + 2\varepsilon^-$	$= UQH_2$	+0.10
cyt. $b^{3+} + \varepsilon^-$	$=$ cyt. b^{3+}	+0.08
$FMN + 2H^+ + 2\varepsilon^-$	$= FMNH_2$	−0.21
$FAD + 2H^+ + 2\varepsilon^-$	$= FADH_2$	−0.22
$NAD+ + 2H^+ + 2\varepsilon^-$	$= NADH + H^+$	−0.32
$NADP+ + 2H^+ + 2\varepsilon^-$	$= NADPH + H^+$	−0.32

Coenzymes: UQ = ubiquinone (coenzyme Q); UQH2 = reduced form. NAD$^+$ = nicotinamide adenine dinucleotide (formerly known as coenzyme I or DPN); NADH = reduced form. NADP$^+$ = nicotinamide adenine dinucleotide phosphate (formerly known as coenzyme II or TPN), NADPH = reduced form.
Prosthetic groups: FMN = flavin mononucleotide; FMNH$_2$ = reduced form. FAD = flavin adenine dinucleotide; FADH$_2$ = reduced form. The value of E_0' for a prosthetic group may differ from that given above for different apoenzymes. For example, the FAD of succinic dehydrogenase has E_0' = −0.03.
Cytochromes: Designated 'cyt' followed by a letter (a, aa_3, b, c, $c1$) with superscript indicating oxidation number of the iron atom. Thus cyt. c^{3+} and cyt. c^{2+} are the oxidized reduced forms of cytochrome c.

Not all the substances shown in *Table 16.1* are involved in the oxidation of all metabolites. Electrons most often pass from NADH or NADPH to one of the flavoproteins and thence via ubiquinone and the cytochromes to molecular oxygen.

All the components of the electron-transport system are present in the mitochondria of eukaryotic cells and some occur also in the general cytoplasmic matrix, associated with soluble enzymes. The oxidation of any metabolite involves the enzymatically catalysed transfer of protons and electrons from substrate to an acceptor:

substrate + acceptor ⇌ oxidized substrate + reduced acceptor
(enzyme)

Commonly the acceptor is a coenzyme such as NAD$^+$ or NADP$^+$ or a prosthetic group such as FMN or FAD. The enzyme catalysing the reaction is then known as a **dehydrogenase**. Such an enzyme (consisting of apoenzyme + oxidized form of the coenzyme) combines specifically with its substrate and renders it highly reactive towards the coenzyme. When the reaction has taken place, the oxidized substrate and the reduced coenzyme part company with the apoenzyme and are then free to enter into other chemical reactions. Specificity for the substrate resides in the apoenzyme, even though the latter cannot bind to its substrate unless it has first combined with the coenzyme.

A simple example of a reaction catalysed by a dehydrogenase is the oxidation of the lactate ion. The enzyme concerned is known as lactate dehydrogenase.

The lactate ion first combines with an enzyme molecule:

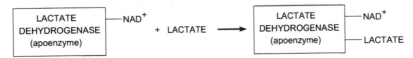

Then, on the surface of the enzyme molecule:

$$\text{LACTATE} + \text{NAD}^+ \longrightarrow \text{PYRUVATE} + \text{NADH} + \text{H}^+$$

and finally:

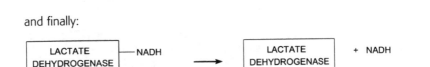

The NADH will subsequently be re-oxidized to NAD^+, when it serves as coenzyme in the enzymatically catalysed reduction of some other substrate. Notice that the acceptor in the oxidation of lactate was NAD^+. The systematic name for lactate dehydrogenase, which identifies both the substrate and the acceptor, is L-lactate:NAD oxidoreductase (E.C. 1.1.1.27). (See Section 14.2 for explanations of formal names of enzymes and Enzyme Commission numbers.) The same enzyme will also catalyse the reduction of pyruvate ions. The direction in which the reversible reaction proceeds is determined by the relative concentrations of the reactants: lactate, pyruvate, NAD^+, NADH, and H^+. Oxidation of lactate occurs when this ion is present in excess and when NADH and H^+ are continuously removed, either by other metabolic activities or by deliberate manipulation of the conditions of the reaction.

The electrons removed from a substance such as lactate, when it has been oxidized, are incorporated into a reduced coenzyme. When this is re-oxidized, the electrons will be transferred to another acceptor, which has a higher oxidation–reduction potential than the coenzyme. Usually the flow of electrons passes via flavoprotein enzymes, ubiquinone, and the cytochrome system to molecular oxygen. For the histochemist, the importance of all this lies in the fact that the flow of electrons may be interrupted by the introduction of an artificial electron-acceptor with an oxidation–reduction potential intermediate between those of any two of the members of the electron transport chain. The **tetrazolium salts**, to be discussed below, are suitable for this purpose because on reduction they are converted to insoluble pigments. Thus, whenever a substrate is oxidized in the presence of a tetrazolium salt, the released electrons will not be transported through the usual sequence of cytochromes, etc., but will be trapped in the formation of a stable, coloured substance.

Not all oxidoreductases make use of the coenzymes NAD^+ and NADP^+; some dehydrogenases are flavoproteins. The most familiar of these is succinate dehydrogenase, whose prosthetic group is FAD. The physiological acceptors associated with the flavoprotein dehydrogenases are not certainly known, though ubiquinone is a likely candidate. Other oxidoreductases use molecular oxygen as an acceptor, thus bypassing all the intermediate components of the electron transport system. These enzymes are known as **oxidases**. Tetrazolium salts cannot be used to detect the activity of oxidases unless they can be made to act as substitutes for oxygen. Other methods are therefore usually needed for these enzymes. The other oxidoreductases considered in this chapter are the **peroxidases**. These catalyse the oxidation of many substances by hydrogen peroxide and are discussed in Section 16.5.

16.4. Histochemistry of dehydrogenases

The dehydrogenases catalyse the general reaction:

(**S** and **SH$_2$** represent oxidized and reduced forms of the substrate. **A** and **AH$_2$** represent oxidized and reduced forms of the acceptor, which is a substance other than O_2 or H_2O_2.)

When the reaction proceeds from left to right, the net effect is the removal of hydrogen (usually two atoms of it) from the substrate. The acceptor is the coenzyme (NAD$^+$ or NADP$^+$) in the case of coenzyme-linked dehydrogenases. These enzymes are detected histochemically by substituting an artificial electron acceptor for the naturally occurring substances constituting the electron transport chain. The artificial substance chosen is one which becomes insoluble and coloured in its reduced state. A visible precipitate forms at sites where hydrogen is given up by an electron carrier whose oxidation reduction potential is negative with respect to that of the artificial hydrogen acceptor.

In the histochemical methods for dehydrogenases, the substrates are the physiological ones, and no attempts are made to trap the products of their oxidation. Instead, a special kind of indicator (the artificial hydrogen acceptor or electron carrier) is used to detect the place in which a biological oxidation is taking place. The substrate is provided in large amounts in the incubation medium. An adequate quantity of the acceptor must also be present, either as coenzyme added to the medium or as intermediate electron carriers already present in the tissue.

16.4.1.
Tetrazolium salts

The artificial hydrogen acceptors of greatest value to the histochemist are the tetrazolium salts. These are heterocyclic compounds (derivatives of tetrazole, CH$_2$N$_4$) which are changed by reduction into insoluble, coloured **formazans**.

$$
\begin{array}{ccc}
\text{tetrazolium} & + \ H^+ \ + \ 2\varepsilon^- \ \rightleftharpoons & \text{formazan} \\
\text{cation} & &
\end{array}
$$

This reaction proceeds from left to right because the formazan is insoluble. Several tetrazolium salts have been used in histochemical methods for dehydrogenases. The ideal one would be stable, not chemically altered by exposure to light, and would be reduced very rapidly to yield a formazan with exceedingly small crystals that were insoluble in lipids and had some substantivity for protein. (Substantivity is explained in Chapter 5 in connection with dyeing, and in Chapter 14 as a desirable property of final reaction products in enzyme histochemistry.) These properties are most closely approached by the cations of some of the ditetrazolium salts, which have the general structure:

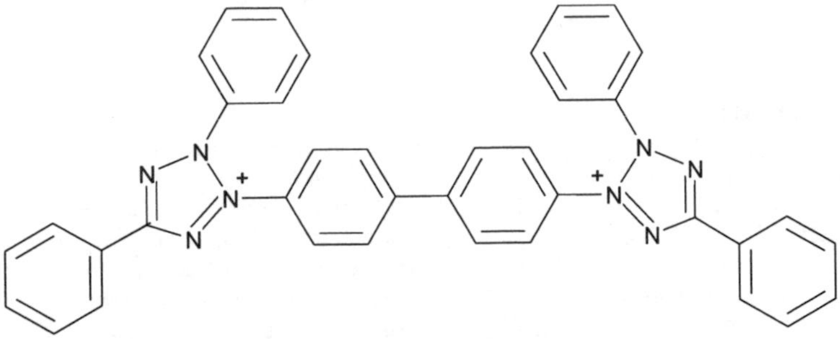

with various substituents on the benzene rings. Monotetrazolium salts, which have only one tetrazole (CN_4) ring in the molecule, are generally less suitable, though some are used as histochemical reagents. When a ditetrazolium salt is reduced, the product may be either a monoformazan in which only one of the tetrazole rings has been opened or a diformazan in which both tetrazole rings have been opened. Monoformazans are usually red, and diformazans are blue, purple, or black. Both the coloured products may be formed in histochemical reactions, though the diformazan is the one desired. Other colours (usually reds) may also result from the presence of monotetrazolium salts as contaminants in samples of ditetrazolium salts.

A list of tetrazolium salts, with some of their properties, is given in *Table 16.2*. For the structural formulae of the compounds other than nitro-BT see pp 157–168 in Horobin and Kiernan (2002).

The most generally useful tetrazolium salt for use in light microscopy is **nitro blue tetrazolium (nitro-BT)**, which has the advantage of forming a diformazan that is not visibly crystalline, is insoluble in water, lipids and organic solvents, and is substantive for protein.

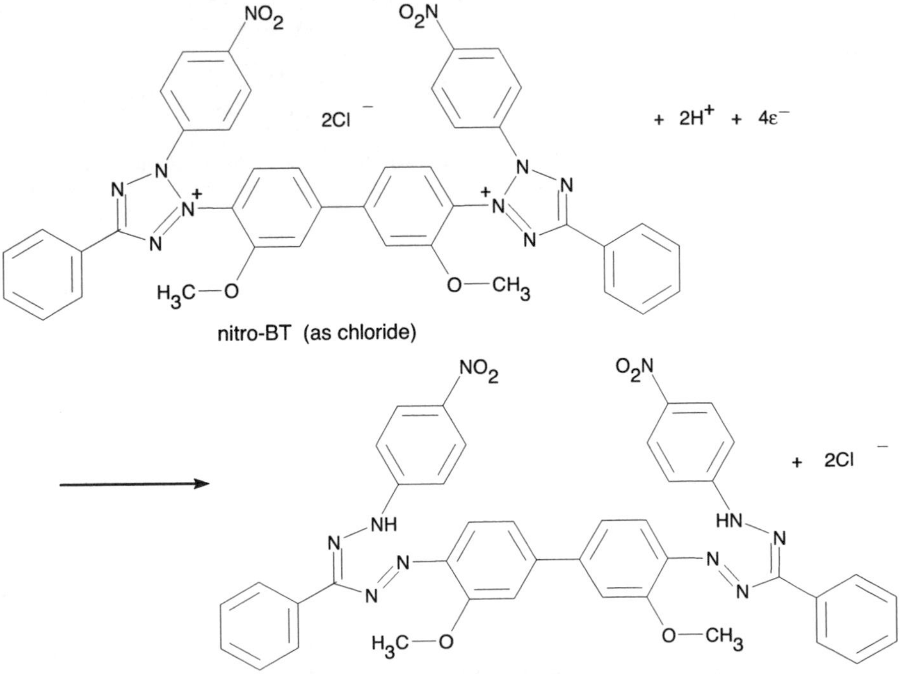

nitro-BT (as chloride)

formazan of nitro-BT

Table 16.2. Properties of some tetrazolium salts and their formazans[a]

Trivial name, abbreviation, and MW	E_0' (V) (pH 7.2; 22°C)	Properties of formazan	Carriers from which electrons are accepted in histochemistry
Monotetrazolium salts			
Triphenyltetrazolium (chloride). TTC (MW 335)	−0.49	Large red crystals. High lipid solubility. Reduction is slow.	cyt. a; cyt. a_3
2,3-p-dinitrotriphenyltetrazolium (chloride). 2,3-p-DNTTC (MW 425)	? −0.05	Small blue crystals. High lipid solubility, but also binds to protein. Reduction is rapid.	Flavoproteins; UQ; cyt. b
m-3-trinitrotriphenyltetrazolium (chloride). 2,3-p-TNTTC (MW 470)	? −0.05	Small red crystals. Lipid-soluble, but also binds to protein. Reduction is very rapid[b].	Flavoproteins; UQ; cyt. b
Tetrazolium violet (chloride). TV (MW 384)	? −0.20	Large dark blue crystals. Pink contaminant. High lipid solubility. Reduction is slow.	
Methylthiazolyldiphenyltetrazolium (bromide). MTT (MW 414)	−0.11	Co^{2+} chelate has small, black crystals. Lipid-soluble but also binds to protein. Reduction rapid.	UQ; cyt. b; cyt. c_1
Iodonitrotetrazolium (chloride). INT (MW 505)	−0.09	Large dark red crystals. Orange contaminant. High lipid solubility. Reduction is rapid.	UQ; cyt. b; cyt. c_1
2-(2-benzothiazolyl-5-styryl-2-(4-phthalylhydrazidyltetrazolium (chloride). BSPT (MW 502)	? −0.10	Purple, amorphous. Used in EM histochemistry. Reduction is rapid.	
Ditetrazolium salts			
Neotetrazolium (dichloride). NT (MW > 668)	−0.17	Dark purple. Small lipid-soluble crystals. Red monoformazan or contaminant. Reduction is rapid.	UQ; cyt. b; cyt. c
Blue tetrazolium (dichloride). BT (MW 728)	−0.16	Small deep blue lipid-soluble crystals. Red monoformazan. Reduction is slow.	
Nitro blue tetrazolium (dichloride). Nitro-BT or NBT (MW 818)	−0.05	Dark blue, amorphous. Slight lipid solubility. Binds to protein. Resists organic solvents. Red monoformazan and contaminant are lipid- and alcohol-soluble. Reduction is rapid.	Flavoproteins; UQ; cyt. b
Tetranitro blue tetrazolium (dichloride). TNBT (MW 908)	? −0.05	Brown, amorphous. Insoluble in lipids and organic solvents. Pink monoformazan or contaminant. Reduction is rapid.	(Probably closely similar to nitro-BT)
Distyryl nitro blue tetrazolium (dichloride). DS-NBT (MW 870)	? −0.10	Amorphous, osmiophilic. Used in EM histochemistry. Reduction is rapid.	

[a]For more information, see Burstone (1962), Lillie & Fullmer (1976), Lillie (1977) and Seidler (1980). The oxidation reduction potentials E'_0 are taken from Pearse (1972). These values of E'_0 may not be accurate, and cannot be compared in a meaningful way with the potentials of systems in which the oxidizing and reducing agents are soluble, for reasons given by Jambor (1954) and Clark (1972). They are useful, however, for comparing one tetrazolium salt with another. (Values of E'_0 marked ? are guessed, on the basis of comparison of histochemical properties with those of tetrazolium salts with known oxidation-reduction potentials.)

[b]A blue-black formazan deposit is formed in injured and diseased cells containing enzymes that bring about reduction of m-3-TNTTC and some other monotetrazolium salts. Seidler (1980) suggests that the blue colour is due to alignment of formazan molecules on abnormal proteins. This explanation is similar to that offered for metachromasia of basic dyes (see Chapter 11).

It will be seen from the above formula that nitro-BT is a ditetrazolium salt in which the radical R″ of the general formula is joined to two substituted tetrazole rings. The oxidation reduction potential of nitro-BT is −0.05V, which lies between that of FAD and that of ubiquinone. This tetrazolium salt can therefore be expected to accept electrons from NADH, NADPH, or $FADH_2$, but not from dihydroubiquinone or from any of the cytochromes. However, studies in which metabolic inhibitors of various components of the electron-transport chain have been used indicate that within mitochondria tetrazolium salts collect electrons from UQH_2 and even from reduced cytochromes (see Burstone, 1962; Seidler, 1979).

Reduction of tetrazolium salts by systems with higher oxidation–reduction potentials would occur if there were large differences between the concentrations of the products and of the reactants. The values of E_0' in *Table 16.1* and *Table 16.2* pertain when [products] = [reactants]. The actual potential for the reduction, at a given temperature and pH, is

$$E = E_0' + \frac{RT}{nF} \log_e \frac{\text{[oxidizing agent]}}{\text{[reducing agent]}}$$

where R is the gas constant, T is the absolute temperature, n is the number of electrons gained by the reduced molecule or ion (usually two), and F is the faraday. $RT/F = 0.026$ at 25°C.

Thus, for a tetrazolium salt E will be higher than E_0' when the concentration of this reagent in the medium exceeds that of the formazan. The concentration of formazan is, of course, always very low on account of its very low solubility. It has been pointed out by Clark (1972) that artificial electron acceptors used in biochemical studies of dehydrogenases commonly react at rates completely out of line with their oxidation–reduction potentials. The values of E_0' apply to systems in true thermodynamic equilibrium, which is not likely to be the state of an experimental system with an excess of oxidizing agent present, or indeed that of the substances in a living cell.

The tetrazolium salt in a histochemical incubation medium is in competition with the naturally occurring electron carriers of the cell. In order to divert electrons from the oxidized substrate to the tetrazolium salt, it is sometimes necessary to inhibit the flow of electrons to oxygen. This may be accomplished either by incubating under strictly anaerobic conditions or, more easily, by adding cyanide ions to the medium. The cyanide inhibits cytochrome oxidase (cyt. a_3). Azide ions act similarly. Cyanide ions can also combine with aldehydes or ketones that are formed in some dehydrogenations, thus enhancing the enzyme-catalysed reaction by removing one of its products.

In ultrastructural cytochemical methods for dehydrogenases, the ferricyanide anion is sometimes preferred to a tetrazolium cation as an artificial electron acceptor (see Benkoel *et al.*, 1976). The phosphate-buffered incubation medium contains, in addition to the substrate and coenzyme, potassium ferricyanide, cupric sulphate and sodium citrate. The citrate ions form a soluble complex with Cu^{2+}, preventing precipitation of the sparingly soluble cupric ferricyanide. Reduction to ferrocyanide results in precipitation of copper ferrocyanide (Hatchett's brown), which is insoluble and electron-opaque.

16.4.2.
Diaphorases

When a tetrazolium salt is reduced by NADH or NADPH, the reaction is catalysed by an enzyme, either NADH-diaphorase or NADPH diaphorase.

These enzymes catalyse the reaction:

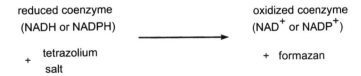

reduced coenzyme (NADH or NADPH) + tetrazolium salt → oxidized coenzyme (NAD^+ or $NADP^+$) + formazan

in which the reduced coenzyme is the substrate and the tetrazolium salt is the acceptor. When a tetrazolium salt is mixed with NADH or NADPH in the absence of a diaphorase apoenzyme, the reaction is very slow. Thus, the coloured product of a histochemical method for a coenzyme-linked dehydrogenase is formed by the catalytic action of another enzyme, the diaphorase. **Consequently, a coenzyme-linked dehydrogenase will be accurately localized only if it occurs in the same place as the diaphorase.** Fortunately, the diaphorases are present in all cells, in mitochondria, and sometimes also in the cytoplasmic matrix. They are rather 'tough' enzymes, unlikely to be inhibited by short fixation in formaldehyde or by other preparative manipulations.

The two histochemically recognized diaphorases represent various enzymes. Much of the NADH-diaphorase activity in animal cells may well be due to lipoamide dehydrogenase (NADH:lipoamide oxidoreductase; E.C. 1.6.4.3), which contains FAD as its prosthetic group and catalyses the reaction:

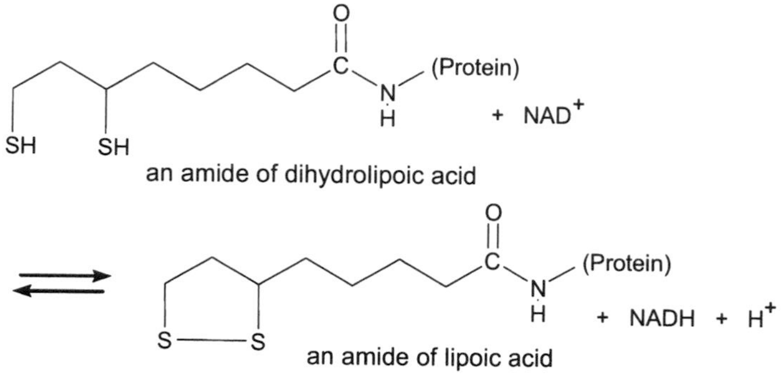

an amide of dihydrolipoic acid

$+ NAD^+$

an amide of lipoic acid

$+ NADH + H^+$

Tetrazolium salts are able to serve as acceptors in the place of the lipoic acid amide when the reaction proceeds from right to left. The properties of NADPH-diaphorase are shared by 'Warburg's old yellow enzyme' (NADPH: (acceptor) oxidoreductase: E.C. 1.6.99.1), which contains FMN. Some NADPH diaphorase activity is due to nitric oxide synthase (E.C. 1.14.13.39). This is a multi-functional oxidoreductase that catalyses a series of reactions in which arginine is oxidized to citrulline, with production of nitric oxide (Marletta et al., 1988; Klatt et al., 1993).

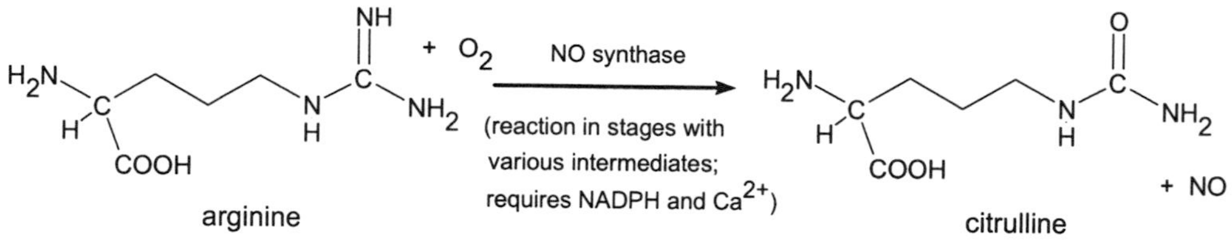

arginine

$+ O_2$ NO synthase
(reaction in stages with various intermediates; requires NADPH and Ca^{2+})

citrulline

$+ NO$

In mammals there are three isoforms of nitric oxide synthase that occur in different cell-types (see Pollock et al., 1995). All have NADPH diaphorase activity (Dawson et al., 1991; Hope et al., 1991) but histochemically detected NADPH diaphorase is not all nitric oxide synthase (Spessert et al., 1994). The diaphorase associated with nitric oxide production can be distinguished from other NADPH-diaphorase activity by optimizing the composition of the incubation medium (Spessert and Claassen, 1998). It is probably best to continue to use the names NADH- and NADPH-diaphorase for the enzymes that catalyse the oxidation of reduced coenzymes by tetrazolium salts, because the histochemical method reveals nothing about the physiological substrates. Names such as 'NADH-tetrazolium reductase' are also used and are acceptable.

The deliberate histochemical localization of the diaphorases is a very simple matter. Sections are incubated in a suitably buffered medium containing a tetrazolium salt and the appropriate **reduced form** of the coenzyme. The general methodological principles applicable to dehydrogenase histochemistry (see below) should also be observed.

In the case of the flavoprotein dehydrogenases, which have prosthetic groups rather than coenzymes, diaphorases cannot be responsible for the production of the formazan deposits. The mechanisms of electron-transfer from enzyme-bound $FADH_2$ or $FMNH_2$ to the tetrazolium salt are thought to involve ubiquinone and cytochromes, as discussed earlier. Some tetrazolium salts are able to accept electrons directly from reduced flavin nucleotides.

16.4.3.
Technical considerations

16.4.3.1. Tissue preparation

Oxidoreductases are generally much more easily inactivated than the hydrolytic enzymes discussed in Chapter 15 (Chalmers and Edgerton, 1989). It is not possible to fix the tissues thoroughly enough to allow the cutting of sections on an ordinary freezing microtome, and embedding in wax is out of the question. Small blocks of tissue may be fixed for 5–10 min in neutral, buffered formaldehyde at 4°C and then sectioned in a cryostat, or fresh frozen sections from the cryostat may be similarly fixed. Unfixed cryostat sections are often used, though meticulous attention to technique is necessary if the cells and their mitochondria are to remain recognizable after incubation (see Chayen and Bitensky, 1991). The two diaphorases and lactate dehydrogenase are notable in that they will survive fixation for several hours in neutral formaldehyde solutions. For the reasons given in Chapter 14, minimal fixation should be employed if possible. Fixation of the sections is more easily controlled than that of blocks. An alternative to formaldehyde is acetone (5 –10 min at 4°C), which also extracts some of the cytoplasmic lipids, to which certain of the formazans may be artifactually bound. Acetone also extracts ubiquinone, which may be a necessary intermediate for the reduction of tetrazolium salts in methods for the flavoprotein enzymes. It has been shown in the case of succinate dehydrogenase that it is necessary to apply UQ to sections that have been treated with acetone in order to be able to detect the enzyme at all sites of activity (Contestabile and Andersen, 1978).

16.4.3.2. Composition of incubation medium

The incubation medium for histochemical localization of a dehydrogenase includes the following:

(1) **Buffer.** The pH of the medium should be 7.0–7.2, even if this is not optimum for the enzyme. At pH values more alkaline than this, there is reduction of NAD^+ or $NADP^+$ even in the absence of a specific substrate. The NADH or NADPH so produced serves as substrate for its appropriate diaphorase, with consequent meaningless deposition of formazan within the section. This artifact, known as **nothing dehydrogenase**, is due partly to the action of lactate dehydrogenase on endogenous lactate ions in the tissue, but mainly to non-enzymatic reduction of the coenzyme by sulphydryl groups of proteins containing cysteine (Frederiks et al., 1989). Nothing dehydrogenase activity is maximal at pH 9.

Incubation media for dehydrogenases often contain cations of divalent metals, so TRIS buffer is usually used. Phosphate buffer is suitable when no metal ions that form insoluble phosphates are present.

(2) **Substrate.** Commonly the substrate is an organic anion and is used as its sodium salt, at a concentration of 0.1 M. Addition of the substrate usually changes the pH of the buffer, which must therefore be adjusted to the correct value by adding a few drops of 1.0 M NaOH or 1.0 M HCl.

(3) **Coenzymes.** The amount of coenzyme contained in a section is usually very small, so for coenzyme-linked dehydrogenases it is necessary to provide an

excess of NAD$^+$ or NADP$^+$ in the incubation medium at a concentration of approximately 0.003 M. For demonstration of diaphorases, the reduced form of the coenzymes (NADH or NADPH) is used.

(4) **Cofactors**. Many dehydrogenases have requirements for traces of divalent metal cations. It is usual to include magnesium chloride (0.005 M) in the medium. This does no harm, but is not necessary for all the enzymes. Magnesium ions probably also help to prevent rupture of mitochondria during incubation (see also (7) below).

(5) **Tetrazolium salt**. The concentration of the tetrazolium salt is not very critical and may range from 10^{-4} to 10^{-3} M. Some samples of nitro-BT and TNBT are difficult to dissolve in water, so they are dissolved in a small volume of an organic solvent before being added to the aqueous medium. The solvent must be one that is not a substrate for dehydrogenases. Ethanol would not be suitable; acetone or N,N-dimethylformamide is satisfactory.

(6) **Electron transport inhibitors**. To suppress aerobic cellular respiration, sodium or potassium cyanide or sodium azide (0.005–0.01 M) is incorporated in the incubation medium. An alternative, but inconvenient technique is to incubate in the complete absence of oxygen. For many enzymes, these precautions are unnecessary when a rapidly reducible tetrazolium salt such as nitro-BT is used.

(7) **Protective agents**. The inclusion of a chemically unreactive synthetic polymer in the medium prevents osmotic damage to mitochondria during incubation and, by increasing the viscosity of the medium, limits the diffusion of soluble enzymes. A protective agent is not always needed if the tissue has been partly fixed, but it is highly desirable when sections of unfixed tissues are used. The polymers employed for this purpose are polyvinylpyrollidone (PVP) (7.5% w/v) and polyvinyl alcohol (PVA) (20% w/v). The molecular weight of PVP used for this purpose is not critical. Chayen and Bitensky (1991) state that PVA should have a MW of 30 000; Nakae and Stoward (1997) used a 70–100 kDa PVA. Addition of these polymers often acidifies the medium and the pH must be adjusted accordingly.

(8) **Intermediate electron acceptors** (see *Fig. 16.1*). It is common practice to add **phenazine methosulphate** (PMS) (10^{-5}–10^{-3} M) to incubation media for dehydrogenases. This easily reduced substance transfers electrons directly from reduced coezymes or other acceptors to tetrazolium salts. The addition of PMS accelerates the reaction and gives more intense staining, but sometimes also causes non-specific deposition of formazan in the sections. this is due to spontaneous, non-enzymatic reduction of the tetrazolium salt by the reduced form of PMS. **Menadione** has also been used for the same purpose, though less often. An oxazine dye, **Meldola's blue** (C.I. 51175; Basic blue 6) has also been proposed as an intermediate electron acceptor in dehydrogenase histochemistry (Kugler and Wrobel, 1978). It is used at a concentration of 10^{-4} M. The effects of Meldola's blue are the same as those of PMS, but the dye, unlike PMS, is not rapidly decomposed by light and causes only slight spontaneous reduction of tetrazolium salts. In a comparison of intermediate electron carriers, Van Noorden and Tas (1982) found that menadione was ineffective, and that Meldola's blue imparted some of its own colour to the cells. They preferred PMS and a related compound, **1-methoxyphenazine methosulphate**.

Intermediate electron acceptors cannot completely replace the naturally occurring diaphorases, and they may work mainly by enhancing the activity of these enzymes (Raap et al., 1983a,b). Inclusion of PMS in the incubation medium can also lead to non-enzymatic formation of formazan. The reduced form of PMS can reduce oxygen (from the atmosphere) to the superoxide ion, $\bullet O_2^-$, a free radical that is able to reduce tetrazolium salts directly (Raap, 1983). False localization from this cause can be prevented by excluding oxygen from the incubation vessel when PMS is used.

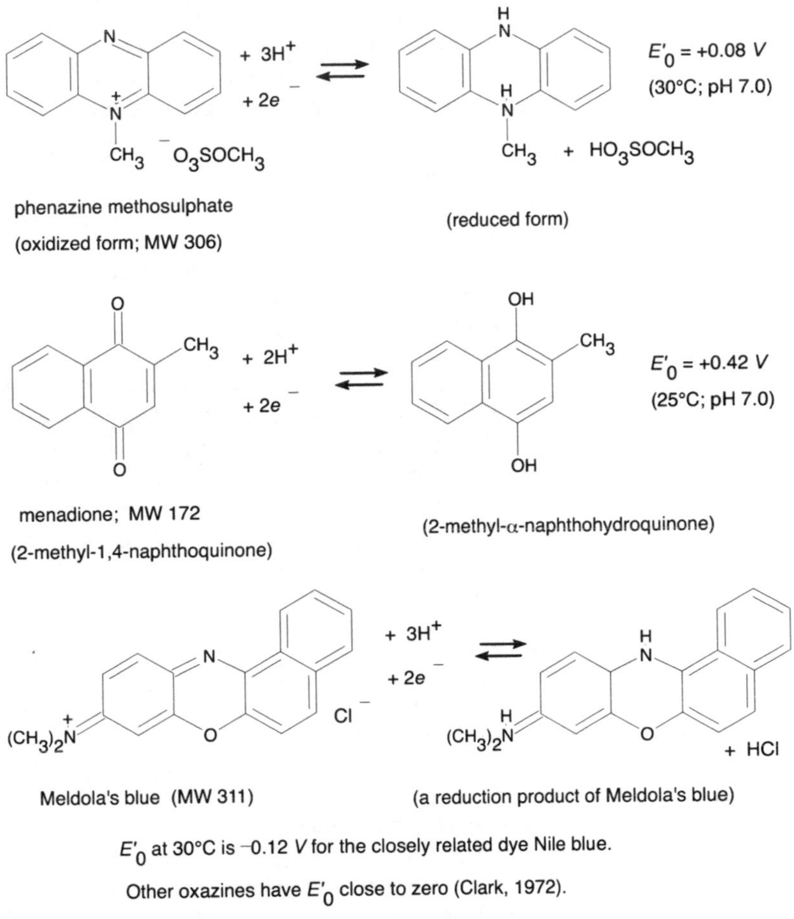
+ 3H+
+ 2e−
CH3 −O3SOCH3
CH3 + HO3SOCH3
E'0 = +0.08 V
(30°C; pH 7.0)
phenazine methosulphate
(oxidized form; MW 306)
(reduced form)
+ 2H+
+ 2e−
E'0 = +0.42 V
(25°C; pH 7.0)
menadione; MW 172
(2-methyl-1,4-naphthoquinone)
(2-methyl-α-naphthohydroquinone)
+ 3H+
+ 2e−
Cl−
(CH3)2N
+ HCl
Meldola's blue (MW 311)
(a reduction product of Meldola's blue)
E'0 at 30°C is −0.12 V for the closely related dye Nile blue.
Other oxazines have E'0 close to zero (Clark, 1972).

Figure 16.1. Intermediate electron acceptors used in enzyme histochemistry.

16.4.3.3. Conditions of reaction

Sections, carried on slides or coverslips, are incubated at room temperature or 37°C for 10–20 min. Chieco *et al.* (1984) recommend treating the sections with a solution of the tetrazolium salt in acetone for 1–2 min before incubating in the complete medium. This manoeuvre gives the least diffusible reactant a chance to permeate into all parts of the section, but is only permissible for enzymes that resist brief fixation in acetone. The histochemical reaction is terminated by transferring the sections to neutral buffered formalin, which may provide some additional fixation and stabilize the tissue for any further manipulations. Counterstains may be applied if desired, in colours that contrast with that of the formazan.

When the tetrazolium salt is nitro-BT or TNBT, the preparations may, with advantage, be dehydrated, cleared, and mounted in a resinous medium. The formazans from other tetrazolium salts are extracted by alcohol, so water-miscible mounting media are necessary. The type of mounting medium will, of course, influence the choice of a counterstain.

16.4.3.4. Controls

When a histochemical method for a dehydrogenase is performed, it is necessary to show that the production of the coloured end-product is brought about as a result of enzymatic oxidation of the substrate, and that the product is present in the same place as the enzyme. The following control procedures will help to establish the biochemical specificity and the accuracy of localization:

(1)   Omit the substrate from the incubation medium. No formazan should be produced.

(2)   Inhibitors are available for some dehydrogenases. They are usually competitive and are used by short pre-incubation followed by addition of the inhibitor to the substrate-containing incubation medium. Fixation of a section in formaldehyde for a few hours inactivates most dehydrogenases and usually spares the diaphorases, but this is a test of low specificity. If available, sections of a tissue known not to contain the enzyme provide valuable negative controls for detecting non-specific tetrazolium reduction.

(3)   In the case of a coenzyme-linked dehydrogenase, carry out the technique for the appropriate diaphorase. This enzyme should be present at the same sites as the dehydrogenase, and will usually be seen in other places too. If there is deposition of formazan from the dehydrogenase medium at sites where there is no diaphorase, the formazan must have diffused away from its place of production. Lipid-soluble formazans are often falsely localized in cytoplasmic lipid droplets. For this reason the ditetrazolium salts whose formazans are substantive for protein are preferred.

(4)   Before accepting a negative result, try the method with PVA or PVP added to the medium, with cyanide or azide added (if not done the first time) and with PMS or Meldola's blue added. Try also with unfixed as well as with briefly fixed material. In the case of flavoprotein dehydrogenases (which have prosthetic groups and do not use coenzymes), replenishment of the section's content of ubiquinone (Sections 16.4.3.1 and 16.4.4) may enable a positive reaction to be obtained.

(5)   It must be remembered that in histochemical demonstrations of dehydrogenases, the production of the final product is a consequence of at least three different chemical reactions. It is optimistically assumed that the intermediate reactants, especially the reduced forms of coenzymes, do not diffuse appreciably during the progress of the incubation. This assumption appears to be justified in the case of some mitochondrial enzymes at the level of resolution of the light microscope. It is not justifiable to draw conclusions concerning the fine structural localization of soluble enzymes other than perhaps to identify the cells in which they occur.

(6)   If possible, along with the sections being investigated incubate sections of one or more tissues in which the distribution of the enzyme is well known (positive controls).

16.4.4. Method for succinate dehydrogenase (Succinate: (acceptor) oxidoreductase; E.C. 1.3.99.1)

Fresh, unfixed tissue should be rapidly frozen and then sectioned at 4–10 µm in a cryostat. The sections, carried on slides or coverslips, may be fixed for 10 min at 0°C in neutral, buffered formaldehyde, or in acetone. The formaldehyde fixative is washed off by rinsing in three changes of 0.06 M phosphate buffer, pH 7.0. Acetone is allowed to evaporate. See also *Note 1* below.

Succinate dehydrogenase is a flavoprotein whose electron-carrying prosthetic group, FAD, is part of the enzyme molecule, so an exogenous coenzyme does not have to be added to the substrate mixture.

Solutions required

A. Incubation medium

0.06 M phosphate buffer, pH 7.0:	50 ml
Nitro blue tetrazolium (nitro-BT):	20 mg
Disodium succinate (hexahydrate):	0.68 g

Prepare just before using. Warming and stirring are sometimes needed, to dissolve the nitro-BT. The final solution should be filtered if it contains any undissolved material.

B. Neutral, buffered 4% formaldehyde (Chapter 2)

Procedure

(1) Incubate sections, prepared as described above, in the medium (solution A) for 10–30 min at room temperature or at 37°C. Cellular regions of the sections should become blue or purple to the unaided eye. Check under a microscope for intracellular deposition of formazan.

(2) Transfer to the fixative (solution B) for 10 min. This will stop the reaction and provide some morphological stabilization of the tissue.

(3) Wash in water, apply a counterstain if desired (e.g. a pink nuclear stain; see Chapter 6), dehydrate through graded alcohols, clear in xylene, and cover, using a resinous mounting medium.

Result

Sites of enzymatic activity (mitochondria) dark blue to purple. Any red mono-formazan that forms is extracted during dehydration.

Notes

(1) Fixation in acetone extracts ubiquinone from the sections. This electron-acceptor may be restored by depositing a thin layer of a 0.1% solution of ubiquinone$_{10}$ (coenzyme Q$_{10}$) in a mixture of equal volumes of ether and acetone on the coverslip or slide (Wattenberg and Leong, 1960) or onto the fixed section (Contestabile and Andersen, 1978) and allowing the solvent to evaporate away. Alternatively, an intermediate electron carrier may be added to the incubation medium (see *Note 3*).

(2) **Controls.** (a) Omit the substrate. A positive reaction in the absence of succinate ions cannot be due to succinate dehydrogenase. (b) Pre-incubate the sections for 5 min in 0.005 M sodium malonate (0.37g of the anhydrous disodium salt in 50 ml of buffer) and add sodium malonate at the same concentration to the complete incubation medium. Malonate is a competitive inhibitor of succinate dehydrogenase.

(3) The incubation time can be shortened by adding 2.0 mg of phenazine methosulphate (PMS) to 50 ml of the incubation medium. The incubation must be carried out in darkness if PMS is used. Meldola's blue (1.5 mg per 50 ml of medium) may be preferable to PMS on account of its greater stability. Do not incubate for more than 10 min if any intermediate electron-acceptor is used, or there may be nonspecific deposition of formazan. The addition of electron-transport inhibitors (CN$^-$ or N$_3^-$) to media for succinate dehydrogenase is not necessary when a rapidly reducible tetrazolium salt such as nitro-BT is used.

16.4.5.
General method for coenzyme-linked dehydrogenases

The following procedure, which is suitable for the demonstration of several dehydrogenases, is based on the techniques described by Pearse (1972), Lojda *et al.* (1979), Van Noorden and Butcher (1984) and Van Noorden and Frederiks (1992, 2002). For individual enzymes the incubation media are made up by adding the tetrazolium salt, the substrate, and the appropriate coenzyme to a previously prepared stock solution containing the stable ingredients. The substrates and coenzymes required by some enzymes are set out in *Table 16.3*.

Stock solution

0.2 M TRIS-HCl buffer, pH7.2:	65 ml
Magnesium chloride (MgCl$_2$.6H$_2$0):	200 mg
Sodium azide (NaN$_3$):	15 mg
Water:	85 ml
Add *either*: Polyvinyl alcohol (MW 30 000):	40 g
or: Polyvinylpyrollidone (MW about 20 000):	15 g

Let the PVA or PVP float on the surface with a magnetic stirrer bar revolving slowly in the bottom of the beaker or flask in which the solution is being prepared. If the powder sinks it will form lumps, which take longer to dissolve.

Adjust to pH7.0–7.2 if necessary by adding 1.0 M sodium hydroxide (4% NaOH). Add water to bring the volume up to 200 ml.

This solution is stable for several weeks at 4°C. The sodium azide, included as an electron-transport inhibitor, also serves to check bacterial and fungal growth. Potassium or sodium cyanide (26 or 20 mg respectively) may be substituted for sodium azide, but the cyanides are less stable, and solutions containing them should be used on the day they are made. All three of these substances are poisonous and must be handled carefully, but the small amounts contained in 200 ml of this solution can safely be discarded by flushing down the sink with plenty of water.

Incubation media

Some of the ingredients, especially the coenzymes, are expensive, so it is usual to prepare only small volumes of incubation media. For each section of tissue, 0.1–0.2 ml of medium will be needed. The following instructions are for the preparation of 5 ml of each medium.

The numbers of atoms of the cation and of molecules of water of crystallization may vary with some of the substrates, so always check the MW shown by the supplier and ensure that the correct number of moles of substrate is taken.

Table 16.3. Some coenzyme-linked dehydrogenases

Trivial name	E.C. Number	Systematic name (indicating substrate and coenzyme)	Product(s) of oxidation of substrate
Alcohol dehydrogenase	1.1.1.1	Alcohol:NAD oxidoreductase	An aldehyde or ketone
Glycerolphosphate dehydrogenase	1.1.1.8	L-glycerol-3-phosphate:NAD oxidoreductase	Dihydroxyacetone phosphate
UDPG dehydrogenase	1.1.1.22	UDP-glucose: NAD oxidoreductase	UDP-glucuronate
Lactate dehydrogenase	1.1.1.27	L-lactate: NAD oxidoreductase	Pyruvate
Glucose-6-phosphate dehydrogenase	1.1.1.49	D-glucose-6-phosphate:NADP oxidoreductase	D-gluconolactone -6-phosphate
Glutamate dehydrogenase	1.4.1.2	L-glutamate: NAD oxidoreductase (deaminating)	2-oxoglutarate + NH$_3$
Glutamate dehydrogenase	1.4.1.3	L-glutamate: NADP oxidoreductase (deaminating)	2-oxoglutarate + NH$_3$

Alcohol dehydrogenase

Stock solution:	5.0 ml
Absolute ethanol: (5×10^{-4} mol):	0.03 ml
Nitro blue tetrazolium:	1.0 mg
Nicotinamide adenine dinucleotide:	1.0 mg

(The small volume of ethanol is more easily measured out by diluting 10 ml of ethanol to 33 ml with water and adding 0.1 ml of the diluted alcohol to the stock solution.)

Glycerolphosphate dehydrogenase

Stock solution:	5.0 ml
Glycerol-3-phosphate, disodium salt (5×10^{-4} mol):	158 mg
Nitro-blue tetrazolium:	1.0 mg
Nicotinamide adenine dinucleotide:	1.0 mg

Check that the pH is 7.0–7.2. Adjust with drops of 1.0 M HCl if necessary.

UDPG dehydrogenase

Stock solution:	5.0 ml
Uridine-5-diphosphate glucose trisodium salt (approx. 1.5×10^{-6} mol):	1.0 mg
Nitro blue tetrazolium:	1.0 mg
Nicotinamide adenine dinucleotide:	1.0 mg

Lactate dehydrogenase

Stock solution:	5.0 ml
Sodium DL-lactate ($NaC_3H_5O_3$) (5×10^{-4} mol):	56 mg
Nitro blue tetrazolium:	1.0 mg
Nicotinamide adenine dinucleotide:	1.0 mg

Glucose-6-phosphate dehydrogenase

Stock solution:	5.0 ml
Glucose-6-phosphate, disodium salt.$3H_2O$ (5×10^{-4} mol):	179 mg
Nitro blue tetrazolium:	1.0 mg
Nicotinamide adenine dinucleotide phosphate, sodium salt:	1.0 mg

Check that the pH is 7.0–7.2. Adjust with drops of 1.0 M HCl if necessary.

Glutamate dehydrogenases

Stock solution:	5.0 ml
Sodium-L-glutamate (5×10^{-4} mol):	85 mg
Nitro blue tetrazolium:	7.0 mg
Either nicotinamide adenine dinucleotide:	1.0 mg
or nicotinamide adenine dinucleotide phosphate, sodium salt:	1.0 mg

Check that the pH is 7.0–7.2. Adjust with drops of 1.0 M HCl if necessary.

Note that a higher than usual concentration of the tetrazolium salt is needed for the demonstration of these enzymes.

Procedure
Fresh tissue is rapidly frozen and sectioned on a cryostat (4–10 μm), the sections being collected onto coverslips or slides. The sections may be fixed for 5–10 min in pre-chilled (4°C) acetone or neutral, phosphate-buffered formaldehyde. Unfixed sections may also be used: the reactions will occur more rapidly but the integrity of the tissue will suffer.

Rinses are carried out in small coplin jars or beakers. The incubation takes place in a closed petri dish with a piece of moist filter paper in the bottom to ensure a humid atmosphere and prevent evaporation of the medium. Read the *Notes* below before carrying out this method.

(1)   (Fixed sections.) Allow acetone to evaporate or rinse the formaldehyde-fixed section in buffer (10–15 s, with agitation). Drain.

(2)   Place slides or coverslips, section uppermost, on the damp filter paper in the bottom of the petri dish. Cover each section with a generous drop of freshly prepared incubation medium. Put the lid on the dish and carefully place it in an oven at 37°C. (Often room temperature is satisfactory.)

(3)   Inspect the sections at 10-min intervals for the formation of blue, intracellular deposits. The time of incubation should not exceed 1 h.

(4)   When staining is judged to be optimum, *either* Rinse in buffer or saline, blot, and allow to dry, *or* Place in neutral, buffered formaldehyde (Chapter 2). This arrests the histochemical reaction and provides further morphological fixation. The time in formaldehyde is not critical: minimum 10 min; can be left overnight.

(5)   Mount air-dried sections in an aqueous medium just before examining them and taking photographs. Rinse fixed sections in water. They may then be counterstained if desired. A pink nuclear stain is suitable (Chapter 6). The sections may then be dehydrated, cleared and mounted in a resinous medium.

Result

Sites of enzymatic activity purple to dark blue. With an aqueous mounting medium, the alcohol-soluble red monoformazan of nitro-BT is not extracted, and it contributes to the observed colour.

Notes

(1)   Lactate dehydrogenase is noteworthy in that it is more resistant to fixation in formaldehyde than the other enzymes. Small blocks may be fixed at 4°C in 2.5–4.0% neutral, buffered formaldehyde and the histochemical method performed on ordinary frozen sections.

(2)   Always remember that the formazan deposit is formed as a result of the activity of a diaphorase, not of the dehydrogenase whose substrate was included in the incubation medium. See also *Note 3*.

(3)   In order to by-pass the diaphorase, an intermediate electron-acceptor may be added to the incubation medium (Section 16.4.3.2 and Fig. 16.1). Immediately before applying the medium to the sections, dissolve in it 0.15 mg of phenazine methosulphate (PMS) per 5.0 ml and incubate in darkness. The time of incubation should not exceed 10 min if PMS is used, or spontaneous reduction of the tetrazolium salt in solution may cause nonspecific precipitation of formazan on the sections. Meldola's blue (0.15 mg per 5.0 ml of medium) may be preferable to PMS, for reasons given in Section 16.4.3.2.

(4)   **Controls**. It is necessary to control for nonenzymatic deposition of formazan and for production of formazan as a result of the activity of enzymes other than the dehydrogenase in which one is interested. The following control procedures are recommended:

(a)   Incubate in a solution containing all the ingredients of the incubation medium except the substrate. No staining should occur. If colour does develop, it may be due to 'nothing dehydrogenase'. See Section 16.4.3.2 (1) and check that the medium is not too alkaline.

(b)   Omit the coenzyme from the incubation medium. If staining is seen in the absence of the coenzyme, the oxidation of the substrate is being catalysed by a dehydrogenase with a prosthetic group. For example, in addition to the glycerolphosphate dehydrogenase shown in *Table 16.3* there is also a mitochondrial flavoprotein (E.C. 1.1.2.1) that catalyses the reaction:

L-glycerol-3-phosphate + (acceptor) $\rightleftharpoons$ dihydroxyacetone phosphate + (reduced acceptor)

No coenzyme is involved, but the reduction of the acceptor (once believed to be cytochrome *c*, but now thought to be ubiquinone) will trigger the transport of electrons to other intermediates of the respiratory chain and to a tetrazolium salt. The mitochondrial flavoprotein glycerolphosphate dehydrogenase can be demonstrated histochemically by using a medium without a coenzyme, though the inclusion of an intermediate electron-acceptor is desirable.

(c) Inhibitors of high specificity are not available for most dehydrogenases. Some of the enzymes (e.g. alcohol, glycerolphosphate, and UDPG dehydrogenases) have sulphydryl groups at their active sites and are inhibited by SH-blocking agents such as PCMB and *N*-ethylmaleimide (10^{-4} to 10^{-3} M). Metal ions (Mg^{2+}, Mn^{2+}, Zn^{2+}) are cofactors for many dehydrogenases, so that chelating agents such as EDTA and 8-hydroxyquinoline (10^{-3} to 10^{-2} M) are inhibitory. A few of the enzymes (e.g. soluble glycerolphosphate dehydrogenase) display increased activity in the presence of chelators.

(d) If an unexpected negative result is obtained, try again with up to 10 times the concentration of the coenzyme. Enzymes that catalyse the hydrolysis of NAD+ and NADP+ are present in some tissues. These coenzymes can also deteriorate on storage in the laboratory.

(5) The histochemical detection of an enzyme requires the penetration of cellular and mitochondrial membranes by all the reagents. Usually freezing and thawing will damage the membranes sufficiently to make them permeable. The glutamate dehydrogenases show increased activity in mitochondria that have been traumatized by rough handling of the tissue (Chayen and Bitensky, 1991).

(6) Although the intensity of the colour of the final reaction product provides an approximate indication of the activity of the enzyme, the concentration of the latter does not vary in direct proportion with the amount of formazan deposited.

16.4.6. Method for diaphorases (tetrazolium reductases)

The presence of these systems of enzymes in tissue is essential for the production of coloured end-products in methods for coenzyme-linked dehydrogenases, except when intermediate electron-acceptors such as PMS are used. In any examination of dehydrogenases whose activities involve NAD^+ or $NADP^+$, the distribution of the appropriate diaphorases should also be ascertained. NADH-diaphorase is located predominantly in mitochondria, whereas NADPH diaphorase is mainly found elsewhere in the cytoplasm. In some cells, notably neurons, NADPH diaphorase activity is due to nitric oxide synthase (Section 16.4.2.) Nakos and Gossrau (1994) state that the NADPH diaphorase method can be made specific for nitric oxide synthase by adding 0.5–1.0% formaldehyde to a phosphate-buffered incubation medium.

Incubation medium

Stock solution (Section 16.4.5):	2 ml
Nitro blue tetrazolium:	0.5 mg
Either nicotinamide adenine dinucleotide, reduced form (disodium salt):	4 mg
or nicotinamide adenine dinucleotide phosphate, reduced form (tetrasodium salt):	4 mg

For NADH-diaphorase, the 'stock solution' may be replaced by TRIS buffer, pH 7.0–7.2. The sodium azide included in the stock solution is also unnecessary, though it does no harm. The incubation medium should be made up immediately before using.

Procedure

(1) Cryostat sections are prepared as for histochemical methods for dehydrogenases.

(2) Incubate in the above medium for 10–30 min at room temperature or at 37°, as described in stages 2 and 3 of the general method for coenzyme-linked dehydrogenases (Section 16.4.5.).

(3) Drain off the incubating medium and transfer the slides or coverslips bearing the sections to neutral buffered formaldehyde for 10–15 min.

(4) Rinse in water, dehydrate through graded alcohols, clear in xylene, and mount in a resinous medium.

Result

Purple to blue–black deposits indicate sites of formazan deposition due to diaphorase activity.

16.5. Histochemistry of peroxidases

The peroxidases catalyse the oxidation of various substances, including reduced coenzymes, fatty acids, amino acids, reduced cytochromes, and many other substances by hydrogen peroxide.

**16.5.1.
Actions and
occurrence**

The name 'peroxidase' (in the singular; donor:H_2O_2 oxidoreductase; E.C. 1.11.1.6) embraces several enzymes of plant and animal origin. They are all iron-containing haemoproteins and they catalyse the reaction:

$$donor + H_2O_2 \longrightarrow reduced\ donor + 2H_2O$$

in which the net effect is the removal of two atoms of hydrogen from each molecule of the donor.

Many organic compounds, including amines, phenols, and the leuco-compounds of dyes, can serve as donors. The substrate is hydrogen peroxide which, when bound to the enzyme, can oxidize other substances much more rapidly than if it were acting alone.

In mammals, peroxidase activity is present in the granules of myeloid leukocytes, in some neurons and some secretory cells (notably in mammary and thyroid glands). A positive histochemical reaction is also given by the haemoglobin of erythrocytes, even in paraffin sections, but this is not considered to be due to truly enzymatic catalysis. The animal enzyme is inhibited by cyanide or azide ions at 10^{-2} M, a concentration higher than that which will inhibit cytochrome oxidase. It is also inhibited by treatment of unfixed cryostat sections with methanol (Streefkerk and van der Ploeg, 1974) but not by brief fixation of tissues in 70% ethanol or 4% formaldehyde. Hydrogen peroxide irreversibly inhibits peroxidase if applied to sections at a concentration of 0.3% (approximately 0.1 M). Complete inhibition of the peroxidase activity of leukocytes and erythrocytes can be achieved by treating formaldehyde or acetone-fixed sections or smears with either 0.024 M HCl in ethanol (Weir et al., 1974) or a solution containing 0.3% H_2O_2 and 0.1% NaN_3 in phosphate-buffered saline, for 10 min (Li et al., 1986). The peroxidase activity of leukocytes survives paraffin embedding, but only if the formaldehyde fixative has been completely washed out of the specimen prior to dehydration. The most popular way to block endogenous peroxidase activity prior to immunoperoxidase staining (Chapter 19) is to immerse the slides for about

10 min in 0.3% hydrogen peroxide in either methanol or phosphate-buffered saline.

Peroxidase histochemistry is important because **HRP**, the enzyme extracted from the root of the horseradish (*Armoracia rusticana*) is extensively used as a reagent in immunohistochemistry (Chapter 19). HRP is also used as an intravital tracer protein in studies of vascular permeability, and in neuroanatomy for both light and electron microscopy. The activity of exogenous HRP in an animal is optimally preserved by brief exposure to a cold glutaraldehyde–formaldehyde mixture (see Section 16.5.4). Inhibition of the endogenous peroxidase of animal tissues is often necessary before applying methods in which HRP is one of the reagents. The blocking procedures mentioned above cannot, however, be used on tissue containing exogenous HRP, because this enzyme is also inhibited by them.

16.5.2.
Histochemical
localization

Histochemical methods for peroxidase are based on the catalysed reactions of hydrogen peroxide with substances that yield insoluble coloured products upon oxidation.

16.5.2.1. Benzidine
In one of the oldest techniques, the donor is benzidine, which is oxidized to a blue substance. The incubation medium contains benzidine and hydrogen peroxide. In this and other methods, the concentration of hydrogen peroxide, the substrate, should not exceed 0.03 M, because higher concentrations inhibit the enzyme.

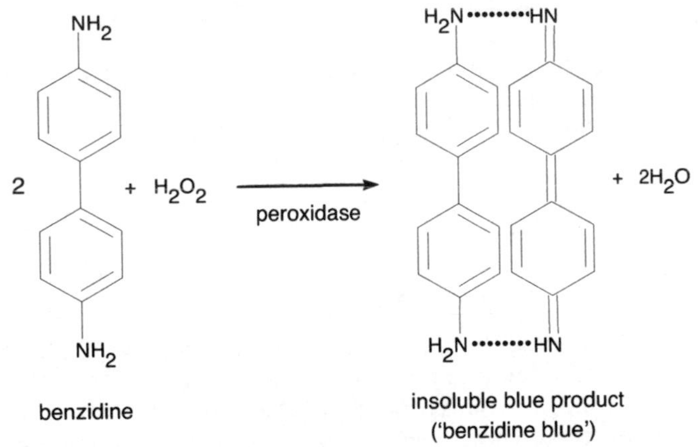

benzidine

insoluble blue product
('benzidine blue')

The blue product is generally believed to have the quinhydrone-like structure shown above. The simple benzidine technique is not often used because the blue crystals are often unduly large and their colour soon fades to a less conspicuous brown. Under some conditions of reaction (pH > 7, temperature > 4°C) a brown product is formed in the first instance. It is probably a polymer derived from condensation of benzidine with its unstable quinone-imine. Various methods are available for the stabilization of benzidine blue, the best-known being treatment of the stained preparations with a concentrated aqueous solution of sodium nitroprusside (sodium nitroferricyanide), $Na_2Fe(CN)_5NO.2H_2O$ (Straus, 1964). However, donors that give more stable products are preferred to benzidine.

The use of HRP as an intravital tracer in neuroanatomical studies has resulted in the development of sensitive techniques for the demonstration of this plant enzyme in animal tissues. The method using DAB (Section 16.5.2.2) has been widely employed, but the sensitivity is greater if the donor is benzidine (Lynch et al., 1973; Mesulam and Rosene, 1977), and greater still if it is **tetramethylbenzidine (TMB)**.

Another advantage of TMB is that, unlike benzidine, it is probably not carcinogenic. Preparations made with TMB as chromogen are sometimes marred by the deposition of large blue crystals at the sites of enzymatic activity and elsewhere (Reiner and Gamlin, 1980). The blue product of oxidation of TMB can be stabilized by treatment with sodium nitroprusside (Mesulam, 1978; Mesulam and Rosene, 1979), ammonium molybdate (Jhaveri et al., 1988), or, after staining, with a solution containing DAB, Co^{2+} ions and H_2O_2 (Rye et al., 1984). The latter technique changes the blue product to a black substance that resists counterstaining and treatment with solvents.

For nitroprusside stabilization the TMB chromogen requires an incubation medium acidic enough (pH 3.3) to disrupt antigen–antibody complexes, and is therefore unsuitable for use in immunohistochemical techniques. With an alternative stabilizing agent, ammonium tungstate, the incubation can be carried out at pH 6 (Weinberg and van Eyck, 1991; Llewellyn-Smith et al., 1993).

16.5.2.2. Diaminobenzidine (DAB)
The electron donor most widely applicable to the histochemical localization of peroxidases is 3,3'diaminobenzidine tetrahydrochloride (DAB), introduced by Graham and Karnovsky (1966):

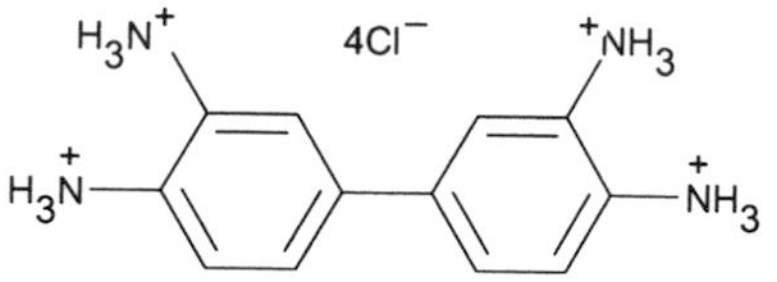

The spontaneous oxidation of this amine by hydrogen peroxide is quite slow, but in the presence of peroxidase an insoluble, amorphous, brown substance is rapidly precipitated. The initial products of oxidation are presumed to be quinone-imines:

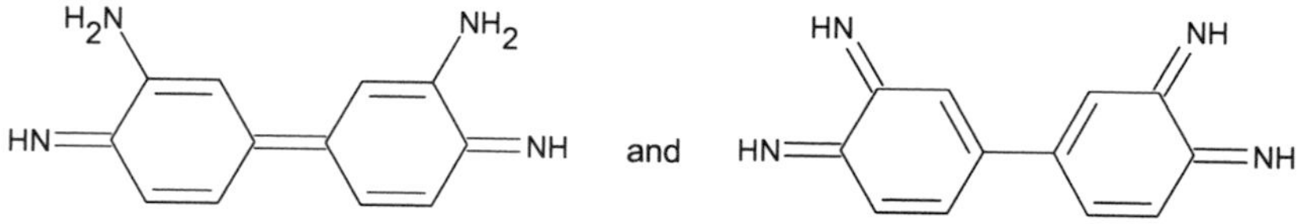

These unstable compounds immediately react with DAB to give polymers, which contain the quinonoid and indamine chromophores. The polymerization, which involves the elimination of hydrogen atoms attached to aromatic rings, is also an oxidation reaction brought about by hydrogen peroxide and catalysed by peroxidase. The polymers are thought to contain such structural arrangements as:

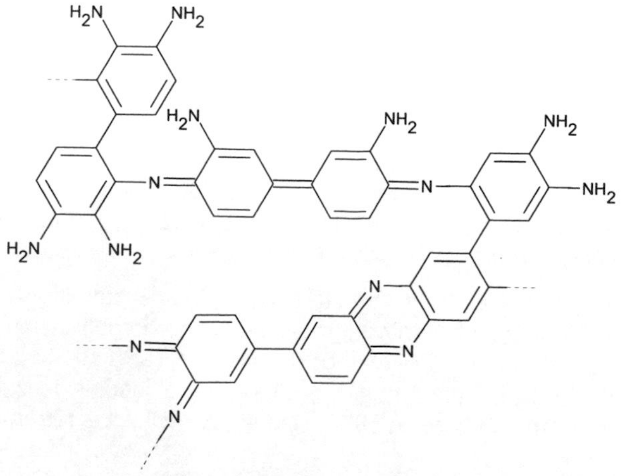

The visibility of this brown, amorphous product can be greatly enhanced by including appropriate blue filters in the light path of the microscope (Gordon, 1988). There are chemical modifications that make the method more sensitive by increasing the darkness of the colour: the inclusion of certain metal ions in the incubation medium results in the formation of blue-black polymers, presumably containing chelated metal ions. Nickel and cobalt salts are particularly effective for this purpose (Adams, 1981; Hsu and Soban, 1982). Nickel is the more popular. Diaminobenzidine brown can be darkened and also rendered electron-opaque by treatment with osmium tetroxide. Even greater intensification is achieved if the postosmication is carried out with an acidified mixture of osmium tetroxide and potassium ferrocyanide (Lascano and Berria, 1988). In recent years, a treatment with 0.02 M copper sulphate, which darkens the brown DAB oxidation product, has been favoured, perhaps because this reagent is less toxic than nickel, cobalt and osmium compounds. For colour photos of the copper-enhanced DAB product, see Heggebo *et al.* (2003).

Physical development, a process in which black metallic silver is deposited (Chapter 18) has also been used to amplify sites of deposition of oxidized DAB (Gallyas *et al.*, 1982; Gallyas and Wolff, 1986; Quinn and Graybiel, 1996). This is particularly effective with the nickel–DAB product (Gallyas and Merchenthaler, 1988; Merchenthaler *et al.*, 1989).

Neither DAB nor its brown oxidation product is fluorescent, but frozen sections of central nervous tissue stained for peroxidase activity using this chromogen exhibit green fluorescence in myelin and in some neuronal cell bodies. This is attributed to combination of DAB with oxidized lipids (Section 12.7).

16.5.2.3. Other chromogens

Other methods for the localization of peroxidase are based on the oxidation and coupling of amines with phenols, quinones, and other substances. The NADI reaction and other methods for cytochrome oxidase (Section 16.6.1) will demonstrate peroxidase if hydrogen peroxide is added to the incubation medium (Burstone, 1962; Lojda *et al.*, 1979). Related methods use combinations of *p*-phenylenediamine with catechol (Hanker *et al.*, 1977), *o*-dianisidine or *o*-tolidine with catechol (Segade, 1987), and catechol with *p*-cresol (Streit and Reubi, 1977). The insoluble products of these methods are probably similar to the 'oxidation colours' used in the dyeing of fur and hair (Chapter 5). The peroxidase-catalysed oxidation of α-naphthol by H_2O_2 yields an anionic polymer that can be stained metachromatically (Chapter 11) with cationic dyes (Mauro *et al.*, 1985).

A popular chromogen for detecting peroxidase-labelled nucleotides and antibodies (Chapters 9 and 19) is **aminoethylcarbazole** (AEC):

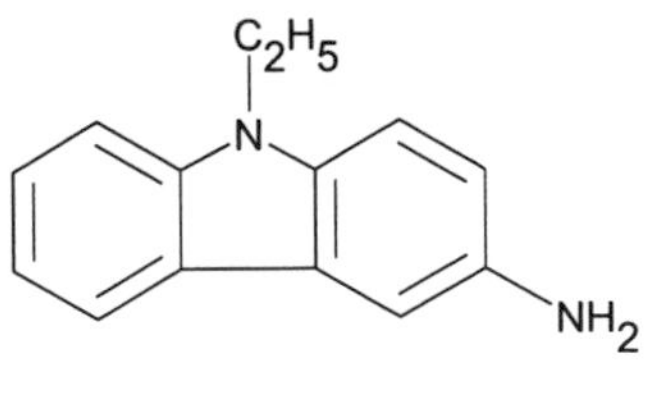

It was introduced by Burstone (1960) in a method for cytochrome oxidase, and then by Graham *et al.* (1965) as a chromogen in peroxidase histochemistry. Methods using AEC are not particularly sensitive; their value lies in the red colour of the oxidation product, which contrasts well with blues and browns from previously or subsequently applied techniques. The red product is insoluble in water but unfortunately it dissolves in alcohol, so an aqueous mounting medium must be used.

Peroxidase catalyzes the reoxidation of leuco compounds (Chapter 5) of many dyes. **Patent blue VF**, an anionic triphenylmethane dye, is the one most frequently used for this purpose.

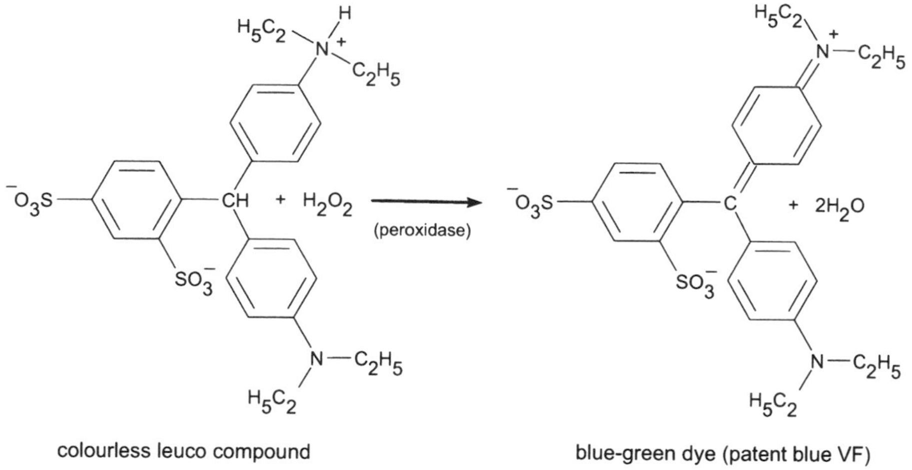

colourless leuco compound   blue-green dye (patent blue VF)

The dye formed by oxidation attaches to protein. The method is used as a stain for haemoglobin and rarely for the myeloperoxidase of leukocytes, but not for HRP. The acidity of the reagent would probably preclude it use for detecting peroxidase-labels in immunohistochemistry.

16.5.3.
Specificity and accuracy of localization

The activities of various enzymes may be expected to cause false-positive reactions in sections stained by histochemical methods for peroxidase. Those most likely to cause confusion are cytochrome oxidase and catalase.

Electron donors such as DAB can be oxidized by cytochrome c in the presence of cytochrome oxidase and oxygen. However, cytochrome oxidase is inactivated by fixatives such as formaldehyde, which are usually employed in the preparation of tissues for the demonstration of peroxidase. With unfixed tissue intended for the localization of cytochrome oxidase, false-positive results can be due to peroxidase, as in the M-NADI reaction (Section 16.6.1). Enough hydrogen peroxide is generated within the tissue to act as substrate for the enzyme. This endogenous substrate can be destroyed, thus eliminating artifacts of the M-NADI type, by adding purified **catalase** to the histochemical incubation medium.

Catalase ($H_2O_2{:}H_2O_2$ oxidoreductase; E.C. 1.11.1.6) catalyses the reaction in which hydrogen peroxide functions as both an oxidizing and a reducing agent:

$$2H_2O_2 \longrightarrow 2H_2O + O_2$$

The enzyme occurs in nearly all cells, in organelles known as **microbodies** or **peroxisomes**. The latter name has persisted despite the fact that the enzyme is not a peroxidase. Its job is to prevent the accumulation of hydrogen peroxide, a potentially toxic metabolite. Peroxisomes also contain a number of oxidases that generate hydrogen peroxide (see Van den Munckhof, 1996). In the presence of catalase the decomposition of hydrogen peroxide occurs exceedingly rapidly. This enzyme can, however, also serve as a peroxidase, catalysing the oxidation of chromogenic donors by H_2O_2. Catalase is specifically inhibited by 3-amino-1,2,4-triazole.

Peroxidase and catalase may also be distinguished by varying the concentration of their substrate. Silveira and Hadler (1978) found that catalase could not be detected (by benzidine and H_2O_2) when the concentration of hydrogen peroxide in the incubation medium was less than about 3×10^{-3} M. The enzymatic activity survived when $[H_2O_2]$ was as high as 4.0 M. Peroxidase, by contrast, was fully active in the presence of 1.5×10^{-3} M H_2O_2, but was inhibited by concentrations greater than about 0.05 M. Silveira and Hadler found that 4.0 M H_2O_2 was necessary for complete inhibition of all peroxidases. The peroxidase-like activity of haemoglobin resembles catalase in that it is not detectable when $[H_2O_2]$ is very low.

The amorphous product of oxidation of DAB is cleanly formed within tiny vesicles and organelles, and is widely believed to localize peroxidase activity accurately even in highly magnified electron micrographs. Some of the other chromogens, notably benzidine and TMB, oxidize to crystalline products that damage the local architecture of the cytoplasm but are nevertheless localized to individual cells and even to small cellular processes such as synaptic terminals. Anionic dyes formed by oxidation of leuco-compounds are soluble in water but become firmly bound to cationic proteins; an acidic medium favours this staining.

16.5.4.
DAB methods
for peroxidase

The endogenous peroxidases of animal cells resist fixation in neutral formaldehyde. Bancroft and Cook (1984) state that animal tissues should not be fixed in formaldehyde for longer than 4 h. The fixative should be thoroughly washed out to terminate its action. Horseradish peroxidase also survives brief fixation in formaldehyde or glutaraldehyde. For optimum preservation of exogenous HRP (Rosene and Mesulam, 1978), the animal should be perfused for 30 min with 0.1 M phosphate buffer, pH 7.4, containing 1% formaldehyde and 1.25% glutaraldehyde. Glutaraldehyde alone (1–2% in the same buffer) is also suitable. Excess fixative is then washed out by perfusing cold (4°C) 10% sucrose in 0.1 M phosphate buffer, pH 7.4, for a further 30 min. The specimens may be stored in phosphate-buffered sucrose solution for up to 7 days at 4°C. Frozen or cryostat sections should be used, either free-floating or mounted on slides or coverslips. Thick frozen sections should be free-floating, to allow penetration by the reagents.

The following procedure is the original method of Graham and Karnovsky (1966), with some optional modifications to increase the sensitivity. It is suitable for the demonstration of endogenous peroxidases of animal tissues and for horseradish peroxidase used as a tracer or as a reagent in immunohistochemical and other techniques. More sensitive methods using TMB (Section 16.5.2.1) are preferred when HRP is used as a tracer in neuroanatomical studies.

Incubation medium
This solution is prepared just before use. Dissolve 25 mg of 3,3'-diaminobenzidine tetrahydrochloride (DAB) in about 2 ml of water and make up to 50 ml with *either* 0.1 M phosphate buffer *or* 0.05 M TRIS buffer, pH 7.3. Before doing this for the first time, read *Note 1* below.

Optionally, add 0.5 ml of the following solution (Adams, 1981):

Cobalt chloride ($CoCl_2.6H_2O$):	2.5 g
Nickel ammonium sulphate ($Ni(NH_4)_2(SO_4)_2.6H_2O$):	2.0 g
Water:	to make 100 ml

This mixture can be stored at room temperature. It does not deteriorate. The effect of either the cobalt or the nickel salt used alone at 2% is almost identical to that of the mixture.

Make a 1% w/v aqueous solution of H_2O_2 *either* by diluting a strong stock solution of hydrogen peroxide (e.g. '100 volumes' = 30% w/w H_2O_2) *or* by dissolving solid urea hydrogen peroxide (which is equivalent to 35% w/w H_2O_2) in water. The 1% solution may be kept for one week.

Caution. Avoid contact of the strong H_2O_2 (or urea hydrogen peroxide) with skin or clothing. H_2O_2 is unstable, so do not use old stock. Decomposition is accelerated by chemical contamination, especially by contact with metals.

Immediately before use (see step 2 of the procedure, and *Note 2* at the end), add 0.5 ml of the 1% hydrogen peroxide to the 50 ml of DAB solution.

Procedure

(1) Incubate the sections in the buffered DAB solution (with or without Co^{2+} and/or Ni^{2+}), without hydrogen peroxide, for 15 min at room temperature.
(2) Add the hydrogen peroxide to the medium. Mix well and wait for a further 5–15 min.
(3) Wash in 3 changes of water, each 1 min.
(4) (Optional) Apply a counterstain if desired.
(5) Dehydrate, clear, and cover, using a resinous mounting medium.

Result

Sites of peroxidase activity are brown if the metal salts are not included in the medium, or blue-black with Co^{2+} and/or Ni^{2+}.

Notes

(1) If the DAB is not first dissolved in a small volume of water the buffered solution will be cloudy. The choice of phosphate or TRIS buffer is not critical; many people prefer TRIS, for a variety of anecdotal reasons. Samples of DAB vary in quality. The compound should be very pale, almost white, and the solution colourless. Darkly coloured material gives nonspecific background staining and weaker specific staining. Brown DAB solutions can be cleaned and made usable by shaking with activated charcoal, 1 mg/ml for 1 min, and filtering (Ros Barcelo *et al.*, 1989). DAB can be bought as tablets and also in in rubber-capped vials, each containing a pre-weighed amount. It is much cheaper to buy a larger amount of the powder, weigh out 25 mg aliquots and keep them in tightly capped tubes at −20°C.
(2) If the sections are thin, they may be put directly into the complete incubation medium. For thicker (> 40 μm) sections or whole-mounts, the pre-incubation is necessary to allow penetration of the DAB, whose molecules are larger and more slowly diffusing than those of hydrogen peroxide.
(3) **Control sections** should be incubated with DAB in the absence of H_2O_2. In unfixed sections a positive reaction in the absence of H_2O_2 can be due to cytochrome oxidase.
(4) Catalase may be inhibited by adding 3-amino-1,2,4-triazole (10^{-2} M) to the incubation medium. Halving the recommended concentration of hydrogen peroxide in the medium should also prevent the formation of coloured products due to catalase.
(5) Some pre-treatments to inhibit endogenous peroxidases of animal tissues are listed in Section 16.5.1.
(6) If nickel or cobalt salts were not included in the incubation medium, the sections may be immersed in 0.5% aqueous copper sulphate ($CuSO_4.5H_2O$) for 3 min after Step 3 to darken the reaction product.
(7) DAB is handled carefully, though it probably is not carcinogenic (see Burns, 1982). Residual DAB can be destroyed by adding a few ml of 5% sodium hypochlorite (household bleach) to the used solution and waiting for an hour before discarding. Lunn and Sansone (1990) preferred to oxidize overnight with acidified potassium permanganate (4% $KMnO_4$, 12% H_2SO_4, in water),

then decolorize the remaining permanganate (by adding solid ascorbic acid), and neutralize the sulphuric acid (with calcium carbonate or some other base).

16.5.5.
AEC method for peroxidase

This is the method of Graham *et al.* (1965), with minor modifications by Boenisch (1989). It is intended for sections of animal tissue that contain horseradish peroxidase (HRP), either administered *in vivo* or applied to sections as part of an immunohistochemical or other labelling method. For notes on fixation, see the first paragraph of the preceding method (Section 16.5.4).

Incubation medium
Instructions for making 1% hydrogen peroxide are given with the previous method (Section 16.5.4).

Dissolve 4 mg of 3-amino-9-ethylcarbazole in 1.0 ml of *N,N*-dimethylformamide. Add 19 ml of 0.05 M acetate buffer, pH 5.0. Filter the solution if is not perfectly clear. Immediately before using, add 0.3 ml of 1% H_2O_2.

Procedure
(1) Immerse the sections in the incubation medium for 2–5 min at room temperature.
(2) Wash in 3 changes of water.
(3) Apply a counterstain if desired. (See Chapter 6. Alcohol must be avoided, and the stain must be one that is stable in water.)
(4) Apply coverslip, using an aqueous mounting medium.

Result
Sites of peroxidase activity are red. Erythrocytes are unstained or only weakly stained with this method.

Note
The pH should not be higher than 6, or the reaction product will deteriorate as it forms, and be brown. Buffers other than acetate may be used, but the concentration of salts in the buffer should not be higher than 0.05 M.

16.5.6.
Leuco-patent blue method

This method is used for demonstrating the peroxidase-like activity of haemoglobin. It also stains certain cytoplasmic particles (myeloperoxidase) in leukocytes (Pearse, 1972). The enzymatic activities of red and white blood cells are demonstrable after fixation in formaldehyde, in frozen or paraffin sections. For notes on the fixation of other animal peroxidases, see the first paragraph of Section 16.5.4.

Incubation medium
A. Stock solution of leuco-patent blue

Patent blue VF (C.I. 42045):	1 g
Water:	100 ml

Dissolve, then add:

Zinc powder:	10 g
Glacial acetic acid:	2 ml

Boil until colourless (or almost so). Cool and filter. This solution can be kept for a week or two at 4°C. It should be replaced if it becomes green or blue. The closely similar dye patent blue V (CI 42051, Acid blue 3) is also used in this technique.

B. Working solution
This is made immediately before use. See under the DAB method (Section 16.5.4) for instructions on making 1% hydrogen peroxide.

Solution A:	30 ml

Glacial acetic acid:	2 ml
1% hydrogen peroxide:	3 ml

Procedure

(1) Immerse frozen sections or hydrated paraffin sections in the working incubation medium (Solution B) for 5 min at room temperature.
(2) Wash in 3 changes of water.
(3) Apply a counterstain if desired. (See Chapter 6. A red nuclear stain is suitable.)
(4) Dehydrate in 3 changes of 100% alcohol, clear in xylene and cover, using a resinous mounting medium.

Result

Haemoglobin and myeloperoxidase granules dark blue-green.

16.6. Histochemistry of oxidases

Oxidases catalyse the general reaction:

$$2 \begin{bmatrix} \text{reduced} \\ \text{substrate} \end{bmatrix} + O_2 \underset{\text{(oxidase)}}{\rightleftharpoons} 2H_2O + 2 \begin{bmatrix} \text{oxidized} \\ \text{substrate} \end{bmatrix}$$

(For convenience it is assumed that each molecule of this generalized substrate loses two hydrogen atoms when oxidized.)

The equation can be derived from two half reactions (Section 16.1):

$$O_2 + 4H^+ + 4\epsilon^- \rightleftharpoons 2H_2O \qquad (E_0 = +0.82)$$

$$(\text{reduced substrate}) + 2\epsilon^- \rightleftharpoons (\text{oxidized substrate}) \qquad (E_0 < +0.82)$$

If the value of E_0' for the second half-reaction is lower (or only slightly higher) than that for the reduction of a tetrazolium salt, it is possible to use a histochemical method similar to those used for the detection of dehydrogenases. The tetrazolium salt will act as a substitute for oxygen and will be reduced to its formazan. The substrates for many oxidases have oxidation–reduction potentials appreciably higher than those of the tetrazolium salts; for such enzymes different histochemical techniques must be used. Some oxidases catalyse the reaction:

$$\text{reduced substrate} + H_2O + O_2 \longrightarrow \text{oxidized substrate} + H_2O_2$$

Histochemical methods for such enzymes are based on **detection of hydrogen peroxide** that is produced. Incomplete reaction of water with an enzyme-reduced substrate complex generates superoxide ions ($\cdot O_2^-$), which are highly reactive free radicals, implicated in a variety of disease processes. To offset the toxic effects of $\cdot O_2^-$ and other oxygen radicals, all cells contain reducing agents (antioxidants, including glutathione, ascorbate and vitamin E) and also enzymes, **superoxide dismutases** (E.C. 1.15.1.1; superoxide:superoxide oxidoreductase) that accelerate the conversion of $\cdot O_2^-$ to O_2. Xanthine oxidase (Section 16.6.4) is an enzyme notable for releasing superoxide ions.

Methods for the localization of four oxidases are discussed in this chapter. Cytochrome oxidase is an indicator of the level of oxygen usage of a tissue. The third enzyme to be discussed (amine oxidase) is one of several oxidases that can be demonstrated by trapping released hydrogen peroxide, and the fourth, xanthine oxidoreductase is an example of an enzyme that is difficult to localize accurately within tissues and is interesting also because it can be both an NAD^+-linked dehydrogenase and a true oxidase.

16.6.1.
Cytochrome oxidase
(Cytochrome $c:O_2$ oxidoreductase; E.C. 1.9.3.1; cytochrome aa_3)

The terminal members of the electron-transport chain are cytochromes a and aa_3, from which electrons are transferred to oxygen. The electrons are derived from cyt. c^{2+}, the reduced form of cytochrome c. Cytochrome oxidase catalyses the net reaction:

$$4 \text{ cyt. } c^{2+} + O_2 + 4H^+ \xrightarrow[\text{(cytochrome oxidase)}]{} 4 \text{ cyt. } c^{3+} + 2H_2O$$

The cytochrome oxidase molecule consists of two linked units, cytochromes a and a_3 (see *Table 16.1*). Each unit contains an iron atom, tightly bound in a haem-like prosthetic group. The enzyme complex is inhibited by cyanide and azide ions and by several other toxic substances, including hydrogen sulphide and carbon monoxide. Cytochrome oxidase occurs in all eukaryotic organisms, and is present in mitochondria. Aerobic prokaryotes have alternative enzyme systems for moving electrons to oxygen.

The histochemical demonstration of cytochrome oxidase activity is useful in several fields of research, as a way to demonstrate populations of cells that are metabolically more active than their neighbours (see Wong-Riley, 1989).

16.6.1.1. The NADI and related reactions

The earliest histochemical reaction for cytochrome oxidase was the **NADI (naphthol–diamine) technique**, investigation of which contributed to the discovery of aerobic metabolic pathways and the functions of mitochondria. In the NADI reaction the formation of an azamethine dye (indophenol blue) from α-naphthol and N-dimethyl-p-phenylenediamine is catalysed in the presence of oxygen and cytochrome c. The last-named substance is naturally present in the tissue. Two oxidation–reduction reactions are involved:

(1)

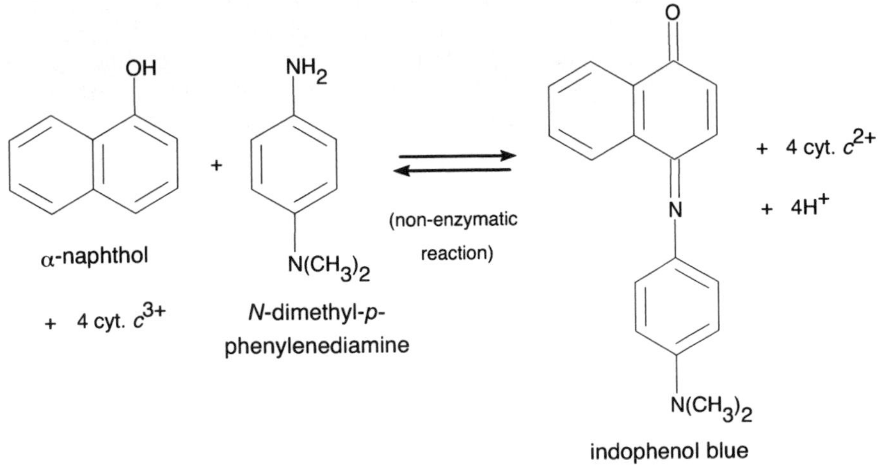

α-naphthol

+ 4 cyt. c^{3+}

N-dimethyl-p-phenylenediamine

(non-enzymatic reaction)

+ 4 cyt. c^{2+}

+ 4H$^+$

indophenol blue

(2)

$$4 \text{ cyt. } c^{2+} + O_2 + 4H^+ \xrightarrow[\text{(cytochrome oxidase)}]{} 4 \text{ cyt. } c^{3+} + 2H_2O$$

Reaction (2) serves to remove cyt. c^{2+} and H^+ from the products of reaction (1), thereby promoting formation of indophenol blue and assuring a continued supply of oxidized cytochrome c. It is the diamine, not the naphthol, that is oxidized by cytochrome c. The unstable product of oxidation of the diamine oxidizes and couples with the naphthol to form the dye. The discovery of cytochrome oxidase was intimately linked with the elucidation of the mechanism of the NADI reaction (Keilin and Hartree, 1938). Inhibition of the NADI reaction by inhibitors of cytochrome oxidase confirms its specificity. In solutions derived from extracted tissues the oxidized form of cytochrome c (cyt. c^{3+}) does not, by itself, cause the oxidation and coupling of α-naphthol and N-dimethyl-p-phenylenediamine to occur as rapidly as is observed in the histochemical NADI reaction. In an intact tissue the cyt. c^{3+} reacts more rapidly, being bound to the cytochrome oxidase aggregate molecule.

The original NADI method is unsatisfactory as a histochemical technique for several reasons. A positive reaction is seen where cytochrome oxidase is not active, as in leukocyte granules in fixed tissues. Indophenol blue fades quite rapidly on exposure to light, is soluble in lipids, and also has no substantivity for protein (Section 14.5.2). Production of indophenol blue in myeloid leukocytes (M-NADI reaction) is catalysed by peroxidase-like proteins. The cytochrome oxidase-catalysed reaction (G-NADI) can be obtained only in unfixed cells and tissues. Improved G-NADI-like methods for cytochrome oxidase were based on the production of dyes (of undetermined composition) from a variety of naphthols, amines, quinones, and quinolines.(see Burstone, 1959, 1962). Cytochrome c was added to the incubation medium, as was catalase. The latter enzyme accelerates decomposition of any H_2O_2 that might be formed by metabolic processes. In the absence of H_2O_2 there can be no peroxidase-catalysed oxidation of the substrate. Organelles with peroxidase activity (notably leukocyte granules) would otherwise give false positive staining for cytochrome oxidase. A major disadvantage of all NADI-derived methods is their sensitivity, which is too low to permit even minimal fixation of the tissue (see Pearse, 1972; Lojda et al., 1979).

16.6.1.2. Methods using DAB

The modern methods for cytochrome oxidase make use of **diaminobenzidine (DAB)**, a reagent that is valuable in many histochemical methods. The oxidation of DAB by cytochrome c is catalysed by cytochrome oxidase, and the product is an insoluble brown polymer, whose colour can be darkened by incorporation of transition metal ions in the incubation medium. The oxidation of DAB was discussed in more detail (Section 16.5.2.2) in connection with methods for peroxidases. In methods for cytochrome oxidase, exogenous cytochrome c is needed, and the medium must also contain catalase, for the reason given in the previous section (16.6.1.1.). The following method (Silverman and Tootell, 1987) was devised for the rat's brain. It is suitable for other organs of small laboratory animals.

Preparation of tissue

An anaesthetized rat is perfused (Chapter 2) for about 15 s with about 50 ml of 0.1 M phosphate buffer, pH 7.4, containing 10% sucrose and 1% sodium nitrite ($NaNO_2$, as a vasodilator), to displace the blood. The fixative, which is 3.5% formaldehyde in phosphate buffer, is then run through for 15 s. The phosphate buffer with sucrose is then perfused for about 15 s, to displace the fixative. The brain is removed, and pieces are rapidly frozen and cut at 20–40 μm with a cryostat. The sections are collected on slides or coverslips that have been subbed with chrome–gelatin (Chapter 4), and quickly dried by placing on a hotplate (50°C) for 10–15 s. The dry sections should be refrigerated if they are not to be stained immediately. See also *Note 1* below.

Solutions required
A. Cold (10°C) acetone

B. Rinsing solution
0.1 M phosphate buffer, pH 7.4 (Chapter 20), containing 10% (w/v) sucrose.

C. Pre-incubation solution

0.05 M TRIS buffer, pH 7.6 (Chapter 20):	99.5 ml
Cobalt chloride ($CoCl_2.6H_2O$):	28 mg
Sucrose:	10 mg
Dimethylsulphoxide (DMSO):	0.5 ml

D. Reaction medium

0.1 M phosphate buffer, pH 7.6:	100 ml
Diaminobenzidine tetrahydrochloride:	50 mg
Cytochrome c:	7.5 mg
Sucrose:	5 g
Catalase:	2 mg
Dimethylsulphoxide (DMSO):	0.25 ml

Before and during use, this solution is maintained at about 40°C, and oxygen is bubbled through it.

E. Final fixative

0.1 M phosphate buffer, pH 7.2–7.6:	90 ml
Sucrose:	10 g
Formalin:	10 ml

Procedure
(1) Immerse the slides (or coverslips) in cold acetone for 5 min. (This is said to improve adhesion; it would also cause further fixation, and extract some lipids.)
(2) Rinse in 3 changes of the rinsing solution (B).
(3) Immerse for 10 min in the pre-incubation solution (C).
(4) Rinse briefly in Solution B.
(5) Place in oxygenated reaction medium (Solution D) at 40°C, for 30 min to 6 h, examining from time to time.
(6) When staining is adequate, transfer to final fixative (Solution E) for 30 min, then dehydrate, clear, and mount, using a resinous medium.

Result
Sites of cytochrome oxidase activity greyish brown to blue-black.

Notes
(1) Alternatively, the brain is removed after perfusion of saline, quickly frozen (in cold isopentane, see Chapter 4) and stored at −20°C. Cryostat sections are fixed for 5 min in 4% formaldehyde.
(2) Greater sensitivity is claimed (Liu *et al.*, 1993) when the pre-incubation is omitted and the incubation medium contains nickel ions.
(3) To inhibit cytochrome oxidase, include 10^{-3} M potassium or sodium cyanide or azide in the incubation medium (Solution D) for control sections.

16.6.2.
Monophenol
monooxygenase

Several names have been applied to the copper-containing enzymes that catalyse the oxidation of *o*-diphenols by oxygen to yield *o*-quinones. These include monophenol mono-oxygenase, catechol oxidase, tyrosinase, phenol oxidase, polyphenol oxidase, and DOPA-oxidase. Dixon and Webb (1979) state that monophenol, DOPA:oxygen oxidoreductase (E.C. 1.14.18.1) is almost indistinguishable from *o*-diphenol:O_2-oxidoreductase (E.C. 1.10.3.1). Histochemical detection of this oxidase activity labels cells that are active in the **synthesis of melanin**. This pigment is produced in melanocytes by a series of enzyme-catalysed and spontaneous reactions. The initial metabolite in the sequence is the amino acid tyrosine. This is first slowly oxidized to dihydroxyphenylalanine (DOPA):

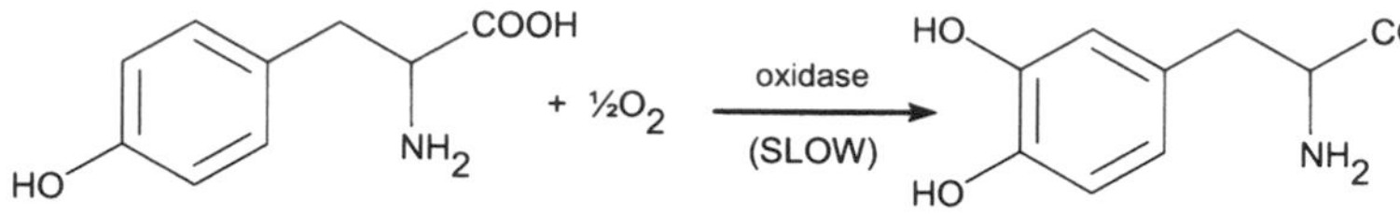
COOH
NH2
HO
+ ½O2
oxidase
(SLOW)
HO
HO
COOH
NH2

Under the catalytic influence of monophenol monooxygenase the DOPA is now rapidly oxidized to DOPA quinone:

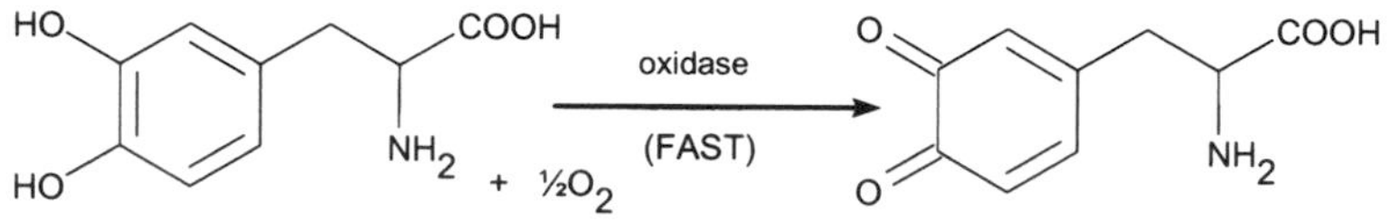
HO
HO
COOH
NH2
+ ½O2
oxidase
(FAST)
O
O
COOH
NH2

The remaining reactions are believed to occur spontaneously:

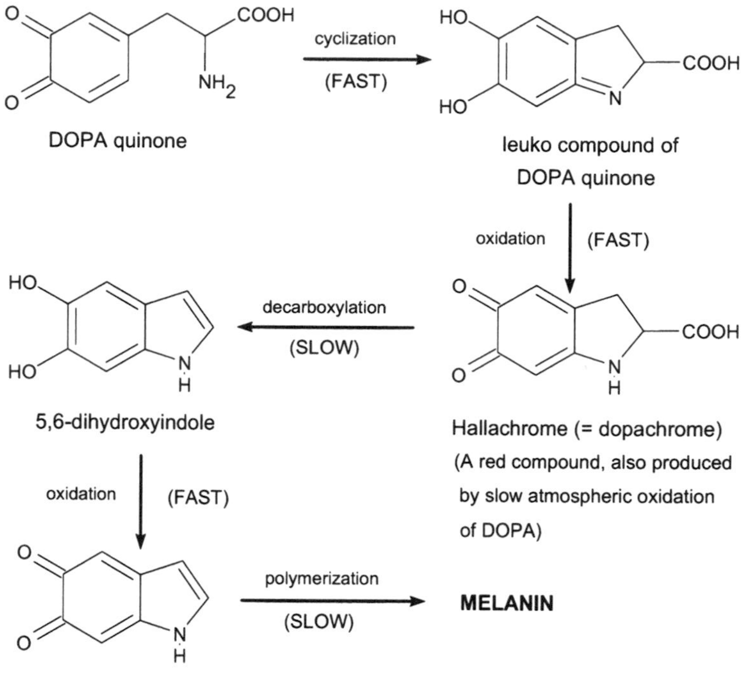
DOPA quinone
cyclization
(FAST)
leuko compound of DOPA quinone
oxidation
(FAST)
Hallachrome (= dopachrome)
(A red compound, also produced by slow atmospheric oxidation of DOPA)
decarboxylation
(SLOW)
5,6-dihydroxyindole
oxidation
(FAST)
polymerization
(SLOW)
MELANIN

Melanin is probably a polymer derived from indole-5,6-quinone:

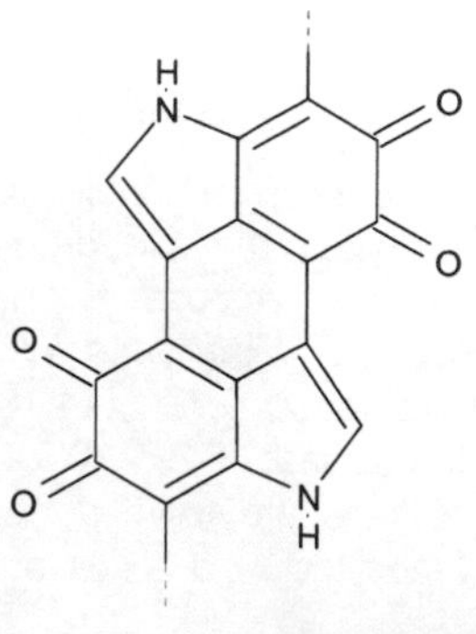

bound to the proteinaceous matrix of the granules in which it occurs. It is a stable, black, insoluble substance.

Monophenol oxygenase is demonstrated histochemically by virtue of its catalysis of the rapid oxidation of DOPA by oxygen, with the ultimate formation of melanin. Several potentially diffusible intermediates are produced in this series of reactions, so it is possible that the final deposits of melanin are not formed in exactly the same sites as those at which the substrate was oxidized. However, the formation of a finely granular pigment in melanocytes, where melanin is normally synthesized, suggests that diffusion does not occur over great distances.

The chemical specificity of the reaction is certainly not complete. Positive staining of erythrocytes and leukocyte granules is probably due to peroxidase activity, with tissue-derived hydrogen peroxide as the substrate and DOPA as the electron-donor (Section 16.5). Inhibitors are of little value because both monophenol monooxygenase and the peroxidases are inhibited by cyanide, azide, and sulphide ions, though lower concentrations (10^{-4} to 10^{-3} M) are effective with the former enzyme. These inhibitors also block the activity of cytochrome oxidase, but this enzyme is unlikely to be involved in the histochemical oxidation of DOPA when formaldehyde-fixed tissue is used. Lillie and Fullmer (1976) state that sodium dithionite ($Na_2S_2O_4$, 5×10^{-3} M) and cysteine (10^{-3} M) enhance the reaction. They might do this by reducing hallachrome to 5,6-dihydroxyindole, thus speeding up the slowest non-enzymatic reaction in the series leading from DOPA to melanin.

The technique for the histochemical demonstration of monophenol monooxygenase is unusual in that the substrate and the product are those naturally used and formed by the enzyme. The method works with cryostat sections of unfixed tissue, with frozen sections of tissue fixed in neutral, buffered 4% formaldehyde for 6–24 h at 4°C, and with paraffin sections of freeze-dried material (Lojda *et al.*, 1979). Small specimens can be stained whole by a slight modification of the technique (see Pearse, 1972; van Noorden and Frederiks, 1992) and then fixed and embedded in wax.

Incubation medium

0.06 M phosphate buffer, pH 7.4:	100 ml
DL-β-dihydroxyphenylalanine (DOPA):	100 mg

Pre-warm the buffer to 37°C. Add the DOPA and place on a magnetic stirrer or shake vigorously for 10–15 min. Any DOPA that has not dissolved after this time should be removed by filtration.

Only L-DOPA is acted upon by the enzyme. The racemic mixture (DL-DOPA) is used because it is cheaper. See also *Note 3* below.

Procedure

(1) Incubate sections in the medium, in darkness, for 60 min at 37°C. After the first 45 min, prepare a fresh batch of incubation medium.
(2) Replace the incubation medium with the new batch and incubate for another 60 min at 37°C.
(3) Wash in three changes of water.
(4) Apply a counterstain (e.g. neutral red or safranine; see Chapter 6) if desired, and rinse in water.
(5) Dehydrate, clear, and mount in a resinous medium.

Result

A dark brown deposit of melanin forms at sites of enzymatic activity (see *Notes* below).

Notes

(1)   It is important to incubate control sections in buffer without added DOPA in order to detect pigments already present in the tissue. In mammalian skin melanin granules are produced in melanocytes (which contain monophenol oxygenase) and then transferred to epidermal cells, which do not contain the enzyme.

(2)   Catechol oxidase is inhibited by cyanide ions, though specificity of the inhibition is low. Sections may be pre-incubated in 10^{-3} M KCN (MW 65) or NaCN (MW 49) for 5 min. The same concentration should also be included in the incubating medium. (**Caution.** Sodium and potassium cyanides are poisonous. They must be handled carefully and not allowed to come into contact with acids. Quantities smaller than 100 mg may safely be discarded by washing down the sink with copious running tap water.)

(3)   Incubation may be prolonged to 6 h if necessary, changing the medium every 45–60 min. White *et al.* (1983) recommended a pH of 6.8 for detecting the enzyme in cell cultures. They used L-DOPA as the substrate, and D-DOPA for the controls.

16.6.3.
Amine oxidase
(Amine:O_2
oxidoreductase
(deaminating)
(flavin-containing);
E.C. 1.4.3.1)

This flavoprotein enzyme is commonly known as **monoamine oxidase** or **MAO**, because it is involved in the metabolism of such compounds as dopamine, noradrenaline, serotonin, tryptamine and tyramine, which contain one amino group. The overall reaction catalysed by MAO is

$$RCH_2CH_2NH_2 + H_2O + O_2 \longrightarrow RCHO + NH_3 + H_2O_2$$

The oxidation is due to removal of two electrons from the carbon atom of $-CH_2NH_2$. (Application of the rules summarized at the beginning of this chapter shows a change in oxidation number from -1 to $+1$.) The electron acceptor is FAD, the prosthetic group of the enzyme. From the reduced FAD, electrons are transferred to the cytochromes and to molecular oxygen.

In early histochemical methods for MAO, the aldehyde product was trapped by a hydroxynaphthoic hydrazide (Chapter 10), and the resulting naphtholic hydrazone converted to a dye by coupling with a diazonium salt. Such methods were unsatisfactory because of diffusion of intermediate products of the reactions and inhibition of the enzyme by some of the reagents. More satisfactory histochemical localization of MAO is obtained by providing a tetrazolium salt to accept electrons from the reduced FAD, thus substituting for the cytochromes and for oxygen. The formazans formed by reduction of tetrazolium salts are coloured and insoluble (Section 16.4.1). Technical instructions for methods of this type are given by Pearse (1972), Lojda *et al.* (1979) and Shannon (1981). It is necessary to use cryostat sections of unfixed tissue for these methods. A third approach to the histochemical localization of this and similar oxidases is to trap the released hydrogen peroxide.

16.6.3.1. Cerium precipitation method

More sensitive techniques for detecting MAO (and other enzymes catalysing reactions that produce H_2O_2) are based on detection of the released hydrogen peroxide. The sensitivity of these methods is high enough to permit the detection of MAO even when much of the enzymatic activity has been inhibited by brief fixation. The accuracy of localization permits their application to slices of tissue cut with a vibrating microtome and subsequently processed for electron microscopy. The simplest way to detect released H_2O_2 is to have cerium(III) ions in the incubation medium. Cerium(IV) perhydroxide, $Ce(OH)_3(OOH)$, is precipitated (Sneed and Brasted, 1955; Briggs *et al.*, 1975).

$$Ce^{3+} + H_2O_2 + 3OH^- \longrightarrow Ce(OH)_3OOH(s) + H^+$$

This is electron dense and can be detected within mitochondria and other organelles (Christie and Stoward, 1982; Angermuller and Fahimi, 1987). The product is not visible in light microscopy, but the deposits can be made visible by further chemical treatment. Cerium perhydroxide oxidizes diaminobenzidine (DAB) to a brown polymer.

$$Ce(OH)_3OOH + DAB \longrightarrow Ce^{3+} + \underset{\text{DAB}}{\text{oxidized}} + H_2O$$

(brown, insoluble)

Further amplification is achieved by including hydrogen peroxide in the DAB solution (Van Noorden and Frederiks, 1993; Halbhuber *et al.*, 1996).

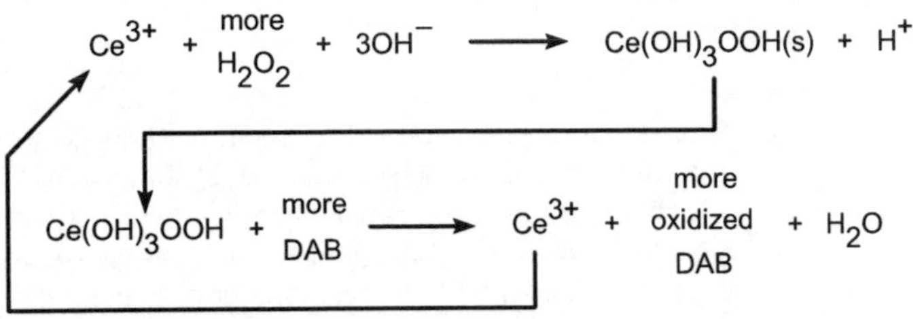

The net result of these reactions is catalysis by $Ce(OH)_3OOH$ of the oxidation of DAB by H_2O_2. If nickel ions are present the colour is blue–black rather than brown. The chemistry of DAB oxidation is discussed in connection with peroxidase histochemistry (Section 16.5.2).

16.6.3.2. Peroxidase-coupled method
The other strategy for detecting newly produced H_2O_2 is to let it be the substrate of another enzyme, peroxidase. The final reaction products in histochemical methods for peroxidase are visible and electron-dense (Section 16.5).

The following method (from Maeda *et al.*, 1987) is one of several 'coupled peroxidatic oxidation' techniques for MAO and for other oxidases that form hydrogen peroxide. As described, the procedure requires free-floating sections cut on a vibrating microtome. However, it should also work with cryostat sections mounted on slides or coverslips.

Solutions required
Phosphate-buffered saline (PBS) (See Chapter 20)
100 ml at room temperature, and 100 ml at 0°C.

Fixative
2–4% formaldehyde with 2–3% glutaraldehyde, in 0.1 M phosphate buffer, pH 7.4 (Chapter 2).

Incubation medium
0.05 M TRIS buffer, pH 7.6, at 4°C (Chapter 20):	10 ml
Diaminobenzidine tetrahydrochloride:	0.5 mg
Horseradish peroxidase:	10 mg
Tyramine hydrochloride:	7.5 mg
Nickel ammonium sulphate:	60 mg
Sodium azide:	6.5 mg

Make up less than 1 h before it is needed. The medium is used at 4°C.

Procedure

(1) Perfuse an anaesthetized rat with 100 ml of PBS at room temperature, followed by 250 ml of the fixative at 4°C. About 250 ml of fixative should be perfused, over the course of 6–7 min.

(2) Remove the brain or other organs to be studied, and cut sections 30 µm thick with a vibrating microtome.

(3) Collect the sections into ice-cold PBS.

(4) Transfer the sections to the cold incubation medium. Agitate occasionally. Examine at hourly intervals for the first 4 h. Longer times (up to 48 h) are sometimes needed.

(5) When staining is satisfactory, rinse the sections in 3 changes of ice-cold PBS.

(6) Mount sections onto slides; leave to dry.

(7) Dehydrate, clear and mount, using a resinous medium.

Result

Sites of MAO activity blue–black. Controls for specificity (see *Note 2* below) are needed.

Notes

(1) Tyramine is the substrate. The sodium azide is necessary to inhibit other enzymes (notably cytochrome oxidase) that would cause oxidation of DAB. The nickel salt must be $Ni(NH_4)_2(SO_4)_2.6H_2O$. It serves to darken the product of the oxidation of DAB (which would otherwise be brown) and to shorten the time required for the development of adequate colour in the sections.

(2) **Controls.** (a) Omit the substrate. (b) Inject a rat with **pargyline hydrochloride**, or **nialamide**, 50 mg/kg body weight intraperitoneally, 2 h before killing it. These drugs inhibit MAO. They may be also added to the incubation medium (10^{-2} M); if this is done, the pH will require adjustment. *To inhibit Type A MAO*, incubate the sections, for 15 min between stages 3 and 4 of the procedure, in 10^{-7}–10^{-5} M **deprenyl** in PBS. *To inhibit Type B MAO*, pre-incubate in 10^{-6}–10^{-4} M **clorgyline**. The Type A enzyme occurs in neuroglia (mainly astrocytes). Type B is found within the cell-bodies, axons and dendrites of neurons that use amines as synaptic transmitters.

(3) This method can also be used in conjunction with electron microscopy. The final reaction product is in the cytoplasmic matrix and mitochondria. It cannot be stated with any confidence that these are the true subcellular sites of monoamine oxidase activity however, because biochemical studies indicate that this is a mitochondrial enzyme. Some diffusion of hydrogen peroxide would be expected to occur prior to the reaction catalysed by the added peroxidase.

16.6.4.
Xanthine oxidoreductase
(xanthine:NAD oxidoreductase, E.C. 1.1.1.204; xanthine:O_2 oxidoreductase, E.C. 1.3.2.2)

This enzyme contains iron and molybdenum and has FAD as a prosthetic group. It exists in two forms: a dehydrogenase that passes electrons to NAD^+, and an oxidase that passes electrons to oxygen. The dehydrogenase form is easily converted to the oxidase form, even during cold storage, by exposure to proteolytic enzymes or organic solvents. This change can be reversed by treating the oxidase with a reducing agent. Both forms of the enzyme exist *in vivo*, though certain tissues contain more of one or the other. This enzyme has more than one substrate: it catalyzes the oxidation of hypoxanthine to xanthine and of xanthine to uric acid:

hypoxanthine   xanthine   uric acid

The prosthetic group of xanthine oxidase adds to the substrate an oxygen atom derived from water, and is itself reduced. The reduced form of the enzyme is then re-oxidized by either NAD^+ (dehydrogenase form) or molecular oxygen (oxidase form). Superoxide ions (Section 16.5) are a product of the oxidase activity. The flow of electrons begins within the reduced enzyme molecule, passing from molybdenum, iron, and FAD to either NAD^+ or O_2 (see Kooij et al., 1991). Electrons can be diverted from this series of acceptors to methoxyphenazine methosulphate (Section 16.4.3.2, paragraph 8), and then to a tetrazolium salt, which is reduced to a coloured, insoluble formazan.

Xanthine oxidase occurs in peroxisomes and probably also in the cytosol. The name peroxisome came from the organelle's histochemical reactivity in methods for peroxidase, but the enzyme was soon found to be catalase, the enzyme that removes hydrogen peroxide from cells (Section 16.5.3).

Xanthine oxidase is inactivated by fixatives but its diffusion can be retarded by an appropriate concentration of PVA (Section 16.4.3.2, paragraph 7). All other components of the incubation medium must also be present at optimal concentrations (Kooij et al., 1991; Van Noorden and Frederiks, 1992). The enzymatic activity in the cut sections deteriorates in less than 30 min, even at $-25°C$, so the incubation medium must be ready to receive the freshly cut sections.

Solutions required
A. 18% Polyvinyl alcohol

Polyvinyl alcohol (average MW 40 000):	18 g
0.1 M phosphate buffer (pH 8.0):	100 ml

Heat on a water bath, with stirring, until the solution is transparent. Store this stock solution in screw-capped 10 ml vials in an oven, at 60°C. Allow a vial to cool to 37°C before using.

Solutions B, C and D are made up an hour or two before using.

B. Hypoxanthine

0.25 M (1% NaOH w/v) sodium hydroxide:	1.0 ml
Hypoxanthine:	6.8 mg

C. Methoxyphenazine

Water:	1.0 ml
1-methoxyphenazine methosulphate:	15.0 mg

D. TNBT

Ethanol:	0.2 ml
N,N-dimethylformamide:	0.2 ml
Tetranitro-blue tetrazolium chloride (may need to be warmed to dissolve):	10 mg

E. Incubation medium
Mix this immediately before cutting the sections. Keep it in a dark place at 37°C.

Solution A:	10 ml
Solution B:	0.1 ml
Solution C:	0.1 ml
Solution D:	0.4 ml (all of it)

See Note below for control media.

F. Hot phosphate buffer
0.1 M phosphate buffer, pH 5.3, kept at 60°C. (This stable solution may be stored indefinitely.)

Procedure

(1) Collect cryostat sections of unfixed tissue onto coverslips or the ends of slides.
(2) Place immediately in the incubation medium (Solution E) and leave for 30 min at 37°C.
(3) Rinse in hot phosphate buffer (Solution F) for 10 s.
(4) Immerse in 10% formalin for 5 min.
(5) Wash in water, 1 min.
(6) Apply a coverslip (or slide), using an aqueous mounting medium.

Result

Sites of enzymatic activity brown. Only activity absent from the same sites in control sections can be attributed to xanthine oxidase. Staining is prominent in endothelial cells, secretory epithelium (mammary gland), intestinal epithelium and hepatocytes of some animals.

Notes

(1) False positive colouration (nothing dehydrogenase) can occur. Control sections should be incubated in (a) medium without hypoxanthine and (b) medium with added **allopurinol** (1.0 mM; 1.4 mg per 10 ml) which competitively inhibits xanthine oxidase.
(2) Xanthine oxidase and hypoxanthine provide a source of superoxide ion in biochemical techniques for assaying superoxide dismutase (SOD) activity. In a histochemical method for SOD, cryostat sections are mounted on a gel that contains xanthine oxidase, and the incubation medium contains hypoxanthine. The activity of SOD generates peroxide, which is precipitated by Ce^{3+} ions (Frederiks and Bosch, 1997).

17 | Methods for soluble organic compounds of low molecular weight

There is a shortage of histochemical techniques for the demonstration of soluble organic compounds of low (<1000) molecular weight. This is due partly to the fact that such substances diffuse rapidly and partly to a lack of suitable chemical reactions. For one group of small molecules, however, there are several satisfactory methods; this is the series of substances known as biogenic amines. Most of the present chapter is concerned with the histochemical study of amines, though several other substances are also discussed.

17.1. Nature and occurrence of biogenic amines

Of the amines occurring in mammalian tissues, it is possible to localize dopamine, noradrenaline, adrenaline, serotonin, and histamine in sections. The structures of these substances are shown in *Fig. 17.1*.

Dopamine (DA) and noradrenaline (NA) are primary monoamines derived from phenylethylamine ($C_6H_5CH_2CH_2NH_2$), whereas adrenaline (ADR) is a secondary amine formed by *N*-methylation of NA. Serotonin (5HT) is another primary monoamine, being an indolylethylamine derivative. Histamine (HIS), an imidazolylethylamine, is usually called a diamine, on account of the basicity of the imidazole ring. All these compounds have fully aromatic rings attached to the ethylamine moieties, and all except HIS are phenols as well as amines.

All the above-mentioned compounds are soluble in water and would therefore be expected to diffuse rapidly from their cellular sites of storage under the ordinary physical conditions of a histochemical technique. Diffusion can be minimized by using freeze-dried material or by the application of a chemical fixative that reacts rapidly with the amine to produce an insoluble compound. Both these approaches are used. The amines are found in two types of site. These are:

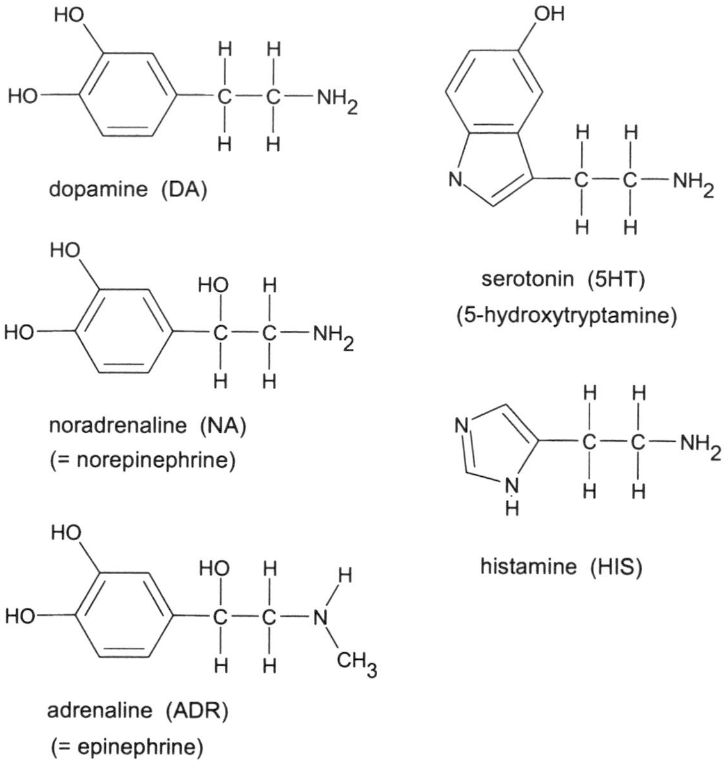

Figure 17.1. Structural formulae of some biogenic amines. The three compounds on the left are called **catecholamines** because their structures include catechol (o-dihydroxybenzene).

(a) In large quantities, in secretory granules of endocrine (or similar) cells. Here, binding to a protein or carbohydrate matrix greatly reduces diffusion of the amines.
   1. Chromaffin cells of the adrenal medulla and related paraganglia (NA and ADR in separate cell-types).
   2. Argentaffin (enterochromaffin) cells of the intestinal mucosa (5HT).
   3. Mast cells (HIS in all mammalian species; also 5HT in rodents, and DA in the lungs of ruminants).
(b) In small quantities as transmitter substances in aminergic neurons. The amines in these sites are easily extracted by water and other solvents.
   1. Most postganglionic sympathetic neurons, their axons and terminal aborizations (NA).
   2. Various systems of neurons in the central nervous system, most conspicuously in the terminal parts of axons (DA, NA, 5HT, ADR and HIS).

In situation (a), where the diffusion of amines is hindered by associated structural macromolecules, the sensitivity of a histochemical method does not need to be as high as for the demonstration of amines in situation (b). Furthermore, the amines in endocrine cells are fairly easily preserved by chemical fixation, but those of neurons are much more labile. This difference is probably also due to stronger binding of the amines to the proteinaceous matrices of the granules of secretory cells than to the synaptic vesicles of neurons.

The histochemical techniques for the biogenic amines (for review, see Hahn von Dorsch *et al.*, 1975; Bjorklund, 1983) depend on the detection *either* of the phenolic groups *or* of ethylamine with an aromatic substituent on the β-carbon atom.

17.2. Histochemical methods for amines in secretory granules

17.2.1.
Serotonin: azo coupling methods

The serotonin-containing cells of the alimentary tract are named 'argentaffin' on account of their ability to reduce ammoniacal or similarly complexed solutions of silver nitrate to the metal. Other presumably endocrine cells found in the gastrointestinal epithelium reduce complex silver ions more weakly and can only be seen if treatment with the silver reagent is followed by the application of a developer, which increases the sizes and densities of the initially deposited metal particles. The latter types of cell are termed 'argyrophil' and the methods for demonstrating them are reminiscent of the methods used for staining axons in the nervous system (see Grizzle, 1996; also Chapter 18). These silver staining methods are useful to histopathologists. The argentaffin reaction is a property of serotonin, and the argyrophil properties of some cells are due, at least in part, to chromogranins, a family of proteins that occur in cytoplasmic vesicles of a variety of peptide-secreting endocrine cells and neurons (Lundqvist *et al.*, 1990).

The most convenient histochemical techniques for argentaffin cells are based on the detection of the phenolic function of serotonin. Phenols couple with diazonium salts in alkaline solution to form coloured azo compounds. Azo-coupling with phenols occurs preferentially *para* to the hydroxyl groups. This position is already occupied in 5HT, so one of the *ortho* sites is used:

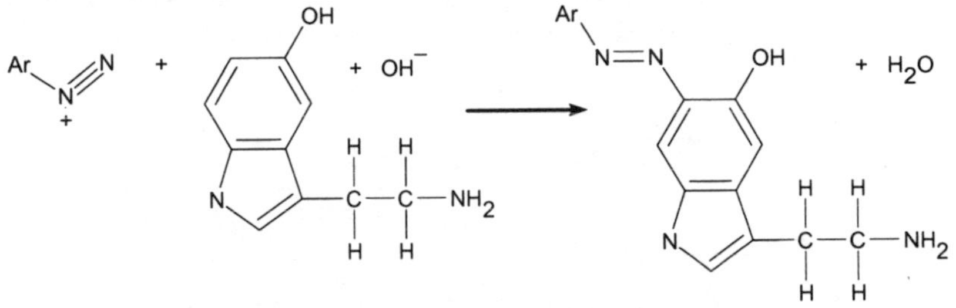

Similar azo-coupling reactions are also to be expected with the aromatic amino acids of all proteins and with any other phenolic compounds present in the tissues. Consequently, generalized 'background' staining occurs if the time of exposure to the diazonium salt is unduly prolonged. The secretory granules of argentaffin cells (and of rodent mast cells) are recognized by virtue of their more intense and more rapidly developing coloration.

The argentaffin cells also give a positive chromaffin reaction (Section 17.2.2), but this is not generally used for their identification.

Fixation and preparation
Use paraffin sections of formaldehyde-fixed material.

Solutions required
A. Diazonium salt solution

Fast red B salt (stabilized diazonium salt from 5-nitroanisidine; Chapter 5):	100 mg
TRIS buffer, pH 9.0:	100 ml

Prepare just before using.

B. A counterstain

A haemalum, used progressively, is suitable.

Procedure

(1) De-wax and hydrate sections (see *Note* below).
(2) Immerse in the diazonium salt solution (A) for 30 s.
(3) Carefully rinse in five changes of water, each 20–30 s, without agitation.
(4) Counterstain nuclei. If a haemalum is used for this purpose, do not wash in running water but 'blue' the sections in water containing a trace of $Ca(OH)_2$.
(5) Dehydrate, clear, and cover, using a resinous mounting medium.

Result

Argentaffin cell granules orange–red; background (protein) yellow; nuclei (if counterstained with alum–haematoxylin) blue.

Note

It may be necessary to cover the sections with a film of nitrocellulose (Chapter 4) to prevent their detachment from the slides during and after treatment with the alkaline Solution A. The film should be removed before clearing. The instructions for stages 3 and 4 allow for more gentle handling of the preparations than is usually necessary.

17.2.2.
The chromaffin reaction

Cytoplasmic granules in the cells of the adrenal medulla assume brown colours after fixation in a solution containing potassium dichromate. Although such cells are said to be 'chromaffin', the coloured product is derived not from the fixative but from the adrenaline and noradrenaline present in the cells. The amines are oxidized by dichromate to coloured quinones. The reaction involves oxidation of the catechol (*o*-diphenol) moiety to a quinone, and oxidative coupling of the amino group to one of the carbon atoms of the ring:

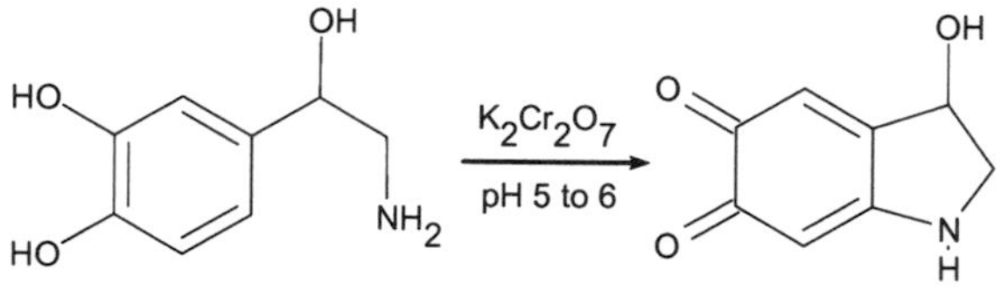

noradrenaline   noradrenochrome

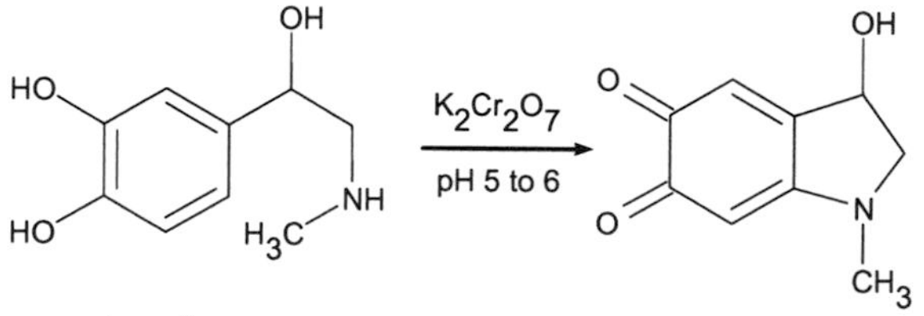

adrenaline   adrenochrome

A similar reaction occurs with DA. It is likely that further oxidations and polymerization take place in the formation of the final brown products, which are insoluble in water or organic solvents. The chromium atoms in the reagent are reduced from oxidation state +6 to +3. The resulting Cr^{3+} ions are bound at the sites of the amine (Lever *et al.*, 1977), and cause increased electron density of the chromaffin granules.

Procedure

This technique is applied to small pieces or thin slices of fresh tissue (e.g. a rat's adrenal gland cut in half).

Solution required

Potassium dichromate ($K_2Cr_2O_7$):	5.0 g
Potassium chromate (K_2CrO_4):	0.45 g
Water:	to make 100 ml

The solution is stable for an indefinitely long time.

Procedure

(1) Fix small pieces of tissue in the above solution (see *Note 1* below) for 24 h.
(2) Wash in running tap water overnight. (See also *Note 2* below.)
(3) Dehydrate, clear, embed in paraffin wax. Cut sections 4–7 μm thick.
(4) De-wax and clear (three changes of xylene) and mount in a resinous medium.

Results

The cytoplasm of cells containing adrenaline (ADR) and noradrenaline (NA) is coloured brown. The product formed from ADR is darker than that from NA.

Notes

(1) A chromate–dichromate mixture is used to obtain a solution of pH 5.5–5.7. Alternatively, one may fix the tissue in a fixative mixture based on potassium dichromate provided that it does not contain acids or other heavy metal ions. Such mixtures are, however, more acid than the optimum pH for the chromaffin reaction.
(2) Step 2 may be followed by a secondary fixation for 12–24 h in 4% formaldehyde if desired. This is necessary if frozen rather than paraffin sections are to be cut.
(3) A counterstain may be applied to the sections if desired. Alum–haematoxylin is suitable for nuclei. Many cationic dyes stain the chromaffin cells, thereby increasing the intensity of their colour in addition to demonstrating nuclei.
(4) The **iodate ion** can oxidize catecholamines in the same way as dichromate though it acts much more rapidly upon NA than upon ADR. Consequently it is possible, using sodium iodate, to stain NA-containing cells selectively. Thin slices of tissue are immersed for 24 h in saturated (10%) aqueous sodium iodate, then post-fixed in formaldehyde and sectioned with a freezing microtome or cryostat.

17.2.3. Catecholamines in glutaraldehyde-fixed tissue

Glutaraldehyde reacts with amino groups probably to form imines:

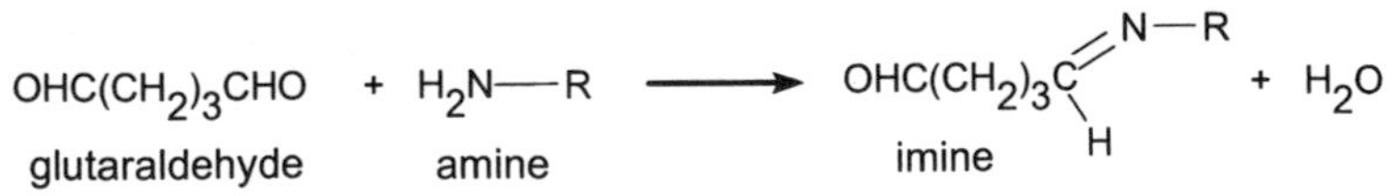

$$OHC(CH_2)_3CHO \;+\; H_2N\!-\!R \;\longrightarrow\; OHC(CH_2)_3C\!\!\underset{H}{\overset{N-R}{<}} \;+\; H_2O$$

glutaraldehyde   amine   imine

Ordinarily an imine such as that shown above will be unstable when, as in the biogenic amines, R is not an aromatic ring. (In aromatic amines, $-NH_2$ is attached directly to an aromatic ring, not to an aliphatic side-chain.) However, in a tissue the other end of the glutaraldehyde molecule is likely to combine similarly with a protein-bound amino group. Extensive cross-linking of the proteinaceous matrix of the tissue probably increases the resistance of the imine linkages to hydrolysis. Primary catecholamines (DA and NA) are bound by their amino groups and are therefore immobilized, but their catechol groups remain free to react with other reagents. Adrenaline, which is a secondary amine, reacts with glutaraldehyde more slowly than NA or DA and is not usually retained in the tissue.

The catechols are strong reducing agents and may be detected by several histochemical methods. A simple procedure is to post-fix the glutaraldehyde-fixed specimens in osmium tetroxide (Coupland *et al.*, 1964), which is reduced to a black material (see also Chapter 2). Alternatively, the catechol-containing site may be made visible by virtue of its ability to reduce silver diammine ions to the metal (Tramezzani et al., 1964; see also Chapter 10, Section 10.10.4). Methods of this type impart optical blackness and electron density to granules containing NA or DA. If adrenaline is to be demonstrated as well, it is necessary to fix the specimens in a solution containing both glutaraldehyde and potassium dichromate at empirically determined optimum concentrations and pH (Coupland et al., 1976; Tranzer and Richards, 1976).

Procedure
Freshly removed specimens are fixed specially for this technique.

Solutions required
A. Fixative

25% aqueous glutaraldehyde:	20 ml
0.1 M phosphate buffer, pH 7.3:	80 ml

Prepare this on day it is to be used.

B. Buffered osmium tetroxide

2% aqueous OsO_4 (stock solution):	5.0 ml
0.1 M phosphate buffer, pH 7.3:	5.0 ml

Stable for about 6 h after addition of the phosphate buffer. A simple 1% aqueous solution of osmium tetroxide, which is stable for several weeks in a clean glass bottle, may be substituted. See Chapter 12 (Section 12.6.1) for notes on the safe handling and disposal of osmium tetroxide.

Procedure
(1)   Fix freshly removed pieces of tissue no more than 2 or 3 mm thick (e.g. halved adrenal gland of a rat) in Solution A for 4 h.
(2)   Rinse specimen in water. Cut frozen sections 10–40 µm thick and collect them into water. Mount onto slides, blot, and allow to dry for 5–10 min. Position the sections near the ends of the slides so that only a small volume of Solution B will be needed.
(3)   Immerse the sections in Solution B in a closed coplin jar for 30 min.
(4)   Wash slides in running tap water for 30 min.
(5)   Dehydrate, clear, and cover, usiing a resinous mounting medium.

Result
Noradrenaline-containing cells black to grey. Osmiophilic lipids (Chapter 12) are also blackened.

Control
Substitute neutral, buffered formaldehyde for Solution A in stage 1 of the method. The osmium tetroxide will now give black products only with lipids.

17.2.4.
Histamine

Various histochemical methods for histamine have been described, but none are very specific (see Pearse, 1985). The least unsatisfactory is based on the formation of a fluorescent adduct with o-phthaldialdehyde (OPT). The method is usually applied to paraffin sections of freeze-dried tissue. Unfortunately, the reagent also forms fluorescent products with many amino acids, and with some proteins (Hakanson et al., 1972) and peptides (Murray et al., 1986). The OPT method has revealed the presence of histamine in cells already suspected of containing this amine, as in the gastric glands (Hakanson et al., 1970) and in atypical mast cells (Kawamura, 1986), but has been of no use for mapping histamine-containing cells and fibres in nervous tissue. Instructions for a simple OPT method (Enerback, 1969) were given in the first edition of this book, but are not repeated here.

Immunohistochemical methods (Chapter 19) are now preferred for examining the distribution of histamine. It is possible to immobilize the amine by fixation in a carbodiimide. Immunoreactivity is seen in all the cell-types known to contain histamine, and in other sites too (Panula *et al.*, 1988; Johansson *et al.*, 1994).

17.3. Sensitive methods for amines in neurons

17.3.1.
Formaldehyde-induced fluorescence

The reactions for noradrenaline and serotonin discussed in Section 17.2 are not sensitive enough to demonstrate aminergic neurons. For this purpose it is necessary to make use of the formation of intensely fluorescent compounds by reaction of the amines with formaldehyde (or any of a few other reagents; see Section 17.3.2 below). These methods, which can detect as little as 5×10^{-16} g of NA or DA, have contributed importantly to knowledge of the anatomy of the central and peripheral nervous systems. Theoretical and practical aspects of the techniques are comprehensively reviewed by Bjorklund (1983).

Formaldehyde reacts with NA, DA, and 5HT by condensation and cyclization to form nonfluorescent compounds. These then undergo either oxidation by atmospheric oxygen or reaction with more formaldehyde, to form brightly fluorescent products. While the first stage of the reaction can occur with formaldehyde in either the liquid or the gaseous phase, the second stage requires an almost dry proteinaceous matrix at 80–100°C. The overall reactions are shown in *Fig. 17.2*.

The reactions are more complicated than is indicated by the equations in *Fig. 17.2*, and the fluorescent products shown are not the only ones formed. Adrenaline yields a product that is only weakly fluorescent. The chemistry of formaldehyde-induced fluorescence is discussed in detail by Corrodi and Jonsson (1967) and Pearse (1985). A simpler account is given by Bjorklund *et al.* (1975).

It is usual to employ freeze-dried tissue in studies of the biogenic amines of the nervous system, though methods have been devised for cryostat sections and for

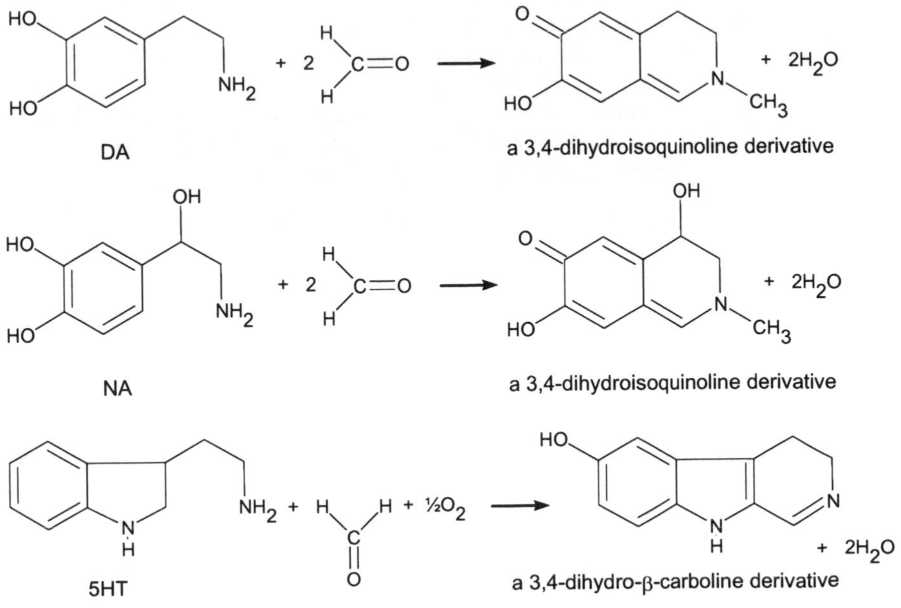

Figure 17.2. Formation of fluorescent products by reaction of monoamines with formaldehyde.

spreads of membranous tissues such as the iris and mesentery. Glyoxylic acid or, alternatively, a formaldehyde and glutaraldehyde (**FAGLU**) mixture (see below) is a more suitable reagent if facilities for freeze-drying are not available. In the simplest form of the method, freeze-dried blocks of tissue are treated with formaldehyde gas, derived from solid paraformaldehyde, under controlled conditions of humidity at about 80°C. The treated blocks are then embedded directly in paraffin wax. The sections must not be exposed to water or alcohols, which remove the fluorophores. There are several modified techniques (e.g. Laties *et al.*, 1967; Watson and Ellison, 1976) in which a buffered solution of formaldehyde is perfused through the vascular system of the animal prior to either freeze-drying or the cutting of cryostat sections. Heating the sections or freeze-dried blocks, with or without paraformaldehyde vapour, effects the second stage of the reaction in which the fluorophores are formed. The most sensitive of the formaldehyde-induced fluorescence techniques is the **ALFA** method, in which the animal is perfused with a solution of an aluminium salt before exposure of the tissue to formaldehyde. The metal ions catalyse the formation of fluorescent derivatives. The ALFA procedure can provide material for freeze-drying and sectioning in paraffin, or for cutting in a cryostat or a vibrating microtome (Loren *et al.*, 1980).

Formaldehyde-induced fluorescence is valuable not only for the identification and morphological study of cells containing biogenic amines, but also for investigating the pharmacological properties of such cells. For example, reserpine depletes cells of their monoamines, and drugs that inhibit monoamine oxidase produce visible increases in the intensity of fluorescence. A pharmacological method for distinguishing between DA and NA was devised by Hess (1978). Animals were treated first with reserpine and then with DOPA, a metabolic precursor of the catecholamines. After a suitable internal of time, only the DA-containing cells exhibited fluorescence in formaldehyde-treated tissues. A much longer time was needed for replenishment of NA. The synaptic axonal varicosities of aminergic neurons normally reabsorb their transmitter substances, and this property is occasionally exploited in order to enhance their formaldehyde-induced fluorescence.

Pearse (1968a) has identified a series of cells that do not normally contain monoamines but which can take up the amino acids DOPA and 5-hydroxytryptophan and decarboxylate them to give DA and 5HT in histochemically demonstrable quantities. He named these cells, most of which have known or suspected endocrine functions, **APUD** (amine precursor uptake and decarboxylation) cells. Some of the APUD cell-types are argentaffin or argyrophil, and most are now known to contain physiologically active peptides.

17.3.2.
Other fluorescent methods for amines

In addition to formaldehyde, several other carbonyl compounds are able to form fluorescent condensation products with biogenic amines. The most valuable is glyoxylic acid:

This substance was introduced as an alternative to formaldehyde by Axelsson *et al.* (1973). It reacts in a similar manner, the fluorescent products being closely similar though obtained in higher yield than with formaldehyde (see Bjorklund *et al.*, 1975).

A major advantage of methods making use of glyoxylic acid is that it is not necessary to prepare the tissue by freeze-drying. Usually the animal is perfused with a buffered aqueous solution of glyoxylic acid. Sections are cut with a vibrating microtome or a cryostat, dried onto slides and heated, either alone or in glyoxylic acid or formaldehyde vapour. It is also possible to use paraffin sections of freeze-dried specimens. Different variations of the method (e.g. Lindvall and Bjorklund, 1974; Furness and Costa, 1975; Bloom and Battenberg, 1976; Loren *et al.*, 1976; Watson and Barchas, 1977) have been developed to give optimum results with different tissues. The fluorescence of amine-containing nerve fibres is brighter after reaction with glyoxylic acid than after reaction with formaldehyde.

In another method (Furness *et al.*, 1977,1978), tissues are treated with an aqueous solution of formaldehyde and glutaraldehyde (**FAGLU**) by immersion or vascular perfusion. Fluorophores are formed with DA, NA, and 5HT, but the chemistry of the technique has not been studied. The fluorescence resists extraction by cold water, alcohols, several other organic solvents, and melted paraffin wax. Unfortunately, the non-specific 'background' fluorescence associated with this technique is brighter than that seen with formaldehyde- or glyoxylic acid-induced fluorescence. For the demonstration of catecholamines, the FAGLU solution is used at pH 7. For serotonin the optimum pH is 10, and the sensitivity can be increased by adding an oxidizing agent, potassium ferricyanide, to the mixture (Wreford *et al.*, 1982).

17.4. Some fluorescence techniques for amines

The methods to be described are suitable, on account of their simplicity, for instructional purposes. In research work it is commonly necessary to use techniques of greater sensitivity; the ALFA method (Loren *et al.*, 1980) is probably the best of these. The use of fluorescence methods for amines fell into decline in the 1980s, and immunohistochemical methods for the enzymes involved in the synthesis of the amines are more popular. The reasons for this change in fashion include the commercial availability of reliable antisera, the fact that the immunohistochemical methods do not require special preparative procedures such as freeze-drying or cutting with a vibrating microtome, and the easy production of permanent non-fluorescent preparations.

17.4.1.
Formaldehyde-induced fluorescence

The technique described below closely resembles the original Falck-Hillarp procedure (Carlsson *et al.*, 1962; Falck *et al.*, 1962).

Preparation of tissues
Alternative methods are prescribed for (a) thin whole-mounts (mesentery, iris, etc.), and (b) solid specimens, no more than 2mm thick.

(a) Stretch pieces of the thin tissue (removed immediately after killing the animal) onto glass slides. Place the slides in a glass rack in a desiccator containing a small beaker, one-third filled with phosphorus pentoxide. Partially evacuate the desiccator and wait for 1 h. Remove the slides and treat with formaldehyde gas as described below.

Caution. P_2O_5 is corrosive. It must not be allowed to come into contact with liquid water with which it reacts violently to form phosphoric acid. To discard used P_2O_5, place the vessel containing it in a safe place, open to the air for 12–24 h. The white powder will then have deliquesced to a syrupy mass, which may be washed down the sink with copious running water.

(b) Rapidly freeze the piece of tissue (by immersion in isopentane cooled by liquid nitrogen) and transfer it to a freeze-drying apparatus. When freeze-drying is complete, treat the specimen with gaseous formaldehyde as described below.

Treatment with formaldehyde vapour
Formaldehyde is generated by the action of heat on solid paraformaldehyde. The moisture content of the latter is a critical factor: the paraformaldehyde should be

equilibrated with air of 50% relative humidity. This can be achieved by storing the powder for 7 days or longer in a desiccator that contains a mixture of concentrated sulphuric acid (specific gravity 1.84), 32 ml, and water, 68 ml. (**Caution.** Add the acid slowly, with stirring, to the water.)

Place about 6 g of the water-equilibrated paraformaldehyde at the bottom of a wide necked jar with a tightly fitting screw cap. Put the slides or freeze-dried specimens into the jar, close it, and maintain at 80°C in an oven for 1 h.

Subsequent processing
Transfer the jar containing formaldehyde vapour to a fume cupboard before opening it.

(a)   Apply coverslips to slides bearing spreads of tissue, using liquid paraffin (mineral oil, heavy, USP) as the mounting medium. Alternatively, rinse in xylene and mount in a non-fluorescent resinous medium such as DPX.

(b)   Embed freeze-dried specimens in paraffin wax (time of infiltration, 15–30 min, with vacuum). Cut sections and mount them onto slides without using water. The slides can be heated to 60°C to melt the wax and flatten the sections. Put drops of liquid paraffin on the sections and apply coverslips. With further warming on the hotplate, the wax dissolves in this mounting medium. Alternatively, remove the wax with xylene or petroleum ether, and apply coverslips with a non-fluorescent resinous mounting medium such as DPX. Clearing and mounting must be carried out very carefully to avoid loss of the sections.

Result
Green fluorescence from noradrenaline and dopamine. Yellow fluorescence from serotonin. The optimum wavelength for excitation is 410nm (violet). Sympathetic nerve fibres are displayed in spreads of iris or mesentery.

If the sections are cleared and mounted in a resinous medium, there is slight suppression of the specific fluorescence, but the preparations are optically superior to those mounted in liquid paraffin.

Sections of freeze-dried blocks commonly contain numerous cracks and other deformities, but the preservation within small areas is satisfactory. In photomicrographs, the physical damage can be hidden by printing the pictures in such a way that the weakly autofluorescent background is black, and only the brighter, specific fluorescence is displayed.

17.4.2.
Glyoxylic acid method

This technique (after Watson and Barchas, 1977) is applicable to cryostat sections of unfixed specimens of central nervous tissue. Each piece of fresh tissue is placed on a cryostat chuck, which is then stood in a slush of dry ice (solid CO_2) and acetone (or in isopentane cooled by liquid nitrogen) until the tissue has frozen.

Materials required
A. Glyoxylic acid solution

0.1 M phosphate buffer, pH 7.0 (approximately) at 0–4°C:	45 ml
Glyoxylic acid (HOOC.CHO.H₂O):	1.0 g
Magnesium chloride (MgCl₂.6H₂O):	0.25 g

Add drops of 1.0 M (4%) sodium hydroxide (NaOH) until the pH is 4.9–5.0, then add:

Water (at 0–4°C):	to make 50 ml

Prepare this solution in a coplin jar immediately before use. Cool it to 0°C by standing the jar in iced water.

B. A hotplate (maintained at 45°C)

C. A dry screw-capped coplin jar
This should contain approximately 2 g of solid glyoxylic acid ($HOOC.CHO.H_2O$), heated to 100°C on a boiling water bath for 30 min prior to use. The lid should be only half-tightened during heating, to allow for expansion of air.

Procedure

(1) Cut cryostat sections at any convenient thickness up to 20 μm. The temperature of the cryostat cabinet should be −17 °C. Collect each section onto a warm (20–25°C) slide, where it will thaw and dry at once. Proceed **immediately** to Stage 2, handling only 1–3 slides at a time.

(2) Place slides in the glyoxylic acid solution (A) and leave them there at 0°C for *either* 12 min (optimum for nerve terminals) *or* 4 min (optimum for cell bodies) *or* 45 s (optimum for some axons).

(3) Remove the slides from Solution A, blot with filter paper, and place on the hotplate at 45°C for about 5 min.

(4) Place the slides in the coplin jar containing solid glyoxylic acid at 100°C for approximately 3 min. (Do this in a fume cupboard.)

(5) Remove the slides and apply coverslips, using liquid paraffin (mineral oil, heavy, USP) as the mounting medium.

Result

Sites of NA and DA emit green fluorescence (optimal excitation by violet–blue light).

Note

Glyoylic acid is deliquescent and may deteriorate with repeated exposures to air. As soon as a bottle is received from the supplier, divide it into aliquots of 1 g and store these in separate vials, **in a desiccator**, below 0°C. Do not allow solid glyoxylic acid to come into contact with the skin; it is irritant and corrosive.

17.4.3.
A formaldehyde–glutaraldehyde (FAGLU) fluorescence method

This technique is based on that of Furness *et al.* (1977). It differs from other aldehyde-condensation methods in that no heating of dry sections is needed. The fixative (Solution A, below) is a satisfactory one for electron microscopy. See also *Note 1* below. For optimum demonstration of serotonin, use the modified FAGLU solution described in *Note 3*.

Solutions required
A. FAGLU reagent

Paraformaldehyde:	12 g
0.1 M phosphate buffer, pH 7.0:	290 ml

Dissolve, with heating to 60°C. Cool to room temperature before adding next ingredient.

25% aqueous glutaraldehyde:	6.0 ml
Water:	to make 300 ml

This solution should be made on the day it is to be used. Both the paraformaldehyde and the glutaraldehyde should be grades marketed as being suitable for electron microscopy.

B. Acidified DMP

2,2-dimethoxypropane (DMP):	25 ml
Concentrated hydrochloric acid:	One drop (about 0.05 ml)

This is prepared as required, but is stable for several hours or possibly for much longer. See Chapter 4 for discussion of DMP as a chemical dehydrating agent.

C. Clearing agent

Chloroform:	50 ml
Benzene or toluene:	50 ml

Procedure

(1) Remove small pieces of fresh tissue, no more than 2 mm thick, and place them in the FAGLU reagent (Solution A) for 3 h. (See also *Note 2* below.)

(2) Blot off excess FAGLU solution with filter paper and immerse the specimen in acidified DMP (Solution B) for 20 min at 20–30°C, with occasional shaking.

(3) Transfer to the clearing agent (Solution C). Shake at intervals of about 3 min until the specimen has sunk to the bottom of the container, then leave for a further 10 min.

(4) Infiltrate with paraffin wax, three changes, each 10 min, in a vacuum-embedding apparatus. Block out. Store the blocks at 4°C until they are to be cut.

(5) Cut sections at a convenient thickness: e.g. 15–25 μm for peripheral tissues; thinner for central nervous system. Mount the sections onto dry slides **without using water**. Place the slides on a hotplate at about 60°C until the wax melts and the sections flatten, then proceed immediately to Step 6.

(6) Remove the slides from the hotplate and put them into a staining rack. Immerse gently in a tank of previously unused xylene. Agitate very gently for 15–20 s and leave for 5 min.

(7) Carefully remove slides individually from the xylene and apply coverslips, using a non-fluorescent mounting medium such as DPX. Place the slides on a hotplate at about 50°C for 5 min, then transfer them to a tray. If they are not to be examined immediately, keep them at 4°C for no more than 1 week.

Result

Sites of NA and DA green. Sites of 5HT yellow. Other components of the tissue also fluoresce but less intensely. Optimum excitation is by blue–violet light: the non-specific background fluorescence then appears as green when an orange–yellow barrier filter is used. If excitation is by broad-band ultraviolet, with a colourless or very pale yellow barrier filter, positively reacting elements appear yellow or greenish yellow against a blue background.

Notes

(1) This technique is valuable on account of its technical simplicity, but the non-specific background fluorescence is more intense than with the two preceding methods. Furness *et al.* (1977) did not provide detailed practical instructions for the preparation of paraffin sections. The procedure described here is effective, but alternative schedules for dehydration and clearing may also be possible. **It is important to avoid flotation of the paraffin sections on warm water**, which results in loss of the specific fluorescence.

(2) For central nervous tissue, Furness *et al.* (1978) recommended perfusion of the animal with a buffered solution containing 4% formaldehyde and 1% glutaraldehyde, followed by sectioning with a vibrating microtome or a cryostat.

(3) The following solution provides maximum fluorescence at sites containing serotonin (Wreford *et al.*, 1982). It should be perfused through the vascular system for 10 min, and fixation continued by immersion at 4°C for 3 h.

Water:	450 ml
Sodium carbonate (Na_2CO_3):	5.85 g
Sodium bicarbonate ($NaHCO_3$):	3.8 g
Paraformaldehyde:	20 g

Heat to dissolve (60°C), then cool to room temperature and add:

25% glutaraldehyde:	10 ml
Water:	to make 500 ml

The pH should be 10.0. Adjust if necessary. Make this solution on the day it is to be used, and keep it at 4°C in a tightly capped bottle.

Immediately before use, add:

Potassium ferricyanide ($K_3Fe(CN)_6$):   2.0 g

17.4.4. Other amines and free amino acids

Acetylcholine. This quaternary ammonium ion can be precipitated by some metal complex anions, including reineckate, $[(NH_3)_2Cr(SCN)_4]^-$ (Gaddum, 1935), silico-tungstate, $[SiO_4(W_3O_9)_4]^{4-}$ (Tsuji and Alameddine, 1981), tungstate and molybdate (Tsuji *et al.*, 1983). These can form electron-dense deposits in synaptic vesicles believed from other lines of evidence to contain acetylcholine. Unfortunately, it is not possible to prove the chemical specificity of such reactions, which can be expected to give electron-dense deposits with many organic bases. It seems probable that precipitants included in the fixative can cleanly precipitate acetylcholine in synaptic vesicles, because it can be detected there immunohistochemically, with an anti-acetylcholine antibody, by light and electron microscopy (Tanaka *et al.*, 1995).

GABA (γ-aminobutyric acid, an inhibitory neurotransmitter) reacts with ninhydrin in octanol to form a fluorescent product. Pharmacological and histochemical studies indicate that this reaction demonstrates GABA in its expected sites in nervous tissue (Wolman, 1971; Gorne and Pfister, 1979), but the method has not often been used. The currently favoured approach to the localization of GABA is immunohistochemical. An antiserum is raised against a conjugate of GABA, glutaraldehyde and a protein such as albumin. The serum contains antibodies that can combine with GABA-glutaraldehyde-protein complexes in fixed tissue (Hodgson *et al.*, 1985). The same type of method has been used for the immunohistochemical staining of **glutamate** and **aspartate** ions (Hepler *et al.*, 1988) which are transmitters at excitatory synapses. Even the smallest amino acid, **glycine**, which is an inhibitory neurotransmitter, can be immobilized by fixation and localized to apparently meaningful subcellular sites (Crooks and Kolb, 1992).

17.5. Ascorbic acid

Ascorbic acid is very soluble in water, so if it is to be localized histochemically it must be immobilized either by quick freezing or by instantaneous chemical precipitation. It is a strong reducing agent, becoming oxidized to dehydroascorbic acid:

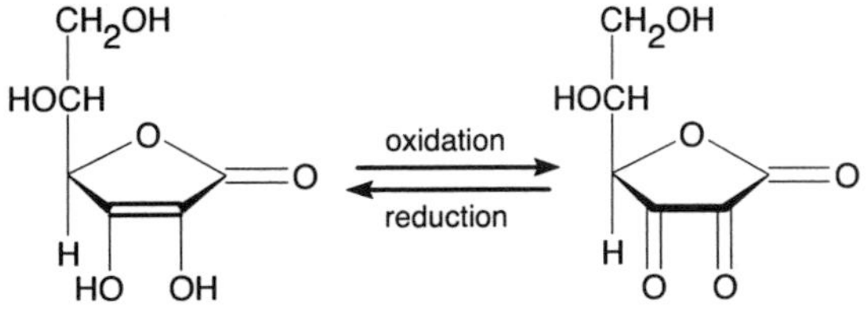

Both forms are likely to be present in tissues. The dehydroascorbic acid can be reduced *in situ* by treating the tissue with gaseous hydrogen sulphide, which is a strong reducing agent. The H_2S can then be removed by partially evacuating the container.

The only histochemical method for the reduced form of ascorbic acid is the acid silver nitrate method of Bourne (1933) and Giroud and Leblond (1934). This method is based on the biochemical observation that ascorbic acid is the only substance in living tissues that rapidly reduces silver nitrate in acid solution:

$$C_6H_8O_6 + 2Ag^+ \longrightarrow C_6H_6O_6 + 2H^+ + 2Ag(s)$$

The high solubility of ascorbic acid makes it unlikely that the silver deposits form in exactly the same subcellular sites. The localization seen within tissues corresponds with that determined by chemical assays (see Pearse, 1985). Only one quarter of tissue-bound silver is attributable to reaction with ascorbic acid (Willis and Kratzing, 1974). The remainder is in unreduced form, bound to protein, and must be removed by treating the specimens, after immersion in $AgNO_3$, with sodium thiosulphate. Otherwise the bound silver would slowly be reduced to the metal on exposure to light. Another possible cause of a false-positive reaction is the presence of phosphate ions (as in bone or other calcified tissues), which might give a von Kossa reaction (Chapter 14). This artifact can be avoided by carrying out the treatment with silver nitrate in darkness.

The procedure described here is based on that of Barnett and Bourne (1941).

Tissue preparation
Freshly removed small organs (less than 2 mm in least dimension) or similarly sized slices or pieces are usually immersed directly in the acidified silver nitrate solution. Bourne (1933) fixed in formaldehyde gas, generated from hot paraformaldehyde, and it is also possible to use paraffin sections of unfixed freeze-dried material. The reagent is applied to the sections before the wax is removed. (See Section 1.6.5 for comments about staining in the presence of wax.)

Solutions required
A. Acidified silver nitrate
Silver nitrate:	0.5 g
Water:	50 ml
Glacial acetic acid:	0.5 ml

Stable, in a brown glass bottle, but it is convenient to make up as required, from an aqueous 1% stock solution of silver nitrate.

B. Sodium thiosulphate solution
Sodium thiosulphate ($Na_2S_2O_3.5H_2O$):	10 g
Water:	to make 200 ml

This solution keeps indefinitely but is used only once.

Procedure
(1) Immerse specimens in the acidified silver nitrate (Solution A), for 1 h, in a dark place. See *Note 1* below.
(2) Rinse in water, then transfer to 5% sodium thiosulphate (Solution B). Leave for 10–60 min.
(3) Wash in 3 changes of water, each 10 min.
(4) Either prepare as a whole mount (thin specimens) or dehydrate, clear, embed in wax, cut sections, remove wax and mount in a resinous medium. See also *Note 2*.

Result
Tiny black granules indicate sites of reduction of silver ions by ascorbic acid. They are typically seen in cytoplasm, subjacent to the cell membrane and around the nucleus. Controls (see *Note 3*) should not show this appearance.

Notes

(1)   The time is not critical, but must be sufficient for penetration of the specimen. 15 min may suffice for thin specimens to be examined as whole mounts. Paraffin sections are left overnight at 37°C, to allow for slow penetration in the presence of wax.

(2)   Sections or whole mounts may be counterstained if desired. Suitable methods are given in Chapter 6.

(3)   Suitable negative controls include specimens soaked in saline or 70% ethanol for 1 h prior to immersion in the acidified silver nitrate, and specimens taken from experimental animals that have been fed a diet deficient in ascorbic acid. See Chapter 20 for positive control tissues.

17.6. Thiamine

Thiamine (vitamin B1) is a quaternary base that is present in many tissues of animals and plants. The thiamine (thiaminium) cation can be oxidized to **thiochrome**, a yellow substance that gives blue fluorescence in response to ultraviolet irradiation.

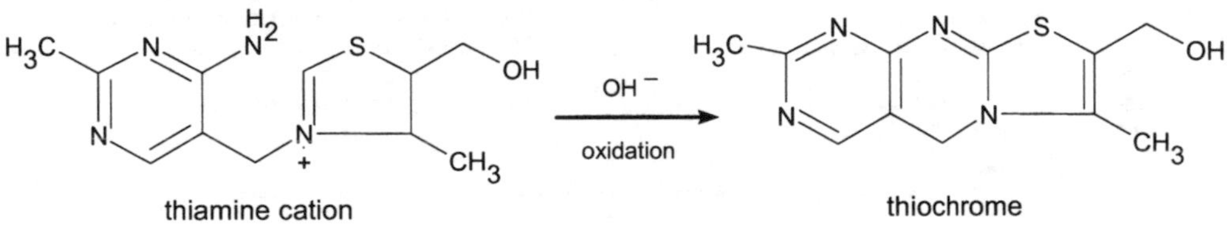

thiamine cation   thiochrome

This reaction is used in chemical assays for thiamine, and has been adapted as a histochemical method. The oxidizing agent may be alkaline potassium ferricyanide (Muralt, 1943) or cyanogen bromide vapour followed by ammonia (Tanaka *et al.*, 1973). Both procedures show an end-product in the myelin sheaths of peripheral nerves.

18 Metal reduction and precipitation methods

The major groups of methods that make use of metal reduction or precipitation are classified and summarized in *Table 18.1*. Many of the items in this table are histochemical and are discussed in other chapters; a few are not considered in this book (see references in the table). The remaining procedures have been developed largely by trial and error, and for most the chemical and physical reasons for their specificity are only partly understood. This chapter is concerned with staining methods that generate deposits of metallic elements or darkly coloured insoluble inorganic compounds. In almost every case the visible product is formed by chemical reduction of a soluble salt or complex of the metal.

These methods provide strong contrast, with the stained structures (black) standing out against a colourless or pale (usually yellowish, light purple or grey) background. They are used principally to demonstrate features that cannot be shown by staining with dyes. The greatest numbers of metal staining methods are for nervous tissue. It has long been recognized that the structure of the nervous system is not adequately revealed by staining methods generally employed to display cells and fibres in other types of tissue. Some of the traditional metal reduction techniques, especially those using silver, can be combined with dye stains or histochemical methods. For critical discussion of all neurohistological methods and their uses and limitations, see Nauta and Ebbesson (1970), Ralis *et al.* (1973), Kiernan and Berry (1975), Santini (1975) and Jones and Hartman (1978).

Metal reduction methods are often said (by those who do not use them frequently) to be unreliable and difficult to do, requiring some kind of magic touch to obtain the desired result. In fact, failures can usually be attributed to not following the instructions accurately and intelligently or to glassware that is not clean enough.

Table 18.1. Metal reduction or precipitation techniques*, classified according to uses

Purpose	Metal reduced or precipitated	Examples of technique
General histology and microbiology:		
Cytoplasmic organelles	Osmium reduction	Mann–Kopsch method (Section 18.4.2)
(especially Golgi apparatus)	Silver reduction	Saxena's method (Section 18.3.4)
Secretory granules (also peripheral nerve endings and others)	Osmium reduction	Iodide–osmium methods (Section 18.4.4)
Nucleolar organizer regions	Silver reduction	AgNOR methods (Chapter 9)
Reticular fibres	Silver reduction	Gordon and Sweets' method (Section 18.3.2)
	Gold reduction	Lynch's bromine–gold method (Section 18.2.3)
Invertebrate organs	Osmium reduction	Osmium-containing fixatives (Chapter 2; also Gray, 1954)
Bacteria (spirochaetes)	Silver reduction	Warthin–Starry method (18.3.3.2)
Fungi	Silver reduction	Grocott's method (18.3.3.1)
Neurohistology:		
Whole cells and their	Silver chromate	Golgi methods (Section 18.5.2)
cytoplasmic processes	Mercury chromate	Golgi–Cox method (Section 18.5.3)
Normal myelin	Osmium reduction	OsO4 fixation or staining (Chapters 2 and 12)
	Palladium reduction	PdCl$_2$ method (Chapter 12)
	Silver reduction	Bromine–silver (Chapter 12)
Degenerating myelin	Osmium reduction	Marchi method (Section 18.4.3)
Normal axons	Silver reduction	Many methods (Section 18.3.1)
Peripheral nerve endings	Gold reduction	Ranvier's method (Section 18.2.1)
	Silver reduction	Many methods (Section 18.3.1)
	Osmium reduction	Iodide–osmium methods (Section 18.4.4)
Degenerating axons	Silver reduction	Nauta and Gygax (1954) and Fink and Heimer (1967) methods (Jones and Hartman, 1967; Switzer, 2000)
Alzheimer's and related lesions in brain	Silver reduction	Gallyas–Braak method (Section 18.3.1.9); Reusche (1991); Garvey *et al.* (1994)
Neuroglial cells	Gold reduction	Cajal's gold-sublimate, for astrocytes (Section 18.2.2)
	Silver reduction	Silver carbonate methods for oligodendrocytes and microglia (Penfield and Cone, 1950; d'Amelio, 1980)
General histochemistry:		
Detection of aldehydes	Silver reduction	Silver diammine (Chapter 10)
Detection of unsaturation in lipids	Osmium reduction	OsO4 fixation and staining (Chapters 2 and 12)
	Palladium reduction	PdCl$_2$ method (Chapter 12)
	Silver reduction	Bromine–silver method (Chapter 12)
Calcium phosphate deposits	Silver reduction	von Kossa's method (Chapter 13)
Detection of serotonin and catecholamines	Silver reduction	Argentaffin reaction (Chapter 17)
Detection of ascorbic acid	Silver reduction	Acid AgNO$_3$ method (Chapter 17)
Enzyme histochemistry:		
Phosphatases	Lead precipitation	Acid phosphatase (Chapter 16)
	Cerium precipitation	Alkaline phosphatase (Chapter 16)
Esterases	Copper precipitation	Choline esterases (Chapter 16)
Oxidoreductases	Cerium precipitation	Discussed in Chapter 16
Amplification of products of histochemical procedures:		
Metal histochemistry	Silver reduction	Timm's sulphide–silver method (Chapter 13)
Nucleic acid hybridization and immunohistochemistry	Silver reduction	Silver enhancement of DaB (Chapters 15, 16) and colloidal gold (Chapter 19)

* Metal ions are used in association with dyes (mordants; see Chapters 5, 6, 8), but in these cases the visible product is not the metal or a simple inorganic compound.

18.1. General practical points

**18.1.1.
Cleaning
glassware**

Gold, silver and osmium are used from solutions that react readily with traces of grease, dust and other organic materials. *Plastic containers must not be used.* The following procedure should be adopted for cleaning all bottles, dishes and other glassware.

(1)   Wash thoroughly in detergent and warm water, using a brush on the inside and the outside of the vessel or container.
(2)   Wash away all the detergent with running tap water.
(3)   Rinse the inside of the object with distilled water.
(4)   Put 3–5 ml of concentrated nitric acid in the container and turn it to allow the acid to pass over the whole inside surface. (This removes traces of reduced silver or osmium. Any dots or marks not removed by nitric acid are likely to be gold. They can be removed with *aqua regia*, which is a freshly made mixture of one part of nitric with three parts of hydrochloric acid.)
      Be careful. Don't splash strong acids around. Avoid inhaling the fumes. Pour the used acid into a large beaker of tap water. Neutralize the water before pouring it down the drain.
(5)   Rinse with *distilled* water, then in copious running tap water. (The first rinse must not contain any chloride or other ions that would precipitate insoluble silver salts from the residual acid.)
(6)   Quarter-fill the vessel with distilled water. Rinse it inside and out by shaking vigorously over a sink. Do this four times.
(7)   Dry the glassware by putting it upside-down on *clean* absorbent paper. This may be in an oven (about 50°C). For rapid drying, rinse with acetone (**Caution.** Highly flammable; miscible with water), which will evaporate more quickly. The glassware must be completely dry before being used for gold, osmium or silver solutions.

**18.1.2.
Handling slides,
sections and
solutions**

Solutions containing compounds of gold, silver or mercury should not come into contact with metal surfaces. Brief contact with stainless steel, however, seems to be harmless. Metal forceps should be briefly dipped in melted wax and allowed to cool, providing an unreactive surface. Racks or trays for holding slides should be made of glass. Free-floating sections are moved with a glass hook. A hook may be quickly made by heating the end of a Pasteur pipette until it bends and the tip seals. A more durable hook is fashioned in a flame from a piece of glass rod. Various shapes and sizes may be needed. Sections are more easily moved with a camel-hair brush, but this is likely to hold solutions, and all sorts of unknown chemical reactions may be taking place on and among the hairs.

Silver nitrate makes black stains (reduction to the metal) on skin and clothing. Be careful, especially with concentrated solutions. Osmium tetroxide also makes black stains, but most who use this compound are careful with it because of its well known hazards (Section 2.4.6). Detailed instructions for safely making an osmium tetroxide solution are given in Chapter 12 (Section 12.6.1).

Compounds of gold, silver and osmium are expensive. Old solutions should be kept for reclamation, not thrown away.

Silver nitrate. Collect old silver solutions in a bottle containing some hydrochloric acid, which precipitates silver chloride. When the bottle is nearly full, neutralize the acid with sodium hydroxide and add more than enough granulated or powdered zinc to react with more than the estimated amount of silver chloride. The zinc metal reduces the silver chloride to silver and is itself oxidized to soluble zinc ions. (1 g of zinc releases the silver originally present in 5.2 g of silver nitrate.) After a few days, decant and discard the supernatant. Add 5% sulphuric acid to dissolve excess zinc. (**Caution.** There is effervescence of hydrogen, though the volume will not be large. No naked flames!) When there is no further effervescence, wash the deposit by repeated shaking with tap water and decantation, until the supernatant is no longer acidic. The crude silver powder can now be collected and dried. Further refining is not possible in a histological laboratory.

Gold chloride. The chemistry of gold chloride is reviewed in Section 18.2. It is easy to reclaim and re-use small quantities (a few grams) of gold chloride in any laboratory. A solution is no longer suitable for use if its colour changes from pure golden yellow to yellow with a green, grey or purple cast. (A colourless solution contains almost no gold and should be discarded.) The gold is reduced to black flakes of metal by boiling with a little NaOH and formalin, washed with ammonia (to extract AgCl) and then with nitric acid (to oxidize organic matter and dissolve Ag). The cleaned gold is then dissolved in the smallest possible volume of *aqua regia*. The concentrated solution is diluted 10–15 times with water and shaken with two changes of an equal volume of diethyl ether. Chlorauric acid moves into the ether layer, which is recovered and allowed to evaporate (**Caution.** No flames or sparks nearby!). For a detailed description of this procedure, see Kiernan (1977).

Osmium tetroxide solutions eventually go black from reduction (by contaminants) to a colloidal form of the hydrated dioxide, $OsO_2.2H_2O$. Old solutions are collected into a bottle that contains some methanol or ethanol. This reduces the remaining OsO_4, thereby making the material safe and preventing evaporative losses. The recovery procedure, carried out in a fume cupboard, typically on about 500 ml of liquid, has 7 stages:

(1) Oxidation by potassium permanganate and H_2SO_4, to convert most of the osmium dioxide to the soluble tetroxide.
(2) Filtration to remove solid MnO_2
(3) Extraction of OsO_4 from the filtrate into carbon tetrachloride.
(4) Precipitation of osmium dioxide powder by adding methanol to the solution in CCl_4
(5) Recovery of the powder by filtration, and drying. The powder is stored in screw-capped vials until needed.
(6) Regeneration of osmium tetroxide by adding an aqueous hydrogen peroxide solution to a weighed amount of osmium dioxide.
(7) Addition of phosphate buffer, which catalyses the decomposition of excess hydrogen peroxide.

A 1% or 2% phosphate-buffered OsO_4 solution is obtained. For a more detailed description of this procedure, see Kiernan (1978). This method is more troublesome than the reclamation of silver or of gold chloride, and it also involves hazardous substances (quite large volumes of osmium tetroxide solution and and carbon tetrachloride), but the financial savings are considerable.

18.2. Gold methods

The techniques considered here have reduction of gold salts as the primary means of introducing contrast into a microscopical preparation. Gold is also used for changing the contrast of silver-stained material (toning; see Section 18.3.1.2), but then it is a secondary reagent.

Auric chloride, $AuCl_3$, which dissolves to form H^+ and $[AuCl_3OH]^-$, is not used in histology and neither is the sparingly soluble aurous chloride, AuCl. Histologists use 'gold chloride' in two forms: sodium tetrachloroaurate ($NaAuCl_4.2H_2O$), which is an orange–yellow solid, and chlorauric acid which is $HAuCl_4$ with 3 or 4 molecules of water of crystallization. Chlorauric acid may be yellow or brown; the colour does not affect the properties. Both dissolve readily in water to give solutions containing chloroaurate anions, $[AuCl_4]^-$

18.2.1.
Peripheral nerve endings (Ranvier's method)

In Ranvier's gold chloride procedure and its more recent modifications (see Cole, 1955; Boyd, 1962; Zacks, 1973), small fragments of fresh tissue are soaked in lemon juice (or in dilute citric or formic acid), followed by a chloroaurate solution and then either formic acid or exposure to bright light. Transparent membranous specimens are mounted whole. Opaque objects are teased to isolate regions of interest. In one variant the stained specimens are embedded in nitrocellulose and sectioned (Koch *et al.*, 1995), and Jacot *et al.* (1995) have described a technique for formaldehyde-fixed tissue.

Ranvier developed this method in 1880 to show epidermal innervation, but it has been used principally to show motor end-plates, muscle spindles and other sensory endings, including those in the cornea. Gold impregnation can reveal very thin axons, and was used in classical studies of axonal sprouting in partly denervated muscles (Hoffman, 1950). The amount of detail visible in the preparations is generally considered to be less, however, than can be seen with a successful silver method. The difference was illustrated by Olkowski and Manocha (1973) in the case of muscle spindles, for which silver methods were also favoured by Swash and Fox (1972).

In solution, citric and formic acids slowly reduce chloroaurate ions, and the colour of the colloidal product, determined by the sizes of the particles, varies with the concentration of the reducing agent (Frens, 1973). The end-product of the Ranvier method is gold formed by reduction of Au(III), presumably by reactive sites in the tissue as well as by the other reagents. It is not known why axons become more darkly coloured than most cells or collagenous fibres.

The following procedure is that of Cole (1943), with notes derived from a thorough study of the Ranvier method made by Boyd (1962), whose paper should be consulted for discussion of technical variations. This method works well with muscle, tendon and cornea. Fresh, unfixed fragments of tissue should be no more than 0.5–1 mm in the smallest dimension. Muscle or tendon has to be shredded (teased) on a glass slide, using glass or stainless steel needles. Further cutting should be avoided, and the pieces of tissue must not be held with forceps. Further teasing and flattening of the specimens is needed at the end of the procedure, before mounting.

Solutions required

A. 1% citric acid

Citric acid:	2 g
Water:	200 ml

Either the anhydrous acid or its monohydrate may be used. The solution can usually be kept for several weeks but must be replaced when it becomes cloudy or contains mould.

See *Note 1* below for alternatives.

B. 1% gold chloride

Chloroauric acid ($HAuCl_4.xH_2O$):	1.0 g
Water:	100 ml

This is stable for several years if it does not become contaminated. A brown bottle is customary, but protection from light is not necessary. Gold chloride solution that has been used for this staining method should not be returned to the stock bottle.

C. 20% formic acid

The exact concentration is not critical. A 1:4 dilution of ordinary concentrated (85–90%) formic acid is satisfactory. It can be kept indefinitely.

D. Glycerol–methanol

A mixture of equal volumes of glycerol and methanol, in which stained specimens are kept. It is stable indefinitely. 50 ml should last a long time. **Glycerol** alone is also needed.

Procedure

(1) Place small fragments of fresh tissue in a small dish of 1% citric acid for 10 min, with occasional agitation. They become transparent. Any object not transparent after 10 min is too big to be stained by this method.

(2) Place the specimens on filter paper and blot gently to remove excess citric acid, then transfer them to 1% gold chloride. The volume of gold chloride solution should be small: about the same as that of the specimens. Cover the container (or place it in a dimly lit place) and wait for 10–60 min. The time is not critical. The specimens should now be bright yellow. Read *Note 2* below before moving on to Step 3.

(3) Remove the specimens onto filter paper and blot to remove excess gold chloride, then transfer to 20% formic acid. Cover to exclude light. The staining develops slowly and may require from 6–48 h. Overnight is often satisfactory. See also *Note 3* below.

(4) Transfer the specimens to glycerol–methanol. They may be kept in this liquid for 6 months.

(5) Tease the stained preparation, using glass needles to flatten membranous structures and separate small bundles of fibres. Examine under a microscope. If the specimen is too thick, squeeze it in glycerol between two slides while examining with a microscope (×10 objective).

(6) Carefully transfer to a small drop of glycerol on a clean slide, apply a coverslip and seal the edges with nail varnish or a resinous mounting medium (see also *Note 4* below). Cleanly made thin preparations are stable for many years.

Result

All parts of the tissue acquire a purple color that varies in intensity. Cells can be recognized, and striations in muscle are clearly shown, as are epithelial cells and larger collagen fibres. Axons are dark red or blue-black.

Notes

(1) Cole (1943) called for 10% citric acid. This may have been an error, because Cole and Mielcarek (1962) prescribed 1% in an otherwise identical procedure. Lemon juice contains about 5% citric acid. Probably the concentration is unimportant. Lemon juice alone is traditional, but Boyd (1962) preferred a 3:1 mixture of filtered lemon juice and concentrated formic acid.

(2) No metal must come into contact with the tissue, the gold chloride solution or the formic acid, or the specimen will be ruined by little black granules of reduced gold. Use plastic forceps (gently) or hooks or needles made by drawing out glass rod in a flame.

(3) Instead of using formic acid, the reduction may be accomplished by putting the pieces in water in a shallow dish under a bright electric light such as an anglepoise or photoflood lamp. The temperature of the water should be kept at 35–40°C by varying the height of the bulb. Examine with a microscope after 30 min. Full development of the stain may require 60 min. The process can be watched under a microscope and arrested by moving the specimens into glycerol (Boyd, 1962).

(4) Glycerol is the customary mountant, and its low refractive index enhances the contrast in the preparation. To make a more stable preparation, place the specimen in sodium thiosulphate (5% aqueous $Na_2S_2O_3.5H_2O$) for 10 min (to remove any residual Au(III) by complexation), wash thoroughly in 3 changes of water, dehydrate, clear and mount in a resinous medium.

18.2.2.
Astrocytes (Cajal's gold-sublimate)

At the beginning of the 20th Century, Santiago Ramon y Cajal and his pupils (notably Pio Del Rio Hortega) developed metal staining methods that defined the different types of non-neuronal cells of the central nervous system. They showed that the neuroglial cells largely filled the spaces not occupied by neurons and their processes. Earlier staining methods using dyes had sugggested that the neuroglia was a connective tissue composed of cells and extracellular fibres. The traditional staining of neuroglial cells depends on impregnation with compounds of silver or gold. **Cajal's gold-sublimate method** for astrocytes, described below, is an example of one of these techniques. It is technically much simpler than the silver methods for glial cells (Penfield and Cone, 1950; Gray, 1954).

The name of the technique is derived from corrosive sublimate, an old synonym for mercuric chloride that is shortened to 'sublimate' in the traditional names of many histological fixatives and stains. Fibrous astrocytes, which occur near the ependyma and pia mater, in white matter, and at sites of injury and disease, are more strongly stained than protoplasmic (or velate) astrocytes, which occur in grey matter. Astrocyte cytoplasm contains intermediate filaments made of glial fibrillary acidic protein (GFAP). The deposition of gold in astrocyte cytoplasm has been verified by electron microscopy (Vaughn and Pease, 1967), which also reveals abundant intermediate filaments in fibrous astrocytes (see Peters *et al.*, 1991). Fibrous astrocytes contain more immunohistochemically demonstrable GFAP than protoplasmic astrocytes (see Jessen *et al.*, 1984). It seems likely that in the presence of $HgCl_2$ colloidal gold is deposited on or near GFAP filaments, but the chemical or physical rationale of this method is not understood. The method is not specific for astrocytes, but they stand out more prominently than other cells.

Fixation is an important factor for the success of this and other metal staining methods for neuroglia. The formal ammonium bromide mixture (FAB) described below is suitable for several such methods. Its properties are probably attributable to its acidity (pH 1.5), rather than to any property of NH_4Br (Lascano, 1946). The acidity is due to reaction of the ammonium ion with formaldehyde. Hexamethylene tetramine is formed and hydrogen ions are released, thus lowering the pH:

$$6HCHO + 4NH_4^+ \longrightarrow C_6H_{12}N_4 + 6H_2O + 4H^+$$

Formalin acidified with sulphuric acid can replace the traditional FAB mixture (Lascano, 1946), but it has been claimed (Polak, 1948) that this simpler formulation is inferior to FAB as a preparation for the silver carbonate methods, which are the traditional staining methods for oligodendrocytes and microglial cells (see Penfield and Cone, 1950).

Solutions required
A. FAB fixative (formal–ammonium bromide)

Formalin (37% HCHO):	15 ml
Ammonium bromide (NH_4Br):	2 g
Water:	to make 100 ml

Prepare before using.

B. Globus's solutions
(See *Note 1*, below. These may not be needed.) Prepare these solutions as required. Both are stable for several weeks in screw-capped bottles.

1. Ammonia–water:

Ammonium hydroxide (SG 0.8–0.9; 27% NH_3):	5.0 ml
Water:	45 ml

2. Globus's hydrobromic acid:

Concentrated hydrobromic acid (47% HBr):	5.0 ml
Water:	45 ml

C. Gold-sublimate mixture

A stock solution of gold chloride (1% aqueous chloroauric acid) is needed. (This should not be a solution that has been previously used for other purposes.)

Working solution

Mercuric chloride ($HgCl_2$):	0.5 g
Water:	45 ml

Dissolve the $HgCl_2$ (warm gently and stir with a glass rod). To this solution, add 10 ml of 1% gold chloride. The mixture should be made just before using. Do not let any metal object come into contact with this solution.

D. 5% sodium thiosulphate (5% w/v aqueous $Na_2S_2O_3.5H_2O$)

Procedure

(1) Fix pieces of tissue up to 5 mm thick in formal–ammonium bromide (Solution A) for 24–48 h. Cut frozen sections (about 20 μm) and collect into water containing a few drops of formalin.

(2) Place about 20 sections in the 10 ml of gold-sublimate mixture (Solution C) for 4–8 h in a Petri dish in the dark. The sections must not be creased or folded. They should be manipulated with a glass hook. The sections in the gold-sublimate solution become purple, and this colour deepens with time. At hourly intervals, starting when the purple coloration appears, remove one or two sections, take them through Steps 3, 4 and 5, and examine under a microscope.

(3) When staining of astrocytes is adequate, pass the remaining sections through two changes of water.

(4) Immerse in 5% sodium thiosulphate (Solution D) for 5 min.

(5) Wash in two changes of water, mount onto slides, dehydrate, clear, and cover, using a resinous mounting medium.

Result

Astrocytes dark red, dark purple, and black. The cytoplasmic processes and perivascular end-feet stain more intensely than the perinuclear parts of the cells. Other cells (notably neurons), blood vessels and connective tissue (meninges) are coloured in lighter shades of purple.

Notes

(1) For material fixed in formaldehyde (without NH_4Br), cut frozen sections and wash them in three changes of water. Place the sections in ammonia–water (Solution B1) overnight in a tightly closed container, then rinse them quickly in two changes of water and put them into Globus's hydrobromic acid (Solution B2) for 1 h at 37°C. Rinse quickly in two changes of water and place the sections in Solution C as Step 2 of the procedure given above.

(2) A modified technique for paraffin sections of formaldehyde-fixed tissue was described by Naoumenko and Feigin (1961).

(3) In diagnostic histopathology, astrocytes are stained by immunohistochemical methods for GFAP applied to routinely prepared paraffin sections of specimens fixed in neutral, buffered formaldehyde. Sections stained by the gold-sublimate technique have value for teaching, because they show, in the normal CNS, the attachments of astrocyte processes (end-feet) to meningeal (pia mater) and vascular elements. The mechanism of contraction of scar tissue in the brain was deduced from studies with Cajal's gold-sublimate method (Penfield, 1927).

**18.2.3.
Reticulin
(Lynch's
bromine–gold
method)**

Reticulin is a form of collagen that occurs in thin fibres and basement membranes (Chapter 8). The neutral carbohydrate molecules asssociated with the collagen protein can be stained with the periodic acid–Schiff method (Chapter 11), but metal reduction methods provide more specific and sensitive demonstration, especially of the thinnest fibres. In these methods, sections are treated with an oxidizing agent and then with a gold- or silver-containing solution. Silver methods are the ones most frequently used, and their mechanism of action has been investigated and is partly understood (Section 18.3.2). The gold reduction method (Lynch, 1965) has received less scrutiny (see *Note 1* below), but is quicker and easier to do than the silver techniques. The method is applied to paraffin sections of formaldehyde-fixed tissue.

Solutions required
A. Bromine solution

Water:	250 ml
Potassium bromide (KBr):	25 mg
Bromine (**Caution!**):	0.5 ml

Bromine is toxic and caustic and has harmful brown vapour. The solution keeps for a few weeks in a glass-stoppered bottle. Keep it in a fume cupboard, and discard it when the colour becomes noticeably paler. Before discarding this solution, add enough 5% aqueous sodium thiosulphate to discharge the colour.

B. Gram's iodine

Potassium iodide (KI):	5 g
Water:	250 ml
Iodine:	2.5 g

In a glass-stoppered bottle, this solution can be kept for many years without deterioration.

C. 1% gold chloride
A 1% stock solution of chloroauric acid (Section 18.2.1).

D. Reducer
This is an aqueous solution: *either* 3% hydrogen peroxide (freshly diluted from 30% H_2O_2) *or* 2% oxalic acid (a stable stock solution). The reducer must be warmed to 37°C in an oven or water bath before it is used.

Procedure
(1) De-wax and hydrate the sections.
(2) Immerse in the bromine solution (A) for 1 h.
(3) Rinse in 3 changes of water, each 3–5 s.
(4) Immerse in Gram's iodine (Solution B) for 5 min.
(5) Rinse in 3 changes of water, each 3–5 s.
(6) Immerse in 1% gold chloride (Solution C) for 5 min.
(7) Rinse in 3 changes of water, each 3–5 s.
(8) Immerse in the reducer (Solution D) at 37°C for 2–4 h.
(9) Wash in running tap water for 1 min, dehydrate, clear and apply coverslips, using a resinous mounting medium.

Result
Reticulin is dark brown to black if the reducer is hydrogen peroxide, or blue if the reducer is oxalic acid. Collagen fibres and cells are light gold–brown or grey.

Notes
(1) In developing this method, Lynch (1965) found that periodic acid, chromic acid and other oxidizing agents used in silver methods for reticulin could not

be substituted for aqueous bromine. These observations seemed to exclude aldehydes as reducing groups generated in the tissue. Oxidation by a permanganate–sulphuric acid mixture allowed specific staining of reticulin with gold, but the intensity was less than after bromine. The iodine treatment before immersion in gold chloride was necessary for reticulin staining.

(2) If this method is applied to the central nervous system, there is staining of fibrous astrocytes in addition to the expected staining of the basement membranes of blood vessels.

18.3. Silver methods

The largest numbers of silver reduction methods are those for nervous tissue. In research laboratories these techniques have been largely replaced by immunohistochemistry. For example there are commercially available antibodies that recognize characteristic proteins of neurons and the different types of neuroglial cell. The great advantage of immunohistochemistry is that of knowing exactly why the staining method works. The disadvantages are that antibodies and other immunological reagents are expensive and they deteriorate with storage. The only neurohistological silver methods discussed in this chapter are the ones for axons, because their mechanisms of action are partly understood and they are still extensively used in histopathology, especially for showing changes in the brain due to Alzheimer's disease and other types of dementia. (Silver nitrate is used in the Golgi method but this is a precipitation, not a reduction technique. See Section 18.5.)

18.3.1
Silver methods for normal axons

The multitude of methods in this category is testimony to the fact that there is no entirely satisfactory way to stain every kind of axon. Even with immunohistochemistry it is not possible to show the terminal parts of all types of axon with a single technique (Karaosmanoglu *et al.*, 1996; Botchkarev *et al.*, 1997). The argyrophilia of normal axons is associated with the neurofilaments. Chemical studies (Gambetti *et al.*, 1981; Phillips *et al.*, 1983) have revealed that the neurofilament proteins are responsible for stainability by at least one of the silver techniques, that of Bodian (1936). Although this technique has sometimes been regarded as histochemically specific for neurofilamentous material (e.g. Duyckaerts *et al.*, 1987), numerous other objects are stained, notably the nuclei of all cells and the cytoplasm of many endocrine cells (Scopsi and Larsson, 1986). Although much is known of the chemical reactions that occur during silver staining, the reason for the specificity of the methods remains obscure. The subject has been reviewed by Kiernan and Berry (1975), Koski and Reyes (1986) and Kiernan (1996a). Even in semi-thin sections of resin-embedded peripheral nerves silver staining cannot reliably reveal unmyelinated axons less than 0.5 μm in diameter (Deprez *et al.*, 1999); electron microscopy is necessary for resolution of the thinnest fibres.

18.3.1.1. Methodology and chemistry

The silver methods for axons all have three features in common. These are:

(1) Treatment of the tissue (blocks or frozen, paraffin or celloidin sections; nearly always after an aldehyde containing fixative) with a solution containing silver ions, whose concentration may vary from about 10^{-5} M to more than 1.5 M.

(2) Subsequent treatment of the specimen with a reducing agent capable of effecting the reaction:

$$Ag^+ + \varepsilon^- \longrightarrow Ag^0(s)$$

(3)   The deposition of a darkly coloured material (consisting mainly or entirely of metallic silver) in the axons, which are said to be argyrophilic.

The chemical reactions involved in selective axonal staining with silver are fairly well understood as the result of the investigations of Holmes (1943), Samuel (1953a), and Peters (1955a,b). These studies were principally concerned with some of the technically simpler procedures applied to paraffin sections. In the first step of such methods, sections are exposed for several hours to a mildly alkaline solution in which the concentration of free silver ions is low (10^{-5} to 10^{-3} M) but in which there is an adequate excess of the silver. The latter condition is attained either by having a large volume of dilute aqueous $AgNO_3$ or by arranging for most of the metal to be present as a complex such as $[Ag(NH_3)_2]^+$ or a silver-protein compound, or by using a saturated solution of a sparingly soluble salt such as Ag_2O, Ag_2CO_3, $AgCl$ or $AgOCN$ in equilibrium with the undissolved solid. Methods in which concentrated silver nitrate solutions are used have not been studied, but it is probable that the same chemical reactions occur. Silver is taken up by the section in two ways. The larger quantity is bound chemically by protein throughout the tissue. This chemically bound silver is not specifically related to axons and can easily be removed by treating the tissue with complexing agents such as ammonium hydroxide, citric acid, or sodium sulphite. A much smaller amount of silver is reduced at sites in the axons and precipitated as tiny 'nuclei' of the metal. These nuclei are too small to be resolved with the electron microscope (Peters, 1955c). Similar nuclei, formed by the action of light upon crystals of silver halides, form the latent image in an exposed but undeveloped photographic emulsion. A latent image nucleus consists of 2–6 atoms of silver (see James, 1977). The nuclei formed in axons may be similar in size. The reduced silver cannot be extracted by NH_4OH or Na_2SO_3.

In the second stage of the method, the sections are transferred to a solution similar to a photographic developer. A commonly used one (Bodian, 1936) contains sodium sulphite and hydroquinone. This mixture is alkaline. The sulphite removes the chemically bound silver, introducing $[Ag(SO_3)_2]^{3-}$ ions into the solution. Hydroquinone reduces this complex ion to silver (metal) on the surfaces of the previously formed nuclei of metallic silver present in the axons. The nuclei are thereby enlarged until they are (in light microscopy) coalescent, and the axons appear as black or brown linear structures. In some techniques the chemically bound silver is removed by treatment with Na_2SO_3 alone and a developer containing a known concentration of silver is used. Such a mixture (known as a **physical developer**) must also contain stabilizing agents to delay the spontaneous reduction of Ag^+ in the solution. Stability is obtained by including in the physical developer a substance that forms a soluble complex with silver, such as citric acid or sodium sulphite, so that the concentration of free silver ions is low. Addition of a macromolecular solute, commonly gelatin, gum acacia or tungstosilicic acid ($H_4[W_{12}SiO_{40}]$, MW 2878), provides additional stabilization.

If the processes of development in histological staining with silver are closely similar to the ones used in photography, it is likely that the silver precipitated as submicroscopic nuclei during the first stage of the procedure serves as a catalyst for reactions of the type:

$$2Ag^+ + \text{hydroquinone} + 2OH^- \longrightarrow 2Ag(s) + \text{p-benzoquinone} + 2H_2O$$

hydroquinone   *p*-benzoquinone

Metallic silver is insoluble, so it accumulates around the particles of the catalyst. Many substances other than silver can catalyse the above reaction, and physical developers have been used to produce visible end-products in a wide variety of histological and histochemical techniques (see Gallyas, 1971b, 1979). The developing agent used in silver-staining methods should be one that is 'weak' or 'slow' by photographic standards. Hydroquinone, pyrogallol and p-hydroxyphenylglycine are suitable, but the more powerful developers such as N-methyl-p-aminophenol (metol, elon) cause excessive deposition of silver, which obscures the histological detail.

18.3.1.2. Gold toning
The coloration of axons impregnated with silver as described above does not always provide adequate contrast under the microscope. This is so also in the case of some other silver methods. Contrast can be improved by adding a third Step of gold toning. The silver-stained sections are immersed in a solution of gold chloride. Sometimes this manoeuvre produces an adequate increase in contrast, but frequently it is necessary to add a further stage of reduction in oxalic acid. Finally, the sections are immersed in aqueous sodium thiosulphate to remove residual silver chloride or protein-bound silver. This last process is analogous to the 'fixing' of a developed photograph. The chemistry of gold toning was rather simply explained by Samuel (1953b) on the basis of the reaction:

$$3Ag \; + \; AuCl_3 \; \longrightarrow \; Au \; + \; 3AgCl$$

This explanation is unsatisfactory because it does not conform with the known chemistry of gold compounds and it assumes that one atom of gold would be optically more conspicuous than three of silver. As explained in Section 18.2, the gold in the 'gold chloride' of histologists is not the cation in $AuCl_3$ but the chloroaurate anion, $[AuCl_4]^-$. This is reduced by silver, with the formation of gold and silver chloride:

$$3Ag \; + \; [AuCl_4]^- \; \longrightarrow \; Au \; + \; 3AgCl \; + \; Cl^-$$

(solid)   (dissolved)   (solid) (solid) (in solution)

The reaction is essentially similar to the one proposed by Samuel (1953b). Silver chloride can be removed by treatment with sodium thiosulphate:

$$AgCl \; + \; 2S_2O_3^{2-} \; \longrightarrow \; [Ag(S_2O_3)_2]^{3-} \; + \; Cl^-$$

(solid)   ($Na_2S_2O_3$ (soluble)   (in solution)
        in solution)

In those techniques in which the toning procedure consists only of treatment with 'gold chloride' followed by sodium thiosulphate, the increased contrast must be due to a reduction in the unwanted argyrophilia of the background rather than to an intensification of the metallic deposits in the axons.

The intensification of gold toning by treatment with oxalic acid is not so easily explained. Oxalic acid is not a photographic developer and it does not reduce AgCl to Ag (which might have accounted for increased metallic deposition), but it does reduce chloroaurate anions to metallic gold. Now the particles of silver in stained axons are very small (Peters, 1955c; Sechrist, 1969), and they may well form, collectively, a colloidal suspension of the metal. After treatment with $HAuCl_4$, the silver is replaced by a mixture of Au and AgCl, presumably also in particles with colloidal dimensions. Many colloids are able to adsorb ions and other molecules, so it is not unreasonable to suppose that $[AuCl_4]^-$ ions are bound by physical forces at the sites of axonal staining. The bound chloroaurate ions would then be reduced on treatment with oxalic acid, in a reaction such as:

$$2[AuCl_4]^- + 3H_2C_2O_4 \longrightarrow 2Au(s) + 6CO_2 + 6H^+ + 8Cl^-$$

Hence, substantial deposits of gold would be precipitated around each original particle of silver. The above speculations are supported by the observations of Zagon *et al.* (1970), who found by electron probe microanalysis that the metallic particles in silver stained and gold-toned protozoa contained considerably more gold than silver.

18.3.1.3. Choice of silver methods

Axons in most parts of the CNS are most easily demonstrated in paraffin sections by methods in which the primary impregnation is with a solution containing a very low concentration of free silver ions, applied for 24–48 h at 37°C. A simple technique is that of Holmes (1943). Another widely used technique is Bodian's (1936) protargol method. Protargol is a silver-protein complex, manufactured for use as an antiseptic, which slowly releases Ag^+ ions. Two types of silver proteinate, designated 'strong' and 'weak', have been used as antiseptics. Only the 'strong' type, which is obsolete as a pharmaceutical product, is suitable for Bodian's technique. The name 'protargol-S' has been adopted by the Biological Stain Commission for silver proteinates tested and certified as satisfactory for the histological demonstration of axons. These procedures are also suitable for paraffin sections of peripheral nerves, but they often fail to demonstrate the innervation of tissues such as skin and viscera.

To stain peripheral nerve endings with silver, thick frozen sections of material thoroughly fixed in formaldehyde should be used. Primary impregnation is accomplished with a concentrated (10–20%) solution of silver nitrate. A simple and versatile technique is Mitchell's modification of the Hirano–Zimmermann procedure. This method can be applied to frozen, paraffin, and celloidin sections, and although it is rather capricious it is usually possible to obtain satisfactory results by varying the times of exposure of sections to the reagents. Cutaneous innervation is notoriously difficult to demonstrate by silver methods, but a simple technique devised by Winkelmann and Schmit (1957) is often satisfactory for this purpose. If it fails, the more troublesome Gros–Schultze method can be tried. The latter procedure is derived from earlier ones introduced by Bielschowsky, and makes use of an ammoniacal silver nitrate solution containing the silver diammine cation, $[Ag(NH_3)_2]^+$. (The chemistry of silver diammine is explained in connection with reticulin staining in Section 18.3.2.1.) The reduction of the $[Ag(NH_3)_2]^+$ complex ion by formaldehyde is probably catalysed by silver nuclei produced in axons during the primary impregnation. Thus, the ammoniacal solution serves the same purpose as a physical developer (Horobin, 1988). Indeed, much of the untrustworthiness of Bielschowsky-type methods disappears when a controlled physical development replaces the alternation of treatments with formalin and silver diammine solutions, as in the physical developer method in Section 18.3.1.8.

For demonstrating lesions in the brain associated with dementia the pathologist needs methods that are reliable and rapid. The technique in Section 8.3.1.9 is widely used. Another simple method (Reusche, 1991) is derived from silver methods for nucleolar organizer regions (Section 9.8).

There are many methods for staining with silver in the block before embedding and sectioning (see Jones, 1950). Excellent results can sometimes be obtained with these methods in both CNS and PNS, but the effects of uneven penetration of the reagents are usually apparent in the sectioned material.

18.3.1.4. Holmes's silver method for axons

Before carrying out this method for the first time, read the general instructions for metal staining (Section 18.1).

The best results are obtained with paraffin sections of tissue from the CNS that has been fixed for 24 h in neutral, buffered formaldehyde. The technique described below differs from the original (Holmes, 1943) only in the addition of a little pyridine to the silver solution, following Holmes (1947). The function of the pyridine is unknown, but if it is omitted there is a reduction in the contrast between the stained axons and their background. Addition of pyridine does not change the pH of the staining solution but it may reduce the concentration of free silver ions by forming complexes such as $[Ag(C_5H_5N)_2]^+$. A preliminary treatment with 20% $AgNO_3$ is often recommended (Holmes, 1947; Luna, 1968). In my experience this is unnecessary.

Solutions required

A. 1% silver nitrate
Keep the stock solution ($AgNO_3$, 1% w/v in water) in a brown glass bottle in subdued light. Replace if it becomes discoloured or contains a precipitate.

B. 1% pyridine
This solution (1% v/v pyridine in water) keeps for several months. (Many people find the odour of pyridine objectionable.)

C. Staining solution
See Chapter 20 for borate buffer. See *Note 2* below for variations in this mixture.

Borate buffer, pH8.4:	100 ml
1% silver nitrate (solution A):	1.0 ml
1% pyridine (solution B):	5.0 ml
Water:	to 500 ml

Mix just before using. For each slide there should be at least 50 ml of this solution.

D. Developer

Hydroquinone (quinol):	2.0 g
Sodium sulphite (Na_2SO_3):	10 g
(or 20 g of $Na_2SO_3.7H_2O$)	
Water:	dissolve and make up to 200 ml

Mix on the day it is to be used. There should be 10 ml or more for each slide, appropriately for the size of the staining vessel.

E. 0.2% gold chloride
May be $NaAuCl_4.2H_2O$ (sodium tetrachloroaurate; yellow) or $HAuCl_4$ (chloroauric acid, with variable water of crystallization; yellow or brown). Dissolve 1 g in 500 ml of water. Keep it in a glass-stoppered bottle. It does not need to be protected from light. This solution can be used repeatedly but should be discarded (and recycled; see Section 18.1.2) when it has a greyish tinge or when there is an appreciable quantity of precipitated material in the bottle.

F. 1% oxalic acid

Oxalic acid ($H_2C_2O_4.2H_2O$):	5 g
Water:	500 ml

This stock solution keeps indefinitely, but should be used only once.

G. 5% sodium thiosulphate

Sodium thiosulphate ($Na_2S_2O_3.5H_2O$):	25 g
Water:	500 ml

The remarks for solution F also apply here.

Procedure

(1) De-wax and hydrate paraffin sections. Wash the sections in three changes of water (which **must** be distilled or de-ionized) for a total of 10 min.

(2) Place the slides, in a glass rack, in the staining solution (C) for 24 h at 37°C. The staining tank must be covered to reduce evaporation and there must be at least 50 ml of the solution for each slide. (A smaller container may be used for the later stages of the method.)

(3) Remove the rack of slides from Solution C and shake off excess liquid, but do not rinse in water. Transfer directly to the developer (Solution D) for 3 min. (See *Note 3* below.)

(4) Rinse in distilled or de-ionized water, then wash for 3 min in running tap water. Rinse again in distilled or de-ionized water.

(5) Immerse in 0.2% gold chloride (Solution E) for 3 min.

(6) Wash in two changes of water.

(7) Immerse in 1% oxalic acid (Solution F) for 3–10 min, until the sections are deep grey. Longer treatment produces a reddish colour and this is best avoided. (See also *Note 3* below.)

(8) Wash in two changes (each 1 min) of tap water.

(9) Immerse in 5% sodium thiosulphate (Solution G) for 5 min.

(10) Wash in three changes of tap water, dehydrate, clear, and mount in a resinous medium.

Result

Axons black. Cell-bodies and nuclei are generally unstained and connective tissue fibres should be no darker than light grey. With over-treatment at Step 7, the grey and black tones are changed to pink and dark red.

Notes

(1) The method as described is nearly always successful with formaldehyde-fixed CNS or peripheral nerve trunks. Peripheral nerve endings, however, are rarely demonstrable by this technique.

(2) If poor results are obtained, variations in the composition of staining Solution C should be tried. The volume of 1% silver nitrate may be halved or doubled. The pH may be varied between 7.0 and 9.0. All other aspects of the technique should be kept constant. The composition of Solution C will usually need to be changed when fixatives other than neutral, buffered formaldehyde are used. Satisfactory results can be obtained with tissue fixed in most of the commonly used mixtures other than those containing potassium dichromate or osmium tetroxide.

(3) The slides **must not be washed in water after Step 2**. It is necessary to carry some silver ions into the developer. The axonal staining is invisible, or at best very faint, after the development at Step 3. The first part of the toning procedure (Step 5) causes the axons to disappear almost completely, but they reappear and become intensely coloured during Step 7 of the method.

18.3.1.5. Mitchell's rapid silver method

This technique (R. Mitchell, personal communication) is described because it is rapid. When it fails, minor variations can be introduced for subsequent sections without wasting too much time. The method is similar to one for celloidin sections described by Hirano and Zimmermann (1962), which can also be used on paraffin sections. Silver nuclei in axons are probably deposited during the impregnation with 20% $AgNO_3$. In the later stages of the method it is likely that a silver diammine complex is transiently formed and then immediately reduced to the metal by formaldehyde at the sites of the silver nuclei.

Material should be fixed in formaldehyde for at least 12 h (a week is recommended) and frozen sections cut (usually 15–25 μm thick) and collected into water. The technique is applicable to any tissue containing nerve fibres.

Solutions required

A. 20% aqueous silver nitrate

Dissolve 20 g of $AgNO_3$ in 100 ml of water in a brown glass-stoppered bottle. See Section 18.2.1 for notes on handling silver nitrate solutions. Filter after use to remove particles derived from sections. The solution may be re-used, and it keeps for several years if it is not contaminated with other substances.

B. Dilute ammonia

Ammonium hydroxide (ammonia solution; SG 0.9, 28% NH_3):	20 drops
Tap water:	50 ml

Make a fresh dilution for each batch of sections.

C. Formalin solution

Formalin (37–40% HCHO):	10 ml
Tap water:	40 ml

Make a fresh dilution for each batch of sections.

Procedure

(1) Rinse the frozen sections in three changes of water (which **must** be distilled or de-ionized). They can be left overnight in water if necessary. The sections must be handled with glass hooks. They are taken individually through the following steps of the method.
(2) Place section in 20% $AgNO_3$ (Solution A) for 10 s.
(3) Transfer (without washing) to the dilute ammonia (Solution B) for 10 s.
(4) Transfer (without washing) to the formalin solution (C) for about 30 s.
(5) Wash section in water (distilled or tap) and either mount in glycerol or dehydrate, clear, and mount in a resinous medium.
(6) Examine the stained section. If it is unsatisfactory, proceed as directed in the *Notes* below.
(7) Once the correct technique has been determined for a particular specimen, sections can be stained (in less than a minute for each) and collected into distilled water for later mounting.

Result

Axons, including fine terminal branches, black. Background (cells, collagen, blood vessels etc.) in shades of yellow, gold, and brown.

Notes

(1) If staining is too light, *either* rinse the section in 3 changes of distilled or deionized water and repeat Steps 2–5, *or* leave a subsequent section longer (up to 30 min) in the 20% $AgNO_3$ at Step 2 and proceed as before.
(2) If staining (especially the background) is too dark, try one of the following modifications on subsequent sections:
    (a) Use a stronger solution of ammonia at Step 3. This variation is more easily controlled than (b) or (c).
    (b) Leave for longer in the dilute ammonia at Step 3.
    (c) Rinse the section in water between Steps 2 and 3.

18.3.1.6. Winkelmann and Schmit method for peripheral nerve endings

Material should be fixed in 4% formaldehyde for several days. Small pieces of tissue are then dehydrated in three changes of ethanol (each 1 h), cleared in xylene (for 1 h), rehydrated, and finally returned to the fixative until they are sectioned (Winkelmann and Schmit, 1957; see also *Note 1* below.)

This method was devised for skin, but axons in other tissues, such as muscle, are also stained by it. Sections can be thicker than for the preceding method. Central nervous tissue gives poor results, and the method does not work with paraffin sections. It is easy to process a batch of 10–12 free-floating frozen sections at the same time.

Solutions required

A. Silver solution

20% aqueous silver nitrate. Keeps indefinitely; may be used repeatedly. See preceding method (Section 18.3.1.5) for advice about using 20% $AgNO_3$.

B. Developer

Hydroquinone:	0.2 g
Sodium sulphite (Na_2SO_3):	1.0 g
Water:	100 ml

Make up before using, and use only once. It can be kept for one or two days in a corked flask, if necessary. Do not use if it goes yellow or brown.

C. 0.2% gold chloride

See *Solution E* of Holmes's method, Section 18.3.1.4.

D. 5% sodium thiosulphate

This is a 5% solution of ($Na_2S_2O_3.5H_2O$) in water. It keeps indefinitely, but is not re-used.

Procedure

(1) Cut frozen sections 50–80 µm thick and collect them into 4% aqueous formaldehyde, in which they may remain for a few days if delay is unavoidable. Take the free-floating sections through Steps 2–10 of the method.
(2) Rinse the sections in three changes of water (**must** be distilled or de-ionized) and leave for 30 min in the last change.
(3) Place sections in 20% silver nitrate (Solution A) for 20 min. The sections should not be creased or folded.
(4) Rinse sections in three changes of water, 3 s in each.
(5) Place sections (avoiding folds and creases) in the developer (Solution B) for 10 min.
(6) Rinse in two changes of water.
(7) Transfer sections to the 0.2% gold chloride solution (C) for 2 min.
(8) Wash in two changes of water.
(9) Immerse sections in 5% sodium thiosulphate (Solution D) for 5 min.
(10) Wash in two changes of water, mount onto slides, dehydrate, clear, and cover, using a resinous medium.

Result

Axons black. Other structures (cells, connective tissue, etc.) in shades of grey.

Notes

(1) The preliminary treatment of the fixed blocks with alcohol and xylene is to remove soluble lipids, especially fat, which can interfere with the penetration of the sections by the reagents. Other solvents (methanol, acetone, etc.) may be substituted. The solvent-extraction of the blocks may be omitted for tis-

sues that contain little or no fat (such as mammalian muscle). Extraction must be omitted if the sections are to be incubated for an enzyme histochemical method before the silver staining.

(2) Many beautiful photomicrographs of the results obtained with this method can be found in Winkelmann (1960). It is important that the sections be adequately thick, so that enough chemically bound silver will be carried through into Step 5 to allow Solution B to function as a physical developer. Thick sections are also needed in order to reveal the full extent of axonal end-formations in skin and other organs.

(3) For staining skeletal muscle, the Winkelmann and Schmit method is carried out after an indigogenic method for esterases (Section 15.2.3) For a detailed description of the dual procedure, see Kiernan (1996a).

18.3.1.7. Gros–Schultze method for axons

This fairly reliable Bielschowsky-type method can be used with frozen or paraffin sections of formaldehyde-fixed material. The procedure described below (based on technical details given by Culling, 1974) is also known as the 'Gros–Bielschowsky' method. The tap water in the formaldehyde reducing solution probably serves to precipitate some silver chloride in and on the sections, increasing the local total silver concentration at the stage of development in the silver diammine solution.

Solutions required

A. 20% aqueous silver nitrate

20% aqueous silver nitrate. Keeps indefinitely; may be used repeatedly. See Mitchell's rapid method (Section 18.3.1.5) for advice about using 20% $AgNO_3$.

B. Formalin solution

Prepare four dishes or staining tanks, each containing a freshly prepared mixture of 20 volumes of formalin (37–40% HCHO) and 80 volumes of tap water.

C. Ammoniacal silver solution

(**Caution.** See *Note 1* below.) To 30 ml of 20% aqueous silver nitrate in a 100 ml conical flask add ammonium hydroxide (strong ammonia solution; SG 0.88–0.91) until the precipitate of brown silver oxide just redissolves. The ammonia should be added drop by drop, with swirling for a few seconds between each addition. About 2.5 ml of strong ammonia solution are needed. When the precipitate has dissolved, add a further 18 drops of the ammonium hydroxide. (A drop is about 0.05 ml.)

D. Dilute ammonia solution

Strong ammonium hydroxide (as above):	5 ml
Water:	95 ml

Make the dilution as needed.

E. Dilute acetic acid

Glacial acetic acid:	1.0 ml
Water:	99 ml

Can be stored indefinitely, but usually diluted as needed.

F. Toning solution

This is 0.02% gold chloride, conveniently made by 10-fold dilution of 0.2% gold chloride (see under Holmes's method, Section 18.3.1.4). This dilute gold chloride should be used for only one or two batches of sections.

G. 5% sodium thiosulphate

5% w/v ($Na_2S_2O_3.5H_2O$) in water. The solution keeps indefinitely, but is used only once.

Procedure

(1) De-wax and hydrate paraffin sections. Collect frozen sections into water. Wash the sections (frozen or paraffin) in three changes of water (**must** be distilled or deionized), for total time of 10 min.

(2) Immerse in 20% silver nitrate (solution A) for 5 min (frozen sections) or 30 min (paraffin sections). (See also *Note 2* below.)

(3) Without washing, transfer the sections directly to the first bath of formalin solution (B). Agitate and transfer the sections or slides successively through the other three formalin baths, allowing about 2 min in each. The last change of formalin solution must be free of turbidity. If it is not, move the sections into one or two more baths of fresh Solution B.

(4) Without washing, transfer sections (or slides) directly into the ammoniacal silver solution (C) for about 20 s. (Slides bearing paraffin sections can be placed in a clean coplin jar and Solution C poured in. Allow about 10 ml for each slide.) The solution becomes grey and turbid and silver mirrors may form on slides and on the inside of the staining vessel. The sections go dark brown. (See also *Notes 2* and *3* below.)

(5) Transfer sections to dilute ammonia (Solution D) for 1 min.

(6) Transfer to dilute acetic acid (Solution E) for 1 or 2 min.

(7) Wash in water for about 30 s.

(8) Immerse in the gold toning solution (F) for 10 min.

(9) Wash in water for about 30 s.

(10) Immerse in 5% sodium thiosulphate (Solution G) for 3–5 min.

(11) Wash in two changes of water, dehydrate, clear, and mount in a resinous medium.

Results

Axons black. In the CNS, fibrillary structures (neurofibrils) in the perikarya and dendrites of some large neurons are also coloured black. Other tissue components are grey or colourless.

Notes

(1) The ammoniacal silver solution should be mixed just before using. The ammonium hydroxide should come from a recently opened stock bottle, because it loses NH_3 on standing. Handle strong ammonia carefully in a fume hood. To dispose of surplus and used solution, acidify with hydrochloric acid until all the silver is precipitated as white AgCl. The precipitate can be collected for reclamation (Section 18.1.2). *All ammoniacal silver solutions are potentially dangerous* because if they evaporate to dryness the deposit may contain fulminating silver, which is probably a mixture of silver amide ($AgNH_2$) and nitride (Ag_3N). Fulminating silver explodes violently when touched. If an ammoniacal solution is to be kept (up to a few days) it should be in a closed flask (a parafilm seal over the top) in a dark place.

(2) The length of time in 20% $AgNO_3$ can be varied if unsatisfactory results are obtained with the times suggested. If no staining at all is obtained, it is likely that Solution C contained too large an excess of ammonia.

(3) Dirty precipitates on the sections can be due to too long a time in the ammoniacal silver solution. They are presumably due to the reaction:

$$2[Ag(NH_3)_2]^{2+} + 2OH^- + HCHO \longrightarrow 2Ag(s) + 4NH_3 + H_2O + HCOOH$$

which should occur only in association with axons and neurofibrils.

18.3.1.8. A physical developer method for axons

This method, which was introduced in the first edition of this book, may be applied to frozen or paraffin sections of any formaldehyde-fixed tissue. Bouin's fluid is also a suitable fixative. This method differs from earlier techniques with physical developers in that (a) the initial impregnation is with a concentrated silver nitrate solution, so only a short time is needed for formation of nuclei within axons; (b) the action of the developer, which is modified from one used in photographic research (Berg and Ford, 1949), is more easily controlled than that of physical developers previously used for histological purposes. Some of the stable physical developers described by Gallyas (1979) can be substituted for the one prescribed below, but with no apparent advantage.

Solutions required

A. 20% aqueous silver nitrate
Keeps for several months and may be used repeatedly. See general notes about silver nitrate solutions (Section 18.1.2).

B. Sodium sulphite solution

Sodium sulphite (Na_2SO_3):	15.0 g
Water:	to 500 ml

Keeps indefinitely, but may be used only once.

C. Stock solution for physical developer

Hydroquinone (quinol):	4.0 g
Citric acid ($C_6H_8O_7.H_2O$):	4.0 g
Gelatin (use a high quality bacteriological grade):	4.0 g
Water:	400 ml
Glacial acetic acid:	20 ml

Dissolve all the above ingredients (30 min with occasional shaking).

Add water:	to make 500 ml

Stable for 4–6 weeks at room temperature. Replace when it goes brown.

D. Physical developer (working solution)

Solution C:	100 ml
Solution A:	8–10 ml

This must be mixed immediately before use (see Step 6 of the procedure). The volume of Solution A in the working solution is not critical, and may be as high as 20 ml (though this wastes an expensive compound).

E. Gold chloride solution
This is a 0.2% aqueous solution of *either* sodium chloroaurate ($NaAuCl_4.2H_2O$) *or* chloroauric acid ($HAuCl_4$ with variable water of crystallization). It may be re-used many times. See Section 18.3.1.4.

F. 1% aqueous oxalic acid
This is 1% w/v ($H_2C_2O_4.2H_2O$) in water. The solution can be kept for many years, but should be used only once. See also Sections 18.1.2 and 18.3.1.4.

G. 5% Sodium thiosulphate
This is 5% w/v $Na_2S_2O_3.5H_2O$ in water. The unused solution can be kept for years. Used solution is discarded.

Procedure
(1) De-wax and hydrate paraffin sections. Attach frozen sections to slides. *Either* Mayer's albumen *or* chrome–gelatin may be used as adhesive. Wash in three changes of water.
(2) Immerse slides in 20% $AgNO_3$ (Solution A) for 15 min (time is not critical and may range from 10 min to 2 h).

(3) Wash in three changes of water.

(4) Immerse in 3% Na_2SO_3 (Solution B) for 5 min. (The slides may remain in this solution for 1 h without ill effect.)

(5) Rinse in three changes of water. Drain.

(6) Mix the working solution of the physical developer (D) and pour it into the vessel containing the slides. The time for development depends on the ambient temperature: usually 4 min at 25°C or 6 min at 20°C. If the developer becomes grey and cloudy, proceed immediately to Step 7, whatever time has elapsed.

(7) Pour off the developer and rinse slides with three changes of water. Examine under a microscope. If axonal staining is adequate, counterstain, dehydrate, clear, and mount. If more intense staining is required, proceed with the remaining stages of the method.

(8) Tone in 0.2% gold chloride (Solution E) for 5 min. Rinse in three changes of water. If staining is now satisfactory, proceed to Step 11. If not, proceed to Step 9.

(9) Immerse in 1% oxalic acid (Solution F) for 5–10 min. The time is not critical.

(10) Rinse in three changes of water.

(11) Immerse in sodium thiosulphate solution (G) for 5 min.

(12) Wash in running tap water for about 2 min.

(13) Apply a counterstain if desired. Neutral red (Chapter 6) is suitable for the CNS; the van Gieson method (Chapter 8) for peripheral tissues.

(14) Wash, dehydrate, clear, and mount in a resinous medium.

Result

Axons black. Other structures are usually completely colourless if the procedure is stopped at Step 7 or Step 8. Treatment with oxalic acid (Step 9) produces a grey background and sometimes causes blackening of connective tissue fibres. If neutral red is used as a counterstain, nuclei, Nissl substance (RNA), proteoglycans and some types of mucus are red. The van Gieson counterstain gives yellow cytoplasm and red collagen.

For some parts of the CNS, including the cerebral and cerebellar cortex, Holmes's method is superior. This method is superior to Holmes's technique for peripheral innervation and for the retina and optic nerve.

18.3.1.9. Gallyas–Braak method for lesions in dementia

In Alzheimer's disease neurofibrillary tangles occur in the cell bodies of neurons of the temporal, parietal and frontal lobes Spherical neuritic plaques are present in the neuropil of the same regions. The plaques are composed of a type of amyloid in which are embedded fragments of neurites (axons and dendrites). The tangles and the neuritic components of the plaques contain an abnormal microtubule-associated protein called p-*tau* and are stainable by a variety of silver methods, including those used for showing normal axons and some that selectively stain the lesions (Gallyas, 1971a; Braak and Braak, 1991; Reusche, 1991; Abe et al., 1994; Garvey et al., 1994; Haga et al., 1994). The lesions are also demonstrable by immunohistochemistry for p-*tau*, and the plaques are stainable by methods for amyloid (Chapter 11). Comparisons of different techniques (Duyckaerts et al., 1987; Vallet et al., 1992; Rosenwald et al., 1993; Sun et al., 2002) favour the silver methods that make use of physical developers. These techniques are useful also for detection of argyrophilic lesions in types of dementia other than Alzheimer's disease (Martinez-Lage and Munoz, 1997; Munoz, 1999).

The following method (Munoz, 1999) is a variant of that of Gallyas (1971a) as modified by Braak and Braak (1991). The basis of the staining may be selective binding of the silver complex AgI_2^- to the p-*tau* protein, with nucleation of silver in

Step 6 of the procedure. Amplification is brought about by physical development followed by gold toning (Sections 18.3.1.1 and 18.3.1.2). A treatment with periodic acid (Step 2) suppresses the argyrophilia of normal brain tissue. This method is applied to mounted paraffin sections (8–15 μm thick) of formaldehyde-fixed brain.

Solutions required

A. 5% Periodic acid

Periodic acid ($HIO_4.2H_2O$):	10 g
Water:	200 ml

Keeps for several weeks and may be used repeatedly, but should be discarded if it goes brown.

B. 0.5% Acetic acid

Water:	398 ml
Glacial acetic acid:	2 ml

Keeps indefinitely, but use only once.

C. 1% silver nitrate

Silver nitrate:	1.0 g
Water:	100 ml

Keeps indefinitely. Used for making Solution D.

D. Silver complex solution
Dissolve 40 g sodium hydroxide in 500 ml of water. Add 100 g potassium iodide; stir until dissolved. *Slowly* add 35 ml of a 1% aqueous solution of silver nitrate. Stir until the solution is clear and make up the volume to 1000 ml. Keep in a dark bottle.

E. Physical developer
The three stock solutions are stable and can be stored in dark bottles. The working developer is made immediately before using.

Stock solution 1
Dissolve 50 g anhydrous sodium carbonate in 1000 ml of water.

Stock solution 2
Consecutively dissolve 2 g ammonium nitrate, 2 g silver nitrate and 10 g tungstosilicic acid in 1000 ml of water.

Stock solution 3
Consecutively dissolve 2 g ammonium nitrate, 2 g silver nitrate, 10 g tungstosilic acid and 7.3 ml of formalin (37–40% HCHO) in 1000 ml of water.

Working developer
Mix in a Coplin jar, in the order stated, immediately before using (Step 6 of the procedure).

Stock solution 2:	9 ml
Stock solution 1:	30 ml
Stock solution 3:	21 ml

F. 0.2% Gold chloride
Either sodium chloroaurate ($NaAuCl_4.2H_2O$) *or* chloroauric acid ($HAuCl_4$ with variable water of crystallization). Dissolve 1.0 g in 500 ml of water. The solution is stable for years and may be re-used many times. See Section 18.3.1.4.

G. 1% Sodium thiosulphate
5% w/v $Na_2S_2O_3.5H_2O$ in water. The solution can be kept for years but is used only once.

H. A counterstain

See Chapter 6 (Section 6.1). Munoz (1999) recommends nuclear fast red.

Procedure

(1) De-wax and hydrate the sections.
(2) Immerse the slides in 5% periodic acid (Solution A) for 5 min.
(3) Wash in 3 changes of water, each 1 min.
(4) Immerse in silver complex solution (D) for 1 min.
(5) Wash in 2 changes of 0.5% acetic acid (Solution B), each 1 min.
(6) Transfer the slides to the freshly made working developer solution for 5–15 min with occasional agitation. A brownish colour indicates sufficient staining.
(7) Wash in 2 changes of 0.5% acetic acid (Solution B), each 1 min.
(8) Wash in 3 changes of water, each 1 min.
(9) Immerse in 0.2% gold chloride (Solution F) for 5 min.
(10) Wash in 3 changes of water, each 1 min.
(11) Immerse in 1% sodium thiosulphate (Solution G) for 5 min.
(12) Rinse in 3 changes of water.
(13) Lightly counterstain nuclei (Solution H)
(14) Dehydrate, clear and mount, using a resinous medium.

Results

Neurofibrillary tangles and neuronal inclusion bodies, neuritic plaques, neuropil threads and argyrophilic grains black.

18.3.2.
Silver methods for reticulin

Reticulin consists of reticular fibres and basement membranes. These are composed of collagen, probably with a higher content of associated carbohydrate than larger collagenous fibres. (For more about the nature of reticulin, see Chapter 8.) Reticulin is stained by virtue of its content of hexose sugars. The simplest method, therefore, is the periodic acid–Schiff (PAS) procedure, which is described, along with other techniques of carbohydrate histochemistry, in Chapter 11. Reticular fibres are also birefringent after picro-sirius red (Section 8.2.2.3.) and, as thin collagen fibres, they are appropriately coloured (though not always easy to see) in trichrome preparations (Sections 8.2.4 and 8.2.5). There are also methods for reticulin in which the fibres and basement membranes are rendered visible by deposition upon them of finely divided metallic silver. These techniques show reticulin in more striking contrast to the background than does PAS or trichrome staining.

18.3.2.1. Chemical principles

The histochemical basis of the silver methods for reticulin is closely similar to that of the PAS procedure (Lhotka, 1956; Velican and Velican, 1970). Adjacent hydroxyl groups of the hexose sugars of the glycoprotein are oxidized to aldehydes by potassium permanganate or periodic acid. The oxidation is sometimes followed by an empirically discovered 'sensitizing' treatment with a ferric or uranyl salt. The chemical rationale of the 'sensitization' is unknown, but the result is enhancement of contrast in the final preparation. The aldehydes then reduce the silver diammine ion, $[Ag(NH_3)_2]^+$, to the metal. Silver diammine is produced by adding ammonium hydroxide to an aqueous solution of silver nitrate. A precipitate of silver oxide is formed, but dissolves as the addition is continued:

$$2NH_4OH + 2AgNO_3 \longrightarrow 2NH_4^+ + NO_3^- + Ag_2O(s) + H_2O$$

$$Ag_2O + 4NH_4OH \longrightarrow 2[Ag(NH_3)_2]^+ + 2OH^- + 3H_2O$$

The sequence of reactions in the silver staining of reticulin is as follows:

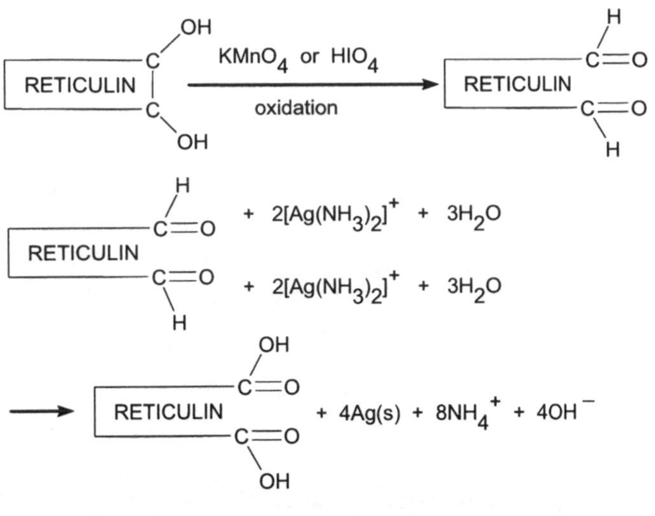

It is to be expected that four atoms of silver will be deposited at the site of each glucosyl, galactosyl, or other reactive sugar residue. This is not enough to provide adequate visibility, but fortunately it is possible to precipitate more silver upon that initially deposited, by a process similar to photographic development. This occurs when the incompletely washed sections are transferred to an aqueous formaldehyde solution. Residual silver diammine ions are reduced to silver by the formaldehyde. Metallic silver catalyses the reaction, so precipitation of the metal due to the action of formaldehyde occurs mainly at the original sites of the sugar molecules of the reticulin. Yet further contrast may be obtained by gold toning (Section 18.3.1.2).

18.3.2.2. Gordon and Sweets' technique

This method (Gordon and Sweets, 1936) is one of many available silver methods for reticulin. The oxidizing agent is $KMnO_4$ rather than HIO_4, probably because the latter was not used in histochemistry when methods of this type were invented. The function of the iron alum is obscure, but it has been shown to improve the histological picture (Velican and Velican, 1972). Any fixative may be used. The sections must be firmly attached to the slides with coagulated albumen or chrome–gelatin if they are to remain in place after treatment with alkaline reagents.

Nearly all fixatives are suitable. After mixtures containing potassium dichromate or chromic acid, it is sometimes necessary to omit the oxidation with potassium permanganate.

Solutions required

A. Acid permanganate

Potassium permanganate ($KMnO_4$):	1.0 g

(*Alternatively*, 17 ml of a stock 6% aqueous $KMnO_4$ solution.)

Water:	95 ml (*or* 78 ml)

Dissolve solid (magnetic stirrer, 30 min) *or* dilute the stock solution.

3% aqueous H_2SO_4:	5 ml

Prepare just before use. May be used repeatedly on the day it is made. The addition of H_2SO_4 is not necessary. If not acidified, permanganate solutions are indefinitely stable if free of contamination. (The bottle cap or stopper may be impossible to remove after a few years!)

B. 1% oxalic acid

Oxalic acid (H₂C₂O₄.2H₂O):	5 g
Water:	to make 500 ml

Keeps indefinitely.

C. Iron alum

Ammonium ferric sulphate (NH₄Fe(SO₄)₂.12H₂O):	10 g
Water:	500 ml

Prepare on the day it is first to be used. The solution is often usable for a few weeks but should be discarded when there is more than a trace of insoluble material. in the bottom of the bottle. *Alternatively*, use a 4% ferric chloride (FeCl₃.6H₂O) solution, which keeps for a year or two without visible change.

D. Ammoniacal silver solution
This unstable reagent is made up from stock solutions.

Stock solutions
(1) **10% aqueous silver nitrate.** Store in a very clean dark glass bottle. Contamination causes black precipitate or a mirror. Clean solutions keep indefinitely (at least 15 years in my experience).
(2) **Ammonium hydroxide (28% NH3)** often called '.880 ammonia'. A full bottle is indefinitely stable, but a stock bottle used only occasionally over the years may not contain enough NH₃ if it is less than about one quarter full. This reagent is not expensive.
(3) **4% aqueous sodium hydroxide.** Insoluble deposits appear in glass bottles of NaOH solutions kept for about 2 years. Replace a solution with anything worse than a trace of insoluble material.

Working solution
Add ammonium hydroxide drop by drop to 10 ml of 10% AgNO₃ until the brown precipitate of Ag₂O is almost (not quite) re-dissolved. Add 7.5 ml of 4% NaOH, followed by a few more drops of ammonium hydroxide, until the newly formed precipitate is just dissolved. Be careful not to add too much ammonia. Swirl the solution for a few seconds after adding each drop, because dissolution of the precipitate is not quite instantaneous. Make up to 100 ml with water. This solution should be made just before using.

Caution. Ammoniacal silver solutions decompose on evaporation to form explosive 'fulminating silver', which is a mixture of silver amide and silver nitride (see Laist, 1954). See *Note 1* at the end of the account of the Gros–Schultze method (Section 18.3.1.7.) for instructions on disposal of used ammoniacal silver solutions.

E. Reducer
A neutralized formalin (made by adding some marble chips to the bought stock bottle) is traditionally recommended for this method.

Formalin (40% HCHO; ideally 'neutralized'):	10 ml
Water:	90 ml

F. Yellow gold chloride (0.2%)

Sodium tetrachloroaurate (NaAuCl₄.2H₂O):	1.0 g
Water:	500 ml

This solution may be re-used repeatedly, often for 10 years. Deterioration is evident when it loses its yellow colour and a deposit, obviously of metallic gold, appears in the bottle.

G. Sodium thiosulphate

Sodium thiosulphate ($Na_2S_2O_3.5H_2O$):	5 g
Water:	to make 500 ml

Keeps indefinitely, but use only once.

Procedure

(1) De-wax and hydrate paraffin sections.
(2) Oxidize for 1 min in acid permanganate (Solution A).
(3) Wash in water.
(4) Immerse in 1% oxalic acid (Solution B) until the sections are white (usually about 30 s).
(5) Wash in water (three changes).
(6) Treat with iron alum (Solution C), 10 min.
(7) Wash in water (three changes).
(8) Immerse slides in the ammoniacal silver solution (Solution D) for 5–10 s.
(9) Rinse in water (once only). See *Note 1* below.
(10) Place in formaldehyde reducer (Solution E), 30 s.
(11) Wash in water (three changes). See *Note 2* below.
(12) Tone by immersing in 0.2% yellow gold chloride (Solution F), for 2 min. (See also *Note 3* below.)
(13) Wash in water (two changes).
(14) Immerse in sodium thiosulphate (Solution G) for 3 min.
(15) Wash in water (three changes).
(16) Dehydrate through graded alcohols, clear in xylene and cover.

Result

Reticulin black. Other components of the tissue in shades of grey-purple. See also *Note 4* below.

Notes

(1) This rinse (Step 9) is a critical component of the method. If the rinse is excessive, staining of reticulin will be inadequate. If the rinse is insufficient there will be non-specific precipitation of silver on the sections. If working with slides in a coplin jar, pour out the ammoniacal silver solution, fill up with water, agitate for about 5 s, pour out the water, and immediately pour in the reducer.

(2) The sections should be examined after Step 11. If staining is excessive, the method should be repeated from Step 6. This will produce an effect equivalent to differentiation. Some of the finely divided metallic silver in the specimen is oxidized to silver ions, which are then precipitated as silver chloride:

$$Ag + Fe^{3+} \longrightarrow Ag^+ + Fe^{2+}$$

$$Ag^+ + Cl^- \longrightarrow AgCl(s)$$

This salt dissolves in the excess of ammonia present in the ammoniacal silver solution:

$$AgCl + 2NH_3 \longrightarrow [Ag(NH_3)_2]^+ + Cl^-$$

Any undissolved silver chloride is removed at Step 14 of the method:

$$AgCl + 2S_2O_3^{2-} \longrightarrow [Ag(S_2O_3)_2]^{3-} + Cl^-$$

(3) Palladium toning (Krikelis and Smith, 1988) is a substitute for gold toning: At Step 12, immerse the slides for 10 min in 0.05% potassium hexachloropal-

ladate (K_2PdCl_6) in 4 M HCl. The silver deposits become uniformly black, without the purplish background associated with gold toning. Palladium toning may therefore be preferable when the preparations are to be photographed. (Do not confuse K_2PdCl_6 with the palladium chloride ($PdCl_2$) used in lipid histochemistry.)

(4) A suitable counterstain is aluminium-nuclear fast red (Chapter 6, Section 6.1.3.7). If this is applied before Step 2 *and* after Step 15, background argyrophilia is suppressed and the specific staining of reticular fibres is intensified (Watson, 2005).

18.3.3.
Silver methods for fungi and bacteria

Most fungi are inconspicuous is sections stained with haemalum and eosin. Some, notably *Candida* and other yeasts, are strongly Gram-positive (Chapter 6). Fungi with capsules of sulphated carbohydrate, notably *Cryptococcus* can be stained with alcian blue (Chapter 11). For a useful table of staining properties of medically significant fungi, see Bancroft and Cook (1984).

The **silver methods for fungi** are similar in principle to the methods for reticulin. Carbohydrates in the cell walls of the organisms are oxidized to generate aldehyde groups, and the aldehydes are detected by reduction of a silver complex. Other carbohydrates that yield aldehydes on oxidation are also stained. These include cellulose, starch, chitin, glycogen, collagen and many types of mucus. These substances are all also stainable by the periodic acid–Schiff method (Chapter 11), which will also demonstrate fungi. Silver stains are preferred in diagnostic pathology because of their potential to show individual fungal hyphae in black against a pale background. All types of fungus are demonstrable.

Silver methods for bacteria are used for demonstrating spirochaetes, which are difficult to detect with dyes. The many techniques, for smears, sections or whole pieces of tissue (see Gray, 1954), have been developed empirically and the histochemical rationale is not known. They are similar to the silver methods for axons, involving typically a treatment with silver nitrate followed by a reducing agent. In some methods the reducing agent is applied first, and in others a silver diammine complex is preferred to silver nitrate. Silver methods are not selective for spirochaetes. Other types of bacteria are also darkly stained. The cells and other components of the host tissue acquire weaker colours (Churukian, 1997). The Warthin–Starry method for spirochaetes in sections, is given here as an example.

18.3.3.1. Grocott's hexamine–silver method for fungi

This is a sensitive method for the cell wall carbohydrates of all kinds of fungi (Grocott, 1955; see also Carson, 1997). The oxidizing agent that generates aldehyde groups is chromium trioxide. The silver complex that detects the aldehydes is made with **hexamethylenetetramine** (also known as **hexamine** or **methenamine**). This compound, $(CH_2)_6N_4$, is the stable product of the reaction of formaldehyde with ammonia. It is a solid that can be weighed accurately (unlike ammonia), and it forms silver complexes that are more stable than the silver diammine ion. The 1:1 complex $[C_6H_{12}N_4.AgNO_3]$ is an insoluble white crystalline compound. It is seen transiently when the hexamine–silver reagent is being made. With an excess of hexamethylenetetramine the complex has the composition $[2C_6H_{12}N_4.3AgNO_3]$ (Walker, 1964). It is soluble in water and the solution can be kept for several weeks in a cool, dark place. The eventual deterioration is due to slow decomposition of hexamethylenetetramine in aqueous solution, yielding ammonia and formaldehyde. The latter reduces the complex, with precipitation of silver.

The hexamethylenetetramine-silver complex shares with silver diammine (Section 10.10.4) the propensity for reduction by aldehydes, yielding black colloidal silver. It's original histochemical application (as Gomori's methenamine–silver) was to detect aldehydes generated by oxidation of glycogen and mucus. Grocott's technique is a technical optimization for the carbohydrates of fungal cell walls.

The method is applied to paraffin sections, usually of specimens fixed in neutral buffered formaldehyde. At least one slide with sections known to contain fungi should be processed alongside the unknowns, as a positive control.

Solutions required
A. 5% chromium trioxide

Chromium trioxide (CrO_3):	5 g
Water:	100 ml

This can be kept indefinitely in a glass-stoppered bottle.

B. 1% sodium metabisulphite

Sodium metabisulphite ($Na_2S_2O_5$):	1 g
Water:	100 ml

This can be kept indefinitely in a screw-capped bottle.

C. Hexamine–silver stock solution
Dissolve 3 g of hexamethylenetetramine (also known as hexamine or methenamine) in 100 ml water. Dissolve 250 mg of silver nitrate in 5 ml of water (or use 5 ml of a 5% aqueous silver nitrate stock solution). Combine the two solutions in a very clean glass bottle and mix thoroughly. (A precipitate forms and redissolves.)

This solution can be kept for about 2 months in a refrigerator. It should be replaced if it becomes turbid or contains a precipitate.

D. 5% borax

Sodium tetraborate ($Na_2B_4O_7.10H_2O$; borax):	1 g
Water:	50 ml

This is usually made as needed, but it can be kept as a stock solution for several years.

E. Hexamine–silver working solution

5% borax (Solution D):	2 ml
Water:	25 ml
Hexamine–silver stock solution (C):	25 ml

This is made immediately before beginning to stain the slides. The staining jar containing the working solution is put in an oven or water bath (in darkness or subdued light) and allowed to heat up to 56°C.

F. Gold chloride toning solution
A 0.2% aqueous solution of chloroauric acid (Solution E of Holmes' method, Section 18.3.1.4) is suitable.

Procedure
(1) De-wax and hydrate paraffin sections.
(2) Immerse in 5% chromium trioxide (Solution A) for 60 min (see.
(3) Wash in water.
(4) Immerse in 5% sodium metabisulphite (Solution B) for about 1 min, to remove brown colour derived from chromium trioxide.
(5) Wash in running tap water for 5–10 min, then in 4 changes of distilled or deionized water.
(6) Place the slides in the working hexamine silver solution (E) at 56°C. Remove a positive control slide after 10 min, rinse in water (must be distilled or

deionized) and check under a microscope. If necessary, prolong the staining up to 30 min, checking at 5-min intervals for black fungal structures.

(7)   Wash in 3 changes of distilled or deionized water.
(8)   Immerse in the gold toning solution (F) for 3 min.
(9)   Wash in 4 changes of water.
(10) Immerse in 5% sodium thiosulphate for 5 min.
(11) Wash in 4 changes of water.
(12) Apply a counterstain if desired (See *Note* below).
(13) Dehydrate, clear, and apply coverlips, using a resinous mounting medium.

Result
Fungi black. Cellulose, starch and chitin are also stained black, if present, as are melanin granules, glycogen and some types of mucus. Connective tissue (collagen, reticulin, elastin) should be unstained or at the most light grey. The counterstain colours all other components of the tissue. In addition to fungi, the cyst walls of *Pneumocyctis carinii* (a unicellular fungus formerly classified as a protozoan) are stained by Grocott's method.,

Note
A counterstain that contrasts well with the gold-toned silver deposit is light green or fast green FCF (Chapter 6). Either of these dyes imparts a green colour to all components of the section.

18.3.3.2. Warthin–Starry method for spirochaetes
Spirochaetes are thread-like Gram-negative bacteria, so thin that they are scarcely visible in material stained by the Gram technique. They include important pathogens in such genera as *Borrelia*, *Helicobacter*, *Leptospira* and *Treponema*, causing Lyme disease, peptic ulceration, Weil's disease and syphilis, respectively. These organisms can be stained with silver methods that are similar in principle to those used for normal axons (Section 18.3.1). The primary treatment with silver ions is at pH 3.6. Silver is nucleated in bacteria at this pH but it is too acidic for much nucleation to occur in most components of animal tissues. The invisible silver nuclei are then enlarged by means of a physical developer (Section 18.3.1.1). For a more detailed review of this method see Kiernan (2002b).

This technique (Warthin and Starry, 1920) is applied to paraffin sections of formaldehyde-fixed tissue. A control known to contain spirochaetes should be stained alongside the test slides.

Solutions required
All the solutions are used hot (55°C). The bottles of stock solutions should be stood in a suitable water bath or oven for an hour or two before using.

A. Acetate buffer, pH 3.6
This is a 0.1 M acetic acid–sodium acetate buffer (Chapter 20. It can be kept for several weeks, but is prone to infection by bacteria and fungi. Do not use if it is cloudy or if any kind of deposit is present in the bottle.

B. Silver solution
Solution A:	50 ml
Silver nitrate (AgNO$_3$):	1.0 g

The silver nitrate can be derived from a stronger stock solution if desired. The final concentration in Solution B is 2% w/v.

C. 5% Gelatin
Gelatin:	10 g
Water:	200 ml

Keeps for a few weeks at 4°C. Warm to about 40°C to melt the solution before using. The solution must not be turbid.

D. Reducer
This is is a physical developer (Section 18.3.1.1). Make up the three solutions while the sections are in the silver solution, and combine them immediately before using.

Hydroquinone:	30 mg

Dissolve in 20 ml water and heat to 55°C.

Silver solution (B):	15 ml

Heat to 55°C.

5% gelatin (Solution C):	37.5 ml

Heat to 55°C.

Combine the three hot solutions in a staining jar immediately before carrying out Step 3 of the procedure.

Procedure
(1)   De-wax and hydrate paraffin sections.
(2)   Dilute the silver solution (B) with an equal volume of acetate buffer (B) and immerse slides in the diluted solution for 60 min at 55°C. Prepare the components of the reducer (Solution C).
(3)   Combine the three components of the reducer (Solution C). Pour off the silver solution from the slides and replace it with reducer. Keep at 55°C until the sections are a gold–brown colour (3–5 min).
(4)   Pour off the reducer and wash at 55°C (running hot tap water is satisfactory) for 5 min.
(5)   Rinse in distilled water, dehydrate, clear and mount in a resinous medium.

Result
Spirochaetes and other bacteria black (ideally) or brown. Tiny gram-negative bacilli, including *Bartonella*, *Campylobacter* and *Legionella* are also blackened. Components of the tissue yellow or light brown.

Note
Bacteria are stained blue by Giemsa's method (Chapter 7), and in fluids spirochaetes can be detected because they display a bright golden yellow colour when examined by dark-field microscopy (Murray *et al.*, 1994). The bacteria cannot be definitively identified by silver or other simple staining methods, but these techniques are useful for detecting organisms in expected sites, especially *Helicobacter* in stomach biopsies.

18.3.4.
A silver method for the Golgi apparatus

Silver and osmium reduction methods allowed the disposition of the Golgi apparatus to be described in various cell-types for more than 50 years before it became possible to study the organelle in detail by electron microscopy. The techniques are of historical interest and may be needed from time to time to prepare slides for teaching purposes. In the classical silver methods, small pieces of tissue were fixed in an aqueous solution containing formaldehyde and one or more other substances that had been found empirically to enhance the argyrophilia of the Golgi apparatus. The fixed specimens were then soaked in silver nitrate, followed by a reducing agent, and were then dehydrated, cleared, and embedded in wax. Thin sections of the block-stained material could be examined directly, or subjected to other procedures such as gold toning and counterstaining.

According to Gabe (1976), Golgi's original method, with an arsenic compound as the 'other substance', gave unpredictable results, and the methods of Cajal (uranyl nitrate), Da Fano (cobalt nitrate) and Aoyama (cadmium chloride) were the most popular ones in middle years of the 20th century. Saxena (1957) compared several additives to a formaldehyde fixative and concluded that chlorides were generally superior to nitrates as promoters of the argyrophilia of the Golgi apparatus, and barium chloride was the most efficacious of the compounds tested. The following method (Saxena, 1957) was developed soon after the discovery of the distinctive ultrastructure of the Golgi apparatus.

Solutions required
A. Fixative

Neutralized formalin:	15 ml
(37–40% formaldehyde that has been stored over	
calcium or magnesium carbonate)	
Barium chloride ($BaCl_2$):	1.0 g
Water:	to make 100 ml

Mix before using, and use only once.

B. 1.5% silver nitrate

Silver nitrate:	1.5 g
Water:	100 ml

Can be kept for several years, in a brown glass-stoppered bottle.

C. Modified Cajal's reducer

Hydroquinone:	1.5 g
Sodium sulphite (Na_2SO_3):	0.5 g
Neutralized formalin (see under Solution A above):	15 ml
Water:	100 ml

Mix before using, and use only once.

Procedure
(1) Fix pieces of tissue (maximum dimension 2 mm or less) in Solution A for 3–6 h. The duration of fixation affects the result (see *Note 1* below).
(2) Rinse in 2 changes of water and place in 1.5% $AgNO_3$ (Solution B), overnight (8–18 h).
(3) Rinse in 2 changes of water and place in modified Cajal's reducer (Solution C) for 5–10 h.
(4) Wash in running tap water for 30 min.
(5) Dehydrate through graded alcohols, clear (cedarwood oil recommended), and embed in paraffin wax.
(6) Cut sections (5 µm or thinner) and mount them on slides. When dry, remove the wax with xylene and apply coverslips, using a resinous mounting medium (see also *Note 2* below).

Result
In a correctly treated preparation the Golgi apparatus is black, and its reticular (net-like, lacy or holey) texture is discernible with an oil-immersion objective. Other components of the cytoplasm, and connective tissue, are yellow or light brown.

Notes
(1) The duration of fixation is critical in all silver methods for the Golgi apparatus (Gabe, 1976). Specimens should be removed at hourly intervals within the prescribed range of times.
(2) Often the resolution of the Golgi apparatus can be improved by gold toning. To do this, dewax and hydrate the sections and treat with gold chloride, followed by sodium thiosulphate, as in Holmes's silver method for axons

(Section 18.3.1.4 of this chapter). Saxena (1957) favoured a more dilute (0.1%) gold chloride solution, applied for a longer time (15–20 min).

(3) In some tissues the Golgi apparatus can be displayed, though not selectively, by simple histochemical methods for lipids (Sudan black B, Chapter 12; also Baker, 1944), carbohydrates (periodic acid–Schiff or affinity for concanavalin A or other lectins, Chapter 11) or enzymes (thiamine pyrophosphatase, Chapter 15).

18.4. Osmium methods

The chemical reactions of osmium tetroxide with lipids and proteins are discussed elsewhere, in the context of fixation (Chapter 2) and lipid histochemistry (Chapter 12). All osmium staining methods are to some extent histochemical, because they result in the deposition of insoluble black compounds of osmium at the sites of reducing agents present in the tissue. Four techniques are considered here: two in which OsO_4 is the sole active component, and two in which other chemically active ingredients contribute to the staining mechanisms.

18.4.1.
Teased whole-mount method for nerve fibres

A nerve fibre is an axon, together with its myelin sheath and the associated neuroglial cells. In a peripheral nerve or a spinal nerve root, the neuroglial cells are Schwann cells, and except at the sites of their nuclei they do do not contribute significantly to the diameters of nerve fibres. The classification of nerve fibres is based on electrophysiological studies of conduction velocity, and on direct measurement of individual fibres in osmicated, teased whole-mounts. The osmium tetroxide, which serves as fixative and stain, is reduced by double bonds in the lipids of the myelin sheath, with deposition of black osmium dioxide. Unmyelinated axons cannot be demonstrated by this method.

It is assumed that the specimen is a nerve no more than 0.5 mm in diameter, displayed by dissection in a terminally anesthetized small animal. Several variations of the method (see *Note* below) are possible.

Solutions required
Normal saline

Sodium chloride:	9.0 g
Water:	to make 1000 ml

Osmium tetroxide
Instructions and associated safety precautions for making a 2% stock solution of osmium tetroxide are given in Chapter 12 (Section 12.6.1).

Procedure
(1) Under a dissecting microscope, use the point of a very sharp blade to make a longitudinal cut in the connective tissue sheath of the nerve.
(2) Remove a length of nerve by cutting with scissors in two places, and put the specimen in a drop of normal saline on a slide.
(3) Place the slide on the stage of an ordinary microscope, under a ×10 objective. Lower the condenser to enhance contrast.
(4) Use fine needles to shred the specimen, so that individual fibers are displayed in large numbers.
(5) Add a drop of osmium tetroxide (1% solution) to the saline, and cover the preparation with an inverted watch glass or petri dish, to maintain humidity and to contain OsO_4 vapour.
(6) After 60 min tilt the slide to pour off the osmium tetroxide solution, taking care not to lose the specimen. Rinse in large drops of water, changed at 10 min intervals, for about 1 h. Further teasing and adjustment of the specimen

is advisable during the later washes. Try to thin out or remove any large opaque parts of the specimen.

(7)   Remove as much water as possible without letting the preparation dry out, and apply a coverslip using an aqueous mounting medium.

Results

All components of the tissue are darkened. Myelin sheaths are black. Nodes of Ranvier are clearly seen in teased whole-mounts of normal nerves, and demyelinated internodes can be seen in some types of peripheral neuropathy. The normal appearances and artifacts due to rough handling are illustrated by Frankl and Denaro (1998).

Notes

(1)   It is also possible to tease individual fibres from small pieces of fixed, post-osmicated nerves (Frankl and Denaro, 1998).

(2)   Sections are sometimes preferable to whole-mounts for examining and measuring myelinated fibres. For quantitative work it is important to standardize all stages of the procedure, so that shrinkage will be the same in all the specimens to be compared. Fixation with the least structural disturbance is achieved by applying a buffered glutaraldehyde–formaldehyde mixture (Chapter 2) to the surgically exposed nerve for 30–60 min (Morris et al., 1972). The specimen is then removed, washed, treated with osmium tetroxide for 30–60 min, and thoroughly washed in water. Embedding should be in a synthetic resin (sections 1 μm thick), though paraffin wax and 4 μm sections may also be used (Stelmack and Kiernan, 1977). The sections may be cleared and coverslipped without further staining, or a counterstain may be applied. In transverse sections each myelinated fibre is seen as a black circle, with the paler axon in its centre. Longitudinally sectioned fibers have a tram-line appearance.

18.4.2.
An osmium method for the Golgi apparatus

Before the introduction of glutaraldehyde into microtechnique in 1962, osmium tetroxide was an essential ingredient of all fixatives that preserved intricate structural detail within cells. Strangeways and Canti (1927) made observations by phase contrast microscopy of cultured cells being fixed by various compounds. They found that osmium tetroxide caused less structural disturbance than any other fixative, and their observations supported the contention that such organelles as mitochondria and the Golgi apparatus existed in living cells and were not artifacts. In the light of modern knowledge, it seems probable that osmium reduction methods demonstrate lipids in the membranes of which the Golgi apparatus is composed. Indeed, it is possible to stain the Golgi apparatus with Sudan black B, a dye that dissolves in lipids (Chapter 12).

According to Gabe (1976), the osmium reduction methods can show the Golgi apparatus in cells of all animals, including marine invertebrates, whereas the silver methods (Section 18.3.4) work well only with tissues of mammals and terrestrial molluscs. The osmium methods demand more time than the silver methods, and OsO_4 is a more expensive and more hazardous reagent than $AgNO_3$.

The following is Cowdry's (1952) modification of Ludford's technique, with notes from Gabe (1976). Small, freshly removed specimens are specially fixed and osmicated before embedding and sectioning. The fixation and postosmication must be carried out in clean glass (not plastic) specimen tubes. The fixative must not come into contact with any metal instrument.

Solutions required
A. Mann's fixative (See Chapter 2; Section 2.5.4.)
This contains osmium tetroxide and mercuric chloride, so be careful with it.

B. 2% osmium tetroxide (See Chapter 12; Section 12.6.1.)
More dilute solutions (1% and 0.5%) are also needed. They are made by diluting
the 2% stock solution with water. **Caution.** Use OsO_4 in a fume cupboard.

C. Turpentine
(This liquid is more correctly called oil of turpentine.) See also *Notes 2* and *3*
below.

Procedure
(1) Fix small specimens (no more than 2 mm in any dimension) by immersion
overnight in Mann's fixative (Solution A).
(2) Wash in 3 changes of water, each 10 min.
(3) Immerse in 2% osmium tetroxide (about 5 ml; enough to cover the specimen) and keep at 30°C for 24 h.
(4) Repeat Step 3 with 1% osmium tetroxide.
(5) Repeat Step 3 with 0.5% osmium tetroxide.
(6) Wash in water at 30°C for 24 h. (Gabe suggests a few hours in running tap
water.)
(7) Dehydrate through graded alcohols, clear and embed in wax. The specimens
are fragile, and according to Gabe (1976) it is essential to use cedarwood oil
(Chapter 4) as the clearing agent.
(8) Cut thin paraffin sections (3 µm if possible; no thicker than 7 µm) and mount
them onto slides. There is likely to be difficulty cutting the sections.
(9) De-wax with xylene. Apply a coverslip to one of the slides and examine it. The
Golgi apparatus, fat and intracellular lipid droplets should be black, on a light
brown background.
(10) If the background is too dark, immerse slides in turpentine for 2 min, rinse in
xylene and examine again. The time in turpentine may be extended to 15
min if necessary, to remove brown and black material from structures other
than the Golgi apparatus. Gabe (1976) states that excessively blackened sections may remain in turpentine for 24 or 48 h. See *Note 3* below for an alternative to turpentine.
(11) When the staining is satisfactory, pass the slides through 2 changes of
toluene or xylene (to remove turpentine) and apply coverslips, using a
resinous mounting medium.

Result
With an oil immersion objective the Golgi apparatus should be seen as an intricate
network of black lines and rings in a distinct region of the cytoplasm.

Notes
(1) Methods of this type are notoriously fickle. Do not be surprised if the staining is either excessive or too weak. The duration of treatment with osmium
tetroxide (Steps 3, 4 and 5) may be increased up to twice the prescribed
times. Other cytological fixatives (Chapter 2, Section 2.5.4) may also be
used. If a mixture containing potassium dichromate or chromium trioxide is
used, the specimens must be washed overnight in running tap water at Step
2, to remove all traces of these compounds.
(2) The mechanism of differentiation by turpentine has not been studied.
According to Baker (1958) some organic solvents can remove bound
osmium (see also Chapter 2), and can also oxidize insoluble black deposits
of OsO_2 to soluble OsO_4. Turpentine is a mixture of terpenes that would be
expected to combine with OsO_4. Possibly it also contains an oxidizing agent.
(3) An alternative to turpentine is hydrogen peroxide, which is much more rapid
in its action. The sections are taken to water and a freshly diluted aqueous
solution containing 0.0004% to 0.0005% H_2O_2 is allowed to act for

15–60 s. The slides are then washed in tap water, dehydrated through graded alcohols, cleared and coverslipped.

18.4.3.
Marchi method for degenerating myelin

When an axon is severed, the part distal to the neuronal cell-body degenerates into a string of tiny fragments. The myelin sheath also undergoes fragmentation, and this process is associated with a change in the component lipids. Phospholipids, which are hydrophilic, predominate in the normal myelin sheath, but hydrophobic esters of cholesterol are the principal lipids of the degenerate fragments (Adams, 1965).

Occasionally, methods for hydrophobic and hydrophilic lipids are used sequentially, to stain degenerating and normal myelin in the same frozen section (Culling, 1974). Such methods, however, are not often used. The degenerating myelin can be seen as birefringent particles when frozen sections are examined with crossed polars, and a fat stain such as Sudan black B enhances the distinction from normal myelin, which is also birefringent (Miklossy and van der Loos, 1991).

The **Marchi method** demonstrates the degenerated remains of myelin sheaths. There are several variations of the technique, but in all of them the tissue is treated simultaneously with OsO_4 (soluble in polar and non-polar substances) and another oxidizing agent, which must be soluble only in polar substances. The polar oxidizing agent in the original method (see Marchi, 1892) was potassium dichromate, which was the principal ingredient of micro-anatomical fixatives prior to the introduction of formaldehyde into histotechnology in 1893. Potassium chlorate (Swank and Davenport, 1935) has been preferred for many years. In degenerating myelin, OsO_4 is bound at sites of double bonds in the unsaturated acyl groups of the hydrophobic cholesterol esters and then reduced to an insoluble black compound, probably $OsO_2.2H_2O$ (Chapter 2 for chemistry). In normal myelin, which is hydrophilic, the polar oxidizing agent prevents the reduction of bound osmium.

Important differences exist between the early and late stages of degeneration of myelin. Strich (1968) and Fraser (1972) have shown that in the early phase (up to about 10 days after injury for PNS or about 100 days for CNS) the products are destroyed by freezing and thawing or by storage for more than 3 weeks in a formaldehyde-containing fixative. They can therefore be demonstrated only by treating blocks of tissue with OsO_4–oxidant mixtures. The products of the late phase of degeneration, however, persist much longer after axonal transection (up to 30 days in the PNS and at least 2 years in the CNS), and are not destroyed by freezing and thawing or removed by prolonged storage of tissues in solutions of formaldehyde. The degenerating myelin of the late phase can therefore be stained either in the block or in frozen sections. For staining in the block, the method of Swank and Davenport (1935) is recommended, and is described below.

The chief advantage of the Marchi method for neuroanatomical tracing is that the length of the time of survival after a destructive lesion is not very critical, so it is possible to apply the technique to human post-mortem material and determine the positions of fibre tracts in the human CNS (e.g. Nathan and Smith, 1955; Nathan *et al.*, 1996). The disadvantages are the impossibility of demonstrating degenerating unmyelinated axons (including all presynaptic branches), and also the occasional blackening of normal myelin sheaths.

Solutions required
A. Fixative
4% formaldehyde (in water, saline or 0.1 M phosphate buffer, pH 7.2–7.6).

B. Staining solution
This keeps for a few months at 4°C in a stoppered bottle.

Potassium chlorate ($KClO_3$):	1.5 g
Water:	200 ml
Osmium tetroxide:	0.5 g
Formalin (37–40% HCHO):	0.5 g
Glacial acetic acid:	2.5 ml

If it is more convenient, the 0.5 g of osmium tetroxide may be added as 25 ml of a stock 2% solution, and the volume of water reduced to 175 ml. See Chapter 12 (Section 12.6.1) for precautions and instructions relating to preparation of OsO_4 solutions.

Procedure

(1) Remove tissue from the central nervous system of an animal with an experimental lesion, or use human post-mortem material from a patient in whom degenerated tracts are expected to be present. The specimens should be no more than 1 cm thick. Fix in Solution A for 2–4 days. (With human tissue it is usually necessary to wait for 2–3 weeks while the whole brain is being fixed by immersion.)

(2) Trim into pieces no more than 3 mm thick, and put these, without washing, into the staining solution (B). The volume of this solution should be approximately 15 times that of the specimens. Leave in a screw capped jar for 7–10 days, with daily agitation to expose all surfaces of the tissue evenly to the reagent.

(3) Wash in running tap water for 24 h. Frozen sections (20–100 µm) may be prepared, if desired: proceed to Step 5a. Otherwise, proceed to Steps 4 and 5b.

(4) Dehydrate in graded alcohols. *Either* embed in nitrocellulose *or* double-embed in paraffin wax; see Chapter 4 for techniques. Cut serial sections 20 µm thick, and mount them onto slides. (With routine paraffin embedding it is more difficult to obtain good sections.)

(5) (a) Mount the frozen sections onto slides and let them air-dry at room temperature. Complete the dehydration in 100% alcohol, clear in 2 changes of xylene, and apply coverslips, using a resinous mounting medium.

   (b) De-wax and clear the sections by passing through 3 changes of xylene. Cover, using a resinous mounting medium.

Result

Degenerating myelinated fibres appear as rows of black dots. The myelin sheaths of occasional normal axons are often stained, but can be recognized by their integrity (rings or tramline appearance). Fat in adipose tissue is also blackened.

Notes

(1) For distinguishing between early and late products of degeneration, see the foregoing discussion of this method.

(2) A counterstain may be applied to some sections, to facilitate topographical orientation. Alum–haematoxylin will stain cell nuclei, but cationic dyes do not work well after fixation in OsO_4.

(3) Swank and Davenport (1935) recommended, for laboratory animals, preliminary fixation by vascular perfusion of a solution of 15 g of $Mg(SO_4)_2.7H_2O$ and 5 g of $K_2Cr_2O_7$ in 250 ml of water.

(4) The Swank and Davenport mixture (Solution B) is also used in methods for staining both normal and degenerating myelin in frozen sections of formaldehyde-fixed nervous tissue. For review, discussion and technical instructions see Adams (1965), Bayliss High (1984) or Kiernan (2007b).

18.4.4.
Iodide–osmium
methods

The innervation of some tissues is shown with striking clarity by using one of the osmium–iodide methods. Specimens are fixed in a solution containing iodide ions and osmium tetroxide, and subsequently are either examined as whole mounts or embedded and sectioned. The cation associated with the iodide was sodium or potassium in the earlier methods of this type (e.g. Champy et al., 1946), but zinc iodide, introduced by Maillet (1963) is now preferred.

The chemistry of the reagent has been partly determined (Gilloteaux and Naud, 1979). When solutions of zinc iodide and osmium tetroxide are mixed, the latter compound is reduced by iodide ions to the osmate(VI) ion:

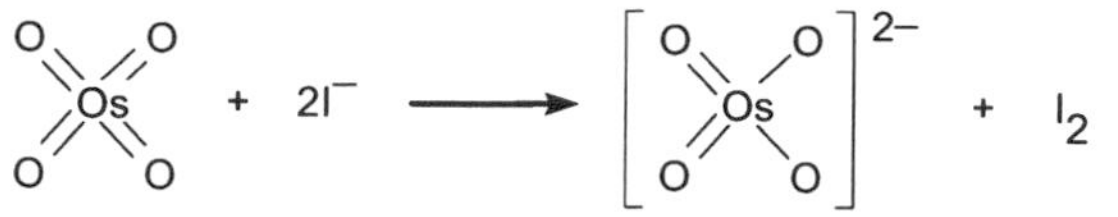

The solution rapidly becomes orange as iodine is liberated. After several hours it turns black; a black precipitate settles out during the next 1–2 weeks. This precipitate is zinc osmate, $ZnOsO_4$. It has been shown to be identical to the black, electron-dense substance formed within tissues fixed in zinc iodide–osmium tetroxide mixtures. Spectroscopic studies of solutions that initially contained osmium tetroxide and iodide ions or iodine indicate that there may also be oxidation of iodine (to iodate, in which the oxidation number of I is +5) by OsO_4, and deposition of metallic osmium:

$$I_2 + 2OsO_4 \longrightarrow 2IO_3^- + 2Os(s) + O_2$$

The sensitivity of the compounds of osmium to reduction by organic material may be regulated by the concentration of elemental iodine, and by the oxidation states of this element in its ions in the staining solution (Carrapico et al., 1984). Reduction of osmium–iodide mixtures occurs more rapidly in tissue than in the solution and may be catalysed at the sites of organic reducing groups such as –SH and –CH=CH–. Gilloteaux and Naud also obtained evidence indicating that deposition of zinc osmate could occur at intracellular sites that, in life, were occupied by calcium ions.

Although several ideas have been suggested and disproved (see Maillet, 1963), there is still no satisfactory explanation for the mechanism of axonal staining by iodide–osmium mixtures. Examination of zinc iodide–osmium-fixed central nervous tissues with the electron microscope has revealed electron-dense deposits within synaptic vesicles (Akert and Sandri, 1968). The reaction in these organelles depends on the presence of free sulphydryl groups in the tissue (Reinecke and Walther, 1978). It is not known whether similarly produced deposits account for the optical blackness of stained peripheral axons. Osmium–iodide reagents also strongly blacken secretory granules containing reducing substances (such as serotonin in enteroendocrine cells, and catecholamines in the adrenal medulla, but this should not be considered a histochemical method (Hillarp, 1959).

Iodide–osmium methods are valuable for the examination of unmyelinated axons and nerve endings in viscera and skeletal muscle. Both autonomic and sensory innervations are demonstrated. Central nervous tissue, which has a high content of osmiophilic membrane-bound lipids, is homogeneously blackened by fixation in iodide–osmium solutions and the preparations are uninformative when examined by light microscopy.

The following procedure is based on a method described by Rodrigo et al. (1970). Pieces of tissue must be taken from a freshly killed animal and should be less than 4 mm thick, preferably only about 1.0mm. Hollow viscera are opened to make flat specimens, which can then be fixed to an improvised glass frame to facilitate penetration of the fixative.

Solutions required

A. 2% osmium tetroxide
Instructions and associated safety precautions for making a 2% stock solution of osmium tetroxide are given in Chapter 12 (Section 12.6.1).

B. Zinc iodide
Put 6 g of zinc powder in a 500 ml conical flask. Add 10 g of iodine (resublimed) and then 200 ml of water. Swirl continuously. The elements combine with evolution of heat and the colour of the solution changes from reddish to grey. Allow the remaining solid material to settle and then filter. This solution should be prepared shortly before use and the excess discarded.

C. Working fixative
Add 25 ml of Solution A to 75 ml of Solution B (or smaller quantities in the same proportions). The mixture is at first yellow, but soon darkens. Mix it immediately before using.

D. 2% potassium permanganate
Potassium permanganate ($KMnO_4$):	2.0 g
Water:	100 ml

Keeps for several months. Filter before using. Alternatively, dilute a stock solution containing 6% $KMnO_4$.

E. 2% oxalic acid
Oxalic acid ($H_2C_2O_4.2H_2O$):	5.0 g
Water:	250 ml

This can be kept indefinitely.

Procedure
(1) Immerse the specimens in at least 20 times their own volumes of Solution C, for 24 h.
(2) Wash in running tap water for 6 h (if frozen sections are to be cut) or for 24 h if the specimens are to be embedded in wax.
(3) Either cut frozen sections or dehydrate, clear, embed in wax, and cut paraffin sections. Mount the sections onto slides and take to water. (See *Note 1* below.)
(4) Examine the sections. If staining is satisfactory, dehydrate, clear, and mount. If the colour is too dark and nerve fibres cannot be distinguished from background, proceed as follows.
(5) To differentiate the stain, pass the slides individually though the following (about 5 s in each):
(a) 2% $KMnO_4$ (Solution D).
(b) Water.
(c) 2% oxalic acid (Solution E).
(d) Water.
Re-examine the sections. Repeat the differentiating procedure until the desired appearance is obtained.
(6) Wash in water, dehydrate through graded alcohols, clear in xylene, and mount in a resinous medium.

Result
Unmyelinated axons and axonal terminals black. Myelin sheaths, fat and some intracellular granules are also blackened. Other components of the tissue appear in shades of yellowish-grey.

Note

(1) Thin specimens can be prepared as whole mounts. It is important to wash out all the osmium tetroxide before dehydrating, because alcohols reduce OsO_4 (See Chapter 2). Sections need to be fairly thick (20–100 μm).

(2) Iodide–osmium staining has been applied to animal organs to display features other than innervation, including cell-types in lymphoid tissues (Dagdeviren *et al.*, 1994; Crivellato and Mallardi, 1997) and the interstitial cells of Cajal in the alimentary tract (Christensen *et al.*, 1987; Zhou and Komuro, 1995). In glutaraldehyde-fixed plant tissues, iodide–osmium solutions blacken vacuoles that contain penolic compounds (Scalet *et al.*, 1989).

18.5. Chromate precipitation methods

Camillo Golgi (1843–1926) discovered his famous method in 1873 when he observed the blackening of occasional whole neurons in dichromate-fixed blocks of tissue that had been subsequently immersed in a solution of silver nitrate (Corsi, 1987). This serendipitous observation permitted description of the morphology of many types of neuron and heralded the development of the neuron theory. The theory was championed by Santiago Ramon y Cajal (1852–1934), who is generally held to be the greatest of all neurohistologists. Although they disagreed bitterly about the structure of the nervous system, the two men shared the Nobel Prize for Physiology or Medicine in 1906.

There are two major groups of chromate precipitation techniques, known respectively as the Golgi (silver chromate) and Golgi–Cox (mercury chromate) methods. With all these procedures, whole neurons (dendrites, perikarya, and axons) and glial cells are coloured in shades of deep reddish-brown or black. The dark material fills the cells, extending into the smallest branches of cytoplasmic processes. Fortunately, only about 1% of the cells in a specimen are stained, so it is possible to see the shapes of the individual cells very clearly, and to examine large dendritic trees in thick (200 μm) sections. Electron microscopy has revealed that the deposits are located mainly within the cytoplasm, and that within individual stained cells the impregnation is sometimes incomplete. The myelinated parts of axons are rarely darkened by Golgi procedures, and these methods are used principally in the study of dendritic morphology and of the relationships between axonal terminals and the cells with which they synapse.

The silver chromate precipitation procedures that differ only in minor technical details from the original are known as **Golgi methods**: pieces of central nervous tissue are treated with silver nitrate after fixation for several days or weeks in potassium dichromate or in a dichromate-osmium tetroxide mixture. In one of his later variants, Golgi used mercuric chloride instead of silver nitrate, and then obtained a black product by treatment with alkali. In 1894 Cox improved and simplified this variant by fixing for several weeks in a stable aqueous solution containing both $K_2Cr_2O_7$ and $HgCl_2$. Sections were then cut and treated with an aqueous alkali to generate a black product in the selectively stained cells. Chromate precipitation techniques using mercury compounds are generally called **Golgi–Cox methods**. Mercuric chloride or nitrate is mixed with or applied or after the dichromate.

Many variants of the Golgi and Golgi–Cox methods are available for use with material that has been fixed in formaldehyde or glutaraldehyde (e.g. Bertram and Ihrig, 1959; Colonnier, 1964; Fairen *et al.*, 1977; Peters, 1981; Gabbott and Somogyi, 1984; Greer and Jen, 1990). Both mercurous and mercuric nitrates have been used instead of mercuric chloride. Some of these techniques can also be used in conjunction with electron microscopy.

Before using a Golgi method for research purposes, the student is advised to read the references cited here and also to consult earlier reviews by Ramon Moliner (1970) and Kiernan and Berry (1975) in which the advantages and disadvantages of the different techniques are evaluated in relation to particular applications.

18.5.1.
Possible staining mechanisms

As the silver nitrate permeates the chromated tissue, submicroscopic crystals of an insoluble substance are precipitated within the cytoplasm of a small proportion of the cells. Often there is also deposition in blood vessels and formation of crystals that are unrelated to the structure of the tissue. Exsanguination (by saline perfusion of the anaesthetized animal) reduces vascular staining. The precipitated substance has been shown to be silver chromate, Ag_2CrO_4 (Chan-Palay 1973), which is the expected product of the reaction of either K_2CrO_4 or $K_2Cr_2O_7$ with $AgNO_3$ (Cotton *et al.*, 1999).

$$CrO_4^{2-} + 2Ag^+ \longrightarrow Ag_2CrO_4(s)$$

$$Cr_2O_7^{2-} + 4Ag^+ + H_2O \longrightarrow 2AgCrO_4(s) + 2H^+$$

This precipitation is prevented in most parts of a specimen processed by the Golgi method, except within the stained cells. Explanations are not yet available for the peculiar specificity of staining achieved with chromate precipitation techniques, but observations and experiments have provided some information about the way the precipitate forms within cells.

Braitenberg *et al.* (1967) noticed that with a Golgi method of the classical (silver chromate) type, staining of neurites was associated with the appearance of filamentous crystals on the surface of the tissue. They suggested that similar linear crystalline growth might occur within the sporadically impregnated cells. This suggestion receives support from light and electron microscopic observations of the early stages of silver impregnation of the chromated tissue (Spacek, 1989). The precipitation of silver chromate begins at randomly distributed sites, some of which are inside neurons. Only those neurons that contain the initial precipitates become filled by subsequent crystalline growth. The enlargement of the deposits is arrested by natural barriers, including the plasmalemma. There can be little doubt that the membrane phospholipids are stabilized by complexation with chromium (Chapter 12) to the extent that they can limit the growth of the intracellular crystalline mass. The pH of the dichromate solution influences the result, and if a satisfactory result is to be obtained it should rise from about 4 to about 6 during the course of the chromation of the tissue (Angulo *et al.*, 1994). Within a specimen being fixed by dichromate, chromium(VI) is reduced to chromium(III), which cross-links the carboxyl groups of proteins (Casselman, 1955; Kiernan, 1985; see also Chapter 2). It has been suggested that dichromate ions are electrostatically attracted to the bound chromium(III) in the cytoplasm, providing numerous intracytoplasmic sites for the subsequent formation of submicroscopic crystals of silver chromate. The pH-dependence of successful impregnation indicates that it may be the $HCrO_4^-$ ion rather than $Cr_2O_7^{2-}$ or CrO_4^{2-} that diffuses within neurites (Stefanovic *et al.*, 1998).

In the mercury-precipitating Golgi–Cox methods a white substance is deposited in a small proportion of the neurons and glial cells. According to Blackstad *et al.*, (1973) this is probably mercurous chromate (Hg_2CrO_4) after $HgNO_3$, or mercuric oxide chromate ($Hg_3O_2CrO_4$, a salt of the oxonium ion $Hg_3O_2^{2+}$) after $Hg(NO_3)_2$. The blackening by alkali indicates the presence of Hg(I) in the initial precipitate. Many mercurous salts are changed to a black mixture of the metal with mercuric oxide when they react with OH^- ions:

$$2Hg^+ + OH^- \longrightarrow Hg + HgO + H^+$$

18.5.2.
A Golgi (silver chromate) method

This method (Gonzalez-Burgos *et al.*, 1992) was designed for formaldehyde-fixed brains of rodents. The blood of an anaesthetized rat is washed out by perfusion from the left ventricle to the right atrium (Chapter 2 for technique) of 50 ml of 0.1 M sodium phosphate buffer (Chapter 20). This is followed followed by 50 ml of phosphate-buffered 4% formaldehyde (Chapter 2), and the brain is then removed and cut into slices 3–4 mm thick, which are immersed in the same fixative for 24 h.

Solutions required
A. Chromating reagent
This is not stable. It is made on the day it is to be used, by adding formalin and glacial acetic acid to a stable stock solution of potassium dichromate: 2% (w/v) $K_2Cr_2O_7$ in water.

2% potassium dichromate:	50 ml
Formalin (37–40% formaldehyde):	10 ml
Glacial acetic acid:	5 ml

Each specimen requires 15 ml of the working solution.

B. 0.75% Silver nitrate

Silver nitrate (AgNO$_3$):	1.0 g
Water:	133 ml

This can be kept for several years in a glass-stoppered brown bottle. Used solution must not be returned to the stock bottle.

Procedure
(1) Place the fixed specimens in the chromating agent (Solution A; 15 ml for each piece) for 48 h in a dark place. Replace the solution after 24 h.
(2) Wash in water (distilled or deionized), 3 changes of 50 ml per specimen, with continuous shaking or frequent agitation, for a total of 30 min.
(3) Place in 0.75% silver nitrate (Solution B), 15 ml per specimen, for 24 h in a dark place.
(4) Wash in water (distilled or deionized), 3 changes, each 30 min.
(5) Dehydrate, clear and embed in paraffin wax. (See Chapter 4 for suggested schedules. See also *Note 1* below). Cut and mount thick (100–150 μm) sections,
(6) Remove the wax with xylene and mount in a resinous medium. See *Note 2* below.

Result
The background is transparent and pale yellow. Sporadic neurons and neuroglial cells are black. Dendritic trees are shown in their entirety and the axons of small (local circuit) neurons are commonly visible.

Notes
(1) Alternatively, embed in nitrocellulose. Following a similar Golgi procedure, Angulo *et al.* (1994) cut sections 200–300 μm thick with a vibrating microtome.
(2) The black deposits in neurons can fade over a period of months to years, possibly by reaction with reducing agents in the mounting medium. Fading can be avoided by applying a viscous resinous mountant without a cover glass (Gray, 1954). The slides must be protected from dust. See also *Note 3* at the end of the next method.

18.5.3.
A Golgi–Cox (mercury chromate) method

Although they are slow, the Golgi–Cox methods are possibly the most reliable of the Golgi techniques, especially for demonstrating the dendritic architecture of neurons in the mammalian CNS. The anaesthetized animal should be perfused with saline to remove blood before removing the brain. The whole brain of a rat or mouse may be immersed in the Golgi–Cox fixative (Step 1 of the procedure below).

Solutions required
A. Golgi–Cox fixative
This is prepared from three stable stock solutions:

(1) 5% aqueous mercuric chloride ($HgCl_2$)
(2) 5% aqueous potassium dichromate ($K_2Cr_2O_7$)
(3) 5% aqueous potassium chromate (K_2CrO_4)

Working solution
Mix in order:

(1):	20 ml
(2):	20 ml
Water:	40 ml
(3):	16 ml

Caution. $HgCl_2$ can cause acute poisoning and chronic disease. Exposure to chromates in industry can cause a variety of serious disorders. The Golgi–Cox fixative must be collected and treated as hazardous waste, in accordance with institutional and governmental regulations.

B. Alkaline developer

Strong ammonia solution (17% NH_3):	5 ml
Water:	95 ml

Mix just before using.

Procedure
(1) Fix pieces of nervous tissue (not more than 10 mm thick) in the working solution of Golgi–Cox fixative. The for 2–8 weeks in a tightly capped container at 37°C. A gauze pad in the bottom of the container facilitates even penetration. Pour off the fixative and replace it with fresh solution after the first day. (See also *Note 1* below.)
(2) Wash in water, many changes, for 6–8 h, then dehydrate and embed in nitrocellulose. (See *Note 2* for quicker, simpler methods.)
(3) Cut sections 100 μm thick. Handle them with glass hooks or wax-coated forceps.
(4) Treat the sections with the alkaline developer (Solution B) for 2 or 3 min.
(5) Wash in two changes of water, dehydrate, clear, and mount in a resinous medium. (See *Note 3* below.)

Result
Some neurons and neuroglial cells, including their cytoplasmic processes are black, on a pale yellow or colourless background. Axons are not usually stained.

Notes
(1) Specimens can be fixed (buffered formaldehyde perfusion, followed by immersion for a few days, and washing in 3 changes of water for at least 6 h altogether to remove formaldehyde. The ideal time in the Golgi–Cox fixative must be determined by trial for each type of tissue. 3 weeks is often long enough for rodent brains.
(2) As an alternative to nitrocellulose embedding, immerse the fixed blocks in 30% aqueous sucrose solution at 4°C until they sink (1 or 2 days), and cut

frozen sections (Kolb and McClimans, 1986; Greer and Jen, 1990). Vibrating microtome sections are also suitable (Gibb and Kolb, 1998), and do not require prior cryoprotection with sucrose. Sections cut with a freezing or vibrating microtome are washed in water mounted onto slides that have been coated with 1% gelatin, and thoroughly dried before moving to Step 4.

(3) For nitrocellulose sections a mixture of chloroform (33 ml), xylene (33 ml), and absolute ethanol (33 ml) is preferred to absolute alcohol for the last stage of dehydration (following 95% alcohol). This can be followed by clearing for 10–15 min in creosote (beechwood) or in cedarwood oil, followed by a rinse in xylene.

The black colour fades with time if a coverslip is applied (see *Note 3* following the previous method). It is usual to mount the sections in **thick** Canada balsam, and allow to set at 40–45°C without a coverslip. Such preparations are stable for many years. If a synthetic mounting medium such as DPX is used, coverslips may be applied, but fading may occur after as little as 6 months. It is possible to modify the Golgi and Golgi–Cox deposits chemically, to produce more stable black substances (see Geisert and Updyke, 1977; Wouterlood *et al.*, 1983, for details).

19 Immunohistochemistry

In the preceding chapters attempts have been made to show how the principles of chemistry and biochemistry are applied for the localization of substances within tissues. This chapter is concerned with methods based on the precepts of immunology. Students totally unfamiliar with this science are advised to read an introductory text such as Bona and Bonilla (1996), Delves *et al.* (2006), or the relevant parts of a textbook of pathology. Fortunately the immunological principles applicable to microscopical techniques are fairly easy to grasp. Books on immunohistochemical techniques by Polak and Van Noorden (1997), Beesley (2001) and Boenisch (2001) are recommended. For simultaneous immunostaining of multiple antigens, see Van der Loos (1999). These methods are employed in many fields of biological research, and are regularly used in diagnostic histopathology. The required reagents are available commercially except for new antibodies used in research, which must be raised in the laboratory.

Immunohistochemical staining is based on **affinity** between antigens and antibodies. Affinity is the attractive force between molecules that causes them to join together and stay joined. In the case of immunological reactions, the forces of affinity are not covalent; they resemble the binding of many dyes by their substrates (Chapter 5), but generally are much more specific. Comparable affinity exists between lectins and the carbohydrates to which they bind (Chapter 11). There are histochemical techniques that exploit biologically important affinities other than those of lectins and antibodies. One such group of methods, the hybridization of nucleic acids, is discussed in Chapter 9.

19.1. Antigens and antibodies

Vertebrate animals are able to defend themselves against the potentially harmful effects of macromolecules derived from other organisms. Any such foreign material that may enter an animal s body is called an **antigen**. When an antigen is introduced into the extracellular fluid of an animal, some of its molecules are carried, by lymph or blood-vessels, to lymph nodes. Here the antigen molecules come into contact with small lymphocytes of the B-type (bone-marrow derived). These react to the encounter by transforming themselves into plasma cells, which synthesize and secrete **antibodies**. These are proteins of the γ-globulin (gamma-globulin) class that can combine specifically with the antigens that evoked their production. It will be noticed that the words 'antigen' and 'antibody' are difficult to define. An antibody is a substance produced in response to the presence of an antigen. The antibodies secreted by plasma cells in lymphoid tissues circulate in the blood plasma and so gain access to all parts of the body including the original sites of introduction of antigens. The combination of an antibody with its antigen commonly results in neutralization of the toxicity or pathogenicity of the latter.

When a molecule of antigen bumps into a molecule of its antibody, the two combine to form an **antigen–antibody complex**. This happens because part of the antibody molecule has been specially tailored to accommodate part of the antigen molecule. The reaction is reminiscent of the 'lock-and-key' mechanism by which an enzyme combines with its substrate. The two components of the complex are held together by non-covalent forces such as ionic attraction, hydrogen bonding, and hydrophobic interaction.

The part of an antigen molecule that joins it to the antibody is known as an **antigenic determinant** or **epitope**. A large protein molecule, or an object such as a bacterium that consists of many different macromolecules, will have many antigenic determinants and will therefore evoke the synthesis of many different species of antibody molecule, all capable of combining with the same antigen. It is, however, a property of all antibodies that they form complexes only with the antigens that stimulated their production. This specificity is fundamental to the techniques of immunohistochemistry.

Although each antibody molecule binds only to its specific epitope, two closely similar proteins may react with an antibody raised to only one of them. Such **cross-reactivity** occurs when the antigenic determinant site is a short sequence of amino acids common to both the proteins. Cross-reactivity is sometimes a source of confusion in the interpretation of immunohistochemically stained preparations because it cannot be detected by the usual controls for specificity. The subject will not be further considered in this introductory account. For discussions concerning specificity see Swaab *et al.* (1977), Hutson *et al.* (1979), and Vandesande (1979).

19.2. Antibody molecules

The antibodies circulating in the blood belong to the γ-globulin class of plasma proteins, and are known as **immunoglobulins**. The most abundant type is immunoglobulin G (IgG). This is not the only kind of immunoglobulin. The other types, however, are relatively unimportant to the immunohistochemist. The IgG molecule consists of two identical subunits joined by a disulphide (cystine) bridge. Each subunit comprises two polypeptide chains: a long one, the heavy (H) chain, and a short one, the light (L) chain. The H chain is joined to the L chain by a disulphide bridge. The structure of IgG is shown diagrammatically in *Fig. 19.1*. It can be seen that the molecule is Y-shaped. The stem of the Y and the proximal parts of the arms have the same amino acid composition in all the IgG molecules of a given species of animal. Specificity for antigens resides in the distal (variable) part of the H and L chains constituting the two limbs of the Y. Each limb is capable of combining with an antigenic determinant and is therefore called an antibody fragment or **Fab**. The stem of the Y, consisting of parts of both H chains, is called the constant fragment or **Fc**. The Fab and Fc fragments can be isolated by collecting the products of digestion of IgG by papain, a proteolytic enzyme. Other fragments have been isolated from the products of attack by other enzymes and by disulphide-splitting reagents.

From the point of view of the immunohistochemist, the IgG molecule has three important features:

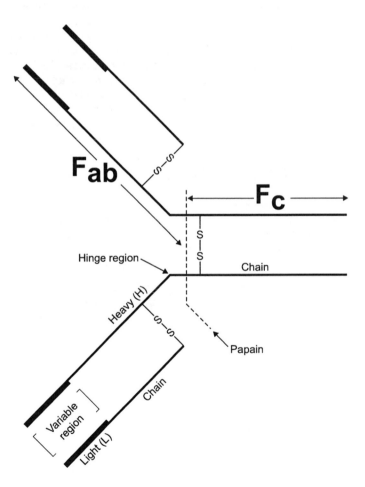

Figure 19.1. Diagram showing the structure of one molecule of immunoglobulin G (IgG). The antibody-combining sites are the variable regions of the two Fab segments. When IgG serves as an antigen in immunohistochemical techniques it is the Fc segment of the molecule that is the antigenic determinant. Each IgG molecule is potentially capable of combining with two specific antigenic determinant sites. The distance between these two sites may vary because there is flexibility at the hinge region of the H chains. Note that papain releases one Fc and two Fab fragments from each IgG molecule. Cleavage of the disulphide bridges yields two H chains and two L chains. Oligosaccharides are attached to the H chains in the Fc segment.

(1)   There are two sites, the ends of the Fab segments, capable of binding to an antigenic determinant. Thus, the antibody molecule is **bivalent**.

(2)   Part of the IgG molecule, the Fc fragment, is common to all antibodies of the animal species concerned and is not involved in combining with antigens.

(3)   Immunoglobulins are themselves macromolecules and as such can behave as antigens when injected into different species of animals. Because the Fc fragment has a constant chemical structure, it is possible to raise in one species antibodies against all the possible immunoglobulins that might be produced by another species of animal. Such antibodies (contained in anti-γ-globulin antisera) are important immunohistochemical reagents. As an antigen, the Fc chain of an IgG molecule may have several antigenic sites and be able to bind more than one molecule of anti-antibody.

Antibody molecules are large: the MW of IgG is 150 000. For this reason it is possible to conjugate some of their amino acid side-chains with other compounds such as fluorochromes or enzymes. This process, known as **labelling**, usually involves the formation of covalent linkages with the ε-amino groups of lysine. The combining properties of an antibody will remain intact provided that the labelling molecule does not sterically obstruct the specific 'keyholes' formed by the distal parts of the Fab segments. In solution, the molecules of a labelling agent react randomly with different parts of the molecules of IgG, so some blocking of the combining sites is inevitable. Consequently the potency of an antibody-containing solution is always reduced by combination with a fluorescent or enzymatic label.

19.3. Antigen–antibody complexes

When a solution containing an antigen is mixed with a solution containing appropriate antibodies, the antigen–antibody complex often precipitates. Insoluble aggregates are formed because each antibody molecule is bivalent and each antigen molecule has multiple determinant sites. If either component of the mixture is present in excess, the aggregates will be smaller and will remain soluble.

If an antigen forms part of a solid structure, such as a cell in a section of a tissue, it is able to bind antibody molecules from an applied solution:

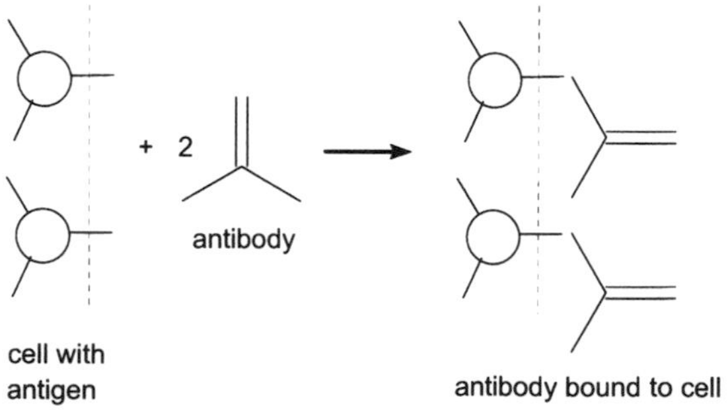

cell with
antigen

antibody

antibody bound to cell

The antibody is quite firmly attached. It is not removed when the preparation is rinsed with saline, though it could be removed by excessive washing. Similar attachment occurs when a dissolved antigen is brought into contact with an object such as a plasma cell which contains appropriate antibodies:

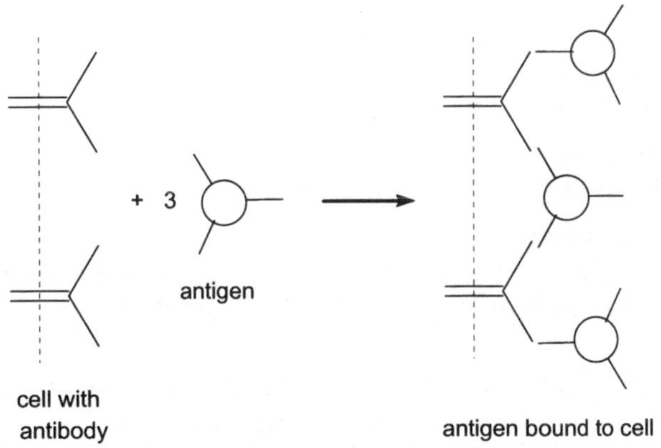

cell with
antibody   antigen bound to cell

The number of molecules bound from an applied solution depends on the abundance of combining sites in the specimen. Steric factors are also important: if in the above example the two antibody molecules were further apart, they would be able to unite with four antigen molecules rather than three.

It is possible to label antibodies by conjugating them with fluorochromes or with histochemically demonstrable enzymes. Consequently, if a solution of a labelled antibody is applied to a section of tissue containing the appropriate antigen, the label will be detected at the sites of antigen–antibody complexes. The techniques of immunohistochemistry are based on the use of labelled antibodies, but the methodology is, unfortunately, not quite as simple as might at first be thought. Technical complexities are introduced by the need to enhance sensitivity and to suppress the attachment of reagents to tissue by mechanisms other than specific antigen–antibody affinity.

19.4. Mini-immunoglossary

The understanding of immunohistochemical methods will be easier if some commonly used terms are first defined.

Absorption
(1)   Neutralization of specific antibody in an antiserum, by adding an excess of the appropriate antigen.
(2)   Removal of unreacted fluorochrome from a solution containing conjugated proteins, by treatment with activated charcoal.
(3)   Treatment of a labelled antiserum with powdered acetone-fixed tissue, such as liver or kidney, in order to remove unwanted labelled proteins that bind to tissues by non-immune mechanisms. The tissue powder must not, of course, contain the antigen to which the antiserum was raised.
(4)   The wavelength of light from a microscope's lamp that stimulates a fluorochrome to emit light of a different colour.

Amplification
The generation of several molecules of a visible substance at the site of detection of each single molecule of interest in a specimen. For example, two antibody molecules might bind to one antigenic site, and each antibody might carry several fluorescent labelling molecules. Enzymatic labels can use indefinite amounts of substrate to generate insoluble, coloured products. A physical developer can deposit black metallic silver on submicroscopic colloidal gold particles, increasing their diameters hundreds of times.

Antiserum

Serum containing antibodies to an antigen. Loosely used also for diluted sera, diluted solutions of the globulin fraction, and solutions of affinity-purified antibodies (Section 19.5.1). Antisera are polyclonal.

Emission

The wavelength of light emitted by a fluorescent substance.

Fluorescence

Immediate emission by a specimen of light that typically is visible and of longer wavelength than the light falling on the specimen.

Globulin

The proteins remaining in serum after removal of the albumin by chromatographic or other separation methods. The γ-globulin fraction, comprising the immunoglobulins, constitutes approximately one-third of the total globulin. The concentration of γ-globulin in whole serum ranges from 7 to 15 mg/ml.

Immunization

Administration of antigen to an animal to evoke the production of antibodies. Originally the word was applied to the induction of immunity to infectious diseases. It now enjoys wider usage. The act of injecting antigenic material is often called **inoculation**.

Immunocytochemistry

Widely used as synonym for **immunohistochemistry** but strictly applicable only when cells or intracellular structures are the objects of interest.

Immunofluorescence

Secondary fluorescence introduced into tissues by the application of immunohistochemical methods in which fluorochromes are used as labels.

Immunostain

A useful verb, meaning to carry out an immunohistochemical procedure.

Label

A molecule artificially attached to a protein, typically by covalent bonding. The type of labelling used in an immunohistochemical method determines the amount of **amplification**, and therefore the sensitivity of the technique. The most frequently used labels are:

Ordinary dyes and **radioactive isotopes**, but these are for applications other than immunohistochemistry.

Fluorescent substances. The absorption and emission spectra of different fluorochromes are exploited when two or more labelled antibodies are applied to the same preparation.

Enzymes for which simple, reliable histochemical methods are available. Horseradish peroxidase (HRP) and alkaline phosphatase are the most popular labels of this type.

Biotin is an easily attached organic label that can be detected by virtue of its specific affinity for **avidin**, a protein that can itself be labelled with fluorochromes or enzymes.

Colloidal gold particles attached to protein molecules are directly detectable by electron microscopy, but to be seen with light they must be enlarged by **physical development**, which is the gold-catalyzed deposition silver from a temporarily stabilized mixture of silver ions with a reducing agent.

Monoclonal antibody (or MAB)

A single species of antibody globulin, produced by the identical cultured descendants (clone) of a single antibody-producing cell. A MAB recognizes a specific epitope, which may be a quite short sequence of amino acids. Most MABs are mouse immunoglobulins.

Phosphorescence

This is similar to **fluorescence**, but there is an interlude of time between the absorption of the exciting light and the radiation of the emitted light. The delay may be measured in microseconds, but it allows electronic instruments to separate nonspecific background fluorescence from the emission of a phosphorescent label.

Plasma

Blood without cells, obtained by preventing coagulation and then removing the cells by centrifugation.

Polyclonal

Describes a reagent that contains antibodies derived from an indefinite number of non-identical antibody-producing cells. Antisera are polyclonal.

Primary

The antibody or antiserum that combines specifically with the antigen of interest. Except in the direct immunofluorescence technique, a primary antibody or antiserum is unlabelled.

Saline

Water is unphysiological and alcohol denatures proteins. Immunological reagents are usually dissolved in a solution of sodium chloride, 0.7–0.9% in a buffer (such as 0.03 M phosphate) at pH 7.2–7.4. Phosphate-buffered saline is commonly called **PBS**. When used as a solvent in immunohistochemical procedures, 'saline' may optionally contain a surfactant and a protein, as explained in Section 19.12. Saline solutions are not necessarily ideal diluents, especially for monoclonal antibodies, which often give superior results when applied from a 0.05 M TRIS buffer, at pH 6.0 or 8.5, without added NaCl (Boenisch, 1999).

Secondary

A secondary antiserum is one that combines with the Fc fragments of previously applied primary antibody molecules whose Fab fragments are bound to antigenic sites in a specimen. The secondary antiserum may or may not be labelled.

Serum

Blood plasma from which the fibrinogen has been removed. Mammalian sera contain about 8% w/v protein, consisting of approximately equal proportions of albumin and globulin.

19.5. Direct fluorescent antibody methods

These are the simplest and oldest immunohistochemical methods. A known antigen in a section or smear of tissue is localized by virtue of its combination with fluorescently labelled molecules of its antibody. The technique has several shortcomings and is not often used, but it will be described in some detail in order to introduce principles that apply also to the more complicated modern methods.

19.5.1.
Antibody
production

It is first necessary to isolate the antigen and purify it as much as possible. An animal (of a species other than that from which the antigen was taken, if the antigen is of animal origin) is then immunized by injecting it, usually on several occasions, with the purified antigen. When the animal has a high circulating level of antibody, blood is collected and the serum, an **antiserum**, is separated. If possible, the globulin or, preferably, the γ-globulin fraction, is isolated from the antiserum. The techniques for purification of antigen, immunization, and isolation of serum proteins require some expertise in practical biochemistry and immunology. Apparatus not usually available in a general histology laboratory is also needed. Very detailed descriptions of most of the practical procedures used in immunology are given by Garvey *et al.* (1977) and Lefkovits and Pernis (1979–1990). Thousands of pure antigenic substances and antisera are available commercially, and the production of antibodies in the laboratory is an activity of research workers investigating new and unusual antigens.

An antiserum may be further purified by **affinity chromatography**. The serum is poured into a column that contains the antigen bound to an insoluble support, and all the unbound components are washed off with saline. The bound antibody is then eluted from the column by an acidic buffer, which weakens the antigen–antibody attraction.

19.5.2.
Fluorescent labelling

The following account applies to attachment of fluorescent labelling molecules to any protein or mixture of proteins. In the present context the material to be labelled is a primary antiserum.

The most frequently used labelling reagents are **fluorescein isothiocyanate** (FITC) and **tetramethylrhodamine isothiocyanate** (TRITC):

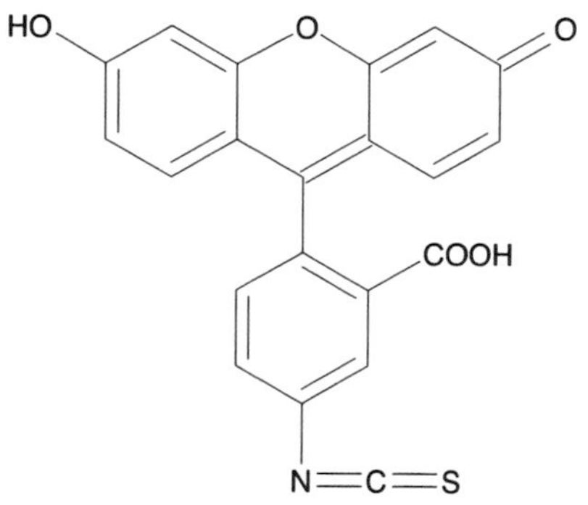

fluorescein isothiocyanate
('isomer 1')

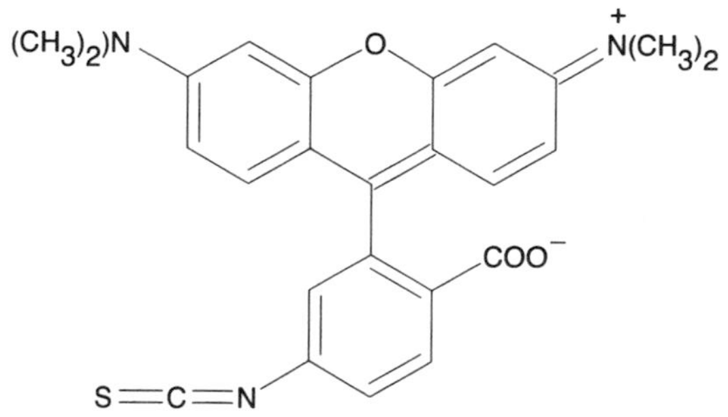

tetramethylrhodamine
isothiocyanate
('R isomer')

In alkaline solution (pH 9–10), these compounds combine covalently with proteins, reacting principally with the ε-amino group of lysine to form thiourea derivatives:

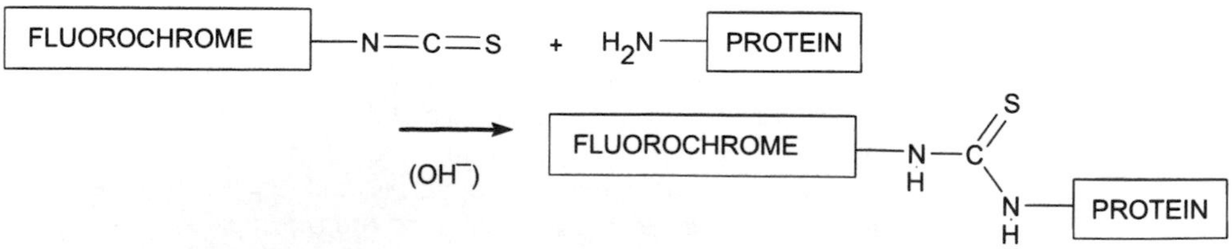

Other reactive groups used for the same purpose are **sulphonyl chloride** ($-SO_2Cl$), which forms sulphonamides:

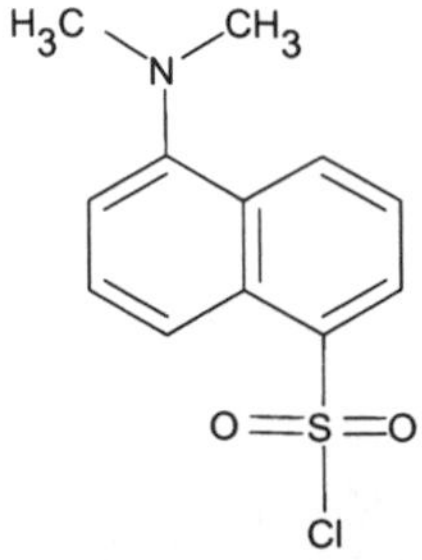

1-dimethylaminonaphthalene-
5-sulphonyl chloride
(dansyl chloride)

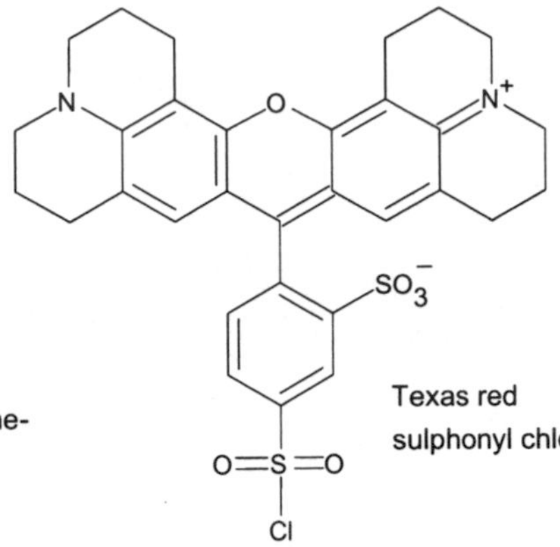

Texas red
sulphonyl chloride

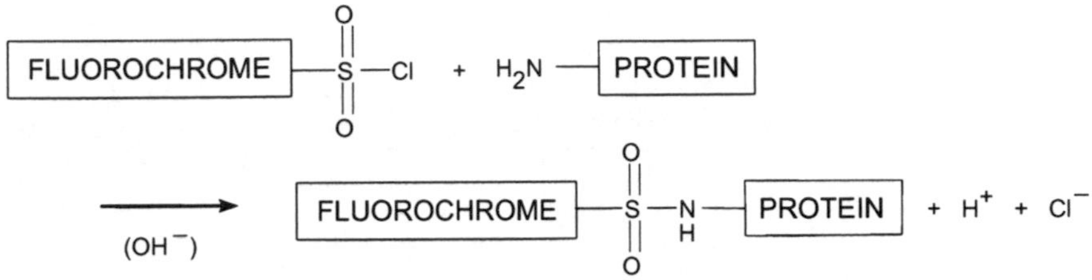

and **dichlorotriazinyl**, which forms stable secondary amine-like compounds with amines:

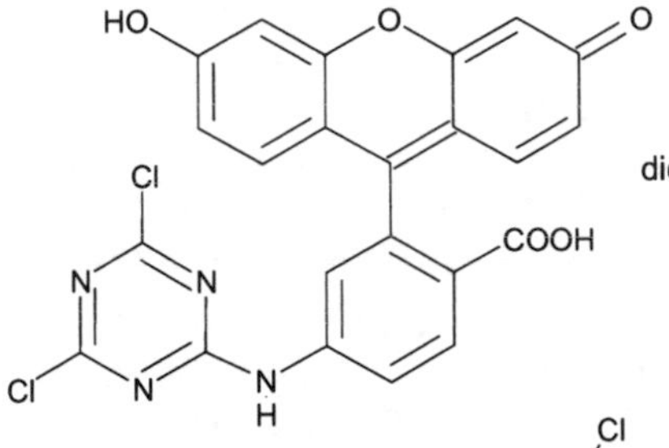

dichlorotriazinylfluorescein
("6-isomer")

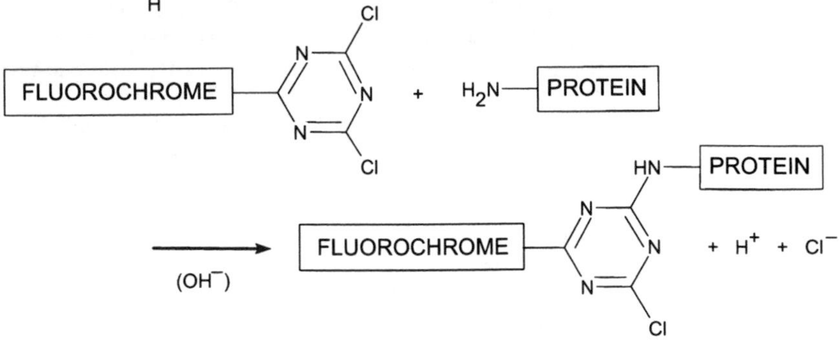

but can combine also with thiol and hydroxyl groups (Section 5.3). The second chlorine atom of the dichlorotriazinyl group is less reactive. It may eventually be replaced by −OH in stored aqueous solutions, but this does not matter. Various **succinimidyl esters** can be attached to fluorescent compounds, and these also react with amino groups to form stable covalent conjugates:

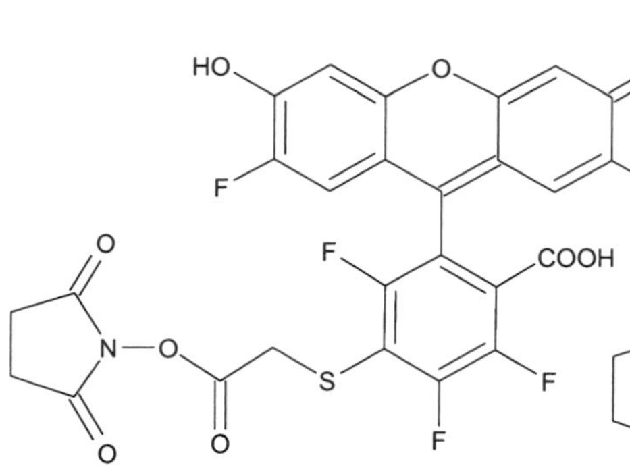

Oregon green 514 succinimidyl ester

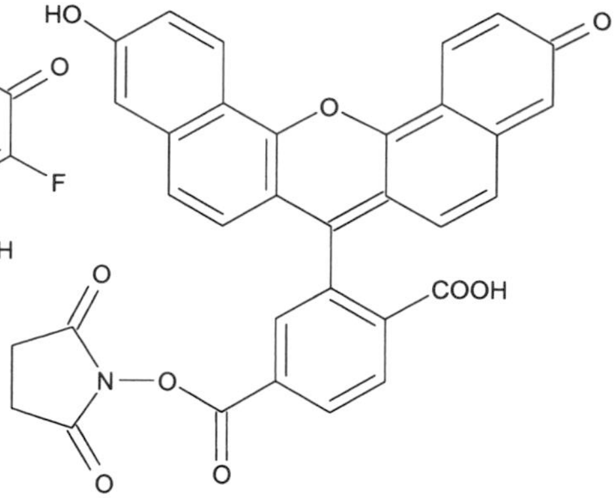

naphthofluorescein succinimidyl ester

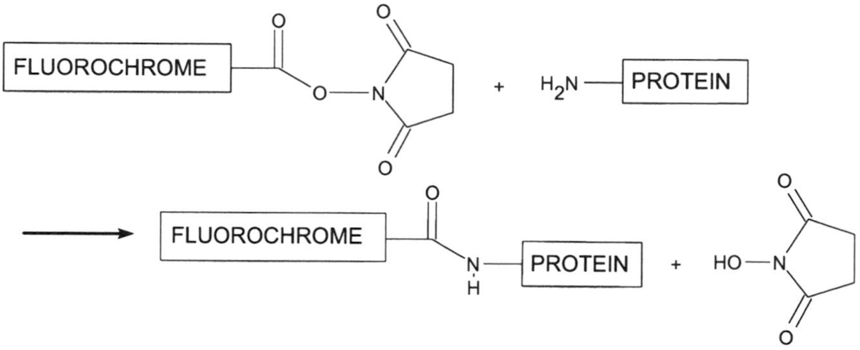

The fluorochrome will, of course, conjugate with all the types of protein present in the serum, not just with the antibody or antibodies of interest. Unbound fluorescent material will also be present because some hydrolysis of the labelling agent occurs in the alkaline medium that is necessary for reaction with amines.

Unconjugated fluorescent material must be removed because it would stain tissues in its own right. The labelled serum is therefore dialysed to remove small molecules (MW below about 5000) and to replace the alkaline solvent with a saline solution of physiological pH. It may also be passed through a gel-filtration column, which retains small molecules, or it may be treated with activated charcoal, which does much the same thing. Sometimes all three methods are used. Finally, the serum is concentrated by dialysis against an inert synthetic polymer such as polyvinylpyrollidone. The labelled antiserum is now ready for use. Practical instructions for preparing labelled proteins are given by Nairn (1976) and Pearse and Stoward (1980).

A different type of fluorescent labelling can be accomplished by tagging proteins with chelates of certain rare earth (lanthanide) metals, notably europium and terbium. These compounds fade less than wholly organic fluorochromes and they are not adversely affected by dehydration and resinous mounting media (Soini *et al.*, 1988; Seveus *et al.*, 1994). Unfortunately, they are commercial products of undisclosed identity. Europium chelates are **phosphorescent labels**: their fluorescence persists for a short time after shutting off the exciting light. With appropriate equipment (laser scanning time-resolved microscopy), the fluorescence of the label can be separated from the autofluorescence of the tissue, and collected by a sensitive video camera (Dehaas *et al.*, 1996). A platinum–porphyrin complex has also been used as a phosphorescent label (Dehaas *et al.*, 1997).

19.5.3.
Immunostaining procedure

Sections of the antigen-containing specimen are cut and mounted onto slides or coverslips. (See Section 19.12.1 for remarks on fixation and tissue processing for immunohistochemistry.) The sections are rinsed with saline and a drop of labelled antiserum is placed on each. Various twofold dilutions of the serum in saline are tried. Dilutions weaker than 1:8 are unlikely to be needed for direct fluorescent anti-body methods. The serum is left in contact with the sections, in a humid atmosphere, for approximately 1 h. It is then washed off with saline and a coverslip is applied. Immunofluorescent preparations are usually mounted in a mixture of glycerol and a somewhat alkaline buffer (Chapter 4, Section 4.3.2.2). Resinous mounting media have been said to weaken the intensity of the fluorescence (Nairn, 1976), but dehydration in alcohol, clearing in xylene and mounting in DPX provides permanent preparations (Espada *et al.*, 2005).

The stained, mounted sections are examined by fluorescence microscopy, with appropriate excitation and filtering for the label that has been used (Section 19.12.6).

19.5.2.
Controls

The following control procedures must be carried out alongside the definitive staining technique.

(1) Incubate in saline alone. The only fluorescence seen will be autofluorescence.

(2) Incubate in a fluorescently labelled nonimmune serum derived from the same species as that in which the antiserum was raised. Any fluorescence seen in this control but not in No. 1 will be due to nonspecific attachment of fluorescent proteins to the section. Absorption of the labelled antiserum with a tissue powder may help to eliminate this artifact.

(3) If possible, incubate with labelled antiserum an identically processed section known not to contain the antigen. (This is possible only when the antigen is one foreign to the tissue, such as bacteria or a foreign protein). The specimens for this control should be of the same tissue as that used for the definitive procedure.

(4) Mix some labelled antiserum with a solution in saline of the purified antigen if this is available. A large excess of the latter should be present in the mixture. The added antigen combines with the antibody and little or no specific fluorescence should be seen in a section stained with this absorbed antiserum.

(5) If possible, stain a section known to contain the antigen of interest.

19.5.3.
Shortcomings of the direct method

With the direct fluorescent antibody method it is not possible to localize antigens present at low concentrations in a tissue. There are two reasons for this lack of sensitivity:

(1) The process of conjugation with a reactive fluorochrome will block the combining sites of some of the antibody molecules, reducing the potency of the antiserum. The likelihood of attachment of label to the combining site will be reduced if the concentration of the labelling agent is low, but then the number of fluorescent groups usefully attached to antibody molecules will also be less. An ideally labelled antiserum has about 10 fluorochrome molecules attached to each molecule of IgG.

(2) The immunological reaction in the direct method is:

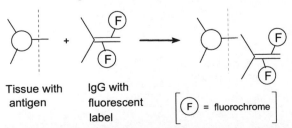

Tissue with antigen   IgG with fluorescent label   [(F) = fluorochrome]

Thus, only one molecule of antibody, with its attached fluorochrome, combines with each antigenic determinant site in the tissue. If the concentration of antigen is low, the density of bound fluorochrome molecules may not be high enough to permit their detection under the microscope. In other methods it is possible to accumulate greater numbers of molecules of visible substances at each antigenic site.

Another objection to the direct method arises from the necessity to label a primary antiserum. Primary antisera are troublesome to prepare or expensive to buy, and often are available only in small quantities. The conjugation also requires time and effort. An investigation of the localizations of several antigens would demand the preparation of as many labelled antisera: an inordinate amount of work and expense. In the methods to be described next, a single labelled antiserum will render visible the sites of localization of any number of different antigens.

19.6. Indirect fluorescence techniques

With indirect methods it is possible to identify either antigens or antibodies (Section 19.10.2) in a tissue. The reagent common to the procedures of this type is a fluorescently labelled antiserum to immunoglobulin: an anti-antibody. The method for demonstration of a tissue antigen will illustrate the principle of the method.

19.6.1.
Method for detection of an antigen

A section containing the antigen is first incubated with a suitable dilution of an appropriate antiserum. This antiserum, which is not labelled, is called the **primary antiserum**:

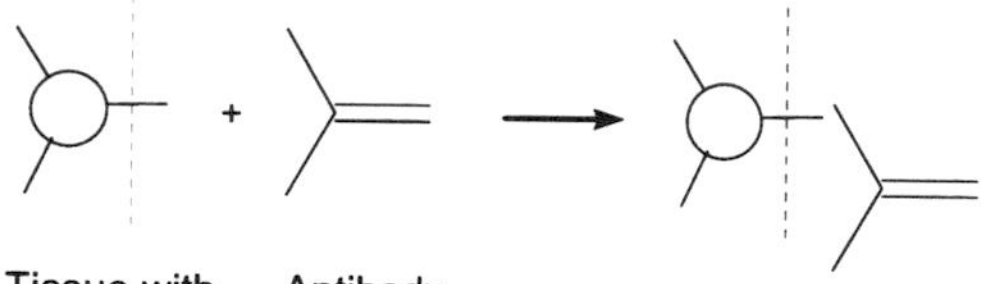

Tissue with   Antibody
antigen   in primary
                 antiserum

The antibody molecules that attach to the antigenic sites in the tissue are immunoglobulins. Their Fc segments are the same as those of all other immunoglobulins of the same species and can themselves serve as antigens. It is possible to raise an anti-immunoglobulin antiserum by injecting into another species of animal some γ-globulin from the blood of the species that was the source of the primary antiserum. This **secondary antiserum** may be labelled by conjugating it with a fluorescent dye. Secondary antisera, unlabelled and labelled, are commercially available and the supplier usually provides suggestions for dilution and times of application in different immunohistochemical techniques.

In the next stage of the staining method, the section is treated with fluorescently labelled secondary antiserum. The anti-IgG molecules in it will bind to the Fc segments of the already attached immunoglobulin molecules derived from the primary antiserum:

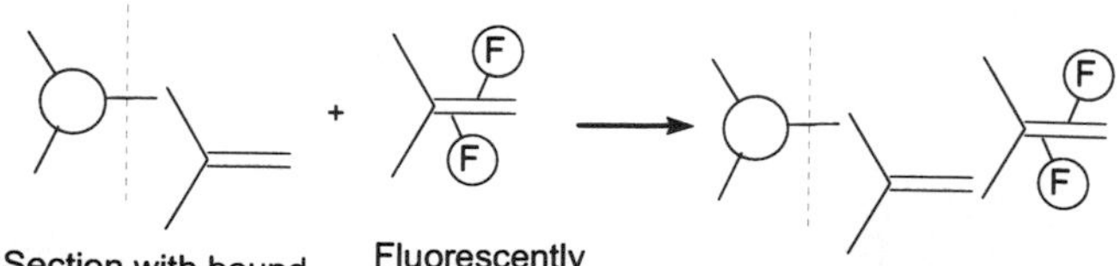

Section with bound   Fluorescently
primary antibody   labelled IgG from
                         secondary
                         antiserum

Thus, the fluorochrome will be seen at the sites occupied by the antigen.

A specific example will further clarify the technique. Let us suppose that a guinea-pig has been given an intravenous injection of egg albumen. Several hours later the foreign protein will be present in the renal tubules. We have available an antiserum to egg albumen raised in a rabbit. This *rabbit anti-(egg albumen)* is the **primary antiserum**. We also have a fluorescently labelled antiserum to rabbit immunoglobulin. The latter antiserum was raised in a goat, so it is *labelled goat anti-(rabbit γ-globulin)*: the **secondary antiserum**. Sections of one of the guinea-pig's kidneys are treated as follows:

(1) Rinse in saline.
(2) Apply rabbit anti-(egg albumen). Use serial twofold dilutions in saline, from 1:10 to 1:160. Leave in contact with the sections for 30 min at room temperature in a humid atmosphere.
(3) Rinse sections with three changes of saline.
(4) Apply labelled goat anti-(rabbit immunoglobulin). Try 1:10 and 1:40 dilutions, for 30 min.
(5) Rinse sections with three changes of saline.
(6) Mount in buffered glycerol (Chapter 4) and examine by fluorescence microscopy.

The sera are diluted in order to minimize nonspecific adherence of protein molecules to the sections. This would result in fluorescence at sites other than those containing the antigen. It is usually necessary also to use one or two of the other tricks that are available to suppress nonspecific binding of immunoglobulins (Section 19.12.3).

Usually the dilution of a primary antiserum is more critical than that of a secondary antiserum. Diluted sera containing 0.1–1.0 mg of total protein per ml are often the most satisfactory for indirect immunofluorescence methods. For a monoclonal antibody or an affinity-purified antiserum, the protein content may be hundreds of times less than this. Vendors of primary antibodies commonly provide leaflets with suggested dilutions; the optimum dilution can be determined only by trials with sections known to contain the antigen.

**19.6.2.
Controls**

As with the direct fluorescent antibody method, control procedures are necessary. These are:

(1) Omit treatment with both sera to reveal the autofluorescence of the tissue.
(2) Omit treatment with the primary antiserum. Incubate with saline instead. Any fluorescence seen cannot be due to the antigen and is either autofluorescence or a result of non-specific binding of fluorescently labelled proteins from the secondary antiserum.
(3) In place of the primary antiserum, use non-immune serum from the same species as that in which the primary antiserum was raised. Ideally this should be a 'pre-immune' serum, which is a sample taken from the individual animal that was later inoculated with the antigen. If fluorescence is seen that does not appear in controls 1 and 2, the primary antiserum used in the definitive method is being bound to the tissue, either by a non-immune mechanism (background fluorescence), or by specific affinity. (The latter might be due to a recent bacterial or viral infection common to the animal from which the tissue was collected and the animal that was used to raise the primary antibody.)
(4) Mix the primary antiserum with an excess of the purified antigen, if this is available. Absent or greatly diminished immunofluorescence should be obtained after application of this absorbed antiserum. This is a negative con-

trol procedure, and it does not prove that the primary antibody will bind to its antigen in cells or tissues (Burry, 2000).

(5) Apply the complete procedure to a section of a tissue known not to contain the antigen. (In the example above, this negative control would be a section of kidney from a guinea-pig that had not been injected with egg albumen.)

(6) Apply the complete procedure to a section of a tissue known to contain the antigen in specific sites: a positive control.

In laboratories with well established procedures, Controls 5 and 6 are sufficient for routine immunostaining. Controls 1, 2, 3 and 4 are necessary for new primary antibodies and for troubleshooting if unexpected results are obtained.

19.6.3
Critique of the method

This technique is superior to the direct immunofluorescent method for two reasons:

(1) It is not necessary to label and thereby reduce the potency of the valuable primary antiserum. Labelled secondary antisera are quite cheap (as laboratory supplies go) and are useful for the detection of any antigen.

(2) The determinant sites of antigens are multiple. This is true of the antigen in the tissue and of the Fc segments of the antibody molecules derived from the primary antiserum. Consequently, more than one molecule of fluorescent antibody from the secondary antiserum will be able to attach to each molecule of the primary antibody. For example, two suitably spaced antigenic determinant sites in a section will bind two antibody molecules from a primary antiserum:

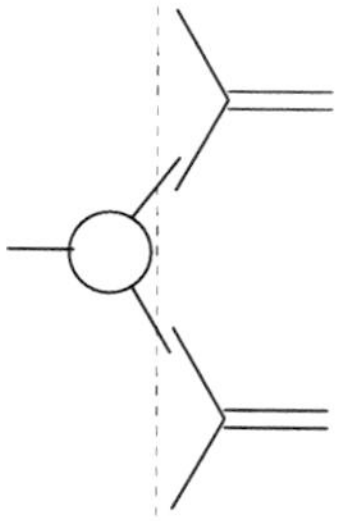

If each of these bound antibody molecules also has two antigenic determinant sites on its Fc segment, four molecules of fluorescent anti-antibody will be bound:

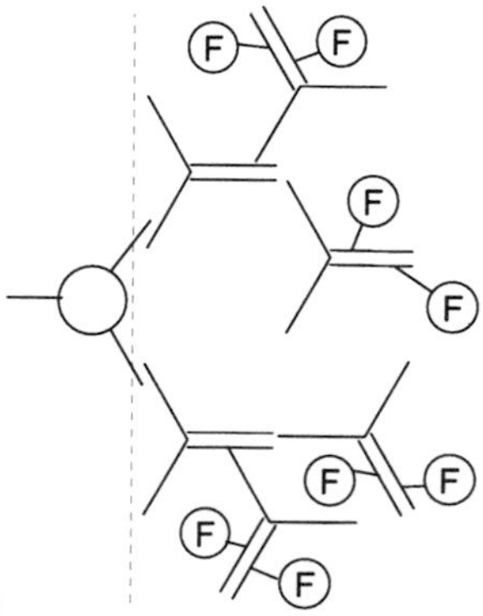

In this example, each antigen molecule has accreted twice as many fluorescent molecules as would have been possible had a direct immunofluorescent method been used. In reality the amplification factor is greater than 2. Indirect immunohistochemical techniques are always more sensitive than direct ones.

The indirect immunofluorescence method is versatile, and has fewer steps than the more sensitive enzymatic procedures discussed in the later sections of this chapter. By using primary antisera raised in different species, it is possible to localize three or four antigens in the same section, by applying secondary antisera conjugated with different fluorochromes (Staines et al., 1988). Multiple labelling procedures have many steps and they are used mainly in research. Confocal microscopy provides high resolution and the ability to collect and electronically manipulate images obtained from specimens that contain different fluorochromes.

19.7. Enzyme-labelled antibody methods

In these techniques antibodies are labelled by conjugation with enzymes. The enzyme currently most in favour is horseradish peroxidase (HRP). Simple and reliable histochemical methods are available for the localization of peroxidases and some of them yield products that can be detected by both light and electron microscopy (Chapter 16).

19.7.1.
Enzyme conjugation

Various methods of conjugation are feasible. A simple one consists of mixing solutions containing the antibody and HRP and then adding a little glutaraldehyde. Cross-linking of protein molecules occurs by the same chemical reactions as those involved in the fixation of tissues by glutaraldehyde (Chapter 2). After reaction the solution can be expected to contain the following:

Unreacted glutaraldehyde
Unreacted HRP
Unreacted antibody
Unreacted other proteins
(Antibody)–$(CH_2)_5$–(Antibody)
(HRP–$(CH_2)_5$–(HRP)
(Antibody)–$(CH_2)_5$–(HRP)
(Other proteins)–$(CH_2)_5$–(Other proteins)
(Other proteins)–$(CH_2)_5$–(HRP)

Larger aggregates derived from three or more protein molecules form a precipitate, which is removed by centrifugation. Any excess of glutaraldehyde is removed by dialysis or gel filtration. Some of the double molecules (Antibody)–$(CH_2)_5$–(HRP) have the structure:

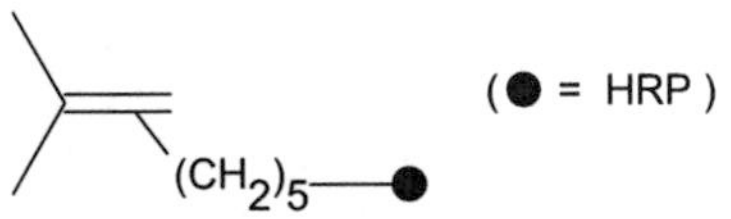

$(\bullet = HRP)$

$(CH_2)_5$—$\bullet$

with the Fc segment labelled and the Fab segments unhindered. This is the only useful component of the solution, but further purification is often not necessary.

In another labelling method, an antibody is conjugated with a polymer macromolecule that is also joined to several molecules of HRP (Chilosi et al., 1994). Amplification from one molecule of immunoglobulin to several of the enzyme is incorporated into a single reagent in this product, which is marketed for 'enhanced polymer one-step staining' (EPOS). The sensitivity achieved with an EPOS secondary antibody is said to be comparable to that of multi-step methods such as those described in Sections 19.8 and 19.9 (Pastore et al., 1995). EPOS reagents that incorporate primary monoclonal antibodies are also available, for direct enzyme-labelled immunostaining of some antigens that are commonly examined in clinical pathology.

19.7.2.
Immunostaining procedure and controls

Enzyme-labelled secondary antisera are sold by many suppliers, and recommendations for dilution and time of application are usually provided. The solution containing an HRP-labelled antibody is used in exactly the same way as a fluorochrome-labelled secondary antiserum. The sites of attachment of HRP to the tissue are detected histochemically, usually by means of the DAB–hydrogen peroxide reaction (Chapter 16). The bound HRP is capable of catalyzing the oxidation of many molecules of DAB by hydrogen peroxide with consequent accumulation of substantial amounts of the insoluble brown product. The apparent size of each antigenic site in the tissue is therefore enlarged until such time as the enzyme is inhibited by the accumulated products of its activity. The amplification factor is greater than can be obtained in fluorescent antibody techniques.

In its simplest form the method is carried out as follows.

(1)   Rinse sections in saline.
(2)   Apply the diluted primary antibody, following the supplier's recommendations if available. Otherwise, use serial twofold dilutions in saline, from 1:20 to 1:320. Leave in contact with the sections for 30–60 min at room temperature in a humid atmosphere.
(3)   Rinse sections with three changes of saline.
(4)   Apply enzyme-labelled secondary antiserum, following the supplier's recommendations if available. Otherwise try 1:20 and 1:80 dilutions, for 30–60 min.
(5)   Rinse sections with three changes of saline.
(6)   Carry out a histochemical method to detect the enzyme label. For HRP, a diaminobenzidine method is most commonly used (Section 16.5.4) because the end-product is stable and insoluble. The aminoethylcarbazole technique is also popular, but its red product is soluble in organic solvents.
(7)   Finish the preparation in a manner appropriate to the enzyme histochemical method that was used in Step 6 (*either* an aqueous mounting medium, *or* dehydration, clearing and a resinous medium).

As with the immunofluorescence methods, control procedures must accompany the use of enzyme-labelled antibodies. Indeed, false-positive results are more likely to be seen with the latter than with the former techniques, because some tissues contain endogenous peroxidases. With the indirect enzyme-labelled antibody methods the following controls are required:

(1)   Omit all immunological reagents. Carry out only the histochemical method for the enzymatic label. This will reveal sites of endogenous enzyme. (A blocking procedure for endogenous peroxidase activity may be applied routinely before Step 1 of the method. See Section 16.5.1.)
(2)   Omit treatment with the primary antiserum. This will reveal any non-specific attachment of enzyme-labelled proteins or of conjugated enzyme. HRP has a rather strong tendency to bind to tissues in this way.
(3)   Substitute non-immune or pre-immune serum for the primary antiserum to detect non-immunological binding of immunoglobulins. See Section 19.12.3 for ways to suppress this type of nonspecific staining. 4. Treat with primary antiserum that has been absorbed with an excess of its antigen. This should result in absent or greatly diminished intensity of staining.

19.7.3.
Enzymatic labels other than HRP

Horseradish peroxidase is the most popular enzymatic label for antibodies, but it is not the only one used. Others include **alkaline phosphatase** (Ponder and Wilkinson, 1981; Cordell *et al.*, 1984; Hohmann *et al.*, 1988), β-**galactosidase** (Bondi *et al.*, 1982) and **glucose oxidase** (Clark *et al.*, 1982). These enzymes can also be used in unlabelled antibody enzyme methods (Section 19.8) and avidin–biotin methods (Section 19.9). One advantage of having a variety of enzymes available as immunohistochemical labels is the possibility of demonstrating more than one antigen in the same section in different colours (Appenteng *et al.*, 1986; van der Loos *et al.*, 1987; Sakanaka *et al.*, 1988).

19.7.4.
Critique of the method

The advantages of this technique (over the indirect fluorescent antibody method) are its higher sensitivity and the permanent nature of the final preparation. The higher probability of obtaining false-positive results is a relative disadvantage. If the secondary antibody is an EPOS reagent rather than a conventionally enzyme-labelled antiserum, the sensitivity of the method is increased to a level comparable to that of the three-stage PAP and ABC methods (Sections 19.8 and 19.9).

When antigenic sites are few and far between, an indirect fluorescent antibody technique is preferred because it is easier to see isolated fluorescent spots on a dark background than to find occasional small accumulations of enzymatic reaction product against a bright background. Histochemical methods yielding fluorescent end-products are available for a few enzymes, including peroxidases (Papadimitriou *et al.*, 1976; see also Section 19.9.3) and alkaline phosphatase (Ziomek *et al.*, 1990; Murray and Ewen, 1992; Larison *et al.*, 1995) but with these have not become popular in conjunction with immunohistochemical methods. Enzyme-labelled antibodies are valuable for ultrastructural immunohistochemistry because the end-products of many histochemical reactions for enzymes, including the DAB–H_2O_2 method for peroxidase, can be detected by electron microscopy.

In all methods based on covalent labelling, the potencies of secondary antibodies are reduced by hindrance of some of the combining sites of their Fab segments. The next methods to be described are much more sensitive than the indirect enzyme-labelled antibody procedure, because secondary antibody molecules are not modified. No chemically labelled proteins are required, and the likelihood of false positive results is no higher than with other techniques.

19.8. The unlabelled antibody–enzyme method

19.8.1.
Principle of the method

Horseradish peroxidase (HRP) can serve as an antigen when it is injected into an animal (usually a rabbit). By careful mixing of the resultant immunoglobulin with HRP it has been possible to isolate a stable, soluble antigen–antibody complex. This is known as **peroxidase–antiperoxidase (PAP)** and has the structure:

(● = HRP)

Two molecules of specific IgG are associated with three of HRP. The complex is available commercially. Combination with antibody does not inhibit the activity of the enzyme. Each complex molecule of PAP has two Fc segments, which are available for attachment to suitable anti-IgG molecules. For example, the F_c segments of rabbit PAP will bind to the F_{ab} segments of the specific IgG in a goat anti-(rabbit γ-globulin). The PAP complex is thus a valuable and versatile immunohistochemical reagent for the detection of the sites of binding of anti-antibodies. A stable **alkaline phosphatase-anti-(alkaline phosphatase) complex (APAAP)** is also sold and may be used instead of PAP in unlabelled antibody–enzyme methods. The final step of the method will then be a histochemical method for alkaline phosphatase, such as one of those described in Chapter 15.

19.8.2.
Procedure for detection of an antigen

Theoretical and practical aspects of the unlabelled antibody–enzyme method will be illustrated by considering the technique for localization of an antigen, 'X', in sections of a tissue. An antiserum to X is raised in a rabbit. The other reagents needed are goat anti-(rabbit immunoglobulin) (ideally an antiserum specific for the Fc segment of IgG), rabbit PAP, and the chemicals required for histochemical demonstration of peroxidase. Both the secondary antiserum and the PAP are available from several commercial suppliers. The procedure is as follows:

(1) Apply rabbit antiserum to X (the primary antiserum) to the sections for 1 h at room temperature. If this primary has not been used before, try several dilutions (in phosphate-buffered saline) from 1:50 to 1:2000. A longer exposure (12–24 h, at 4°C) is advantageous when a very dilute (1:2000–1:10 000) primary antiserum is used, or if the investigation requires the use of thick (50–150 μm) sections.

(2) Rinse in three changes of phosphate-buffered saline.

(3) Apply the secondary antiserum, goat anti-(rabbit immunoglobulin), for 30 min at room temperature. A 1:10 to 1:40 dilution of this serum is used. The concentration is not critical but it must be much higher than that of the primary antiserum or the PAP.

(4) Rinse in three or four changes of phosphate-buffered saline.

(5) Apply rabbit peroxidase–antiperoxidase (rabbit PAP) for 30 min at room temperature. This reagent is supplied as a stock solution, typically containing 1.0 mg protein per ml. It is diluted 1:50 with phosphate-buffered saline, unless the supplier suggests otherwise.

(6) Rinse in three or four changes of phosphate-buffered saline.

(7) Incubate for demonstration of peroxidase activity (Chapter 16). The DAB–H_2O_2 method is usually used with the incubation medium buffered to pH 7.6. Aminoethylcarbazole (AEC) is another acceptable chromogen.

(8) Wash in water. If DAB was used, dehydrate, clear, and mount in a resinous medium. An aqueous mounting medium must be used after the AEC–H_2O_2 method for peroxidase.

A three-layered 'sandwich' is built up by the three reagents employed:

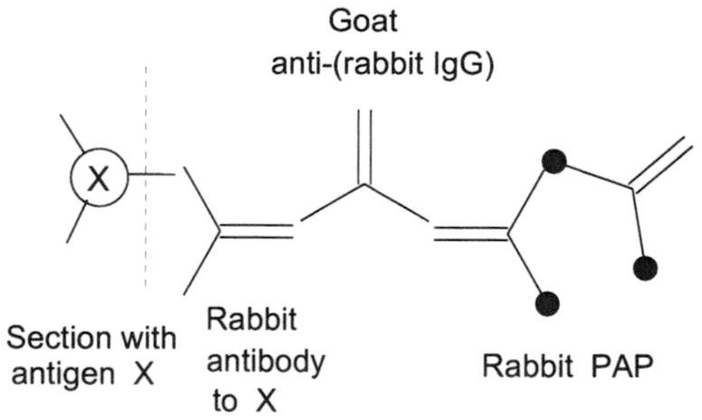

Because the goat anti-(rabbit IgG) is bivalent, its molecules attach to the Fc segments of the primary rabbit anti-X antibodies *and* to those of the rabbit antiperoxidase antibodies in the PAP complex. The product of the histochemical reaction for HRP therefore accumulates at the sites of the antigen X.

The intensity of the colour of the end-product is influenced by the dilution of the primary antiserum. When the antigen is present at high concentration in the tissue, the density of the final product is higher after the application of more dilute solutions of the primary antiserum. The probable reason for this apparently paradoxical effect is given in *Fig. 19.2.*

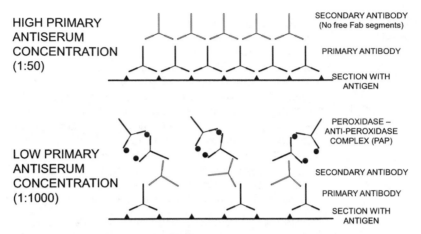

Figure 19.2. Effects of different primary antiserum concentrations on the staining of tissue with high density of antigenic sites by the unlabelled antibody–enzyme (PAP) method. High concentration of primary antiserum *(above)* results in binding of the secondary antibody by both its Fab segments, so that neither is free to combine with the PAP reagent. With low concentrations of primary antiserum *(below)* the Fc segments of the primary antibody molecules are further apart, and each binds only one Fab segment of the secondary antibody. The other Fab segments of the secondary antibody molecules are therefore free to combine with the Fc segments of the PAP complex. If antigenic determinants are close together in the tissue, the strongest staining is obtained with a greatly diluted primary antiserum, whereas no staining may be obtained after application of a more concentrated primary antiserum. (From Bigbee *et al.*, 1977, reproduced with permission of the authors. Copyright 1977. The Histochemical Society Inc.)

19.8.3.
Controls

The following control procedures should accompany any investigation in which the PAP method (or any other unlabelled antibody–enzyme procedure) is used for the localization of an antigen in a tissue:

(1) Omit treatment with both the antisera and the PAP. Incubate for peroxidase to demonstrate the endogenous enzymatic activity of the tissue. (In most laboratories a blocking procedure for endogenous peroxidase activity is applied routinely before Step 1 of the method. See Section 16.5.1.)

(2) Omit treatment with the primary antiserum. Any staining then observed cannot be due to the antigen.

(3) Substitute a non-immune serum for the primary antiserum (e.g. normal rabbit serum, in the method for antigen X described above). This control will reveal any non-immunological attachment of γ-globulins to the tissue. (See Section 19.12.3 for strategies to minimize this type of nonspecific staining.)

(4) Omit treatment with both the primary and the secondary antisera. Non-specific binding of PAP, should it occur, will then be demonstrated. If non-specific binding is a function of the HRP moiety of PAP, it can be prevented by treating the sections (before Step 1 of the above procedure) with a solution of HRP, followed by 1% H_2O_2 in 30% methanol, which irreversibly inhibits the enzymatic activity of the bound HRP (Minard and Cawley, 1978).

(5) Mix the primary antiserum or antibody solution with an excess of the purified antigen and apply this mixture to the sections in Step 1 of the method. Greatly diminished staining should be observed. Absorbed antisera will seldom cause complete inhibition of staining by the PAP method.

(6) For a positive control, carry out the complete immunostaining procedure on a section or cell culture known to contain the antigen.

19.8.4.
Critique of the method

The main advantage of the unlabelled antibody–enzyme method is its great sensitivity. Positive results can often be obtained with sections of tissues fixed and processed by methods that denature most of the antigen present. It is even possible to use old H and E-stained slides from which the coverslips, mounting media, and dyes have been removed. The high sensitivity is due to the attachment of three molecules of peroxidase at each site of binding of the PAP complex. Amplification due to multiplicity of antigenic sites on the Fc segment of the primary antibody may also occur, as with indirect immunofluorescence techniques. The large size of the PAP complex molecule limits the amount of PAP binding to the secondary antibody. Although control procedures are necessary in order to exclude non-specific staining, this is a 'cleaner' method than most others, probably because the PAP reagent is a pure antigen–antibody complex, unlikely to associate itself with proteins other than its own specific antibodies. With some tissues and some antibodies, there is even less non-specific background staining with the ABC method (Section 19.9.2) than with PAP.

It has been pointed out that the intensity of staining is commonly increased when the primary antiserum is diluted. Consequently it is not possible when using the PAP method to draw even approximate conclusions concerning the quantity of antigen in a specimen or even to make meaningful comparisons between strongly and weakly stained regions within a single section. It can only be concluded that an antigen is either present or undetectable. With other immunohistochemical methods, especially those involving fluorescently labelled antibodies, it is widely assumed that the intensity of the observed staining has some quantitative significance.

19.9. Avidin–biotin methods

19.9.1.
Useful properties of avidin and biotin

Biotin (MW 244.3), a metabolite of many kinds of microorganism, is a vitamin that forms the coenzyme or prosthetic group of several enzymes that transfer carboxyl groups.

Avidin (MW 70 000) is a glycoprotein of egg white. Each molecule consists of four identical subunits, each capable of binding a molecule of biotin. The affinity between biotin and avidin is very high, even though no covalent bonds are formed, so the binding occurs rapidly and is reversible only in extreme conditions, such as strong acidity or aqueous 6 M guanidine. (Administration of large quantities of egg white to laboratory animals results in sequestration of the biotin produced by intestinal bacteria, and causes deficiency of the vitamin. The investigation of this apparent toxicity of egg white led to the discovery of biotin and avidin.) **Streptavidin** (MW 60 000) is a microbial protein that contains no carbohydrate. Its properties are similar to those of avidin. The two proteins are used for the same purposes, but streptavidin is about five times as expensive as avidin.

It is possible to conjugate proteins and other large molecules with biotin. This reaction is known as **biotinylation**. A typical reactive derivative of biotin is the sodium salt of sulpho-*N*-succinimidobiotin, shown over. This combines with amino groups of protein, to which biotin becomes joined by an amide linkage:

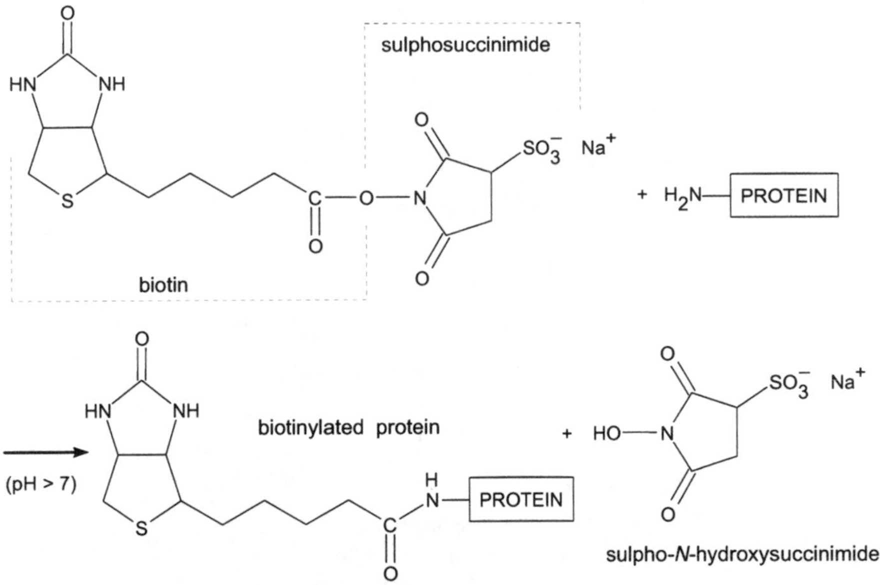

The sulphonic acid group of the reagent makes it soluble in water. Several other reactive derivatives of biotin are available, for labelling proteins, carbohydrates and nucleic acids.

The biotin molecule is small enough not to interfere with the biological activity of the macromolecule that it labels, and its reactivity with avidin is unchanged. Many biotinylated antisera and enzymes are commercially available.

The first methods to make use of biotin and avidin for immunohistochemical detection of antigens (Guesdon, Ternynck and Avrameas, 1979) consisted of either three or four stages, separated by washes in PBS.

19.9.1.1. Labelled avidin–biotin procedure

(1) Application of a primary antiserum (for example, rabbit antibody to the antigen in the tissue).

(2) Application of a biotinylated secondary antiserum (for example, biotinylated goat anti-rabbit IgG).

(3) Application of a solution of avidin that has been covalently conjugated with a fluorochrome or a histochemically demonstrable enzyme such as horseradish peroxidase. The enzyme is then localized histochemically in the usual way.

The final complex has the form:

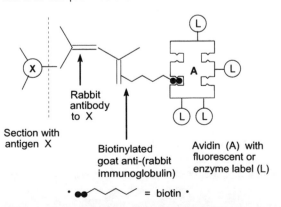

Section with antigen X

Rabbit antibody to X

Biotinylated goat anti-(rabbit immunoglobulin)

Avidin (A) with fluorescent or enzyme label (L)

= biotin

19.9.1.2 Bridged avidin–biotin procedure

The first two steps are the same as those of the previous procedure. Then:

(3) Application of a solution of unlabelled avidin to the section.
(4) Application of a solution of a biotinylated enzyme, such as a conjugate of biotin with horseradish peroxidase.
(5) The bound enzyme is then demonstrated histochemically.

In this case, the final complex is:

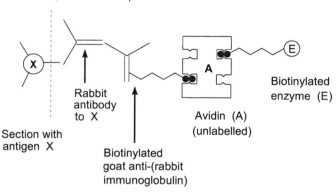

19.9.2.
The 'ABC' method

Sensitivity greater than that of the preceding two methods is achieved by using as the detecting agent a freshly prepared **avidin–biotin complex (ABC)**, made by mixing a solution of avidin with one of biotinylated HRP (Hsu *et al.*, 1981). The structure of the final product with the ABC method is:

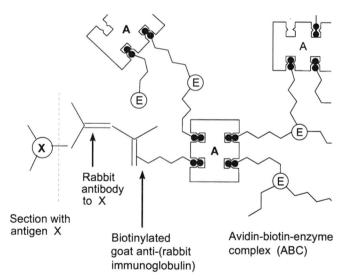

This looks like the product of the bridged avidin–biotin procedure, but differs in that the preformed avidin–biotin–HRP complex is an enormous cross-linked molecule containing many more than three HRP molecules per free biotin-binding site. The size of this complex may restrain its diffusion into the section. The technical details of the ABC method are described and discussed in the next subsection.

19.9.2.1. Procedure for detection of an antigen

The following procedure is that of Hsu and Raine (1981), incorporating the optional modifications of Cattoretti *et al.* (1988). Fixation and processing are determined by the nature of the antigen, as with other immunohistochemical methods. The sections are hydrated and equilibrated with PBS, which is also the solvent for all the reagents. Control procedures are outlined in Section 19.9.2.2.

Solutions required
A. Phosphate-buffered saline
PBS is used as solvent for all immunological reagents, and for all aqueous washes. See Chapter 20 for saline solutions. This saline may optionally contain a surfactant and a protein, as explained in Section 19.12.

B. Antisera
(1)   A **primary antiserum** that will combine with the antigen being sought.
(2)   A **biotinylated secondary antiserum** that will combine with immunoglobulins of the species in which the primary antiserum was raised.

C. An avidin solution
This typically contains 10 µg of avidin per ml, in PBS. See also *Note 1* below.

D. A solution of biotinylated horseradish peroxidase (typically 2.5 µg/ml), in PBS.

E. ABC
This is made by combining solutions **C** and **D** (typically 1:4 volumes; see also *Note 2* below). Mix 15–20 min before it is needed: see Step 7 of the method.

F. Reagents for demonstration of peroxidase activity at neutral pH
See Chapter 17. The DAB–H_2O_2 method is the most popular one. The AEC technique is also suitable.

G. Counterstain
Any dye solutions needed to provide a **counterstain** appropriate to the tissue and the reason for demonstrating the antigen. Many of the methods in Chapters 6 and 7 can be used. See also *Note 3* below.

Procedure
Rinses and washes are done in generous quantities of saline (Solution A). Each 'rinse' is about 30 s, with constant agitation. A 'wash' is about 5 min, with agitation at 1-min intervals. See *Note 4* below.

(1)   (Optional) Inhibit endogenous peroxidase by treating sections for 30 min with 0.3% hydrogen peroxide in PBS, followed by two washes in PBS. (See Section 16.5.1 for discussion of endogenous peroxidase inhibition.)
(2)   (Optional) Block non-specific background staining by treating the sections for 30 min with a 10% dilution of serum from a species of animal different from that in which the primary antiserum was raised. Other proteins can also be used (Section 19.12.3). Rinse in PBS.
(3)   Incubate in suitably diluted primary antiserum (e.g. rabbit antiserum to 'antigen X'). The range of dilution may vary between 1:200 and 1:6400, and the optimum should be determined by trial, as with the PAP method. Long incubations (12–48 h) at 4°C are preferred for thick (50–150 µm) free-floating sections. Shorter incubation (such as 1 h) at room temperature is satisfactory for mounted paraffin sections (less than 15 µm).
(4)   Rinse in 3 changes of PBS.
(5)   Incubate in biotinylated secondary antiserum (e.g. goat antiserum to rabbit IgG). for 30–60 min at room temperature. A 1:10 to 1:40 dilution is usual, but some workers use greatly diluted serum at 4°C for 12–48 h, especially for thick sections.
(6)   Before moving the sections on to Step 6, make the **working ABC solution** by mixing the recommended volumes of avidin and biotinylated HRP stock solutions.

(7) Rinse in 3 changes of PBS.
(8) Incubate sections in the working ABC solution for 60 min at room temperature.
(9) Rinse in 3 changes of PBS.
(10) (Optional) At this stage of the procedure, optionally carry out the additional amplification steps listed in *Note 3* below.
(11) Carry out a histochemical method for peroxidase activity.
(12) Wash in water, counterstain as desired (*Note 4*), and make a permanent preparation in a mounting medium appropriate to the counterstain.

Results

Sites of immunoreactivity recognized by the primary antiserum are brown (simple DAB–H_2O_2 method), black, (Co^{2+}- or Ni^{2+}-enhanced DAB–H_2O_2 method) or red (AEC–H_2O_2 method). Other structures may be counterstained in contrasting colours.

Notes

(1) Solutions of biotinylated secondary antiserum, avidin and biotinylated HRP are commercially available, often in proprietary kits such as the 'Vectastain' system. The measurements, dilutions and other instructions that accompany commercial products or kits are usually applicable to paraffin sections 5–10 μm thick, and they should be followed, even if they differ from the suggestions given here or in other publications. Variations are likely to be needed for thicker sections, as indicated in the preceding instructions.

(2) Solutions C, D and E should be made up in plain PBS, without any added protein such as serum or casein (Section 19.12.3) because these materials can contain small amounts of biotin, and this would reduce the efficacy of the avidin-containing reagents.

(3) To introduce more peroxidase into sites of immunoreactivity in the section, a biotin-rich **complex of biotin–peroxidase and avidin (CBA)** may be applied after Step 8, and the preparation can be treated with alternating applications of ABC and CBA. The CBA contains five times as much biotinylated HRP as the regular ABC reagent. Thus, with the 'Vectastain' product ABC is made by mixing 4 volumes of the avidin solution with 1 volume of the biotinylated HRP solution. For CBA, the proportions are 4:5. Cattoretti *et al.* (1988) recommended three treatments with ABC and two with CBA:

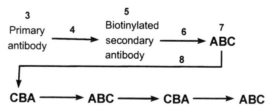

with a rinse in PBS after each application. (Numbers are of the steps in the regular ABC method.)

    The amplification of staining intensity is due to the affinity between ABC and CBA, which results in the accumulation of increasing amounts of the labelling enzyme.

(4) **Counterstaining.** It is advisable to leave at least one section (for the complete procedure and each control) not counterstained, to allow proper assessment of the intensities of the specific immunostaining and of any artifacts or nonspecific 'background' revealed in the controls.

    The principles of staining are explained throughout this book, but especially in Chapter 6. At Step 11 of the ABC method, the requirements of a counterstain are that it contrasts with and is less conspicuous than the final immunohistochemical reaction product.

If the immunohistochemical reaction product is a polymer that resists extraction by organic solvents (DAB methods for peroxidase), appropriately coloured cationic and anionic dyes can provide a wide range of colours. There are fewer options if the enzymatic end-product is alcohol-soluble (as with the AEC chromogen for peroxidase and many of the methods for alkaline phosphatase). A simple haemalum stain for cell nuclei (Chapter 6) is stable in aqueous mounting media (AEC chromogen) and is not weakened by dehydration (DAB methods).

(5) Excessive washing can break the bonds between antigen and antibody molecules if the affinity, however specific, is weak. This risk is greatest for the binding of the primary antibody to the tissue. This tissue-to-primary binding could be broken by too much washing at any later stage in the procedure. All reagents other than the primary antibody are articles of commerce that are sold in large quantities for many purposes, in a competitive market. The common reagents should not give any trouble, but this assumption does not absolve the user of responsibility for dedicating many more sections to controls than to the definitive procedure.

19.9.2.2. Controls

For the reader who has read the chapter up to this point, the controls for specificity of the ABC method should be obvious. The specimen should have no endogenous activity of the labelling enzyme (usually peroxidase). There should be no staining if the primary antiserum is omitted, and staining should be reduced by prior absorption of the primary antiserum with purified antigen. There should be no evidence of non-immune binding of the secondary antiserum or of the avidin–biotin–enzyme complex to the section. Occasionally a tissue is encountered that contains cells with enough endogenous biotin to give confusing results with ABC methods (Bhattacharjee et al., 1997). This biotin is released from mitochondrial pyruvate carboxylase, especially when microwave heating is used to accelerate immunostaining (Miller and Kubier, 1997). For blocking endogenous biotin, see Section 19.12.4.

Whenever possible a section known to contain the antigen of interest should be immunostained alongside the unknowns, as a positive control to ensure that all the reagents are working properly.

19.9.2.3. Critique of the method

The regular ABC and PAP methods are probably of approximately equal sensitivity (Hsu and Raine, 1981). In both procedures, large complex molecules are used to introduce the detecting enzyme into the sites where antibodies are bound. It is therefore often necessary to treat the preparations, before staining, by one of the methods for increasing permeability (Section 19.12.2) of the tissue. According to Sternberger and Sternberger (1986), non-immune binding of reagents is more likely to occur with the ABC system than with the PAP method, at least with nervous tissue. The ABC technique is, however, widely respected for giving 'clean' preparations. Some workers claim that the results are cleaner with streptavidin than with avidin.

When high sensitivity is not needed, as in the staining of cytoskeletal proteins, the indirect immunofluorescence techniques are often preferred to those in which the last step is the histochemical demonstration of an enzyme, especially by research workers. Immunoenzyme methods that provide permanent preparations are preferred by pathologists.

19.9.3. Amplification with biotinylated tyramine

In the procedures known as **CARD** (catalyzed reporter deposition) or **TAT** (tyramine amplification technique), a peroxidase label catalyzes the oxidation by H_2O_2 of a labelled derivative of tyramine. The product of the enzymatic reaction retains the label and immediately binds covalently to protein. In the first of these methods to be introduced into immunohistochemistry the reagent was biotinylated tyramine:

sulpho-*N*-succinimidobiotin

tyramine

biotinyltyramide
(= biotinylated tyramine)

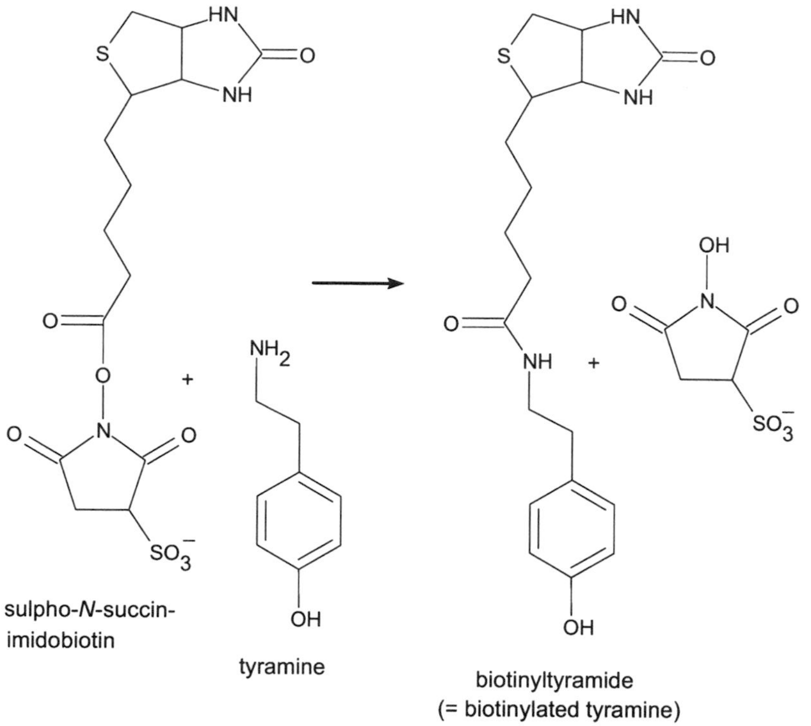

In the presence of peroxidase, hydrogen peroxide oxidizes the phenolic (lower) end of this molecule. The immediate product of oxidation is believed to be a free radical (Bobrow *et al.*, 1989), which immediately forms a covalent bond to part (possibly the phenolic side-chain of tyrosine) of a nearby protein molecule. Each deposited molecule of the oxidized tyramine derivative has an intact biotinyl group that is able to bind avidin or streptavidin (see *Fig 19.3*). For example, HRP-labelled streptavidin may be applied, followed by histochemical detection of HRP with DAB and H_2O_2 (Adams, 1992; Werner *et al.*, 1996). Fluorescently labelled avidin is also used (Dehaas *et al.*, 1996). Tyramine itself can be fluorescently labelled; the product of peroxidase-catalysed oxidation retains the fluorescent tag and is firmly bound to the tissue (van Gijlswijk *et al.*, 1997). Simple methods for laboratory synthesis of labelled tyramides are described by Hopman *et al.* (1998).

The labelled tyramine amplification techniques are sensitive histochemical methods for peroxidase activity. They are mentioned here because immunohistochemistry is one of their principal applications. The high sensitivity is not always an advantage, however, and tyramine amplification procedures can give patchy results or extreme overstaining (Mengel *et al.*, 1999). Fluorescent tyramine derivatives are also used in fluorescent *in situ* hybridization (FISH) techniques (Section 9.6.3). With different fluorescent labels it is possible to impart different colours to individual chromosomes or to the sites of different DNA sequences.

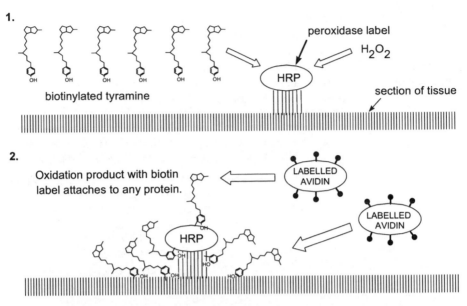

Figure 19.3. Tyramine amplification (CARD or TAT) at a site where horseradish peroxidase (HRP) is present in a section. The label (•) attached to avidin (or streptavidin) may be a fluorochrome or a histochemically demonstrable enzyme such as HRP or alkaline phosphatase.

19.10. Other immunohistochemical methods

The techniques described so far are those most widely used for the demonstration of antigens in tissues. Other techniques also exist for the localization of both antigens and antibodies. Some of these will now be briefly described, to give the reader an idea of the scope and versatility of immunohistochemical methodology.

19.10.1. Sandwich technique for antibody in tissue

Antibodies in a tissue are demonstrated by applying the purified antigen followed by a fluorescently labelled antiserum to the antigen. The method is often used with impression smears of cells from lymph nodes and with cryostat sections. Unfixed tissue is used because the Fab segments of antibody molecules cannot be expected to retain their properties after coagulation or chemical cross-linking. For example, a section of human tissue containing antibodies to an antigen Y could be treated with a solution of Y, followed by a fluorescently labelled rabbit antiserum to Y.

This is a method for demonstrating specific antibodies. Antibodies in general (i.e. immunoglobulins) are detected by considering them to be antigens. Human immunoglobulin G, for example, can be localized in sections with rabbit anti-(human IgG) followed by a labelled goat antiserum to rabbit immunoglobulins.

19.10.2.
Detection of antibody in serum

In some autoimmune diseases the blood contains circulating antibodies to certain components of a patient's or an animal's own tissues. The existence and specificity of such autoantibodies can be detected immunohistochemically by applying the suspect serum (usually as a 1:10 dilution in saline) to unfixed cryostat sections of tissues known to contain appropriate auto-antigens. Different tissues serve as controls. The sites of binding of antibodies to the sections are made visible by the application of a fluorescently or enzymatically labelled antiserum to the immunoglobulins of the species from which the serum under test was obtained.

For example, to test human serum for antibodies against thyroglobulin one requires some sections of normal human thyroid gland and a fluorescently labelled rabbit anti-(human γ-globulin). The stained preparation has the structure:

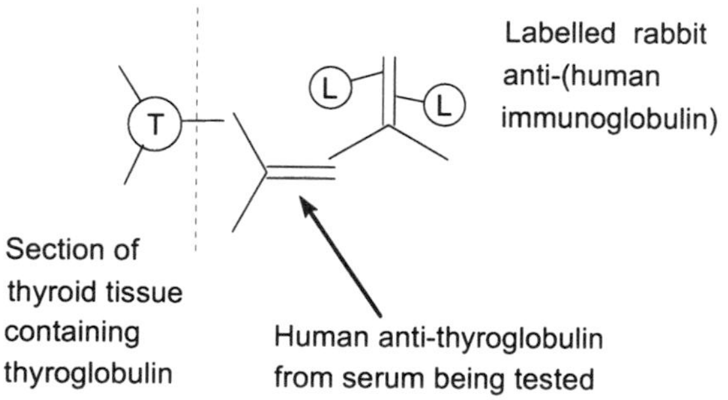

Labelled rabbit anti-(human immunoglobulin)

Section of thyroid tissue containing thyroglobulin

Human anti-thyroglobulin from serum being tested

A positive result appears as fluorescence in the thyroid follicles. Serum from someone with normal thyroid function provides a necessary negative control. Sections of other human organs (liver, kidney, etc.) serve as a controls for organ-specificity.

Often the sections used are composite blocks containing several tissues, so that it is possible to seek the presence of several autoantibodies in a single drop of serum.

19.10.3.
Methods using staphylococcal protein A

The cell-wall of *Staphylococcus aureus*, a common pathogen, contains a component known as **protein A** that is able to bind to the Fc segments of most types of mammalian IgG molecule. The binding is non-immune but results from an affinity similar to that existing between antigens and antibodies. The molecule of protein A is bivalent and can therefore be made to serve as a bridge between the Fc portions of IgG molecules of different kinds. It is also possible to label protein A with fluorochromes or with HRP (Dubois-Dalcq *et al.*, 1977). Thus, protein A may be used for the same purposes as an antiserum to IgG. Solutions containing protein A must not be mixed with any kind of serum to suppress non-specific binding to tissue (Section 19.12.3) because it would combine with the IgG in the serum. Casein or albumin may be used instead for this purpose.

A conjugate of protein A with HRP is employed in a technique closely similar to an enzyme-labelled antibody method. The specific primary antiserum is applied to a section of tissue and followed by HRP–protein A conjugate:

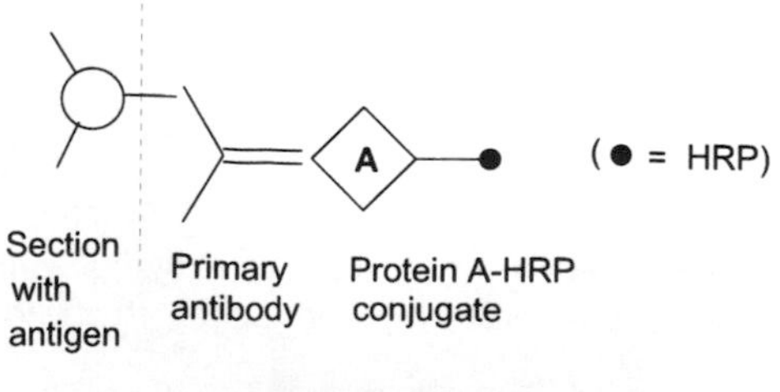

(● = HRP)

Section with antigen

Primary antibody

Protein A-HRP conjugate

The sites of bound HRP are demonstrated histochemically in the usual way. This method sometimes provides 'cleaner' staining, with less non-immunological background coloration, than the equivalent enzyme-labelled antibody technique.

Protein A has also been employed instead of a secondary antiserum in the unlabelled antibody–enzyme method. Application of a specific primary antiserum is followed by protein A and then by PAP:

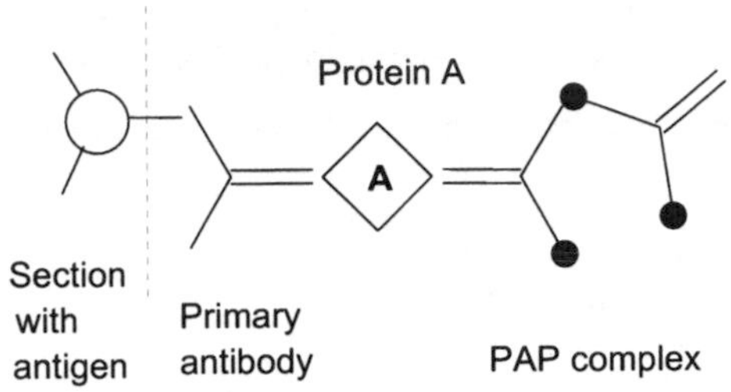

Section with antigen | Primary antibody | Protein A | PAP complex

This technique, however, is somewhat less sensitive than those in which secondary anti-immunoglobulin sera are used (Celio *et al.*, 1979). Some other immunohistochemical applications of protein A were described by Notani *et al.* (1979). Obviously protein A is not suitable for use with any specimen that already contains IgG.

The main advantage of protein A is that it is able to combine with IgG of all mammals, so that it has a greater number of potential uses than an antiserum to the immunoglobulin of a single species. Before accepting a negative result, it is necessary to confirm that protein A does bind to the primary antibody, especially if this is a monoclonal antibody. Protein A binds only to some subtypes of IgG. Protein G is another bacterial product, with different IgG-binding specificities.

19.10.4.
Use of mouse antibodies on mouse tissues

Most monoclonal antibodies (MABs) are immunoglobulins produced by cultured cells derived from mice. The ordinary way to detect a MAB bound to a section is to apply an anti-(mouse immunoglobulin) that was raised in some other species such as the rabbit. Sometimes a MAB must be used to detect an antigen in sections of a specimen taken from a mouse. The secondary antibody is then likely to be bound by the immunoglobulins normally present in extracellular fluids and leukocytes of the mouse tissue, causing strong nonspecific background staining and obscuring the sites of attachment of the MAB molecules. The following procedure (Hierck *et al.*, 1994) allows the use of many (but not all) mouse MABs to detect antigens in mouse tissues.

The reagents needed to stain for an antigen 'X' are:

(1) Primary antibody to X (a mouse MAB): mouse anti-X. This is a diluted solution, perhaps 1:1000, determined to be optimal for immunohistochemical staining of tissues from animals other than the mouse.
(2) HRP-labelled rabbit antiserum to mouse serum proteins: rabbit anti-(mouse serum).
(3) Normal mouse serum.
(4) Reagents for histochemical detection of peroxidase activity.

The method is as follows.

(1) Add 1 volume of HRP-labelled rabbit anti-(mouse serum) to 200 volumes of diluted mouse anti-X, and leave at 4°C overnight. All the MAB molecules will attach to rabbit anti-(mouse IgG) molecules, and there will be an excess of rabbit antibody molecules that are capable of binding to mouse serum proteins.

(2) Add 1 volume of normal mouse serum to the mixture, and leave for 2 h at 4°C. Molecules of mouse IgG and other serum proteins will attach to (block) all the free anti-(mouse serum) Fab segments of the rabbit antiserum.

(3) Apply the mixture to sections for 4 h. The Fab segments of the MAB molecules will attach to the antigen in the tissue, but the HRP-labelled rabbit anti-(mouse) antibodies will not be bound by the tissue because they are already blocked by mouse serum proteins.

(4) Rinse in 3 changes of PBS.

(5) Carry out the histochemical method for peroxidase.

The structure of the immune complex formed in this method is:

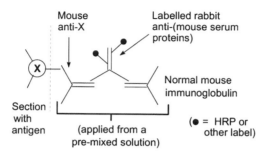

The times allowed for formation of immune complexes in the preparation of the reagent are probably unduly long, because reactions between antibodies and antigens in solution occur almost instantaneously. Labels other than peroxidase might also be used in methods of this kind.

Nonspecific background staining can also been suppressed by pretreating sections of mouse tissue with a mixture of Fab and Fc fragments derived from papain digestion of unlabelled anti-(mouse immunoglobulin). This is followed by the primary mouse monoclonal antibody and then by a labelled anti-(mouse immunoglobulin) (Lu and Partridge, 1998).

19.10.5.
Labelling with colloidal gold

It is quite easy to make a colloidal suspension (sometimes called a sol) of gold, containing particles of known diameter in the range 20–150 nm (Frens, 1973). In order to prevent the suspended particles from clumping together and sinking, the sol contains a macromolecular stabilizing agent, which coats the surfaces of the particles. If this stabilizing agent is or includes a protein with specific affinity, such as a lectin or an immunoglobulin, the metal will serve as a label, in much the same manner as a fluorescent dye or a histochemically demonstrable enzyme (Geoghegan and Ackerman, 1977; Horisberger and Rosset, 1977). Typically either an anti-IgG serum or staphylococcal protein A is bound to gold particles in this way, and used to identify sites of attachment of a primary antibody (Roth et al., 1978a; Bendayan, 1981b; Fujimori, 1999). Avidin can also be used to coat colloidal gold particles (see van den Pol, 1984). These methods have two advantages over those that use HRP:

(a) The colloidal gold particles will stick to antigenic sites on the surface of an ultrathin section of plastic-embedded tissue. (If enzyme-labelled antibody methods are to be used in conjunction with electron microscopy, the immunostaining must be done on thick sections cut with a vibrating microtome, before embedding in plastic.)

(b) It is possible to have antibodies labelled with gold particles of different size, and thereby identify more than one antigen in the same section.

The colloidal gold methods were introduced for use in conjunction with electron microscopy. The sols are strongly coloured, but the bound quantities are small, so they produce only faint staining for light microscopy (Roth, 1982). It is possible to enlarge the particles by treating the sections with a physical developer until dense, optically visible deposits are formed (Holgate *et al.*, 1983; Danscher and Norgaard, 1985). The principle of physical development is explained in Chapter 18. The protein that labels the gold particles can also be made visible by any appropriate immunohistochemical method.

Protein–gold sols can be made and combined with protein in the laboratory, or the gold-labelled reagents may be purchased. The production of gold-labelled proteins requires meticulous attention to technique, and is not practised in general histological laboratories. For details of their preparation and uses, see Polak and Varndell (1984), Bendayan and Duhr (1986) and Birrell *et al.* (1987).

19.11. Non-immunological affinity techniques

Specific attachments between molecules are by no means confined to the reactions of antigens with antibodies. The affinities of other biologically significant substances for one another have been exploited in a variety of histochemical methods. The following types of technique are worthy of mention.

(1) The hybridization of **nucleic acids** (Chapter 9).
(2) The use of **lectins** in carbohydrate histochemistry (Chapter 11). GM1 ganglioside, a glycolipid component (Chapter 12) of cell membranes, can be localized by virtue of its specific affinity for **choleragenoid**, which is the non-toxic (cell-binding) portion of the cholera toxin molecule. The choleragenoid may be unlabelled and detected immunohistochemically (Willinger and Schachner, 1980), or biotinylated and detected with avidin–HRP (Asou *et al.*, 1983).
(3) The use of labelled or fluorescent inhibitors for the localization of **enzymes** or their substrates (Chapter 14).
(4) The use of labelled drugs and hormones to bind to physiologically or pharmacologically defined **receptors** in tissues. For example, fluorescently labelled α-bungarotoxin (from a snake venom) has been used to demonstrate receptors for acetylcholine, including those at neuromuscular junctions (Anderson and Cohen, 1974). The binding of drugs is studied mainly with radioactive labelling and autoradiographic techniques. Simple visible labelling is possible for some hormones. Thus, oestrogen or progesterone have been conjugated to fluorescently labelled albumin (Bergqvist *et al.*, 1984), and parathyroid hormone to biotin. (Niendorf *et al.*, 1988). These techniques are of interest in research, but caution is needed in interpreting the results. With some fluorescent derivatives of drugs the microscopically observed binding has been shown not to coincide with the sites of pharmacological action (Correa *et al.*, 1980).
(5) Natural affinities between proteins can be exploited. For example, the filamentous protein **actin**, which mediates contraction and locomotion of cells, selectively binds heavy meromyosin, which is isolated from the actomyosin of striated muscle. The binding results in thickening ('decoration') of the actin filaments, observable by electron microscopy. For light microscopy, heavy meromyosin can be fluorescently labelled (Sanger, 1975) or detected immunohistochemically. **Phalloidin**, a fungal toxin that binds to actin, can be biotinylated and used for affinity staining in light and electron microscopy (Faulstich *et al.*, 1989).
(6) Connective tissue matrix contains proteoglycans and glycoproteins that bind specifically to **hyaluronic acid**. This affinity has been exploited for the histochemical detection of hyaluronic acid (Ripellino *et al.*, 1985; Girard *et al.*, 1986).

19.12. Miscellaneous practical considerations

This chapter concludes with a few technical tips of a general nature.

19.12.1.
Preservation of structure and antigenicity

There is no ideal way to fix and section tissues for immunohistochemistry. Buffered formaldehyde is suitable for many purposes, though a coagulant agent is advantageous for some antigens, in which distortion is necessary in order to expose the epitopes. Antigenicity is suppressed more by alcoholic formaldehyde solutions such as AFA (Chapter 2) than by aqueous formaldehyde, but it can be restored by antigen retrieval (Zhang et al., 1998). Some other fixatives often used for immunohistochemical work are described in Chapter 2 (Section 2.5.5). A popular one is that of Stefanini et al. (1967) containing formaldehyde and neutral picrate ions. Glutaraldehyde is sometimes added to such mixtures (Newman et al., 1982; Somogyi and Takagi, 1982), especially if ultrastructural preservation is required. A fixative mixture containing 4% $HgCl_2$ and 8% HCHO (from formalin) was recommended by Hickey et al. (1983). After vascular perfusion or immersion for 24 h, sections were cut with a vibrating microtome and collected into TRIS buffer. TRIS is a primary amine, and combines rapidly with aldehydes, so it terminates the fixation and ensures that the primary antiserum will not react with formaldehyde that leaches out of the tissue. The toxicity of mercury is avoided by using a zinc–formalin fixative, such as 1% zinc sulphate in 4% formaldehyde (Herman et al., 1988; see also Sections 2.4.3 and 2.5.2).

Many antigens survive embedding in wax but some do not. The optimum treatment for every tissue and antigen has to be found by trial and error. Chemical fixation is unlikely to remove or irreversibly alter all the antigen present in a specimen, but chemical cross-linking and other changes can impede the movements of large molecules such as antibodies, and prevent the intimate contact that is needed for combining with antigens. Antigen retrieval (Section 19.12.2) should therefore be attempted if an expected result cannot be obtained with fixed material.

Some soluble antigens, including serum proteins, may diffuse from their normal loci in the tissue during the course of freezing or cutting of unfixed material (Sparrow, 1980) or in the interval between death and chemical fixation of tissue (Banks, 1979; Mori et al., 1991), giving rise to artifactual false-positive localizations in the stained preparations (Mason and Biberfeld, 1980; Fabian, 1992; Loberg and Torvik, 1992). Errors from this cause should be suspected when an antigen is detected in unexpected places, especially when one of the more sensitive immunohistochemical techniques, such as the unlabelled antibody–enzyme method, is used. Antigens are least likely to diffuse in the tissues of animals fixed by vascular perfusion.

19.12.2.
Improving the access of antibodies to antigens

Failure to demonstrate the presence of an antigen in a tissue does not necessarily mean the antigen is not there. It may be masked by other molecules that obstruct the access of the antibody molecules in the primary antiserum. The most obvious barriers to penetration are lipoprotein membranes (fixed or unfixed), and matrices of cytoplasmic or extracellular material that have been tightly cross-linked by an aldehyde or a chromium-containing fixative. There are several ways to increase the permeability of a tissue to large molecules; some were mentioned in connection with nucleic acid hybridization. The first methods to be used were pre-treatment of the sections with either a surfactant or a proteolytic enzyme. These procedures are critically discussed by Horobin (1982) and Feldmann et al. (1983). Various high temperature treatments, known as antigen retrieval, are preferred for paraffin sections of formaldehyde-fixed tissue. For a brief review of these methods see Kiernan (2005).

A suitable **proteolytic enzyme** is trypsin. A convenient solution is one containing 0.01–0.1% (w/v) enzyme in 0.1 M $CaCl_2$, adjusted to pH 7.4 with a little 0.1 M NaOH. Sections are incubated for 10–60 min, at room temperature or 37°C. The optimum conditions can be determined only by trial. Most antigens are proteins or peptides, so it is important not to overdo a proteolytic digestion. A pH well removed from the optimum for the enzyme (as in the trypsin solution above) helps to moderate the destructive action. Proteolytic digestion is damaging to structure, so it is used only when necessary, as when demonstrating types I, III and IV collagen (Chapter 8) in paraffin sections (Bedossa et al., 1987).

Surfactants (detergents) emulsify the lipid components of membranes, making holes through which large molecules can pass. Non-ionic surfactants are used because they do not impart electrical charge, which might cause nonspecific protein binding to the specimen. Digitonin, saponin, and the synthetic compound known as Triton X-100 are all suitable. The surfactant is applied to the section as a pre-treatment or, more commonly, it is added to the antibody and saline washing solutions, in a concentration of 0.05–1.0% (w/v). Saponin may even be added to fixative mixtures for light microscopy (Pignal et al., 1982), but it damages the ultrastructure of cell membranes and changes the distributions cytoskeletal proteins (Baumann et al., 2000). Surfactants are often necessary for immunostaining frozen or cryostat sections, in which the lipoprotein membranes have not been attacked by organic solvents. Hausen and Dreyer (1982) pre-incubated sections for 5 min in 5 M (30% w/v) urea. This is not a surfactant but it changes the shapes of protein molecules by interfering with hydrogen bonding.

Antigen retrieval is a term applied to several procedures in which sections of formaldehyde-fixed specimens are treated with water, usually at or above 100°C. Shi et al. (1991) heated the slides in aqueous zinc sulphate or lead thiocyanate solution, in a microwave oven. In later work, hot buffers (pH 3.5–9.5), aqueous urea (0.8–3.0 M) and EDTA were used (Shi et al., 1993, 1994, 1995, 1996; Beckstead, 1994; Balaton et al., 1995), and simple autoclaving was also found to be effective (Bankfalvi et al., 1994; Hunt et al., 1996). It is now apparent that high temperature antigen retrieval is achieved primarily by water. In comparative studies it has been found that most antigens are effectively unmasked by heating for 2 min in either 0.1 M citrate buffer (pH 6) or 1 mM EDTA (pH 8), in a domestic pressure cooker. For some particular antigens the pH needs to be higher or lower (Taylor et al., 1996a,b; Pileri et al., 1997). Ultrasound treatment before paraffin embedding has been used to retrieve certain antigens in formaldehyde-fixed specimens (Gimeno et al., 1998). The boiling solutions used for antigen retrieval can damage sections or remove them from the slides. A lower temperature (80°C) is less harmful, but a longer time (overnight) is needed to achieve the same effects (Koopal et al., 1998).

Namimatsu et al. (2005) introduced **citraconic anhydride** as a 'universal antigen retrieval method'. Sections were treated with a 0.05% aqueous solution of this compound, buffered to pH 7.4, for 45 min at 98°C. Their procedure has been used in other published investigations (e.g. Ho et al., 2007; Shi et al. 2007). Biochemists use 1% citraconic anhydride, at pH 8–9, at either room temperature or 0°C. The reagent combines with $-NH_2$ of lysine side-chains:

citraconic
anhydride

citraconylated protein

The reaction is complete in 10 min and is slowly reversible (several hours) when the pH is lowered to 3.5 (Dixon and Perham, 1968; Atassi and Habeeb, 1972). The replacement of $-NH_2$ groups by citraconyl anions can destabilize the tertiary structure of proteins, because of repulsive forces between the negative charges (Batra, 1991). In biochemical procedures a large excess of the reagent (800 mol/mol of protein, added gradually over 30 min) is needed for all the lysines to react (Mir et al., 1992).

Yamashita (2007) has suggested that such changes may expose masked epitopes when citraconic anhydride is used in hot antigen retrieval solutions. Namimatsu et al. (2005) suggested that citraconic anhydride attacked cross-links due to formaldehyde fixation.

Citraconic anhydride reacts readily with water even at room temperature (see Blatt, 1943), being completely converted to citraconic acid in about 12 h. At 98°C the same reaction can be expected to occur in about 5 min. A hot solution buffered to pH 7.4, will then contain only the anions of citraconic acid.

citraconic
anhydride

citraconic acid

The possible role of citraconic anhydride or the citraconate ion in high temperature antigen retrieval clearly requires further investigation. Hot water on the alkaline side of neutrality retrieves or unmasks the epitopes of most formaldehyde-fixed antigens (see Yamashita, 2007).

Some antigen retrieval procedures use multiple treatments. An extreme example is autoclaving, followed by treatments with 88% formic acid and 4 M guanidine thiocyanate, to enable immunostaining of the bovine spongiform encephalopathy prion in sections of human brain (Everbroek et al., 1999).

The fact that there is no single, best technique of antigen retrieval indicates that more than one mechanism is at work (see Yamashita, 2007). Removal of methylol ($-CH_2OH$) groups and hydrolysis of methylene bridges derived from formaldehyde (Chapter 2 and Walker, 1964) are the presumed effects of exposure to hot water, undoing some of the chemical changes of formaldehyde fixation (Yamashita and Okada, 2005a). The released peptide chains can be expected to change their conformations (i.e. denaturation or coagulation) quickly at 100°C, exposing previously inaccessible antigenic determinant sites (Emoto et al., 2005; see also Kiernan, 2005). Proteolytic enzymes achieve a similar effect by breaking some peptide linkages and allowing more freedom of movement of the polypeptide chains, but with hot water there is less risk of digesting the epitopes that are to be stained. Citrate and EDTA are complexing agents, and Jasani et al. (1997) suggested that calcium ions might contribute in some way to the masking of anigens. Later work indicates that chelation of calcium is not involved in the retrieval of most antigens (Yamashita and Okada, 2005b).

19.12.3.
Reduction of non-specific binding of immunoglobulins

Tissue-bound aldehyde groups, which can combine covalently with all proteins, including antibodies, are a major source of trouble when the fixative contains **glutaraldehyde**. Although glutaraldehyde is best avoided for immunohistochemical work, it is necessary for satisfactory preservation of ultrastructure, and also for the immobilization of some soluble substances (Chapter 17). The aldehyde groups should be converted to unreactive hydroxyls by **reduction with sodium borohydride** before attempting any immunohistochemical procedure on glutaraldehyde-fixed material (Willingham, 1983; see also Section 10.10.6 for practical instructions).

The other way to reduce non-specific sticking of protein molecules to sections is to **treat with a solution of a protein** that will not interfere in any way with the staining method to be used. This will block all nonspecific binding sites, so that subsequently applied antibodies will adhere only to their antigens, for which they have high affinity. It is usual to use a 1:100 to 1:10 dilution in saline (the concentration is not critical) of a normal (i.e. non-immune) serum from the species in which the secondary antiserum was raised. Thus, if the secondary antibody is goat anti-(rabbit IgG), all the solutions used could contain 1–10% serum from a goat that has not been immunized against any rabbit proteins. **The use of non-immune serum in this way is desirable as a routine measure, whatever fixative has been used**, especially with sensitive methods like the PAP or ABC procedures.

A whole serum should not be used to block nonspecific antibody attachment if the bridging reagent is staphylococcal protein A (Section 19.10.3), because the protein A would bind to the IgG of the blocking serum, and everything would end up being stained by the secondary antibody. If protein A is to be used, the blocking protein should not contain IgG from any species. **Bovine serum albumin** and **casein** are proteins that meet this requirement. Skimmed milk powder (1% in saline) is a cheap source of casein; even though the solution is opalescent it works well.

Blocking proteins are likely to contain traces of biotin, and for this reason they should not be mixed with avidin-containing reagents (Section 19.9).

19.12.4.
Blocking
endogenous
biotin

Tissues contain biotin, which is largely covalently bound as prosthetic groups of enzymes in mitochondria. This biotin can be split off during heat-induced antigen retrieval procedures and it then attaches nonspecifically to other parts of the tissue (Section 19.9.2.2), where it can bind avidin or streptavidin. To block this endogenous biotin, hydrated sections are treated with avidin and then with biotin to block unoccupied binding sites of avidin. Unbound biotin is then washed off. Diluted egg white and skimmed milk are recommended as a cheap sources of avidin and biotin respectively (Miller *et al.*, 1999).

Procedure
(1) Add the white of one egg to 100 ml water and immerse the hydrated sections in this solution for 10 min.
(2) Wash thoroughly in water.
(3) Immerse in skimmed milk for 10 min.
(4) Wash thoroughly in water, and proceed with the immunohistochemical procedure.

19.12.5.
Economizing
with expensive
reagents

Many antisera and monoclonal antibodies are available only in small quantities. It is seldom possible to use large excesses of solutions, as is the custom when carrying out ordinary staining techniques. Often they are made in the laboratory with great expenditure of effort, or obtained from commercial sources for high prices. Reagents common to many methods, such as FITC-conjugated goat anti-(rabbit immunoglobulin) or rabbit PAP, are less expensive, but still costly enough to justify parsimony in their use. An antibody or antiserum is received from the supplier in either liquid or freeze-dried form, with instructions for reconstitution. Repeated freezing damages antibody molecules. It is therefore advisable to divide the stock into aliquots of 0.1–0.2 ml, and freeze these in micro centrifuge tubes. One aliquot is used, diluted, for each immunostaining session, so that there is only one episode of freezing and thawing.

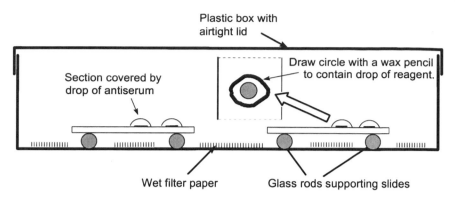

Figure 19.4. A simple arrangement for staining mounted sections with small drops of a reagent such as an antiserum. The wet filter paper ensures a humid atmosphere, preventing evaporation of the reagent.

When about 0.05 ml of a diluted reagent is available for each section, the slides are placed horizontally in an atmosphere saturated with water vapour, and a drop of the solution is deposited on each section (*Fig. 19.4*).

If the available volume of diluted antiserum is less than 0.05 ml, a tiny drop is applied to a section beneath the smallest possible coverslip (or piece of glass broken from a coverslip). A large drop of mineral oil is then put on top of and around the small coverslip, and covered again with a large coverslip. Thus, the expensive reagent is kept in contact with the slide, and evaporation is prevented. This procedure is often used with nucleic acid probes (Angerer *et al.*, 1987). Another method is to smear Vaseline thinly on both surfaces of a piece of Parafilm, and then make a hole, slightly larger than the section, in the middle. Two slides, each bearing a section, are applied to the greased surfaces to make the roof and floor of the incubation chamber. A drop of antiserum or other expensive reagent (about 20 µl/cm² of area) is applied to one of the sections before the chamber is assembled (Abbuhl and Velasco, 1985). Slides with a 75 µm layer of paint at each corner are commercially available. Capillary action draws a drop of reagent into the 150 µm space between an opposing pair of such slides (Kumar, 1989).

The value of prolonged incubation in very dilute antiserum has already been mentioned. This manoeuvre increases the sensitivity of immunohistochemical methods (Brandtzaeg, 1981) and often allows staining by immersion of slides. Sofroniew and Schrell (1982) found that diluted antisera could be kept in coplin jars for several weeks at 4°C. They recommended a solvent that contained 30 mM sodium azide to inhibit the growth of bacteria and fungi. Thiomersal (thimerosal), 10^{-3} M (405 mg of the sodium salt per litre), can be substituted for sodium azide. A 4% aqueous solution of thiomersal can be kept for at least a year in the refrigerator, and one drop (0.05 ml) of this will disinfect about 5 ml of diluted serum. My experience has been that diluted antisera stored in this way lose their efficacy after about 2 weeks, and probably should not be kept for more than one week.

19.12.6.
Optical properties of some common fluorochromes

For **FITC conjugates** the **optimum wavelength** for excitation is 490 nm (blue). The maximum emission is at 550 nm (green-yellow). Exciting light of 320 nm (in the near ultraviolet) may also be used, but the emission will be less intense. However, with ultraviolet excitation and a colourless barrier filter it is easier to distinguish between the specific emission of FITC and the blue autofluorescence of the specimens. When blue exciting light is used, a yellow or orange barrier filter is necessary and the autofluorescence appears to be green. This colour is sometimes difficult to distinguish from the specific emission of FITC. **Rhodamine B derivatives** and **Texas red** are optimally excited by green light (540–590 nm) and have orange-red emissions (580–615 nm). **Dansylated** proteins absorb in the ultraviolet and emit blue-green light. The properties of these and some other fluorochromes are summarized in Chapter 6 (*Table 6.1*). Data for numerous fluorochromes are given by Herman *et al.* (1998, Appendix E).

20 Miscellaneous data

20.1 Buffer solutions

A buffer is chosen for (a) its efficacy in the required pH range, and (b) the absence of components that would react undesirably with other substances in the solution to be buffered. Prescriptions for the commonly used buffers follow. The pH values are given to the nearest 0.1 pH unit; greater accuracy is rarely required in histochemistry. For more extensive tables of buffers, see Pearse (1968b), Perrin and Dempsey (1974) or Lillie and Fullmer (1976). Some useful practical information concerning the preparation of buffers is given by Kalimo and Pelliniemi (1977). Variations in temperature affect the pH of any solution, but most of the buffers given below should be accurate to ±0.1 pH unit over the range 15–25°C.

The pH of a mixture containing a buffer should be checked with a pH meter. The meter must be calibrated, using at least two buffers of known pH, every time it is used. It is usual to standardize a pH meter against buffer solutions obtained from a chemical supply house. The following standard solutions, however, are easily made in the laboratory:

0.05 M Potassium hydrogen phthalate
The solid salt should be dried in an oven (110°C) for 2 h and stored in a desiccator.

$KHC_8H_4O_4$:	10.21 g
Water:	to make 1000 ml
Thymol:	1 crystal, to discourage mould growth

The pH is 4.0 from 0°C to 40°C.

Although it was recommended by Lillie and Fullmer (1976) this solution should not be used as a solvent for dyes because it inhibits staining, even when 4.0 is the optimum pH, and it sometimes modifies the colour. These undesirable effects might be due to a combination of ionic and non-ionic attraction between the aromatic phthalate ion and the dye molecules.

0.01 M Borax
To avoid loss of water, the solid salt must not be heated above room temperature. The solution of borax should be used within 10 min of removal from its securely capped bottle because absorption of atmospheric CO_2 can lower its pH.

Na$_2$B$_4$O$_7$.10H$_2$O:	3.81 g
Water:	to make 1000 ml

The pH is 9.3 from 10°C to 15°C; 9.2 from 20°C to 25°C; 9.1 from 30°C to 35°C.

20.1.1.
pH 0.7–5.2:
Acetate-
hydrochloric
acid buffer

The buffer is compatible with all reagents other than salts of metals whose chlorides are insoluble (e.g. Ag, Pb).

Stock solutions
A. 1.0 M sodium acetate

Either CH$_3$COONa:	82.04 g
or CH$_3$COONa.3H$_2$O:	136.09 g
Water:	to 1000 ml

B. 1.0 M hydrochloric acid (Section 20.3)

pH	A ml 1.0 M sodium acetate	B ml 1.0 M HCl	Water: to make total volume (ml)
0.7	50	95	250
0.9	50	80	250
1.1	50	70	250
1.2	50	65	250
1.4	50	60	250
1.7	50	55	250
1.9	50	53	250
2.3	50	51	250
3.2	50	48	250
3.6	50	45	250
3.8	50	42.5	250
4.0	50	40	250
4.2	50	35	250
4.4	50	30	250
4.6	50	25	250
4.8	50	18	250
4.9	50	15	250
5.2	50	10	250

The final volume of 250 ml must include all other ingredients of a buffered mixture. It is important to check the final pH with a meter. The buffering capacity is poor between pH1.8 and 3.5.

20.1.2.
pH 3.6–5.6:
Acetate–acetic
acid buffer

This buffer is compatible with all commonly used reagents.

The instructions here are for preparation of a 0.1 M buffer. Some techniques require 0.2 M acetate buffer, so it is convenient to keep 0.2 M stock solutions, with double the strengths of those described below. (See also *Note* following the table.)

Stock solutions
A. 0.1 M sodium acetate

Either CH$_3$COONa:	8.2 g
or CH$_3$COONa.3H$_2$O:	13.61 g
Water:	to 1000 ml

B. 0.1 M acetic acid (Section 20.3)

pH	A ml 0.1 M sodium acetate	B ml 0.1 M acetic acid
3.6	15	185
3.8	24	176
4.0	36	164
4.2	53	147
4.4	74	126
4.6	98	102
4.8	120	80
5.0	141	59
5.2	158	42
5.4	171	29
5.6	181	19

Note

This buffer may also be made up with 0.2 M, 0.05 M, or 0.01 M reagents, but the pH values for the proportions given in the table are not accurate for concentrations other than 0.1 M. Check with a meter and adjust the pH when making acetate buffer at strengths other than 0.1 M.

20.1.3.
pH 2.7–7.7:
phosphate–
citrate buffer

This buffer is effective over a wide range. It should not be used in the presence of metal ions that form complexes with citric acid or have insoluble phosphates (e.g. Ag, Al, Ba, Ca, Co, Cu, Fe, Mg, Mn, Ni, Pb, Zn).

Stock solutions

A. 0.2 M disodium hydrogen phosphate (sodium phosphate, dibasic)

Either Na_2HPO_4:	28.39 g
or $Na_2HPO_4.2H_2O$:	35.60 g
or $Na_2HPO_4.7H_2O$:	53.61 g
or $Na_2HPO_4.12H_2O$:	71.62 g
Water:	to 1000 ml

The dihydrate is the most stable form because it is neither hygroscopic nor efflorescent.

B. 0.1 M citric acid

Either $C_6H_8O_7$ (anhydrous):	19.21 g
or $C_6H_8O_7.H_2O$:	21.01 g
Water:	to 1000 ml

The monohydrate is the form of citric acid most commonly used.

pH	A ml 0.2 M Na_2HPO_4	B ml 0.1 M citric acid
2.6	22	178
2.8	32	168
3.0	41	159
3.2	49	151
3.4	57	143
3.6	64	136
3.8	71	129
4.0	77	123
4.2	83	117

4.4	88	112
4.6	93.5	106.5
4.8	99	101
5.0	103	97
5.2	107	93
5.4	111	89
5.6	116	84
5.8	121	79
6.0	126	74
6.2	132	68
6.4	138.5	61.5
6.6	145.5	54.5
6.8	154.5	45.5
7.0	165	35
7.2	174	26
7.4	182	18
7.6	187	13
7.8	191.5	8.5

20.1.4.
pH 3.0–6.2: Citrate–citric acid buffer

Citrate forms complexes with many metals, including calcium.

Stock solutions
A. 0.1 M citric acid

Either Citric acid (anhydrous):	19.21 g
or Citric acid (monohydrate):	21.01 g
Water:	to make 1000 ml

This can be kept for several weeks. Discard if it shows signs of infection.

B. 0.1 M sodium citrate

Sodium citrate ($C_6H_5O_7Na_3.2H_2O$):	29.41 g
Water:	to make 1000 ml

pH	A ml 0.1 M citric acid	B ml 0.1 M sodium citrate
3.0	46.5	3.5
3.2	43.7	6.3
3.4	40.0	10.0
3.6	37.0	13.0
3.8	35.0	15.0
4.0	33.0	17.0
4.2	31.5	18.5
4.4	28.0	22.0
4.6	25.5	24.5
4.8	23.0	27.0
5.0	20.5	29.5
5.2	18.0	32.0
5.4	16.0	34.0
5.6	13.7	36.3
5.8	11.8	38.2
6.0	9.5	41.5
6.2	7.2	42.8

20.1.5.
**pH 5.3–8.0:
phosphate
buffer**

The table gives quantities for preparing 0.1 M sodium phosphate buffer solutions. These may be diluted with water to obtain weaker solutions (e.g. 0.06 M, 0.05 M, etc.). Twofold dilution increases the pH by approximately 0.05. Phosphate buffers cannot be used in the presence of those metal ions that would be precipitated as insoluble phosphates (i.e. all common cations other than Na^+, K^+, and NH_4^+). Equimolar quantities of potassium salts may be substituted for the sodium phosphates prescribed here. (Sodium ions provide a closer approximation to animal extracellular fluids.)

Stock solutions
A. 0.1 M sodium dihydrogen phosphate (sodium phosphate, monobasic; sodium acid phosphate)

Either NaH_2PO_4:	12.00 g
or $NaH_2PO_4.H_2O$:	13.80 g
or $NaH_2PO_4.2H_2O$:	15.60 g
Water:	to 1000 ml

The dihydrate is preferred because it is neither hygroscopic nor efflorescent.

If **potassium dihydrogen phosphate** is preferred, its 0.1 M solution contains KH_2PO_4 (anhydrous): 13.61 g in 1000 ml.

B. 0.1 M disodium hydrogen phosphate (sodium phosphate, dibasic)

Either Na_2HPO_4:	14.20 g
or $Na_2HPO_4.2H_2O$:	17.80 g
or $Na_2HPO_4.7H_2O$:	26.81 g
or $Na_2HPO_4.12H_2O$:	35.81 g
Water:	to 1000 ml

The dihydrate is preferred because it is neither hygroscopic nor efflorescent.

pH	A ml 0.1 M $Na_2H_2PO_4$	B ml 0.1 M Na_2HPO_4
5.3	192	8
5.5	188	12
5.7	184	16
5.8	180	20
5.9	174	26
6.0	168	32
6.1	162	38
6.2	154	46
6.3	146	54
6.4	136	64
6.5	128	72
6.6	112	88
6.7	104	96
6.8	96	104
6.9	82	118
7.0	68	132
7.1	56	144
7.2	48	152
7.3	40	160
7.4	34	166
7.5	28	172
7.6	23	177
7.7	17	183
7.8	12	188
7.9	8	192

20.1.6.
pH 6.8–8.2:
HEPES buffer

HEPES (N[2-hydroxyethyl]piperazine-N'-2-ethanesulphonic acid) is a zwitterionic amino acid that does not complex with the physiologically important ions Ca^{2+}, Mg^{2+} and Mn^{2+}. It is used in tissue culture media and in a few histochemical procedures.

Stock solutions
A. 0.05 M HEPES (See above for full name. Use the acid, not its sodium salt.)

HEPES:	11.92 g
Water:	to make 1000 ml

B. 1.0 M Sodium chloride (NaCl, 58.44 g/l)

C. 1.0 M Sodium hydroxide (NaOH, 40.00 g/l)

pH	A ml	B ml	C ml
6.8	100	9.25	0.75
7.0	100	8.90	1.10
7.2	100	8.46	1.54
7.4	100	7.93	2.07
7.6	100	7.36	2.64
7.8	100	6.80	3.20
8.0	100	6.31	3.69
8.2	100	5.91	4.09

It is important to check the pH with an accurately calibrated meter, because slight inaccuracy with ingredient C will give a buffer with the wrong pH.

20.1.7.
pH 7.2–9.0: TRIS
buffer

This is a 0.05 M TRIS buffer. It is compatible with salts of all heavy metals other than those with insoluble chlorides (e.g. Ag, Pb). The amino group of TRIS reacts with aldehydes, so these buffer solutions are **not used in fixatives**. The effective concentrations of some metal ions may be reduced by complex formulation with TRIS.

Stock solutions
A. 0.2 M TRIS

Tris(hydroxymethyl)aminomethane, $(CH_2OH)_3CNH_2$:	24.2 g
Water:	to make 1000 ml

B. 0.1 M hydrochloric acid (Section 20.3)

pH (See *Note*)	A ml 0.2 M TRIS	B ml 0.1 M HCl	Water: to make total volume (ml)
7.2	50	89.5	200
7.4	50	84	200
7.6	50	77	200
7.8	50	69	200
8.0	50	58.5	200
8.2	50	46	200
8.4	50	35	200
8.6	50	25	200
8.8	50	17	200
9.0	50	11.5	200

Note
TRIS buffers are more strongly affected by temperature than most others. The pH values in this table are correct at 25°C. For each degree C below 25°C the pH will be higher by 0.03. Thus, the mixture in the eighth line of the table (pH 8.6 at 25°C) will have pH 8.75 at 20°C and pH 8.39 at 32°C.

20.1.8
**pH 5.0–7.4:
Cacodylate–
hydrochloric
acid buffer**

This buffer (Plumel, 1948) is much used in fixatives for electron microscopy, but it is doubtful whether it has any advantage over cheaper, less toxic buffers. Sodium cacodylate, an arsenic compound, is expensive and is even more poisonous by mouth than by intravenous injection. Used solutions must be disposed of safely, following local laws and regulations.

Stock solutions

A. 0.2 M sodium cacodylate

$Na(CH_3)_2AsO_2.3H_2O$:		2.14 g
Water:		to make 50 ml

B. 0.2 M hydrochloric acid (See Section 20.3)

pH	A ml 0.2 M sodium cacodylate	B ml 0.2 M HCl	Water: to make total volume (ml)
5.0	50	47	200
5.2	50	45	200
5.4	50	43	200
5.6	50	39	200
5.8	50	35	200
6.0	50	29.5	200
6.2	50	24	200
6.4	50	18.5	200
6.6	50	13.5	200
6.8	50	9.5	200
7.0	50	6.5	200
7.2	50	4.2	200
7.4	50	2.5	200

20.1.9.
**pH 7.4–9.0:
Borate buffer**

This buffer (Holmes, 1943), which is compatible with low concentrations of silver nitrate, should not be confused with other borax-containing buffers.

Stock solutions

A. 0.2 M boric acid

H_3BO_3:		12.37 g
Water:		to 1000 ml

Takes 1–2 h to dissolve, with vigorous magnetic stirring.

B. 0.05 M borax

$Na_2B_4O_7.10H_2O$:		19.07 g
Water:		to 1000 ml

Dissolves easily.

pH	A ml 0.2 M boric acid	B ml 0.05 M borax
7.4	180	20
7.6	170	30
7.8	160	40
8.0	140	60
8.2	130	70
8.4	110	90
8.7	80	120
9.0	40	160

20.1.10.
pH 7.0–9.6:
Barbitone buffer

This is compatible with most commonly used reagents. Barbitone sodium (also known as barbital sodium, sodium diethylbarbiturate, veronal, and medinal) is a toxic substance and is subject to dangerous drug control legislation in most countries. It is seldom necessary to use barbitone buffer, because there are other buffer systems that cover the same pH range.

Stock solutions

A. 0.1 M barbitone sodium

Barbitone sodium ($C_8H_{11}O_3N_2Na$):	20.62 g
Water:	to 1000 ml

B. 0.1 M hydrochloric acid (See Section 20.3)

pH	A ml 0.1 M barbitone sodium	B ml 0.1 M HCl
7.0	107	93
7.2	111	89
7.4	116	84
7.6	123	77
7.8	132.5	67.5
8.0	143	57
8.2	154	46
8.4	164.5	35.5
8.6	174	26
8.8	181.5	18.5
9.0	187	13
9.2	190.5	9.5
9.4	195	5
9.6	197	3

20.1.11.
pH 8.5–12.8:
glycine–sodium
hydroxide buffer

Stock solutions

A. 0.1 M glycine with 0.1 M sodium chloride

Glycine (aminoacetic acid; H_2NCH_2COOH):	7.51 g
Sodium chloride (NaCl):	5.84 g
Water:	to make 1000 ml

B. 0.1 M sodium hydroxide (See Section 20.3)

pH	A ml 0.1 M glycine + NaCl	B ml 0.1 M NaOH
8.5	190	10
8.8	180	20
9.2	160	40
9.6	140	60
10.0	120	80
10.3	110	90
10.9	102	98
11.1	100	100
11.4	98	102
11.9	90	110
12.2	80	120
12.5	60	140
12.7	40	160
12.8	20	180

20.1.12.
pH 9.2–10.6:
Carbonate–
bicarbonate
buffer

Stock solutions

A. 0.2 M sodium carbonate

Sodium carbonate (Na_2CO_3): 21.2 g

Water: to 1000 ml

B. 0.2 M sodium bicarbonate

Sodium bicarbonate ($NaHCO_3$): 16.8 g

Water: to 1000 ml

pH	A ml 0.2 M Na_2CO_3	B ml 0.2 M $NaHCO_3$	Water: to make total volume (ml)
9.2	4	46	200
9.4	9.5	40.5	200
9.6	16	34	200
9.8	22	28	200
10.0	27.5	22.5	200
10.2	33	17	200
10.4	38.5	11.5	200
10.6	42.5	7.5	200

20.2 Physiological solutions

A physiological solution is one in which the structural and functional integrity of a living tissue is sustained for several hours after removal from the body. Physiological solutions, also called **balanced salt solutions**, mimic the extracellular fluids and have similar ionic composition, pH and osmotic pressure. They may also contain glucose and other simple nutrients such as glutamate, lactate and pyruvate. They are not tissue culture media, however, and they do not accommodate prolonged life or growth *in vitro*.

The following mixtures are derived largely from the data of Dawson *et al.* (1969). **Each ingredient should be weighed and dissolved in 50–100 ml of the water. These solutions should then be added, *in the order given*, to the remaining water.** Precipitation of insoluble salts will thus be avoided. The solutions can be kept until signs of infection are seen; cloudiness or mould usually appears after 2 days at 20°C or 2 weeks at 4°C.

20.2.1.
Normal saline

Sodium chloride (NaCl): 9.0 g

Water: to make 1000 ml

This is the simplest isotonic solution. It will not cause osmotic damage to mammalian or avian cells. For use with unfixed material, a buffered solution containing potassium and calcium ions (such as Ringer-Locke, Section 20.2.4, or Dulbecco's BSS, Section 20.2.6) is preferable for all but the briefest rinses.

For tissues of cold-blooded animals, the concentration of NaCl should be reduced to 0.6–0.65%. (See also Section 20.2.3.)

20.2.2.
Phosphate-
buffered saline
(PBS)

This is not a truly physiological solution because it is decidedly hypertonic. It is widely used for rinsing unfixed tissue, and for diluting antibodies and other reagents used in immunohistochemistry.

0.1 M phosphate buffer, pH7.4: 1000 ml

Sodium chloride (NaCl): 9 g

Keep at 4°C or room temperature. Discard if there are signs of infection.

20.2.3.
Amphibian
Ringer

This, which is the fluid developed by Ringer (1893), differs from the mammalian solution (Section 20.2.4, below) in containing only 6.5 g NaCl/l, and no glucose. The addition of glucose was found by Locke (1895) to prolong the active life of the isolated frog's heart from 5 h to 24 h.

20.2.4.
Mammalian
Ringer-Locke

Sodium chloride (NaCl):	9.0 g
Potassium chloride (KCl):	0.25 g
Calcium chloride (CaCl$_2$):	0.30 g
Sodium bicarbonate (NaHCO$_3$):	0.5 g
Glucose (C$_6$H$_{12}$O$_6$):	1.0 g
Water:	to make 1000 ml

20.2.5.
Krebs
bicarbonate-
phosphate
Ringer

Sodium chloride (NaCl):	6.9 g
Potassium chloride (KCl):	0.4 g
Calcium chloride (CaCl$_2$):	0.3 g
Potassium phosphate, monobasic (KH$_2$PO$_4$):	0.2 g
Magnesium sulphate (MgSO$_4$.7H$_2$O):	0.3 g
Sodium bicarbonate (NaHCO$_3$):	2.1 g
Water:	to make 1000 ml

This solution is isotonic with mammalian tissues. It can also be made by mixing 0.154 M aqueous solutions of the 6 solutes in the following proportions by volume: NaCl 100; KCl 4; CaCl$_2$ 3; KH$_2$PO$_4$ 1; NaHCO$_3$ 21 (Total = 129 volumes). If the salts are to be kept as stock solutions they should be stored in concentrated form (1.0 M or higher) to inhibit microorganisms, and diluted to 0.154 M before mixing.

20.2.6.
Dulbecco's
balanced salt
solution

Sodium chloride (NaCl):	8.0 g
Potassium chloride (KCl):	0.2 g
Sodium phosphate, dibasic (Na$_2$HPO$_4$):	1.15 g
Potassium phosphate, monobasic (KH$_2$PO$_4$):	0.2 g
Calcium chloride (CaCl$_2$):	0.1 g
Magnesium chloride (MgSO$_4$.6H$_2$O):	0.1 g
Water:	to make 1000 ml

This solution was devised for washing tissue cultures (Dulbecco and Vogt, 1954), but it is suitable for vascular perfusion and many other purposes requiring a buffered, isotonic solution. It contains no bicarbonate, so it is not suitable for prolonged maintenance of isolated organs.

20.3 Dilution of acids and alkalis

The simplest way to express the concentration of a substance is as **molarity** (number of mol/l of the solution; not to be confused with the much less often used **molality**, which is the number of mol/kg of solution). Concentrations of acids and bases are still quite commonly expressed as **normality**, however, following an older convention.

A normal solution of an acid or alkali contains the equivalent weight of the substance in a volume of 1 l.

$$\text{Equivalent weight} = \frac{\text{Molecular weight}}{\text{Number of available H}^+ \text{ or OH}^- \text{ ions per molecule}}$$

Thus, the equivalent weight of NaOH (MW 40) is 40 ÷ 1 = 40, so that a 1.0 N solution contains 40 g of NaOH per litre and is also 1.0 M. For sulphuric acid (H$_2$SO$_4$, MW 98.1) the equivalent weight is 98.1 ÷ 2 = 49.05, so a 1.0 N solution will solution will contain 49.05 g of 100% H$_2$SO$_4$ per litre, and will be 0.5 M.

The common laboratory acids are liquids, so it is convenient to dispense them by volume rather than by weight. The bottle in which a concentrated acid is supplied bears a label on which will be found the molecular weight, the density (specific gravity, SG), and the w/w percentage assay (g of 100% acid per 100 g of the liquid in the bottle). From these data, a solution of any normality may be prepared by calculating the volume of the acid needed to make 1 l of the solution.

$$V = \frac{100MN}{BPD}$$

where V is the required volume of concentrated acid (**in ml**) to make 1 l of the diluted acid; N is the desired normality of the solution; M is the molecular weight; P is the percentage assay of concentrated acid (**w/w**); D is the density (**g/ml**) of the concentrated acid; **B** is the basicity (i.e. number of available H^+ per molecule). The only common mineral acid whose basicity is greater than 1 is H_2SO_4 ($B = 2$). For all organic acids and for weak inorganic acids (such as phosphoric) the concentration should always be expressed as molarity, not as normality.

Table 20.1 is useful when preparing 1.0 N or 1.0 M solutions of common acids and alkalis, but only when the density and percentage assay stated on the label are the same as those listed in the table.

Table 20.1. Data for preparation of 1 l of 1.0 N or 1.0 M solutions of some acids and alkalis (add the quantity required to 800 ml water, mix well and then add water to 1000 ml)

Name	Concentrated product Assay (w/w) (%)	SG	Normality or molarity	Quantity required	Strength of dilute solution
Hydrochloric acid	36	1.18	12 N (12 M)	83 ml	1.0 N (1.0 M)
Hydrobromic acid	40	1.38	6.8 N (6.8 M)	147 ml	1.0 N (1.0 M)
Nitric acid	71	1.42	16 N (16 M)	63 ml	1.0 N (1.0 M)
Perchloric acid	60	1.54	9.2 N (9.2 M)	109 ml	1.0 N (1.0 M)
Sulphuric acid	96	1.84	36 N (18 M)	28 ml	1.0 N (0.5 M)
Acetic acid	99.5	1.05	17.4 M (17.4 N)	57 ml	1.0 M (1.0 N)
Formic acid	90	1.20	23.4 M (23.4 N)	42.5 ml	1.0 M (1.0 N)
Sodium hydroxide	100 (solid)	(2.13)	–	40 g	1.0 N (1.0 M)
Potassium hydroxide	100 (solid)	(2.04)	–	56 g	1.0 N (1.0 M)
Ammonium hydroxide	27% NH_3	0.901	14.3 M	70 ml	1.0 M
(ammonia water)	35% NH_3	0.880	18.2 M	55 ml	1.0 M

Notes

(1) **Caution.** Always add the concentrated acid slowly to the larger volume of water, stirring thoroughly to avoid overheating. This warning applies most strongly to sulphuric acid. Sodium or potassium hydroxide should also be added to water in the same way.

Concentrated HCl, HBr, HNO_3, CH_3COOH, HCOOH, and NH_4OH have pungent vapours. They should be poured in a fume cupboard.

All the concentrated acids and alkalis in the table are caustic. Avoid contact with skin. If you get concentrated acid on your skin it must be washed off with copious running tap water within 5–15 s if burning is to be prevented.

Never pipette acids or alkalis by mouth. Better still, don't pipette *any* chemicals by mouth!

(2) **Accuracy**. Concentrated solutions of gases (HCl, HBr, and especially, NH_3) lose potency after the bottles have been opened. When reagent from an old, two-thirds-empty bottle is used in the preparation of a buffer solution, it is more than usually important to check the pH with a meter. Be sure that the meter has been standardized against a reliable buffer solution.

Not all concentrated solutions are the same as those in *Table 20.1*. Check the label on the bottle; if necessary, use the formula to calculate the dilution.

20.4. Atomic weights

Table 20.2 may be used in calculating molecular weights (formula weights) of compounds. In histology and histochemistry, molecular weights accurate to the nearest whole number are adequate. The values of atomic weights in this table are approximated to the first decimal place.

Table 20.2. Approximate atomic weights of the commoner elements, radicals and ions

Element Name	Symbol	Atomic weight			
			Potassium	K	39.1
			Ruthenium	Ru	101.1
Aluminium	Al	27.0	Selenium	Se	79.0
Antimony	Sb	121.8	Silicon	Si	28.1
Arsenic	As	74.9	Silver	Ag	107.9
Barium	Ba	137.3	Sodium	Na	23.0
Beryllium	Be	9.0	Strontium	Sr	87.6
Bismuth	Bi	209.0	Sulphur	S	32.1
Boron	B	10.8	Tellurium	Te	127.6
Bromine	Br	79.9	Thallium	Tl	204.4
Cadmium	Cd	112.4	Thorium	Th	232.0
Calcium	Ca	40.1	Tin	Sn	118.7
Carbon	C	12.0	Titanium	Ti	47.9
Cerium	Ce	140.1	Tungsten	W	183.9
Chlorine	Cl	35.5	Uranium	U	238.0
Chromium	Cr	52.0	Vanadium	V	50.9
Cobalt	Co	58.9	Zinc	Zn	65.4
Copper	Cu	63.5	Zirconium	Zr	91.2
Fluorine	F	19.0			
Gold	Au	197.0	**Radical or ion**	**Molecular weight**	
Hydrogen	H	1.0			
Iodine	I	126.9	CH_2	14.0	
Iron	Fe	55.8	CH_3	15.0	
Lanthanum	La	138.9	C_2H_5	29.1	
Lead	Pb	207.2	C_6H_5	77.1	
Lithium	Li	6.9	CN	26.0	
Magnesium	Mg	24.3	H_2O	18.0	
Manganese	Mn	54.9	NH	15.0	
Mercury	Hg	200.6	NH_2	16.0	
Molybdenum	Mo	95.9	NH_3	17.0	
Nickel	Ni	58.7	NH_4	18.0	
Nitrogen	N	14.0	NO_2	46.0	
Osmium	Os	190.2	NO_3	62.0	
Oxygen	O	16.0	OH	17.0	
Palladium	Pd	106.4	PO_4	95.0	
Phosphorus	P	31.0	SO_3	80.1	
Platinum	Pt	195.1	SO_4	96.1	

20.5 Suitable tissues for histochemical techniques

This list includes some mammalian tissue with which positive histochemical reactions may easily be obtained. For a longer list, including invertebrate material, see Gabe (1976). For botanical materials, see Jensen (1962) and Klein and Klein (1970).

Nucleic acids

DNA	Any cellular tissue (nuclei)
RNA	Brain, spinal cord, ganglia (Nissl substance of neurons); glands (e.g. salivary glands, pancreas, stomach, intestine, pituitary); active lymph nodes (plasma cells).

Proteins and functional groups

Protein	Any tissue (cytoplasm, collagen)
Arginine	Intestine (Paneth cells); lymphoid tissue; any tissue with many nuclei
Tryptophan	Pancreas (exocrine cells, A-cells of islets); amyloid; fibrin
Cysteine	Skin (hair follicles)
Cystine	Skin (stratum corneum, hair shafts; pituitary (neurosecretory material); pancreas (B-cells of islets)
Aldehyde groups	Arterial elastic laminae in young rodents; any tissue fixed in glutaraldehyde (especially cytoplasm and collagen)

Carbohydrates

Glycogen	Liver (hepatocytes)
Glycosaminoglycans:	
Hyaluronic acid	Umbilical cord (Wharton's jelly); eye (vitreous); joints (synovial fluid)
Chondroitin sulphates	Cartilage matrix
Dermatan sulphate	Skin (dermis); tendon; lung (connective tissue)
Keratan sulphates	Cornea
Heparin	Mast cells (e.g. in skin, tongue, mesentery); blood basophils
Neutral glycoproteins	Stomach (surface mucus); thyroid (follicular cells); salivaryglands (serous cells); collagen, reticulin
Acid glycoproteins:	
Sulphated	Rat or mouse tongue (mucous glands); rat or mouse duodenum (Brunner's glands, goblet cells)
With sialic acids labile to neuraminidase	Rat or mouse rectum (goblet cells); mouse sublingual salivary gland (mucous cells)
With sialic acids labile to neuraminidase only after saponification	Rat sublingual salivary gland (mucous cells)

Lipids

Neutral fats	Adipose connective tissue
Phospholipids	Brain, peripheral nerve (myelin); heart, kidney (mitochondria); erythrocytes
Cholesterol esters	Degenerating myelin (2–4 weeks after transection of axons or destruction of neuronal somata in CNS); atherosclerotic lesions in human arteries
Steroids	Adrenal cortex; testis (Leydig cells)
Cholesterol	Brain (myelin)

Inorganic ions

Calcium
(phosphate
and carbonate)
Sites of pathological or senile calcification (kidney, tendons, human pineal gland); incompletely decalcified bones or teeth

Calcium
(soluble salts)
Kidney, muscle, nervous tissue; cell cultures

Iron
Liver, spleen, bone marrow (phagocytic cells); any tissue at site of old injury or haemorrhage

Zinc
Blood, haemopoietic tissue (granular leukocytes); prostate gland (cells or ducts); pancreas (B-cells of islets); brain (neuropil of hippocampus)

Enzymes

Acid phosphatase
Kidney (proximal tubule epithelium); liver (hepatocytes, phagocytic cells); prostate; intestine (cytoplasm of epithelial cells)

Alkaline
phosphatase
Kidney (brush-border of proximal tubules); intestine (brush-border of epithelium); rat brain (endothelium)

Esterases
(non-specific)
Liver (hepatocytes); kidney (tubules); brain (neuroglia, pericytes); blood (neutrophils, monocytes)

Acetyl-
cholinesterase
Muscle (motor endplates); brain (some neurons, neuropil, and axons)

Cholinesterase
(non-specific
or pseudo-
cholinesterase)
Brain (some neurons, capillary endothelium in rat)

Dehydro-genases
Liver, kidney, heart, intestine, etc. (cytoplasm, mitochondria)

Cytochrome
oxidase
Liver, kidney, heart, intestine, etc. (mitochondria); brain (stripes in cerebral cortex)

Monophenol
oxygenase
Skin (melanocytes in epidermis and dermis); eye (retina choroid, iris). Do not use an albino animal.

Peroxidase
Blood, haemopoietic tissue (granular leukocytes). Exogenous HRP in motor neurons 24–48 h after injection into muscle, or in phagocytes 1 h after intravenous injection. Erythrocytes exhibit peroxidase-like activity due to haemoglobin. Horseradish (*Armoracia rusticana*) root is the source of HRP.

Amines

Serotonin
Intestine (large amounts in argentaffin cells of epithelium); rat or mouse mast cells (large amounts in granules). Brain (small amounts in some neuronal somata in and near midline of brain stem, and in axons throughout CNS)

Noradrenaline
Adrenal medulla (large amounts in some chromaffin cells); brain (small amounts in some axons); ductus deferens (sympathetic axons)

Adrenaline
Adrenal medulla (large amounts in some chromaffin cells)

Dopamine
Mast cells in lungs of ruminants (large amounts); Ventral midbrain (any mammal, neurons in substantia nigra)

Histamine
Mast cells (any species); stomach of rat (small amounts in endocrine cells in mucosa of fundus)

Bibliography

Abbuhl, M.F. and Velasco, M.E. (1985). An economical minichamber for immunohistochemical incubation. *Journal of Histochemistry and Cytochemistry* **33**: 162–164.

Abe, H., Mehraein, P. and Weis, S. (1994). A modified NOR-silver impregnation technique for amyloid plaques and neurofibrillary tangles: comparative assessment. *Neuropathology and Applied Neurobiology* **20**: 478–486.

Abiko, Y., Kutsuzawa, M., Kowashi, Y., Kaku, T. and Tachikawa, T. (1999). *In situ* detection of gelatinolytic activity in developing craniofacial tissues. *Anatomy and Embryology* **200**: 283–287.

Abrahart, E.N. (1968). *Dyes and their Intermediates*. Oxford: Pergamon Press.

Acarin, L., Vela, J.M., Gonzalez, B. and Castellano, B. (1994). Demonstration of poly-*N*-acetyl lactosamine residues in ameboid and ramified microglial cells in rat brain by tomato lectin binding. *Journal of Histochemistry and Cytochemistry* **42**: 1033–1041.

Accini, L., Hsu, K.C., Spiele, H. and De Martino, C. (1974). Picric acid–formaldehyde fixation for immunoferritin studies. *Histochemistry* **42**: 257–264.

Achar, B.N., Bhandari, J.M. and Urs, H.G.V.G. (1993). A rapid safranin–metal phthalocyanine double staining technique for plants. *Biotechnic and Histochemistry* **68**: 127–131.

Adams, C.W.M. (1965). Histochemistry of lipids. In Adams, C.W.M. (ed.), *Neurohistochemistry*, pp. 6–66. Amsterdam: Elsevier.

Adams, C.W.M. and Bayliss, O.B. (1962). The release of protein, lipid and polysaccharide components of the arterial elastica by proteolytic enzymes and lipid solvents. *Journal of Histochemistry and Cytochemistry* **10**: 222–226.

Adams, C.W.M. and Bayliss, O.B. (1968). Reappraisal of osmium tetroxide and OTAN histochemical reactions. *Histochemie* **16**: 162–166.

Adams, C.W.M. and Sloper, J.C. (1955). Technique for demonstrating neurosecretory material in the human hypothalamus. *Lancet* **1**: 651–652.

Adams, C.W.M. and Tuqan, N.A. (1961). The histochemical demonstration of protease by a gelatin–silver film substrate. *Journal of Histochemistry and Cytochemistry* **9**: 469–472.

Adams, C.W.M., Abdullah, Y.H. and Bayliss, O.B. (1967). Osmium tetroxide as a histochemical and histological reagent. *Histochemie* **9**: 68–77.

Adams, J.C. (1981). Heavy metal intensification of DAB-based HRP reaction product. *Journal of Histochemistry and Cytochemistry* **29**: 775.

Adams, J.C. (1992). Biotin amplification of biotin and horseradish peroxidase signals in histochemical stains. *Journal of Histochemistry and Cytochemistry* **40**: 1457–1463.

Afzelius, B.A. (1992). Section staining for electron microscopy using tannic acid as a mordant: a simple method for visualization of glycogen and collagen. *Microscopy Research and Technique* **21**: 65–72.

Akert, K. and Sandri, C. (1968). An electron microscopic study of zinc iodide–osmium impregnation of neurones. I. Staining of synaptic vesicles and cholinergic junctions. *Brain Research* **7**: 286–295.

Aldridge, W.N. (1993). The esterases: perspectives and problems. *Chemico-Biological Interactions* **87**: 5–13.

Alers, J.C., Krijtenburg, P.J., Vissers, K.J. and van Dekken, H. (1999). Effect of bone decalcification procedures on DNA *in situ* hybridization and comparative genomic hybridization: EDTA is highly preferable to a routinely used acid decalcifier. *Journal of Histochemistry and Cytochemistry* **47**: 703–709.

Allen, D.T. (1992). *Blood–nervous tissue barriers in the peripheral nervous system*. PhD Dissertation, Department of Anatomy, University of Western Ontario, London, Canada.

Allen, D.T. and Kiernan, J.A. (1994). Permeation of proteins from the blood and peripheral nerves into ganglia. *Neuroscience* **99**: 755–764.

Allen, R.D. (1987). The microtubule as an intracellular engine. *Scientific American* **256**: 42–49.

Allen, R.L.M. (1971). *Colour Chemistry*. London: Nelson.

Allison, R.T. (1978). The crystaline nature of histology waxes: a preliminary communication. *Medical Laboratory Sciences* **35**: 355–363.

Allison, R.T. (1979). The crystaline nature of histology waxes: the effects of microtomy on the micro-structure of paraffin wax in sections. *Medical Laboratory Sciences* **36**: 359–372.

Allison, R.T. (1987). The effects of various fixatives on subsequent lectin binding to tissue sections. *Histochemical Journal* **19**: 65–74.

Allison, R.T. (1995). Picro-thionin (Schmorl) staining of bone and other hard tissues. *British Journal of Biomedical Science* **52**: 162–164.

Allison, R.T. (2002). Tissue processing and sectioning. In Kiernan, J.A. and Mason, I. (eds), *Microscopy and Histology for Molecular Biologists. A User's Guide*, pp. 145–169. London: Portland Press.

Allison, R.T. and Bryant, D. (1998). Effects of processing at 45°C on staining. *Biotechnic and Histochemistry* **73**: 128–136.

Allison, R. and Tanswell, S. (1993). Unexpected results of trichrome staining of quenched epithelial tissue following delayed fixation. *Journal of Histotechnology* **16**: 343–348.

Anatech Ltd (2002). Brazilliant! and brazilin. Available from: http://www.anatechltdusa.com/Innovators/7_Innsummaryofstains.html [accessed June 2007].

An, Y.H. and Martin, K.L. (2004). *Handbook of Histology Methods for Bone and Cartilage*. Totowa, NJ: Humana Press.

Anderson, M.J. and Cohen, M.W. (1974). Fluorescent staining of acetylcholine receptors in vertebrate skeletal muscle. *Journal of Physiology* **237**: 385–400.

Andersson, H., Baechli, T., Hoechl, M. and Richter, C. (1998). Autofluorescence of living cells. *Journal of Microscopy* **191**: 1–7.

Angerer, L.K., Cox, K.H. and Angerer, R.C. (1987). Demonstration of tissue-specific gene expression by *in situ* hybridization. *Methods in Enzymology* **152**: 649–661

Angermuller, S. and Fahimi, H.D. (1987). Electron microscopic cytochemical localization of oxidases with the cerium technique. *Journal of Anatomy* **155**: 222–223.

Angulo, A., Merchan, J.A. and Molina, M. (1994). Golgi–Colonnier method: correlation of the degree of chromium reduction and pH change with quality of staining. *Journal of Histochemistry and Cytochemistry* **42**: 393–403.

Appenteng, K., Batten, T.F.C. and Oakley, B.A. (1986). An alternative method for visualization of immunohistochemical reactions in HRP-labelled neurones. *Journal of Physiology* **382**: 179P.

Archimbaud, E., Islam, A. and Preisler, H.D. (1986). Alcian blue method for attaching glycol methacrylate sections to glass slides. *Stain Technology* **61**: 121–123.

Arnold, J. (1898). Ueber Structur und Architectur der Zellen. I. Mitteilung. *Archiv für mikroskopische Anatomie und Entwicklungsgeschichte* **52**: 134–151.

Arnold, M.M., Srivastava, S., Fredenburgh, J., Stockard, C.R., Myers, R.B. and Grizzle, W.E. (1996). Effects of fixation and tissue processing on immunohistochemical demonstration of specific andigens. *Biotechnic and Histochemistry* **71**: 224–230.

Arnold, N., Seibl, R., Kessler, C. and Weinberg, J. (1992). Nonradioactive *in situ* hybridization with digoxigenin labeled DNA probes. *Biotechnic and Histochemistry* **67**: 59–67.

Aschoff, A., Jantz, M. and Jirikowski, G.F. (1996). In-situ end labelling with bromodeoxyuridine – an advanced technique for the visualization of apoptotic tells in histological specimens. *Hormone and Metabolic Research* **28**: 311–314.

Ashton, A.R. (1984). An affinity label for the regulatory dithiol of ribulose-5-phosphate kinase from maize (*Zea mays*). *Biochemical Journal* **217**: 79–84.

Ashwood-Smith, M.J. (1971). Radioprotective and cryoprotective properties of DMSO. In Jacob, S.W., Rosenbaum, E.E. and Wood, D.C. (eds), *Dimethyl Sulfoxide*, Vol. 1, pp. 147–187. New York: Marcel Dekker.

Asou, H., Brunngraber, E.G. and Jeng, I. (1983). Cellular localization of GM-1 ganglioside with biotinylated choleragen and avidin peroxidase in primary cultured cells from rat brain. *Journal of Histochemistry and Cytochemistry* **31**: 1375–1379.

Atassi, M.Z. and Habeeb, A.F.S.A. (1972). Reaction of proteins with citraconic anhydride. *Methods in Enzymology* **25**: 546–553.

Axelsson, S., Bjorklund, A., Falck, B., Lindvall, O. and Svensson, L.-A. (1973). Glyoxylic acid condensation: a new fluorescence method for the histochemical demonstration of biogenic monoamines. *Acta Physiologica Scandinavica* **87**: 57–62.

Babal, P. and Gardner, W.A. (1996). Histochemical localization of sialylated glycoconjugates with *Tritrichomonas mobilensis* lectin (TLM). *Histology and Histopathology* **11**: 621–631.

Baccari, G.C., Marmorino, C., Minucci, S., Dimatteo, L., Varriale, B., Distria, M. and Chieffi, G. (1992a). Mallory stain may indicate differential rates of RNA synthesis. 1. A seasonal cycle in the Harderian gland of the green frog (*Rana esculenta*). *European Journal of Histochemistry* **36**: 81–90.

Baccari, G.C., Marmorino, C., Minucci, S., Dimatteo, L. and Distria, M. (1992b). Mallory stain may indicate differential rates of RNA synthesis. 2. Comparative observations in vertebrate nuclei. *European Journal of Histochemistry* **36**: 187–196.

Backstrom, G., Hallen, A., Hook, M., Jansson, L. and Lindahl, U. (1975). Biosynthesis of heparin. *Advances in Experimental Medicine and Biology* **52**: 61–72.

Bahr, G.F. (1954). Osmium tetroxide and ruthenium tetroxide and their reactions with biologically important substances. *Experimental Cell Research* **7**: 457–479.

Bailey, A.J. (2003). Restraining cross-links in elastomeric proteins. In Shewry, P.R., Tatham, A.S. and Bailey, A.J. (eds), *Elastomeric Proteins: Structures, Biomechanical Properties, and Biological Roles*, pp. 321–337. Cambridge: Cambridge University Press.

Baker, J.R. (1944). The structure and chemical composition of the Golgi element. *Quarterly Journal of Microscopical Science* **85**: 2–71 (and Plates 1,2).

Baker, J.R. (1946). The histochemical regognition of lipine. *Quarterly Journal of Microscopical Science* **87**: 441–470.

Baker, J.R. (1947). The histochemical recognition of certain guanidine derivatives. *Quarterly Journal of Microscopical Science* **88**: 115–121.

Baker, J.R. (1956). The histochemical recognition of phenols especially tyrosine. *Quarterly Journal of Microscopical Science* **97**: 161–164.

Baker, J.R. (1958). *Principles of Biological Microtechnique* (reprinted 1970, with corrections). London: Methuen.

Baker, J.R. (1960). Experiments on the action of mordants. 1. 'Single-bath' mordant dyeing. *Quarterly Journal of Microscopical Science* **101**: 255–272.

Baker, J.R. (1962). Experiments on the action of mordants. 2. Aluminium–haematein. *Quarterly Journal of Microscopical Science* **103**: 493–517.

Baker, J.R. and Williams, E.G.M. (1965). The use of methyl green as a histochemical reagent. *Quarterly Journal of Microscopical Science* **106**: 3–13.

Balaton, A.J., Vaury, P., Baviera, E.E., Vuong, P.N. and Galet, B.A. (1995). Protocole "EDTA-autocuiseur." Une technique immunohistochimique performante. *Annales de Pathologie* **15**: 295.

Bald, W.B. (1983). Optimizing the cooling block for the quick freeze method. *Journal of Microscopy* **131**: 11–23.

Baluk, P., Hirata, A., Thurston, G., Fujiwara, T., Neal, C.R., Michel, C.C. and McDonald, D.M. (1997). Endothelial gaps: time course of formation and closure in inflamed venules of rats. *American Journal of Physiology – Lung Cellular and Molecular Physiology* **16**: L155–L170.

Bancroft, J.D. and Cook, H.C. (1984). *Manual of Histological Techniques*. Edinburgh: Churchill-Livingstone.

Bancroft, J.D. and Gamble, M. (eds) (2002). *Theory and Practice of Histological Techniques*, 5th edn. London: Churchill-Livingstone.

Bancroft, J.D. and Stevens, A. (eds), *Theory and Practice of Histological Techniques*. Edinburgh: Churchill-Livingstone.

Bangle, R. (1954). Gomori's paraldehyde-fuchsin stain. I. Physico-chemical and staining properties of the dye. *Journal of Histochemistry and Cytochemistry* **2**: 291–299.

Bangle, R. and Alford, W.C. (1954). The chemical basis of the periodic acid Schiff reaction of collagen fibers with reference to periodate consumption by collagen and insulin. *Journal of Histochemistry and Cytochemistry* **2**: 62–76.

Bankfalvi, A., Riehemann, K., Ofner, D., Checci, R., Morgan, J.M., Piffko, J., Bocker, W., Jasani, B. and Schmid, K.W. (1994). Feuchtes Autoklavieren. Der einfachere Weg zur Antigendemaskieren. *Pathologe* **15**: 345–349.

Banks, P.M. (1979). Diagnostic applications of an immunoperoxidase method in hematopathology. *Journal of Histochemistry and Cytochemistry* **27**: 1192–1194.

Barbosa, P. and Peters, T.M. (1971). The effects of vital dyes on living organisms with special reference to methylene blue and neutral red. *Histochemical Journal* **3**: 71–93.

Bardosi, A., Dimitri, T., Wosgien, B. and Gabius, H.-J. (1989). Expression of endogenous receptors for neoglycoproteins, especially lectins, that allow fiber-typing on formaldehyde-fixed, paraffin-embedded muscle biopsy specimens. A glycohistochemical, immunohistochemical and glycobiochemical study. *Journal of Histochemistry and Cytochemistry* **37**: 989–998.

Barka, T. and Anderson, P.J. (1963). *Histochemistry. Theory, Practice and Bibliography*. New York: Harper & Row.

Barnett, S.J. and Bourne, G. (1941). Use of silver nitrate for the histochemical demonstration of ascorbic acid. *Nature* **147**: 542–543.

Barrett, A.J. (1971). The biochemistry and function of mucosubstances. *Histochemical Journal* **3**: 213–221.

Barrnett, R.J. and Seligman, A.M. (1958). Histochemical demonstration of protein-bound alpha-acylamido carboxyl groups. *Journal of Biophysical and Biochemical Cytology* **4**: 169–176.

Barszcz, C.A. (1976). Use of zinc chloride in Zenker-type fixatives. *Histo-Logic* **6**: 87.

Bartholomew, J.W. (1962). Variables influencing results, and the precise definition of steps in Gram staining as a means of standardizing the results obtained. *Stain Technology* **37**: 139–155.

Baschong, W., Suetterlin, R. and Laeng, R.H. (2001). Control of autofluorescence of archival formaldehyde-fixed, paraffin-embedded tissue in confocal laser scanning microscopy (CLSM). *Journal of Histochemistry and Cytochemistry* **49**: 1565–1571.

Batra, P.P. (1991). Conformational stability of citraconylated ovalbumin. *International Journal of Biochemistry* **23**: 1375–1384.

Battaglia, M., Pozzi, D., Grimaldi, S. and Parasassi, T. (1994). Hoechst 33258 staining for detecting mycoplasma contamination in cell cultures: a method for reducing fluorescence photobleaching. *Biotechnic and Histochemistry* **69**: 152–156.

Baumann, E., Stoya, G., Volkner, A., Richter, W., Lemke, C. and Linss, W. (2000). Hemolysis of human erythrocytes with saponin affects the membrane structure. *Acta Histochemica* **102**: 21–35.

Bayliss, O.B. and Adams, C.W.M. (1972). Bromine–Sudan black: a general stain for lipids including free cholesterol. *Histochemical Journal* **4**: 505–515.

Bayliss, O.B. and Adams, C.W.M. (1979). The pH dependence of borohydride as an aldehyde reductant. *Histochemical Journal* **11**: 111–116.

Bayliss High, O. (1984). *Lipid Histochemistry (Royal Microscopical Society: Microscopy Handbooks 06)*. Oxford: Oxford University Press.

Bayliss High, O.B. and Lake, B. (1996). Lipids. In Bancroft, J.D. and Stevens, A. (eds), *Theory and Practice of Histological Techniques*, pp. 213–242. Edinburgh: Churchill-Livingstone.

Beckmann, H.-J. and Dierichs, R. (1982). Lipid extracting properties of 2,2-dimethoxypropane as revealed by electron microscopy and thin layer chromatography. *Histochemistry* **76**: 407–412.

Beckstead, J.H. (1994). A simple technique for preservation of fixation-sensitive antigens in paraffin-embedded tissues. *Journal of Histochemistry and Cytochemistry* **42**: 1127–1134.

Beckstead, J.H. (1995). A simple technique for preservation of fixation-sensitive antigens in paraffin-embedded tissues: addendum. *Journal of Histochemistry and Cytochemistry* **43**: 345.

Bedossa, P., Bacci, J., Lemaigre, G. and Martin, E. (1987). Effects of fixation and processing on the immunohistochemical visualization of type-I, -III and -IV collagen in paraffin-embedded tissue. *Histochemistry* **88**: 85–89.

Beecken, H., Gottschalk, E.M., von Gizycki, U., Kramer, H., Maassen, D., Matthies, H.G., Musso, H., Rathjen, C. and Zdhorsky, U.I. (2003). Orcein and litmus. *Biotechnic and Histochemistry* **78**: 289–302.

Beesley, J.E. (ed.) (2001). *Immunocytochemistry and In Situ Hybridization*. Boston: Birkhauser.

Bell, M.A. and Scarrow, W.G. (1984). Staining for microvascular alkaline phosphatase in thick celloidin sections of nervous tissue: morphometric and pathological applications. *Microvascular Research* **27**: 189–203.

Bendayan, M. (1981a). Electron microscopical localization of nucleic acids by means of nuclease–gold complexes. *Histochemical Journal* **13**: 699–710.

Bendayan, M. (1981b). Ultrastructural localization of actin in insulin-containing granules. *Biology of the Cell* **41**: 157–160.

Bendayan, M. and Duhr, M.-A. (1986). Modification of the protein A–gold immunocytochemical technique for the enhancement of its efficiency. *Journal of Histochemistry and Cytochemistry* **34**: 569–575.

Benhamou, N., Gilboa-Garber, N., Trudel, J. and Asselin, A. (1988). A new lectin–gold complex for ultrastructural localization of galacturonic acids. *Journal of Histochemistry and Cytochemistry* **36**: 1403–1411.

Benkoel, L., Chamlian, A., Barrat, E. and Laffargue, P. (1976). The use of ferricyanide for the electron microscopic demonstration of dehydrogenases in human steroidogenic cells. *Journal of Histochemistry and Cytochemistry* **24**: 1194–1203.

Bennett, H.S., Wyrick, A.D., Lees, S.W. and McNeil, J.H. (1976). Science and art in preparing tissues embedded in plastic for light microscopy, with special reference to glycol methacrylate, glass knives and simple stains. *Stain Technology* **51**: 71–79.

Bennion, P.J., Horobin, R.W. and Murgatroyd, L.B. (1975). The use of a basic dye (azure A or toluidine blue) plus a cationic surfactant for selective staining of RNA: a technical and mechanistic study. *Stain Technology* **50**: 307–313.

Bensley, S.H. (1952). Pinacyanol erythrosinate as a stain for mast cells. *Stain Technology* **25**: 269–273.

Berg, W.F. and Ford, D.G. (1949). Latent image distribution as shown by physical development. *Photographic Journal* **89B**: 31–36.

Bergeron, J.A. and Singer, M. (1958). Metachromasy: an experimental and theoretical reevaluation. *Journal of Biophysical and Biochemical Cytology* **4**: 433–457.

Bergqvist, A., Carlstrom, K. and Ljungberg, O. (1984). Histochemical localization of estrogen and progesterone receptors: evaluation of a method. *Journal of Histochemistry and Cytochemistry* **32**: 493–500.

Berlyn, G.P. and Miksche, J.P. (1976). *Botanical Microtechnique and Cytochemistry*. Ames, IA: Iowa State University Press.

Bernhard, G.R. (1974). Microwave irradiation as a generator of heat for histological fixation. *Stain Technology* **49**: 215–224.

Berry, J.P., Hourdry, J., Sternberg, M. and Galle, P. (1982). Aluminum phosphate visualization of acid phosphatase activity: a biochemical and X-ray microanalysis study. *Journal of Histochemistry and Cytochemistry* **30**: 86–90.

Bertalanffy, F.D. (1964). Tritiated thymidine versus colchicine technique in the study of cell population cytodynamics. *Laboratory Investigation* **13**: 871–886.

Bertalanffy, L.V. and Bickis, I. (1956). Identification of cytoplasmic basophilia (ribonucleic acid) by fluorescence microscopy. *Journal of Histochemistry and Cytochemistry* **4**: 481–493.

Bertram, E.G. and Ihrig, H.K. (1959). Staining formalin-fixed nerve tissue with mercuric nitrate stain. *Stain Technology* **34**: 99–108.

Berube, G.R. and Clark, G. (1964). The cationic chelate of chromium and aluminon as a selective nuclear stain. *Stain Technology* **39**: 337–338.

Berube, G.R., Powers, M.M., Kerkay, J. and Clark, G. (1966). The gallocyanin–chrome alum stain: influence of methods of preparation on its activity and separation of the active staining compound. *Stain Technology* **41**: 73–81.

Bettinger, C. and Zimmermann, H.W. (1991a). New investigations on hematoxylin, hematein, and hematein–aluminium complexes. 1. Spectroscopic and physico-chemical properties of hematoxylin and hematein. *Histochemistry* **96**: 279–288.

Bettinger, C. and Zimmermann, H.W. (1991b). New investigations on hematoxylin, hematein, and hematein–aluminium complexes. 2. Hematein–aluminium complexes and hemalum staining. *Histochemistry* **96**: 215–228.

Beveridge, T.J. and Davies, J.A. (1983). Cellular responses of *Bacillus subtilis* and *Escherischia coli* to the Gram stain. *Journal of Bacteriology* **173**: 130–140.

Beveridge, T.J. and Schultze-Lam, S. (1996). The response of selected members of the archaea to the Gram stain. *Microbiology UK* **142**: 2887–2895.

Bhattacharjee, J., Cardozo, B.N., Kamphuis, W., Kamermans, M. and Vrensen, G.F.J.M. (1997). Pseudo-immunolabelling with the avidin–biotin–peroxidase complex (ABC) due to the presence of endogenous biotin in retinal Muller cells of goldfish and salamander. *Journal of Neuroscience Methods* **77**: 75–82.

Bigbee, J.W., Kosek, J.C. and Eng, L.F. (1977). Effects of primary antiserum dilution on staining of 'antigen-rich' tissues with the peroxidase-antiperoxidase technique. *Journal of Histochemistry and Cytochemistry* **25**: 443–447.

Bilinski, S.M. and Bilinska, B. (1996). A new version of the Ag-NOR technique. A combination with DAPI staining. *Histochemical Journal* **28**: 651–656.

Billman, J.H. and Diesing, A.C. (1957). Reduction of Schiff bases with sodium borohydride. *Journal of Organic Chemistry* **22**: 1068–1070.

Bina-Stein, M. and Tritton, T.R. (1976). Aurintricarboxylic acid is a nonspecific enzyme inhibitor. *Molecular Pharmacology* **12**: 191–193.

Bird, C.L. and Boston, W.S. (eds) (1975). *The Theory of Coloration of Textiles*. Bradford: Dyers' Company Publication Trust.

Birrell, G.B., Hedberg, K.K. and Griffith, O.H. (1987). Pitfalls of immunogold labeling: analysis by light microscopy, transmission electron microscopy, and photoelectron microscopy. *Journal of Histochemistry and Cytochemistry* **35**: 843–853.

Bjorklund, A. (1983). Fluorescence histochemistry of biogenic amines. In Bjorklund, A. and Hokfelt, T. (eds), *Handbook of Chemical Neuroanatomy*, Vol. 1, pp. 50–121. Amsterdam: Elsevier.

Bjorklund, A., Falck, B. and Lindvall, O. (1975). Microspectrofluorometric analysis of cellular monoamines after formaldehyde or glyoxylic acid condensation. In Bradley, P.B. (ed.), *Methods in Brain Research*, pp. 249–294. London: Wiley.

Blackstad, T.W., Fregerslev, S., Laurberg, S. and Rokkedal, K. (1973). Golgi impregnation with potassium dichromate and mercurous or mercuric nitrate: identification of the precipitate by X-ray diffraction methods. *Histochemie* **36**: 247–268.

Blank, K. and McCarthy, P.L. (1950). A general method for preparing histologic sections with a water-soluble wax. *Journal of Laboratory and Clinical Medicine* **36**: 776–781.

Blatt, A.H. (ed.) (1943). *Organic Syntheses. Collective*, Vol. 2. New York: Wiley.

Bloom, F.E. and Battenberg, E.L.F. (1976). A rapid, simple and sensitive method for the demonstration of central catecholamine-containing axons. II. A detailed description of methodology. *Journal of Histochemistry and Cytochemistry* **24**: 561–571.

Bobrow, M.N., Harris, T.D., Shaugnessy, K.J. and Litt, G.J. (1989). Catalyzed reporter deposition, a novel method of signal amplification. Application to immunoassays. *Journal of Immunological Methods* **125**: 279–285.

Bodian, D. (1936). A new method for staining nerve fibers and nerve endings in mounted paraffin sections. *Anatomical Record* **65**: 89–97.

Boenisch, T. (1989). Basic enzymology. In Naish, S.J. (ed.), *Immunochemical Staining Methods*, pp. 9–12. Carpinteria, CA: DAKO Corporation.

Boenisch, T. (1999). Diluent buffer ions and pH: their influence on the performance of monoclonal antibodies in immunohistochemistry. *Applied Immunohistochemistry and Molecular Morphology* **7**: 300–306.

Boenisch, T. (ed.) (2001). *Immunochemical Staining Methods*, 3rd edn. Carpinteria, CA: DakoCytomation. Available from: http://www.ihcworld.com/_books/Dako_Handbook.pdf [accessed June 2007].

Bona, C.A. and Bonilla, F.A. (1996). *Textbook of Immunology*, 2nd edn. Netherlands: Harwood.

Bondi, A., Chieregatti, G., Eusebi, G., Fulcheri, E. and Bussolati, G. (1982). The use of β-galactosidase as a tracer in immunocytochemistry. *Histochemistry* **76**: 153–158.

Bonilla, E. and Prelle, A. (1987). Application of Nile blue and Nile red, two fluorescent probes, for detection of lipid droplets in human skeletal muscle. *Journal of Histochemistry and Cytochemistry* **35**: 619–621.

Boon, M.E. (1990). Special issue: application of microwaves. *Histochemical Journal* **22**: 311–393.

Boon, M.E. and Drijver, J.S. (1986). *Routine Cytological Staining Techniques. Theoretical Background and Practice*. New York: Elsevier.

Boon, M.E. and Kok, L.P. (1991). Formalin is deleterious to cytoskeletal proteins: do we need to replace it by formalin-free Kryofix? *European Journal of Morphology* **29**: 173–180.

Boon, M.E., Vanderpoel, H.G., Tan, C.J.A. and Kok, L.P. (1994). Effect of embedding methods versus fixative type on karyometric measures. *Analytical and Quantitative Cytology and Histology* **16**: 131–136.

Bornig, H. and Geyer, G. (1974). Staining of cholesterol with the fluorescent antibiotic "filipin". *Acta Histochemica* **50**: 110–115.

Bosch, M.M.C., Walspaap, C.H. and Boon, M.E. (1996). Lessons from the experimental stage of the two-step vacuum–microwave method for histoprocessing. *European Journal of Morphology* **34**: 127–130.

Bosman, F.T., Visser, B.C. and Vanoeveren, J. (1996). Apoptosis: pathophysiology of programmed cell death. *Pathology Research and Practice* **192**: 676–683.

Botchkarev, V.A., Eichmuller, S., Peters, E.M.J., Pietsch, P., Johansson, O., Maurer, M. and Paus, R. (1997). A simple immunofluorescence technique for simultaneous visualization of mast cells and nerve fibers reveals selectivity and hair cycle-dependent changes in mast cell–nerve fiber contacts in murine skin. *Archives of Dermatological Research* **289**: 292–302.

Bottcher, C.J.F. and Boelsma-Van Houte, E. (1964). Method for the histochemical identification of choline-containing compounds. *Journal of Atherosclerosis Research* **4**: 109–112.

Bourne, G. (1933). Vitamin C in the adrenal gland. *Nature* **131**: 874.

Boyd, I.A. (1962). Uniform staining of nerve endings in skeletal muscle with gold chloride. *Stain Technology* **37**: 225–230.

Boyd, W.C. (1970). Lectins. *Annals of the New York Academy of Sciences* **169**: 168–190.

Braak, H. and Braak, E. (1991). Demonstration of amyloid deposits and neurofibrillary changes in whole brain sections. *Brain Pathology* **1**: 213–216.

Bradbury, S. (1973). *Peacock's Elementary Microtechnique*, 4th edn. London: Edward Arnold.

Braitenberg, V., Guglielmotti, V. and Sada, E. (1967). Correlation of crystal growth with the staining of axons by the Golgi procedure. *Stain Technology* **42**: 277–283.

Brandes, G. and Reale, E. (1990). The reaction of acridine orange with proteoglycans in the articular cartilage of the rat. *Histochemical Journal* **22**: 106–112.

Brandtzaeg, P. (1981). Prolonged incubation time in immunocytochemistry: effects on fluorescence staining of immunoglobulins and epithelial components in ethanol- and formaldehyde-fixed paraffin-embedded tissues. *Journal of Histochemistry and Cytochemistry* **29**: 1302–1315.

Breuer, A.C., Eagles, P.A., Lynn, M.P., Atkinson, M.B., Gilbert, S.P., Weber, L., Leatherman, J. and Hopkins J.M. (1988). Long-term analysis of organelle translocation in isolated axoplasm of *Myxicola infundibulum*. *Cell Motility and the Cytoskeleton* **10**: 391–399.

Bridges, J.W. (1968). Fluorescence of organic compounds. In Bowen, E.J. (ed.), *Luminescence in Chemistry*, pp. 77–115. London: van Nostrand.

Briggs, R.T., Drath, D.B., Karnovsky, M.L. and Karnovsky, M.J. (1975). Localization of NADH oxidase on the surface of human polymorphonuclear leukocytes by a new cytochemical method. *Journal of Cell Biology* **67**: 566–586.

Britton, H.T.S. (1956). *Hydrogen Ions*. 4th edn, 2 vols. London: van Nostrand.

Bronner, R. (1975). Simultaneous demonstration of lipids and starch in plant tissue. *Stain Technology* **50**: 1–4.

Brooker, L.G.S. (1966). Sensitizing and desensitizing dyes. In James, T.H. (ed.), *The Theory of the Photographic Process*, pp. 198–232. New York: Macmillan.

Brooks, S.A., Leathem, A.J.C. and Schumacher, U. (1997). *Lectin Histochemistry: A Concise Practical Handbook*. Oxford: Bios.

Brown, G.G. (1978). *An Introduction to Histotechnology*. New York: Appleton-Century-Crofts.

Buehner, T.S., Nettleton, G.S. and Longley, J.B. (1979). Staining properties of aldehyde fuchsin analogs. *Journal of Histochemistry and Cytochemistry* **27**: 782–787.

Buesa, R.J. (2000). Mineral oil: the best xylene substitute for tissue processing yet? *Journal of Histotechnology* **23**: 143–149.

Bullock, G.R. (1984). The current status of fixation for electron microscopy: a review. *Journal of Microscopy* **133**: 1–15.

Bulmer, D. (1962). Observations on histological methods involving the use of phosphotungstic and phosphomolybdic acids, with particular reference to staining with phosphotungstic acid/haematoxylin. *Quarterly Journal of Microscopical Science* **103**: 311–323.

Bu'Lock, A.J., Vaillant, C., Dockray, G.J. and Bu'Lock, J.D. (1982). A rational approach to the fixation of peptidergic nerve cell bodies in the gut using parabenzoquinone. *Histochemistry* **74**: 49–55.

Burnell, J.N. (1988). An enzymic method for measuring the molecular weight exclusion limit of plasmodesmata of bundle sheath cells of C_4 plants. *Journal of Experimental Botany* **39**: 1575–1580.

Burness, D.M. and Pouradier, J. (1977). The hardening of gelatin and emulsions. In James, T.H. (ed.), *The Theory of the Photographic Process*, pp. 77–87. New York: Macmillan.

Burns, J. (1982). The unlabelled antibody peroxidase-anti-peroxidase method (PAP). In Bullock, G.R. and Petrusz, P. (eds), *Techniques in Immunocytochemistry*, Vol. 1, pp. 91–105. London: Academic Press.

Burns, J. and Whitehead, R. (1966). Staining of Paneth cells with thioflavine T. *Nature* **211**: 769–771.

Burns, V.W.F. (1972). Location and molecular characteristics of fluorescent complexes of ethidium bromide in the cell. *Experimental Cell Research* **75**: 200–206.

Burry, R.W. (2000). Specificity controls for immunocytochemical methods. *Journal of Histochemistry and Cytochemistry* **48**: 163–165.

Burstone, M.S. (1959). New histochemical techniques for the demonstration of tissue oxidase (cytochrome oxidase). *Journal of Histochemistry and Cytochemistry* **7**: 112–122.

Burstone, M.S. (1960). Histochemical demonstration of cytochrome oxidase with new amine reagents. *Journal of Histochemistry and Cytochemistry* **8**: 63–70.

Burstone, M.S. (1962). *Enzyme Histochemistry*. New York: Academic Press.

Butcher, L.L. (1983). Acetylcholinesterase histochemistry. In Bjorklund, A. and Hokfelt, T. (eds), *Handbook of Chemical Neuroanatomy, Vol. 1. Methods in Chemical Neuroanatomy*, pp. 1–49. Amsterdam: Elsevier.

Cain, A.J. (1947). Use of Nile blue in the examination of lipoids. *Quarterly Journal of Microscopical Science* **88**: 383–392.

Cainelli, G. and Cardillo, G. (1984). *Chromium Oxidations in Organic Chemistry*. Berlin: Springer-Verlag.

Callis, G. (2002). Bone. In Bancroft, J.D. and Gamble, M. (eds), *Theory and Practice of Histological Techniques*, 5th edn, pp. 269–301. London: Churchill-Livingstone.

Campbell, K.P., NacLennan, D.H. and Jorgensen, A.O. (1983). Staining of the Ca^+-binding proteins calsequestrin, calmodulin, troponin C, and S-100, with the cationiccarbocyanine dye "stains-all". *Journal of Biological Chemistry* **258**: 11267–11273.

Campbell, S.S., Crawford, B.J. and Reimer, C.L. (1991). A simple ethanol-based freeze-substitution technique for marine invertebrate embryos which allows retention of antigenicity. *Journal of Microscopy* **164**: 197–215.

Cannon, H.G. (1937). A new biological stain for general purposes. *Nature* **139**: 549.

Cares, R. (1945). A note on stored formaldehyde and its easy reconditioning. *Journal of Technical Methods and Bulletin of the International Association of Medical Museums* **25**: 67–70.

Carlquist, S. (1982). The use of ethylenediamine in sectioning hard plant structures for paraffin sectioning. *Stain Technology* **57**: 311–317.

Carlsson, A., Falck, B. and Hillarp, N.-A. (1962). Cellular localization of brain monoamines. *Acta Physiologica Scandinavica* **54(Suppl. 196)**: 1–28.

Carrapico, F., Madalena-Costa, F. and Pais, M.S.S. (1984). Impregnation of biological material by ZnI_2–OsO_4, KI–OsO_4 and NaI–OsO_4 mixtures for electron microscopic observations: chemical interpretation of the reaction. *Journal of Microscopy* **134**: 193–202.

Carri, N.G. and Ebendal, T. (1989). Staining of developing neurites with coomassie blue. *Stain Technology* **64**: 50–52.

Carson, F.L. (1997). *Histotechnology. A Self-Instructional Text*, 2nd edn. Chicago: ASCP Press.

Carson, F.L., Martin, J.H. and Lynn, J.A. (1973). Formalin fixation for electron microscopy: a re-evaluation. *American Journal of Clinical Pathology* **59**: 365–373.

Carter, H.E., Glick, F.J., Norris, W.P. and Phillips, G.E. (1947). Biochemistry of the sphingolipides. III. The structure of sphingosine. *Journal of Biological Chemistry* **170**: 285–294.

Cason, J.E. (1950). A rapid one-step Mallory–Heidenhain stain for connective tissue. *Stain Technology* **25**: 225–226.

Casselman, W.G.B. (1955). Cytological fixation by chromic acid and dichromates. *Quarterly Journal of Microscopical Science* **96**: 203–222.

Cattoretti, G., Berti, E., Schiro, R., D'Amato, L., Valeggio, C. and Rilke, F. (1988). Improved avidin–biotin–peroxidase complex (ABC) staining. *Histochemical Journal* **20**: 75–80.

Cawood, A.H., Potter, U. and Dickinson, H.G. (1978). An evaluation of coomassie brilliant blue as a stain for quantitative microdensitometry of protein in section. *Journal of Histochemistry and Cytochemistry* **26**: 645–650.

Chaberek, S. and Martell, A.E. (1959). *Organic Sequestering Agents*. New York: Wiley.

Chadwicke, D.O. and Goode, J.A. (eds) (1995). *The Molecular Biology and Pathology of Elastic Tissues. Ciba Foundation Symposium 192*. Chichester: Wiley.

Chalmers, G.R. and Edgerton, V.R. (1989). Marked and variable inhibition by chemical fixation of cytochrome oxidase and succinate dehydrogenase in single motoneurons. *Journal of Histochemistry and Cytochemistry* **37**: 899–901.

Champy, C., Coujard, R. and Coujard-Champy, C. (1946). L'innervation sympathétique des glandes. *Acta Anatomica* **1**: 233–283.

Chan-Palay, V. (1973). A brief note on the chemical nature of the precipitate within nerve fibers after the rapid Golgi reaction: selected area diffraction in high voltage electron microscopy. *Zeitschrift fur Anatomie und Entwicklungs-Geschichte* **139**: 115–117.

Chang, H., Sander, C.S., Muller, C.S.L., Elsner, P. and Thiele, J.J. (2002). Detection of poly(ADP-ribose) by immunohistochemistry: a sensitive new method for the early identification of UVB- and H_2O_2-induced apoptosis in keratinocytes. *Biological Chemistry* **383**: 703–708.

Chaplin, A.J. (1985). Tannic acid in histology: an historical perspective. *Stain Technology* **60**: 219–231.

Chaplin, M.F. (1999). A proposal for the structuring of water. *Biophysical Chemistry* **83**: 211–221.

Chapman, D.M. (1977). Eriochrome cyanin as a substitute for haematoxylin and eosin. *Canadian Journal of Medical Technology* **39**: 65–66.

Chapman, D.M. (1982). Localization of methylene blue paramolybdate in vitally stained nerves. *Tissue and Cell* **14**: 475–487.

Chatton, R. (1923). Technique de double inclusion à l'agar et à la paraffine pour microtomie, avec orientation ou en masse, d'objets très petits. *Comptes Rendus Hebdomadaires des Séances et Mémoires de la Société de Biologie et de ses Filiales* **88**: 199–202.

Chayen, J. and Bitensky, L. (1991). *Practical Histochemistry*, 2nd edn. Chichester: Wiley.

Checler, F., Grassi, J. and Vincent, J.P. (1994). Cholinesterases display genuine arylacylamidase activity but are totally devoid of intrinsic peptidase activities. *Journal of Neurochemistry* **62**: 756–763.

Chemical Rubber Company (eds) (2007). *CRC Handbook of Chemistry and Physics*, 87th edn. Cleveland, OH: CRC Press.

Chen, G., Hanson, C.L. and Ebner, T.J. (1998). Optical responses evoked by cerebellar surface stimulation *in vivo* using neutral red. *Neuroscience* **84**: 645–668.

Chieco, P., Normanni, P. and Boor, P.J. (1984). Improvement in soluble dehydrogenase histochemistry by nitroblue tetrazolium preuptake in sections: a qualitative and quantitative study. *Stain Technology* **59**: 201–211.

Chilosi, M., Lestani, M., Pedron, S., Montagna, L., Benedetti, A., Pizzolo, G. and Menestrina, F. (1994). A rapid immunostaining method for frozen sections. *Biotechnic and Histochemistry* **69**: 235–239.

Christensen, J., Rick, G.A. and Soll, D.J. (1987). Intramural nerves and interstitial cells revealed by the Champy–Maillet stain in the opossum esophagus. *Journal of the Autonomic Nervous System* **19**: 137–151.

Christie, K.N. and Stoward, P.J. (1982). Distribution of endogenous hydrogen peroxide in cardiac muscle. *Journal of Anatomy* **135**: 837–838.

Chubb, I.W., Hodgson, A.J. and White, G.H. (1980). Acetylcholinesterase hydrolyses substance P. *FEBS Letters* **113**: 173–176.

Christie, R.M., Mather, R.R. and Wardman, R.H. (2000). *The Chemistry of Colour Application*. Oxford: Blackwell.

Churukian, C.J. (2000). *Manual of the Special Stains Laboratory*, 2000 edn. Rochester, NY: University of Rochester Medical Center.

Churukian, C.J. (1999). Lillie's oil red O method for neutral lipids. *Journal of Histotechnology* **22**: 309–311.

Churukian, C.J., Frank, M. and Horobin, R.W. (2000). Alcian blue pyridine variant – a superior alternative to alcian blue 8GX: staining peformance and stability. *Biotechnic and Histochemistry* **75**: 147–150.

Ciapetti, G., Granchi, D., Verri, E., Savarino, L., Cavedagna, D. and Pizzo-Ferrato, A. (1996). Application of a combination of neutral red and amido black staining for rapid, reliable cytotoxicity testing of biomaterials. *Biomaterials* **17**: 1259–1264.

Clark, C.A., Downs, E.C. and Primus, J.F. (1982). An unlabeled antibody method using glucose oxidase–antiglucose oxidase complexes (GAG). *Journal of Histochemistry and Cytochemistry* **30**: 27–34.

Clark, G. (ed.) (1973). *Staining Procedures Used by the Biological Stain Commission*, 3rd edn. Baltimore, MD: Williams & Wilkins.

Clark, G. (1979a). Displacement. *Stain Technology* **54**: 111–119.

Clark, G. (1979b). Staining with chromoxane cyanine R. *Stain Technology* **54**: 337–344.

Clark, G. (1981). *Staining Procedures used by the Biological Stains Commission*, 4th edn. Baltimore, MD: Williams & Wilkins.

Clark, P.G. (1954). A comparison of decalcifying methods. *American Journal of Clinical Pathology* **24**: 1113–1116.

Clark, W.M. (1972). *Oxidation–reduction Potentials of Organic Systems*. Huntington, NY: R.E. Krieger.

Clasen, R.A., Simon, G., Scott, R.V., Pandolfi, S. and Lesak, A. (1973). The staining of the myelin sheath by Luxol dye techniques. *Journal of Neuropathology and Experimental Neurology* **32**: 271–283.

Cleland, W.W. (1964). Dithiothreitol, a new protective reagent for SH groups. *Biochemistry* **3**: 480–482.

Clonis, Y.D., Atkinson, T., Bruton, C.J. and Lowe, C.R. (1987). *Reactive Dyes and Enzyme Technology*. Basingstoke: Macmillan.

Cole, E.C. (1943). Studies on hematoxylin stains. *Stain Technology* **18**: 125–142.

Cole, W.V. (1955). Motor endings in the striated muscle of vertebrates. *Journal of Comparative Neurology* **102**: 671–716.

Cole, W.V. and Mielcarek, J.E. (1962). Fluorochroming nuclei of gold chloride-stained motor endings. *Stain Technology* **37**: 35–39.

Collins, J.A., Schandl, C.A., Young, K.K., Vesely, J. and Willingham, M.C. (1997). Major DNA fragmentation is a late event in apoptosis. *Journal of Histochemistry and Cytochemistry* **45**: 923–934.

Collins, J.S. and Goldsmith, T.H. (1981). Spectral properties of fluorescence induced by glutaraldehyde fixation. *Journal of Histochemistry and Cytochemistry* **29**: 411–414.

Colonnier, M. (1964). The tangential organization of the visual cortex. *Journal of Anatomy* **98**: 327–344.

Combs, J.W., Lagunoff, D. and Benditt, E.P. (1965). Differentiation and proliferation of embryonic mast cells of the rat. *Journal of Cell Biology* **25**: 577–592.

Conger, K.A., Garcia, J.H., Lossinsky, A.S. and Kauffmann, F.C. (1978). The effect of aldehyde fixation on selected substrates for energy metabolism and amino acids in mouse brain. *Journal of Histochemistry and Cytochemistry* **26**: 423–433.

Conn, H.J. (1933). *The History of Staining*. Geneva, NY: Biological Stain Commission.

Conn, H.J. (1980–1981) The history of the Stain Commission (in 4 parts). *Stain Technology* **55**: 327–352; **56**: 1–17, 59–66, 135–142.

Connor, J.R., Pavlick, G., Karli, D., Menzies, S.L. and Palmer, C. (1995). A histochemical study of iron-positive cells in the developing rat brain. *Journal of Comparative Neurology* **355**: 111–123.

Contestabile, A. and Andersen, H. (1978). Methodological aspects of the histochemical localization of some cerebellar dehydrogenases. *Histochemistry* **56**: 117–132.

Conway, K. and Kiernan, J.A. (1999). Chemical dehydration of specimens with 2,2-dimethoxypropane (DMP) for paraffin processing of animal tissues: practical and economic advantages over dehydration in ethanol. *Biotechnic and Histochemistry*. **74**: 20–26.

Cook, G.M.W. (1995). Glycobiology of the cell surface: the emergence of sugars as an important feature of the cell periphery. *Glycobiology* **5**: 449–458.

Cook, G.M.W. and Stoddart, R.W. (1973). *Surface Carbohydrates of the Eukaryotic Cell*. London: Academic Press.

Cook, H.C. (1974). *Manual of Histological Demonstration Methods*. London: Butterworths.

Corbett, J.F. (1971). Hair dyes. In Venkataraman, K. (ed.), *The Chemistry of Synthetic Dyes*, Vol. 5, pp. 475–534. New York: Academic Press.

Cordell, J.L., Falini, B., Erber, W.N., Ghosh, A.K., Abdulaziz, Z., Macdonald, S., Pulford, K.A.F., Stein, H. and Mason, D.Y. (1984). Immunoenzymatic labeling of monoclonal antibodies using immune complexes of alkaline phosphatase and monoclonal anti-alkaline phosphatase (APAAP complexes). *Journal of Histochemistry and Cytochemistry* **32**: 219–229.

Correa, F.M.A., Innis, R.B., Rouot, B., Pasternak, G.W. and Snyder, S.H. (1980). Fluorescent probes of α- and β-adrenergic and opiate receptors: biochemical and histochemical evaluation. *Neuroscience Letters* **16**: 47–53.

Corrodi, H. and Jonsson, G. (1967). The formaldehyde fluorescence method for the histochemical demonstration of biogenic monoamines. *Journal of Histochemistry and Cytochemistry* **15**: 65–78.

Corsi, P. (1987). Camillo Golgi's morphological approach to neuroanatomy. In Masland, R.L., Portera-Sanchez, A. and Toffano, G. (eds), *Neuroplasticity: A New Therapeutic Tool in the CNS Pathology*, pp. 1–7. Berlin: Springer.

Costello, D.P. and Henley, C. (1971). *Methods for obtaining and handling marine eggs and embryos*. Woods Hole, MA: Marine Biological Laboratory. Available from: http://www.mbl.edu/BiologicalBulletin/EGGCOMP/pages/02.html [accessed April 2007].

Cotton, F.A., Wilkinson, G., Murillo, C.A. and Bochmann, M. (1999). *Advanced Inorganic Chemistry*, 6th edn. New York: Wiley.

Coupland, R.E., Kobayashi, S. and Crowe, J. (1976). On the fixation of catecholamines including adrenaline in tissue sections. *Journal of Anatomy* **122**: 403–413.

Coupland, R.E., Pyper, A.S. and Hopwood, D. (1964). A method for differentiating between noradrenaline- and adrenaline-storing cells in the light and electron microscope. *Nature* **201**: 1240–1242.

Couteaux, R. and Bourne, G.H. (1973). Motor end plate structure. In Bourne, G.H. (ed.), *The Structure and Function of Muscle*, Vol. 2, pp. 483–530. New York: Academic Press.

Cowden, R.R. and Curtis, S.K. (1970). Demonstration of protein-bound sulphydryl and disulphide groups with fluorescent mercurials. *Histochemie* **22**: 247–255.

Cowden, R.R. and Curtis, S.K. (1974). Use of a fluorescent probe for hydrophobic groups, anilinonaphthalene sulphonic acid, in the supravital study of unusual slug oocyte nuclei. *Histochemical Journal* **6**: 447–450.

Cowdry, E.V. (1952). *Laboratory Technique in Biology and Medicine*, 3rd edn. Baltimore, MD: Williams & Wilkins.

Cowen, T., Haven, A.J. and Burnstock, G. (1985). Pontamine sky blue: a counterstain for background autofluorescence in fluorescence and immunofluorescence histochemistry. *Histochemistry* **82**: 205–208.

Cox, B.A., Shackleford, J.M. and Yielding, L.W. (1982). Histochemical application of two phenanthridium compounds. *Stain Technology* **57**: 211–218.

Crivellato, E. and Mallardi, F. (1997). Stromal cell organisation in the mouse lymph node. A light and electron microscopic investigation using the zinc iodide–osmium technique. *Journal of Anatomy* **190**: 85–92.

Crooks, J. and Kolb, H. (1992). Localization of GABA, glycine, glutamate and tyrosine hydroxylase in the human retina. *Journal of Comparative Neurology* **315**: 287–302.

Culling, C.F.A. (1974). *Handbook of Histopathological and Histochemical Techniques*, 3rd edn. London: Butterworths.

Culling, C.F.A. and Reid, P.E. (1977). The apparent failure of sodium borohydride reduction to block further PAS reactivity in rat epithelial mucins. *Histochemical Journal* **9**: 781–785.

Culling, C.F.A., Reid, P.E. and Dunn, W.L. (1976). A new histochemical method for the identification and visualization of both side chain acylated and nonacylated sialic acids. *Journal of Histochemistry and Cytochemistry* **24**: 1225–1230.

Culling, C.F.A., Allison, R.T. and Barr, W.T. (1985). *Cellular Pathology Technique*, 4th edn. London: Butterworths.

Cunningham, L. (1967). Histochemical observations of the enzymatic hydrolysis of gelatin films. *Journal of Histochemistry and Cytochemistry* **15**: 292–298.

Cupo, D.Y. and Wetterhahn, K.E. (1985). Binding of chromium to chromatin and DNA from liver and kidney of rats treated with sodium dichromate and chromium(III) chloride *in vivo*. *Cancer Research* **45**: 1146–1151.

Dagdeviren, A., Alp, H. and Ors, U. (1994). New applications for the zinc iodide–osmium technique. *Journal of Anatomy* **184**: 83–91.

Danielli, J.F. (1947). A study of techniques for the cytochemical demonstration of nucleic acids and some components of protein. *Symposia of the Society for Experimental Biology* **1**: 11–113.

Danscher, G. (1996). The autometallographic zinc-sulphide method. A new approach involving *in vivo* creation of nanometer-sized zinc sulphide crystal lattices in zinc-enriched synaptic and secretory vesicles. *Histochemical Journal* **28**: 361–373.

Danscher, G. and Norgaard, J.O.R. (1985). Ultrastructural autometallography: a method for silver amplification of catalytic metals. *Journal of Histochemistry and Cytochemistry* **33**: 706–710.

Danscher, G. and Stoltenberg, M. (2005). Zinc-specific autometallographic *in vivo* selenium methods: tracing of zinc-enriched (ZEN) terminals, ZEN pathways, and pools of zinc ions in a multitude of other ZEN cells. *Journal of Histochemistry and Cytochemistry* **53**: 141–153.

Danscher, G. and Zimmer, J. (1978). An improved Timm sulphide–silver method for light and electron microscopic localization of heavy metals in biological tissues. *Histochemistry* **55**: 27–40.

Dapson, J.C. and Dapson, R.W. (2005). *Hazardous Materials in the Histopathology Laboratory. Regulations, Risks, Handling and Disposal*. Battle Creek, MI: Anatech Ltd.

Dapson, R.W. (1993). Fixation for the 1990s: a review of needs and accomplishments. *Biotechnic and Histochemistry* **68**: 75–82.

Dapson, R.W. (2005a). Dye–tissue interactions: mechanisms, quantification and bonding parameters for dyes used in biological staining. *Biotechnic and Histochemistry* **80**: 49–72.

Dapson, R.W. (2005b). A method for determining identity and relative purity of carmine, carminic acid and aminocarminic acid. *Biotechnic and Histochemistry* **80**: 201–205. (See also *Biotechnic and Histochemistry* **81**: 55 (2006) for a corrected illustration.)

Dapson, R.W., Feldman, A.T. and Wolfe, D. (2006). Glyoxal fixation and its relationship to immunohistochemistry. *Journal of Histotechnology* **29**: 65–76.

Dapson, R.W., Framk, M. and Kiernan, J.A. (2007). Revised procedures for the certification of carmine (CI 75470, Natural red 4) as a biological stain. *Biotechnic and Histochemistry* **82**: 13–15.

Darzynkiewicz, Z. and Li, X. (1996). Measurements of cell death by flow cytometry. In Cotter, T.G. and Martin, S.J. (eds), *Techniques in Apoptosis*, pp. 71–106. London: Portland Press.

Davey, H.M. and Kell, D.B. (1997). Fluorescent brighteners: novel stains for the flow cytometric analysis of microorganisms. *Cytometry* **28**: 311–315.

Davis, R.P. and Janis, R. (1966). Free aldehydic groups in collagen and other tissue components. *Nature* **210**: 318–319.

Davison, F.D., Groves, M. and Scaravilli, F. (1995). The effects of formalin fixation on the detection of apoptosis in human brain by *in situ* end-labelling of DNA. *Histochemical Journal* **27**: 983–988.

Davoli, M.A., Lamplugh, L., Beauchemin, A., Chan, K., Mordier, S., Mort, J.S., Murphy, G., Docherty, A.J.P., Leblond, C.P. and Lee, E.R. (2001). Enzymes active in areas undergoing cartilage resorption during the development of the secondary ossification center in the tibiae of rats aged 0–21 days: II. Two proteinases, gelatinase B and Collagenase-3, are implicated in the lysis of collagen fibrils. *Developmental Dynamics* **222**: 71–88.

Dawson, R.M.C., Elliott, D.C., Elliott, W.H. and Jones, K.M. (1969). *Data for Biochemical Research*, 2nd edn. Oxford: Oxford University Press.

Dawson, T.M., Bredt, D.S., Fotuhi, M., Hwang, P.M. and Snyder, S.H. (1991). Nitric oxide synthase and neuronal NADPH diaphorase are identical in brain and peripheral tissues. *Proceedings of the National Academy of Sciences of the United States of America* **88**: 7797–7801.

Day, F.A. and Neufeld, D.A. (1997). Use of enzyme overlay membranes to survey proteinase activity in frozen sections: cathepsin-like and plasmin-like activity in regenerating newt limbs. *Journal of Histochemistry and Cytochemistry* **45**: 779–783.

De, A.K., Khopkar, S.M. and Chalmers, R.A. (1970). *Solvent Extraction of Metals*. London: van Nostrand-Reinhold.

Dean, J.A. (ed.) (1999). *Lange's Handbook of Chemistry*, 15th edn. New York: McGraw-Hill.

De Bruijn, W.C., Memelink, A.A. and Riemersma, J.C. (1984). Cellular membrane contrast and contrast differentiation with osmium triazole and tetrazole complexes. *Histochemical Journal* **16**: 37–50.

De Capoa, A., Ferraro, M., Avia, P., Pelliccia, F. and Finazzi-Agro, A. (1982). Silver staining of the nucleolus organizer regions (NOR) requires clusters of sulfhydryl groups. *Journal of Histochemistry and Cytochemistry* **30**: 908–911.

De Fazio, A., Leary, J.A., Hedley, D.W. and Tattersall, M.H.N. (1987). Immunohistochemical detection of proliferating cells *in vivo. Journal of Histochemistry and Cytochemistry* **35**: 571–577.

Dehaas, R.R., Verwoerd, N.P., Vandercorput, M.P., Vangijlswijk, R.P., Siitari, H. and Tanke, H.J. (1996). The use of peroxidase-mediated deposition of biotin–tyramide in combination with time-resolved fluorescence imaging of europium chelate label in immunohistochemistry and *in situ* hybridization. *Journal of Histochemistry and Cytochemistry* **44**: 1091–1099.

Dehaas, R.R., Vangijlswijk, R.P.M., Vandertol, E.B., Zijlmans, H.J.M.A.A., Bakkerschut, T., Bonnet, J., Verwoerd, N.P. and Tanke, H.J. (1997). Platinum porphyrins as phosphorescent label for time-resolved microscopy. *Journal of Histochemistry and Cytochemistry* **45**: 1279–1292.

Deierkauf, F.A. and Heslinga, F.J.M. (1962). The action of formaldehyde on rat brain lipids. *Journal of Histochemistry and Cytochemistry* **10**: 79–82.

De Jong, J.P., Voerman, J.S.A., Leenen, P.J.M., Van Der Sluijs-Gelling, A.J. and Ploemacher, R.E. (1991). Improved fixation of frozen lympho-haemopoietic tissue sections with hexazotixed pararosaniline. *Histochemical Journal* **23**: 392–401.

Delves, P.J., Martin, S.J., Burton, D.R. and Roitt, I.M. (2006). *Roitt's Essential Immunology*, 11th edn. Malden, MA: Blackwell.

Demalsy, P. and Callebaut, M. (1967). Plain water as a rinsing agent preferable to sulfurous acid after the Feulgen method. *Stain Technology* **42**: 133–136.

DePalma, L. (1996). The effect of decalcification and choice of fixative on histiocytic iron in bone marrow core biopsies. *Biotechnic and Histochemistry* **71**: 57–60.

Deprez, M., Ceuterick de Groote, C., Fumal, A., Reznik, M. and Martin, J.J. (1999). A new combined Bodian–luxol technique for staining unmyelinated axons in semithin, resin-embedded peripheral nerves: a comparison with electron microscopy. *Acta Neuropathologica* **98**: 323–329.

Derenzini, M., Romagnoli, T., Mingazzini, P. and Marinozzi, V. (1988). Interphasic nucleolar organizer region distribution as a diagnostic parameter to differentiate benign from malignant tumors of human intestine. *Virchows Archiv B* **54**: 334–340.

Derenzini, M. (2000). The AgNORs. *Micron* **31**: 117–120.

Dermietzel, R., Leibstein, A., Siffert, W., Zamboglou, N. and Gros, G. (1985). A fast screening method for histochemical detection of carbonic anhydrase. *Journal of Histochemistry and Cytochemistry* **33**: 93–98.

Diaspro, A. (ed.) (2002). *Confocal and Two-Photon Microscopy: Foundations, Applications and Advances.* New York: Wiley-Liss.

Dickson, G.R. (1984). *Methods of Calcified Tissue Preservation.* New York: Elsevier.

Dinsdale, D. (1984). Ultrastructural localization of zinc and calcium within the granules of rat Paneth cells. *Journal of Histochemistry and Cytochemistry* **32**: 139–145.

Distl, R., Meske, V. and Ohm, T.G. (2001). Tangle-bearing neurons contain more free cholesterol than adjacent tangle-free neurons. *Acta Neuropathologica* **101**: 547–554.

Dixon, H.B. and Perham, R.H. (1968). Reversible blocking of amino groups with citraconic anhydride. *Biochemical Journal* **109**: 312–314.

Dixon, M. and Webb, E.C. (1979). *Enzymes*, 3rd edn. New York: Academic Press.

Dodt, H.U. and Zieglgansberger, W. (1998). Visualization of neuronal form and function in brain slices by infrared videomicroscopy. *Histochemical Journal* **30**: 141–152.

Dobkin, G. and Troyer, D. (2003). Preparing tissue sections using the RAMP technique. *Vet Technician* **24**: 777–780.

Doinikow, B. (1913). Zur Histopathologie der Neuritis mit besonderer Berucksichtigung der Regenerationsvorgange. *Deutsche Zeitschrift fur Nervenheilkunde* **46**: 20–42.

Drachenberg, C.B., Ioffe, O.B. and Papadimitriou, J.C. (1997). Progressive increase of apoptosis in prostatic intraepithelial neoplasia and carcinoma: comparison between *in situ* end-labeling of fragmented DNA and detection by routine hematoxylin–eosin staining. *Archives of Pathology and Laboratory Medicine* **121**: 54–58.

Drury, R.A.B. and Wallington, E.A. (1980). *Carleton's Histological Technique*, 5th edn. Oxford: Oxford University Press.

Drzeniek, R. (1973). Substrate specificity of neuraminidases. *Histochemical Journal* **5**: 271–290.

Dubois-Dalcq, M., McFarland, H. and McFarlin, D. (1977). Protein A–peroxidase: a valuable tool for the localization of antigens. *Journal of Histochemistry and Cytochemistry* **25**: 1201–1206.

Dujindam, W.A.L. and Van Duijn, P. (1975). The interaction of apurinic aldehyde groups with pararosaniline in the Feulgen–Schiff and related staining procedures. *Histochemistry* **44**: 67–85.

Dulbecco, R. and Vogt, M. (1954). Plaque formation and isolation of pure lines with poliomyelitis viruses. *Journal of Experimental Medicine* **99**: 167–182.

Dunnavant, W.R. and James, F.L. (1956). Molecular rearrangements. I. The base-catalyzed condensation of benzil with urea. *Journal of the American Chemical Society* **78**: 2740–2743.

Dux, M. and Jancso, G. (1994). A new technique for the direct demonstration of overlapping cutaneous innervation territories of peptidergic C-fibre afferents of rat hindlimb nerves. *Journal of Neuroscience Methods* **55**: 47–52.

Duyckaerts, C., Brion, J.P., Hauw, J.-J. and Flament-Durand, J. (1987). Quantitative assessment of the density of neu-rofibrillary tangles and senile plaques in senile dementia of the Alzheimer type. Comparison of immunocytochem-istry with a specific antibody and Bodian's protargol method. *Acta Neuropathologica* **73**: 167–170.

Dvorak, A.M. and Morgan, E.S. (1998). Ribonuclease–gold labels chondroitin sulphate in guinea pig basophil granules. *Histochemical Journal* **30**: 603–608.

Edwards, R. and Price, R. (1982). Butvar B-98 resin as a section adhesive. *Stain Technology* **57**: 50.

Eggert, F.M. and Germain, J.P. (1979). Rapid demineralization in acidic buffers. *Histochemistry* **59**: 215–224.

Eggert, F.M., Linder, J.E. and Jubb, R.W. (1981). Staining of demineralized cartilage. 1. Alcoholic versus aqueous dem-ineralization at neutral and acidic pH. *Histochemistry* **73**: 385–390.

Ehrlich, P. (1886). Die von mir herrührende Hämatoxylinlösung. *Zeitschrift für wissenschaftliche Mikroskopie* **3**: 150.

Einarson, L. (1951). On the theory of gallocyanin–chromalum staining and its application for quantitative estimation of basophilia. A selective staining of exquisite progressivity. *Acta pathologica et microbiologica scandinavica* **28**: 82–102.

Elftman, H. (1954). Controlled chromation. *Journal of Histochemistry and Cytochemistry* **2**: 1–8.

Elghetany, M.T. and Saleem, A. (1988). Methods for staining amyloid in tissues: a review. *Stain Technology* **63**: 201–212.

Elias, J.M. (1982). *Principles and Techniques in Diagnostic Histopathology*. Park Ridge, NJ: Noyes Publications.

Elleder, M. and Lojda, Z. (1970). Studies in lipid histochemistry. III. Reaction of Schiff's reagent with plasmalogens. *Histochemie* **24**: 328–335.

Elleder, M. and Lojda, Z. (1971). Studies in lipid histochemistry. VI. Problems of extraction with acetone in lipid histo-chemistry. *Histochemie* **28**: 68–87.

Elleder, M. and Lojda, Z. (1972). Studies in lipid histochemistry. IX. The specificity of Holczinger's reaction for fatty acids. *Histochemie* **32**: 301–305.

Elmes, M.E. and Jones, J.G. (1981). Paneth cell zinc: a comparison of histochemical and microanalytical techniques. *Histochemical Journal* **13**: 335–337.

Emerman, M. and Behrman, E.J. (1982). Cleavage and cross-linking of proteins with osmium(VIII) reagents. *Journal of Histochemistry and Cytochemistry* **30**: 395–397.

Emmel, V.M. and Stotz, E.H. (1986). Certified biological stains: a stability study. *Stain Technology* **61**: 385–387.

Emoto, K., Yamashita, S. and Okada, Y. (2005). Mechanisms of heat-induced antigen retrieval: does pH or ionic strength of the solution play a role for refolding antigens? *Journal of Histochemistry and Cytochemistry* **53**: 1311–1321.

Enerback, L. (1969). Detection of histamine in mast cells by o-phthalaldehyde reaction after liquid fixation. *Journal of Histochemistry and Cytochemistry* **17**: 757–759.

Engel, U., Breborowicz, D., Boghansen, T. and Francis, D. (1997). Lectin staining of renal tubules in normal kidney. *APMIS* **105**: 31–34.

Engen, P.C. and Wheeler, R. (1978). N-butyl methacrylate and paraffin as an embedding medium for light microscopy. *Stain Technology* **53**: 17–22.

Epstein, E.H., Munderloh, N.H. and Fukuyama, K. (1979). Dithiothreitol separation of newborn rodent dermis and epi-dermis. *Journal of Investigative Dermatology* **73**: 207–210.

Erenpreisa, J., Freivalds, T., Roach, H. and Alston, R. (1997). Apoptotic cell nuclei favour aggregation and fluorescence quenching of DNA dyes. *Histochemistry and Cell Biology* **108**: 67–75.

Erley, D.S. (1957). 2,2-dimethoxypropane as a drying agent for preparation of infrared samples. *Analytical Chemistry* **29**: 1564.

Espada, J., Juarranz, A., Galaz, S., Canete, M., Villanueva, A., Pacheco, M. and Stockert, J.C. (2005). Non-aqueous per-manent mounting for immunofluorescence microscopy. *Histochemistry and Cell Biology* **123**: 329–334.

Everbroek, B., Pals, P., Martin, J.J. and Cras, P. (1999). Antigen retrieval in prion protein immunohistochemistry. *Journal of Histochemistry and Cytochemistry* **47**: 1465–1470.

Everett, M.M. and Miller, W.A. (1974). The role of phosphotungstic and phosphomolybdic acids in connective tissue staining. *Histochemical Journal* **6**: 25–34.

Fabian, R.H. (1992). Poor reliability of immunocytochemical localization of IgG in immersion-fixed tissue from the cen-tral nervous system. *Journal of Histochemistry and Cytochemistry* **40**: 987–991.

Fadok, V.A., Voelker, D.R., Campbell, P.A., Cohen, J.J., Bratton, D.L. and Henson, P.M. (1992). Exposure of phos-phatidylserine on the surface of apoptotic lymphocytes triggers specific recognition and removal by macrophages. *Journal of Immunology* **148**: 2207–2216.

Fahy, E., Subramanian, S., Brown, H.A., Glass, C.K., Merrill, A.H., Murphy, R.C., Raetz, C.R.H., Russell, D.W., Seyama, Y., Shaw, W., Shimizu, T., Spener, F., van Meer, G., VanNieuwenhze, M.S., White, S.H., Witztum, J.L. and Dennis, E.A. (2005). A comprehensive classification system for lipids. *Journal of Lipid Research* **46**: 839–861.

Fairen, A., Peters, A. and Saldanha, J. (1977). A new procedure for examining Golgi impregnated neurons by light and electron microscopy. *Journal of Neurocytology* **6**: 311–337.

Falck, B., Hillarp, N.-A., Thieme, G. and Torp, A. (1962). Fluorescence of catechol amines and related compounds con-densed with formaldehyde. *Journal of Histochemistry and Cytochemistry* **10**: 348–354.

Faulstich, H., Zobeley, S., Bentrup, U. and Jockusch, B.M. (1989). Biotinylphallotoxins: preparation and use as actin probes. *Journal of Histochemistry and Cytochemistry* **37**: 1035–1045.

Feigl, F. (1960). *Spot Tests in Organic Analysis*, 6th edn, transl. R.E. Oesper (ed.). Amsterdam: Elsevier.

Feigl, F. and Anger, V. (1972). *Spot Tests in Inorganic Analysis*, 6th English edn, transl. R.E. Oesper (ed.). Amsterdam: Elsevier.

Feirabend, H.K.P., Ploeger, S., Kok, P. and Choufoer, H. (1993). Does microwave irradiation have other than thermal effects on histological staining of the mammalian CNS? A light microscopical study of microwave stimulated staining under isothermal conditions in man and rat. *European Journal of Morphology* **30**: 312–327.

Feldmann, G., Maurice, M., Bernuau, D., Rogier, E. and Durand, A.M. (1983). Penetration of enzyme-labelled antibodies into tissues and cells: a review of the difficulties. In Avrameas, S., Druet, P., Masseyeff, R. and Feldmann, G. (eds), *Immunoenzymatic Techniques*, pp. 3–15. Amsterdam: Elsevier.

Fensel, K., Kroncke, K.D., Kolb, H. and Kolb-Bachofen, V. (1994). *In situ* nick translation detects focal apoptosis in thymuses of glucocorticoid- and lipopolysaccharide-treated mice. *Journal of Histochemistry and Cytochemistry* **42**: 613–619.

Ferrari, F.A., Maccario, R., Marconi, M., Vitiello, M.A., Ugazio, A.G., Burgio, V. and Siccardi, A.G. (1980). Reliability of alpha-naphthyl acetate esterase staining of blood smears for the enumeration of circulating human T lymphocytes. *Clinical and Experimental Immunology* **41**: 358–362.

Fink, R.P. and Heimer, L. (1967). Silver impregnation of degenerating nerve endings, 2 methods. *Brain Research* **4**: 369–374.

Fink, S. (1987). Some new methods for affixing sections to glass slides. II. Organic solvent-based adhesives. *Stain Technology* **62**: 93–99.

Fischer, J.M.C., Peterson, C.A. and Bols, N.C. (1985). A new fluorescent test for cell vitality using calcofluor white M2R. *Stain Technology* **60**: 69–79.

Fish, P.A. (1895). The use of formalin in neurology. *Transactions of the American Microscopical Society* **17**: 319–330.

Fitzgerald, M.J.T. and Fitter, W.F. (1971). Significance of pH in staining cutaneous nerves with methylene blue. *Laboratory Practice* **20**: 783–800.

Fowler, S.D. and Greenspan, P. (1985). Application of Nile red, a fluorescent hydrophobic probe, for the detection of neutral lipid deposits in tissue sections: comparison with oil red O. *Journal of Histochemistry and Cytochemistry* **33**: 833–836.

Fox, C.H., Johnson, F.B., Whiting, J. and Roller, R.P. (1985). Formaldehyde fixation. *Journal of Histochemistry and Cytochemistry* **33**: 845–853.

Fraire, A.E., Kemp, B., Greenberg, S.D., Kim, H.S., Estrada, R. and McBride, R.A. (1996). Calcofluor white stain for the detection of Pneumocystis carinii in transbronchial lung biopsy specimens: a study of 68 cases. *Modern Pathology* **9**: 861–864.

Frangioni, G. and Borgioli, G. (1979). Polystyrene embedding: a new method for light and electron microscopy. *Stain Technology* **54**: 167–172.

Frank, M., Dapson, R.W., Wickersham, T.W. and Kiernan, J.A. (2007). Certification procedures for nuclear fast red (Kernechtrot), CI 60760. *Biotechnic and Histochemistry* **82**: 35–39.

Frankl, S.M. and Denaro, F.J. (1998). Peripheral nerve teasing: two protocols for diagnosis and research. *Journal of Histotechnology* **21**, 39–43.

Franklin, A.L. and Filion, W.G. (1985). A new technique for retarding fading of fluorescence: DPX–BME. *Stain Technology* **60**: 125–135.

Franklin, W.A. and Locker, J.D. (1981). Ethidium bromide: a nucleic acid stain for tissue sections. *Journal of Histochemistry and Cytochemistry* **29**: 572–576.

Franzblau, C. and Faris, B. (1981). Elastin. In Hay, E.D. (ed.), *Cell Biology of the Extracellular Matrix*, pp. 65–93. New York: Plenum Press.

Fraser, F.J. (1972). Degenerating myelin: comparative histochemical studies using classical myelin stains and an improved Marchi technique minimizing artifacts. *Stain Technology* **47**: 147–154.

Frederik, P.M., Bomans, P.H.H., Busing, W.M., Odselius, R. and Hax, W.M.A. (1984). Vapor fixation for immunocytochemistry and X-ray microanalysis on cryoultramicrotome sections. *Journal of Histochemistry and Cytochemistry* **32**: 636–642.

Frederiks, W.M. (1977). Some aspects of the value of Sudan black B in lipid histochemistry. *Histochemistry* **54**: 27–37.

Frederiks, W.M. and Bosch, K.S. (1997). Localization of superoxide dismutase activity in rat tissues. *Free Radical Biology and Medicine* **22**: 241–248.

Frederiks, W.M., Marx, F. and Myagkaya, G.L. (1989). The 'nothing dehydrogenase' reaction and the detection of ischaemic damage. *Histochemical Journal* **21**: 565–573.

Frens, G. (1973). Controlled nucleation for the regulation of the particle size in monodisperse gold suspensions. *Nature Physical Science* **241**: 20–22.

Fried, B., Gilbert, J.J. and Feese, R.C. (1976). Mercuric bromophenol blue to reveal gelatin substrates for protease. *Stain Technology* **51**: 140–141.

Friedberg, S.H. and Goldstein, D.J. (1969). Thermodynamics of orcein staining of elastic fibres. *Histochemical Journal* **1**: 261–376.

Friedrich, K., Seiffert, W. and Zimmermann, H.W. (1990). Romanowsky dyes and Romanowsky–Giemsa effect. 5. Structural investigations of the purple DNA–AB–EY dye complexes of Romanowsky–Giemsa staining. *Histochemistry* **93**: 247–256.

Fujimori, O. (1999). Protein A–gold/silver staining method: a review of a highly sensitive technique for light microscopic immunohistochemistry. *Applied Immunohistochemistry and Molecular Morphology* **7**: 280–288.

Furness, J.B. and Costa, M. (1975). The use of glyoxylic acid for the fluorescence histochemical demonstration of peripheral stores of noradrenaline and 5-hydroxytryptamine in whole-mounts. *Histochemistry* **41**: 335–352.

Furness, J.B., Costa, M. and Wilson, A.J. (1977). Water-stable fluorophores, produced by reaction with aldehyde solutions, for the histochemical localization of catechol- and indolethylamines. *Histochemistry* **52**: 159–170.

Furness, J.B., Heath, J.W. and Costa, M. (1978). Aqueous aldehyde (Faglu) methods for the fluorescence histochemical localization of catecholamines and for ultrastructural studies of central nervous tissue. *Histochemistry* **57**: 285–295.

Gabbott, P.L. and Somogyi, J. (1984). The 'single' section Golgi-impregnation procedure: methodological description. *Journal of Neuroscience Methods* **11**: 221–230.

Gabe, M. (1976). *Histological Techniques*, English edn, transl. E. Blackith and A. Kavoor. Paris: Masson.

Gaddum, J.H. (1935). Choline and allied substances. *Annual Review of Biochemistry* **4**: 311–330.

Gallyas, F. (1971a). Silver staining of Alzheimer's neurofibrillary changes by means of physical development. *Acta Morphologica Academiae Scientiarum Hungaricae* **19**: 1–8.

Gallyas, F. (1971b). A principle for silver staining of tissue elements by physical development. *Acta Morphologica Academiae Scientiarum Hungaricae* **19**: 57–71.

Gallyas, F. (1979). Light insensitive physical developers. *Stain Technology* **54**: 173–176.

Gallyas, F. and Merchenthaler, I. (1988). Copper–H_2O_2 oxidation strikingly improves silver intensification of the nickel-diaminobenzidine (Ni-DAB) end-product of the peroxidase reaction. *Journal of Histochemistry and Cytochemistry* **36**: 807–810.

Gallyas, F. and Wolff, J.R. (1986). Metal-catalysed oxidation renders silver intensification selective. Applications for the histochemistry of diaminobenzidine and neurofibrillary changes. *Journal of Histochemistry and Cytochemistry* **34**: 1667–1672.

Gallyas, F., Gorcs, T. and Merchenthaler, I. (1982). High-grade intensification of the end-product of the diaminobenzidine reaction for peroxidase. *Journal of Histochemistry and Cytochemistry* **30**: 183–184.

Galvez, J.J. (2006). Microwave tissue processing techniques: their evolution and understanding. *Microscopy and Analysis* **20**: 15–16.

Gambetti, P., Autilio-Gambetti, L. and Papasozomenos, S.C. (1981). Bodian's silver method stains neurofilament polypeptides. *Science* **213**: 1521–1522.

Ganter, P. and Jolles, G. (1969,1970). *Histochimie Normale et Pathologique*, 2 vols. Paris: Gaulthier-Villars.

Gao, K. (ed.) (1993). *Polyethylene Glycol as an Embedment for Microscopy and Histochemistry*. Boca Raton, FL: CRC Press.

Gao, K. and Godkin, J.D. (1991). A new method for transfer of polyethylene glycol-embedded tissue sections to silanated slides for immunocytochemistry. *Journal of Histochemistry and Cytochemistry* **39**: 537–540.

Gardiner, W. (1898). Methods for the demonstration of 'connecting threads' in the cell wall. *Proceedings of the Cambridge Philosophical Society* **9**: 504–512.

Garvey, J.S., Cremer, N.E. and Sussdorf, D.H. (1977). *Methods in Immunology*, 3rd edn. Reading, MA: W.A. Benjamin.

Garvey, W. (1991). Modification of the Mayer hematoxylin stain. *Journal of Histotechnology* **14**: 163–165.

Garvey, W., Fathi, A. and Bigelow, F. (1994). Demonstration of senile plaques and neurofibrillary tangles in Alzheimer's disease with uranyl and silver nitrates. *Journal of Histotechnology* **17**: 353–356.

Gatenby, J.B. and Beams, H.W. (eds) (1950). *The Microtomist's Vade-mecum (Bolles Lee)*, 11th edn. London: Churchill.

Gavrieli, Y., Sherman, Y. and Ben-Sasson, S.A. (1992). Identification of programmed cell death *in situ* via specific labeling of nuclear fragmentation. *Journal of Cell Biology* **119**: 493–501.

Geisert, E.E. and Updyke, B.V. (1977). Chemical stabilization of Golgi silver chromate impregnations. *Stain Technology* **52**: 137–141.

Geoghegan, W.D. and Ackerman, G.A. (1977). Adsorption of horseradish peroxidase, ovomucoid and anti-immunoglobulin to colloidal gold for the indirect detection of concanavalin A, wheat germ agglutinin and goat anti-human immunoglobulin G on cell surfaces at the electron microscopic level: a new method, theory and application. *Journal of Histochemistry and Cytochemistry* **25**: 1187–1200.

Gibb, R. and Kolb, B. (1998). A method for vibratome sectioning of Golgi–Cox stained whole rat brain. *Journal of Neuroscience Methods* **79**: 1–4.

Gilad, G.M. and Gilad, V.H. (1981). Cytochemical localization of ornithine decarboxylase with rhodamine or biotin-labeled α-difluoromethylornithine. An example for the use of labeled irreversible enzyme inhibitors as cytochemical markers. *Journal of Histochemistry and Cytochemistry* **29**: 687–692.

Giles, C.H. (1975). Dye-fibre bonds and their investigation. In Bird, C.L. and Boston, W.S. (eds), *The Theory of Coloration of Textiles*, pp. 41–110. Bradford: Dyers' Company Publication Trust.

Gill, G.W., Frost, J.K. and Miller, K.A. (1974). A new formula for a half-oxidized hematoxylin solution that neither overstains nor requires differentiation. *Acta Cytologica* **18**: 300–311.

Gill, J.E. and Jotz, M.M. (1976). Further observations on the chemistry of pararosaniline–Feulgen staining. *Histochemistry* **46**: 147–160.

Gilloteaux, J. and Naud, J. (1979). The zinc iodide–osmium tetroxide staining-fixative of Maillet. Nature of the precipitate studied by X-ray microanalysis and detection of Ca^{2+}-affinity subcellular sites in a tonic smooth muscle. *Histochemistry* **63**: 227–243.

Gimeno, E.J., Massone, A.R. and Portiansky, E.L. (1998). Preembedding epitope retrieval – an ultrasound-based method for unmasking desmin in tissue blocks. *Applied Immunohistochemistry* **6**: 35–41.

Girard, N., Delpech, A. and Delpech, B. (1986). Characterization of hyaluronic acid on tissue sections with hyaluronectin. *Journal of Histochemistry and Cytochemistry* **34**: 539–541.

Giroud, A. and Leblond, C.-P. (1934). Etude histochimique de la vitamine C dans la glande surrenale. *Archives d'Anatomie Microscopique* **30**: 105–129.

Gitirana, L.de B. and Trindade, A.V. (2000). Direct blue staining plus polarization microscopy: an alternative dye for polarization method for collagen detection in tissue sections. *Journal of Histotechnology* **23**: 347–349.

Glazer, A.N. (1976). The chemical modification of proteins by group-specific reagents. In Neurath, H. and Hill, R.L. (eds), *The Proteins*, Vol. 2, pp. 1–103. New York: Academic Press.

Glegg, R.E., Clermont, Y. and Leblond, C.P. (1952). The use of lead tetraacetate, benzidine, *o*-anisidine and a 'film test' in investigating the periodic acid–Schiff technique. *Stain Technology* **27**: 277–305.

Glenn, J.A., Sonceau, J.B., Wynder, H.J. and Thomas, W.E. (1993). Histochemical evidence for microglia-like macrophages in the rat trigeminal ganglion. *Journal of Anatomy* **183**: 475–481.

Glenner, G.G., Pinho e Costa, P. and Falcao de Freitas, A. (eds) (1980). *Amyloid and Amyloidosis (Proceedings of the Third International Symposium on Amyloidosis)*. Amsterdam: Exerpta Medica.

Glenner, G.G. (1957). The histochemical demonstration of indole derivatives by the rosindole reaction of E. Fischer. *Journal of Histochemistry and Cytochemistry* **5**: 297–304.

Glomb, M.A. and Monnier, V.M. (1995). Mechanism of protein modification by glyoxal and glycolaldehyde, reactive intermediates of the Maillard reaction. *Journal of Biological Chemistry* **270**: 10017–10026.

Goland, P., Grand, N.G. and Katele, K.V. (1967). Cyanuric chloride and *N*-methylmorpholine in methanol as a fixative for polysaccharides. *Stain Technology* **42**: 41–51.

Gold, H. (1971). Fluorescent brightening agents. In Venkataraman, K. (ed.), *The Chemistry of Synthetic Dyes*, Vol. 5, pp. 535–679. New York: Academic Press.

Gold, R., Schmied, M., Rothe, G., Zischler, H., Breitschopf, H., Wekerle, H. and Lassmann, H. (1993). Detection of DNA fragmentation in apoptosis: application of *in situ* nick translation to cell culture systems and tissue sections. *Journal of Histochemistry and Cytochemistry* **41**: 1023–1030.

Gold, R., Schmied, M., Giegerich, G., Breitschopf, H., Hartung, H.P., Toyka, K.V. and Lassmann, H. (1994). Differentiation between cellular apoptosis and necrosis by the combined use of *in situ* tailing and nick translation techniques. *Laboratory Investigation* **71**: 219–225.

Goldfischer, S., Kress, Y., Coltoff-Schiller, B. and Berman, J. (1981). Primary fixation in osmium-potassium ferrocyanide: the staining of glycogen, glycoproteins, elastin, an intranuclear reticular structure, and intercisternal trabeculae. *Journal of Histochemistry and Cytochemistry* **29**: 1105–1111.

Goldstein, D.J. (1962). Ionic and non-ionic bonds in staining, with special reference to the action of urea and sodium chloride on the staining of elastic fibres and glycogen. *Quarterly Journal of Microscopical Science* **103**: 477–492.

Goldstein, D.J. (1963). An approach to the thermodynamics of histological dyeing, illustrated by experiments with azure A. *Quarterly Journal of Microscopical Science* **104**: 413–439.

Goldstein, D.J. (1964). Relation of effective thickness and refractive index to permeability of tissue components in fixed sections. *Journal of the Royal Microscopical Society* **84**: 43–54.

Goldstein, D.J. and Horobin, R.W. (1974). Rate factors in staining by alcian blue. *Histochemical Journal* **6**: 157–174.

Goldstein, I.J. and Poretz, R.D. (1986). Isolation, physicochemical characterization, and carbohydrate-binding specificity of lectins. In Liener, I.E., Sharon, N. and Goldstein, I.J. (eds), *The Lectins. Properties, Functions and Applications in Biology and Medicine*, pp. 35–248. Orlando, FL: Academic Press.

Gonzalez-Burgos, I., Tapia-Arizmendi, G. and Feria-Velasco, A. (1992). Golgi method without osmium tetroxide for the study of the central nervous system. *Biotechnic and Histochemistry* **5**: 288–296.

Goodpasture, C. and Bloom, S.E. (1975). Visualization of nucleolar organizer regions in mammalian chromosomes using silver staining. *Chromosoma* **53**: 37–50.

Goodrich, E.S. (1919). The pseudopodia of the leucocytes of the invertebrates. *Quarterly Journal of Microscopical Science* **64**: 19–26.

Goodrich, E.S. (1942). A new method of dissociating cells. *Quarterly Journal of Microscopial Science* **64**: 19–26.

Goodwin, A.E. and Grizzle, R.M. (1994). Endogenous enzymes cause structural and chemical artifacts in methacrylate- and celloidin-embedded sections of unfixed freeze-dried tissues. *Journal of Histochemistry and Cytochemistry* **42**: 109–114.

Gorbsky, G. and Borisy, G.G. (1986). Reversible embedment cytochemistry (REC): a versatile method for the ultrastructural analysis and affinity labeling of tissue sections. *Journal of Histochemistry and Cytochemistry* **34**: 177–188.

Gordon, H. and Sweets, H.H. (1936). A simple method for the silver impregnation of reticulum. *American Journal of Pathology* **12**: 545–552.

Gordon, P.F. and Gregory, P. (1983). *Organic Chemistry in Colour*. Berlin: Springer-Verlag.

Gordon, S.R. (1988). Use of selected excitation filters for enhancement of diaminobenzidine photomicroscopy. *Journal of Histochemistry and Cytochemistry* **36**: 701–704.

Gorne, R.C. and Pfister, C. (1979). Pharmakologische Beeinflussung der γ-aminobuttersaure-(GABA)-Fluoreszenz in Hirnstrukturen der Ratte, mit Bemerkungen zum Chemismus der Nachweisreaktion. *Acta Histochemica* **65**: 168–183.

Goss, G., Petras, R.E., Perkins, A. and Miller, M. (1992). Effects of refixation and reprocessing on the quality of slides prepared from paraffin embedded tissues. *Journal of Histotechnology* **15**: 43–47.

Gown, A.M. and Willingham, M.C. (2002). Improved detection of apoptotic cells in archival paraffin sections: immunohistochemistry using antibodies to cleaved caspase 3. *Journal of Histochemistry and Cytochemistry* **50**: 449–454.

Goyer, R.A. and Cherian, M.G. (1977). Tissue and cellular toxicology of metals. In Brown, S.S. (ed.), *Clinical Chemistry and Chemical Toxicology of Metals*, pp. 89–103. Amsterdam: Elsevier-North Holland.

Graham, E.T. and Joshi, P.A. (1995). Novel fixation of plant tissue, staining through paraffin with alcian blue and hematoxylin, and improved slide preparation. *Biotechnic and Histochemistry* **70**: 263–266.

Graham, E.T. and Joshi, P.A. (1996). Plant cuticle staining with Bismarck brown Y and azure B or toluidine blue O before paraffin extraction. *Biotechnic and Histochemistry* **71**: 92–95.

Graham, R.C. and Karnovsky, M.J. (1966). The early stages of absorption of injected horseradish peroxidase in the proximal tubules of mouse kidney, ultrastructural cytochemistry by a new technique. *Journal of Histochemistry and Cytochemistry* **14**: 291–302.

Graham, R.C., Lundholm, U. and Karnovsky, M.J. (1965). Cytochemical demonstration of peroxidase activity with 3-amino-9-ethylcarbazole. *Journal of Histochemistry and Cytochemistry* **13**: 150–152.

Grand, R.J.A., Milner, A.E., Mustoe, T., Johnson, G.D., Owen, D., Grant, M.L. and Gregory, C.D. (1995). A novel protein expressed in mammalian cells undergoing apoptosis. *Experimental Cell Research* **218**: 439–451.

Gray, P. (1954). *The Microtomist's Formulary and Guide*. New York: Blakiston.

Green, F.J. (1990). *The Sigma–Aldrich Handbook of Stains, Dyes and Indicators*. Milwaukee, Wisconsin: Aldrich Chemical Company.

Green, M.R. and Pastewka, J.V. (1974a). Simultaneous and differential staining by a cationic carbocyanine dye of nucleic acids, proteins and conjugated proteins. I. Phosphoproteins. *Journal of Histochemistry and Cytochemistry* **22**: 767–773.

Green, M.R. and Pastewka, J.V. (1974b). Simultaneous and differential staining by a cationic carbocyanine dye of nucleic acids, proteins and conjugated proteins. II. Carbohydrate and sulfated carbohydrate-containing proteins. *Journal of Histochemistry and Cytochemistry* **22**: 774–781.

Green, M.R. and Pastewka, J.V. (1979). The cationic carbocyanine dyes stains-all, DBTC, and ethyl stains-all, DBTC-3,3′,9 triethyl. *Journal of Histochemistry and Cytochemistry* **27**: 797–799.

Greenspan, P. and Fowler, S.D. (1985). Spectrofluorometric studies of the lipid probe, Nile red. *Journal of Lipid Research* **26**: 781–789.

Greenspan, P., Mayer, E.P. and Fowler, S.D. (1985). Nile red: a selective fluorescent stain for intracellular lipid droplets. *Journal of Cell Biology* **100**: 965–973.

Greer, E.R. and Jen, C.K. (1990). Modified Golgi method for whole rat brain. *Stain Technology* **65**: 155–157.

Gregory, P. (1990). Classification of dyes by chemical structure. In Waring, D.H. and Hallas, G. (eds), *The Chemistry and Application of Dyes*, pp. 17–47. New York: Plenum Press.

Gregory, R.E. (1980). Alcoholic Bouin fixation of insect nervous systems for Bodian silver staining. II. Modified solutions. *Stain Technology* **55**: 151–160.

Gregory, R.E., Greenway, A.R. and Lord, K.A. (1980). Alcoholic Bouin fixation of insect nervous systems for Bodian silver staining. I. Composition of 'aged' fixative. *Stain Technology* **55**: 143–149.

Griffith, W.P. (1967). *The Chemistry of the Rarer Platinum Metals (Os, Ru, Ir and Rh)*. London: Wiley.

Grizzle, W.E. (1996). Theory and practice of silver staining in histopathology. *Journal of Histotechnology* **19**: 183–195.

Grocott, R.G. (1955). Stain for fungi in tissue sections and smears using Gomori's methenamine–silver nitrate technic. *American Journal of Clinical Pathology* **24**: 975–979.

Grosman, J. and Vardaxis, N.J. (1997). Aluminum acid alizarin violet: a general purpose nuclear fluorochrome. *Biotechnic and Histochemistry* **72**: 299–303.

Guesdon, J.-L., Ternynck, T. and Avrameas, S. (1979). The use of avidin–biotin in immunoenzymatic techniques. *Journal of Histochemistry and Cytochemistry* **27**: 1131–1139.

Guiot, Y. and Rahier, J. (1995). The effects of varying key steps in the non-radioactive *in situ* hybridization protocol: a quantitative study. *Histochemical Journal* **27**: 60–68.

Gunstone, F.D., Harwood, J.L. and Padley, F.B. (eds) (1986). *The Lipid Handbook*. London: Chapman and Hall.

Guntern, R., Bouras, C., Hof, P.R. and Vallet, P.G. (1992). An improved thioflavine S method for staining neurofibrillary tangles and senile plaques in Alzheimer's disease. *Experientia* **48**: 8–10.

Gurr, E. (1971). *Synthetic Dyes in Biology Medicine and Chemistry*. London: Academic Press.

Gurr, E., Anand, N., Unni, M.K. and Ayyangar, N.R. (1974). Applications of synthetic dyes to biological problems. In Venkataraman, K. (ed.), *The Chemistry of Synthetic Dyes*, Vol. 7, pp. 277–351. New York: Academic Press.

Gurrieri, S., Wells, K.S., Johnson, I.D. and Bustamante, C. (1997). Direct visualization of individual DNA molecules by fluorescence microscopy: characterization of the factors affecting signal/background and optimization of imaging conditions using YOYO. *Analytical Biochemistry* **249**: 44–53.

Gustavson, K.H. (1956). *The Chemistry of Tanning Processes*. New York: Academic Press.

Gutierrez, M. (1991). Reaccion quimica del bloqueo del grupo guanidilo de la arginina. *Anales de la Real Academia Medicina y Cirurgia de Cadiz* **27**: 143–147.

Haas, F. (1992). Serial sectioning of insects with hard exoskeleton by dissolution of the exocuticle. *Biotechnic and Histochemistry* **67**: 50–54.

Hadler, W.A. and Silveira, S.R. (1978). Histochemical technique to detect choline-containing lipids. *Acta Histochemica* **63**: 265–270.

Hadler, W.A., Lucca, O.de, Ziti, L.M. and Patelli, A.S. (1969). An analysis of the effect of some fixatives on the histochemical distribution of nonhaem ferric iron in spleen sections. *Revista Brasileira de Pesquisas Medicas e Biologicas* **2**: 378–383.

Hahn von Dorsch, H., Krause, R., Fehrmann, P. and Sulzmann, R. (1975). Histochemische Nachweismethoden für biogene Amine. *Acta Histochemica* **52**: 281–302.

Haga, C., Ikeda, K., Iwabuchi, K., Akiyama, H., Kondoh, H. and Kosaka, K. (1994). Methenamine–silver staining: a simple and sensitive method for senile plaques and neurofibrillary tangles. *Biotechnic and Histochemistry* **69**: 295–300.

Hakanson, R., Owman, C.H., Sjoberg, N.O. and Sporrong, B. (1970). Amine mechanisms in enterochromaffin-like cells of gastric mucosa in various mammals. *Histochemie* **26**: 189–220.

Hakanson, R., Owman, C. and Sundler, E. (1972). *O*-Phthalaldehyde (OPT). A sensitive detection reagent for glucagon, secretin and vasoactive intestinal peptide. *Journal of Histochemistry and Cytochemistry* **20**: 138–140.

Halbhuber, K.-J., Gossrau, R., Muller, U., Hulstaert, C.E., Zimmermann, N. and Feverstein, H. (1988a). The cerium perhydroxide–diaminobenzidine (Ce–H_2O_2–DAB) procedure. New methods for light microscopic phosphatase histochemistry and immunohistochemistry. *Histochemistry* **90**: 289–297.

Halbhuber, K.-J., Zimmermann, N. and Linss, W. (1988b). New, improved lanthanide-based methods for the ultrastructural localization of acid and alkaline phosphatase activity. *Histochemistry* **88**: 375–381.

Halbhuber, K.J., Hulstaert, C.E., Gerrits, P., Moller, U., Kalicharan, D. and Feuerstein, H. (1991). Cerium as amplifying agent: an improved cerium–perhydroxide–DAB–nickel (Ce/Ce–H_2O_2–DAB–Ni) method for the visualization of cerium phosphate in resin sections. *Cellular and Molecular Biology* **37**: 295–307.

Halbhuber, K.J., Scheven, C., Jirikowski, G., Feuerstein, H. and Ott, U. (1996). Reflectance enzyme histochemistry (REH): visualization of cerium-based and DAB primary reaction products of phosphatases and oxidases in cryostat sections by confocal laser scanning microscopy. *Histochemistry and Cell Biology* **105**: 239–249.

Hanker, J.S., Thornburg, L.P. and Yates, P.E. (1973). The demonstration of cholinesterases by the formation of osmium blacks at the sites of Hatchett's brown. *Histochemie* **37**: 223–242.

Hanker, J.S., Yates, P.E., Metz, C.B. and Rustioni, A. (1977). A new specific, sensitive and non-carcinogenic reagent for the demonstration of horseradish peroxidase. *Histochemical Journal* **9**: 789–792.

Hansch, C. and Leo, A. (1995). *Exploring QSAR. Fundamentals and Applications in Chemistry and Biology*, Vol. 1. Washington, DC: American Chemical Society.

Harris, C.M. and Livingstone, S.E. (1964). Bidentate chelates. In Dwyer, F.P. and Mellor, D.P. (eds), *Chelating Agents and Metal Chelators*, pp. 95–141. New York: Academic Press.

Hascall, V.C. and Hascall, G.K. (1981). Proteoglycans. In Hay, E.D. (ed.), *Cell Biology of the Extracellular Matrix*, pp. 39–63. New York: Plenum Press.

Hasegawa, J. and Hasegawa, J. (1977). Substrate limitations of the color film technique for the localization of proteases. *Journal of Histochemistry and Cytochemistry* **25**: 234.

Haugland, R.P. (2002). *Handbook of Fluorescent Probes and Research Chemicals*, 9th edn. Eugene, OR: Molecular Probes Inc.

Hauke, C. and Korr, H. (1993). RCA-I lectin histochemistry after trypsinisation enables the identification of microglial cells in thin paraffin sections of the mouse brain. *Journal of Neuroscience Methods* **50**: 273–277.

Hausen, P. and Dreyer, C. (1981). The use of polyacrylamide as an embedding medium for immunohistochemical studies of embryonic tissues. *Stain Technology* **56**: 287–293.

Hausen, P. and Dreyer, C. (1982). Urea reactivates antigens in paraffin sections for immunofluorescent staining. *Stain Technology* **57**: 321–324.

Hawkins, N.J., Lees, J. and Ward, R.L. (1997). Detection of apoptosis in colorectal carcinoma by light microscopy and *in situ* end labelling. *Analytical and Quantitative Cytology and Histology* **19**: 227–232.

Hayat, M.A. (ed.) (1973–1977). *Electron Microscopy of Enzymes. Principles and Methods*, Vols 1–5. New York: van Nostrand-Reinhold.

Hayat, M.A. (1975). *Positive Staining for Electron Microscopy*. New York: van Nostrand-Reinhold.

Hayat, M.A. (1981). *Principles and Techniques of Electron Microscopy. Biological Applications*, 2nd edn, Vol. 1. Baltimore, MD: University Park Press.

Hayat, M.A. (1993). *Stains and Cytochemical Methods*. New York: Plenum Press.

Hayes, B.L. (2002). *Microwave Synthesis: Chemistry at the Speed of Light*. Matthews, NC: CEM Publishing.

Hayhoe, F.G.J. and Quaglino, D. (1988). *Haematological Cytochemistry*, 2nd edn. Edinburgh: Churchill-Livingstone.

Heath, I.D. (1962). Observations on a highly specific method for the histochemical detection of sulphated mucopolysaccharides, and its possible mechanisms. *Quarterly Journal of Microscopical Science* **103**: 457–475.

Heggebo, R., Gonzalez, L., Press, C.M., Gunnes, G., Espines, A. and Jeffrey, M. (2003). Disease–associated PrP in the enteric nervous system of scrapie-affected Suffolk sheep. *Journal of General Virology* **84**: 1327–1338.

Heidemann, E. (1988). The chemistry of tanning. In Nimni, M.E. (ed.), *Collagen*, Vol. 3, pp. 39–61. Boca Raton, FL: CRC Press.

Heinicke, E.A., Kiernan, J.A. and Wijsman, J. (1987). Specific, selective, and complete staining of neurons of the myenteric plexus, using cuprolinic blue. *Journal of Neuroscience Methods* **21**: 45–54.

Helander, K.G. (1987). Studies on the rate of dehydration of histological specimens. *Journal of Microscopy* **145**: 351–355.

Helander, K.G. (1994). Kinetic studies of formaldehyde binding in tissue. *Biotechnic and Histochemistry* **69**: 177–179.

Helander, K.G. (1999). Formaldehyde binding in brain and kidney: a kinetic study of fixation. *Journal of Histotechnology* **22**: 317–318.

Hendrickson, J.B., Cram, D.J. and Hammond, G.S. (1970). *Organic Chemistry*, 3rd edn. New York: McGraw-Hill.

Henkel, A.W., Lubke, J. and Betz, W.J. (1996). FM1–43 dye ultrastructural localization in and release from frog motor nerve terminals. *Proceedings of the National Academy of Sciences of the United States of America* **93**: 1918–1923.

Henwood, A. (2002). Mast cell staining with alcian blue tetrakis(methylpyridinium) chloride. *Biotechnic and Histochemistry* **77**: 93–94.

Henwood, A. (2003). Current applications of orcein in histochemistry. A brief review with some new observations concerning influence of dye batch variation and aging of dye solutions on staining. *Biotechnic and Histochemistry* **78**: 303–308.

Henzen-Longmans, M.H., Tadema, T.M., Mol, J.J. and Meijer, C.J. (1985). Influence of fixation and decalcification on the immunohistochemical staining of cell-specific markers in paraffin-embedded human bone biopsies. *Journal of Histochemistry and Cytochemistry* **33**: 1103–1109.

Hepler, J.R., Toomim, C.S., McCarthy, C., Conti, F., Battaglia, G., Rustioni, A. and Petrusz, P. (1988). Characterization of antisera to glutamate and aspartate. *Journal of Histochemistry and Cytochemistry* **36**: 13–22.

Herman, G.E., Chlipala, E., Bochenski, G., Sabin, L. and Elfont, E. (1988). Zinc formalin for automated tissue processing. *Journal of Histotechnology* **11**: 85–89.

Heslinga, and Deierkauf, F.A. (1961). The action of histological fixatives on tissue lipids. Comparison of the action of several fixatives using paper chromatography. *Journal of Histochemistry and Cytochemistry* **9**: 572–577.

Hess, A. (1978). A simple procedure for distinguishing dopamine from noradrenaline in peripheral nervous structures in the fluorescence microscope. *Journal of Histochemistry and Cytochemistry* **26**: 141–144.

Hickey, W.F., Lee, V., Trojanowski, J.Q., McMillan, L.J., McKearn, T.J., Gonatas, J. and Gonatas, N.K. (1983). Immunohistochemical application of monoclonal antibodies against myelin basic protein and neurofilament triple protein subunits. Advantages over antisera and technical limitations. *Journal of Histochemistry and Cytochemistry* **31**: 1126–1135.

Hicks, D.J., Johnson, L., Mitchell, S.M., Gough, J., Cooley, W.A., La Ragione, R.M., Spencer, Y.I. and Wangoo, A. (2006). Evaluation of zinc salt based fixatives for preserving antigenic determinants for immunohistochemical demonstration of murine immune system cell markers. *Biotechnic and Histochemistry* **81**: 23–30.

Hierck, B.P., Iperen, L.V., Gittenberger-de Groot, A.C. and Poelmann, R.E. (1994). Modified indirect immunodetection allows study of murine tissue with mouse monoclonal antibodies. *Journal of Histochemistry and Cytochemistry* **42**: 1499–1502.

Highman, B. (1946). Improved methods for demonstrating amyloid in paraffin sections. *Archives of Pathology* **41**: 559–562.

Hillarp, N.A. (1959). On the histochemical demonstration of adrenergic nerves with the osmic acid–sodium iodide technique. *Acta Anatomica* **38**: 379–384.

Hilwig, I. and Gropp, A. (1972). Staining of constitutive hetreochromatin in mammalian chromosomes with a new fluorochrome. *Experimental Cell Research* **75**: 122–126.

Hilwig, I. and Gropp, A. (1975). pH-dependent fluorescence of DNA and RNA in cytologic staining with 33258 Hoechst. *Experimental Cell Research* **91**: 457–460.

Hippe-Sanwald, S. (1993). Impact of freeze substitution on biological electron microscopy. *Microscopy Research and Technique* **24**: 400–422.

Hirano, A. and Zimmermann, H.M. (1962). Silver impregnation of nerve cells and fibers in celloidin sections. *Archives of Neurology* **6**: 114–122.

Hixson, D.C., Yep, J.M., Glenney, J.R., Hayes, T. and Walberg, E.F. (1981). Evaluation of periodate/lysine/paraformaldehyde fixation as a method for cross-linking plasma membrane glycoproteins. *Journal of Histochemistry and Cytochemistry* **29**: 561–566.

Ho, M., Bera, T.K., Willingham, M.C., Onda, M., Hassan, R., FitzGerald, D. and Pastan, I. (2007). Mesothelin expression in human lung cancer. *Clinical Cancer Research* **13**: 1571–1575.

Hodgson, A.J., Penke, B., Erdei, A., Chubb, I.W. and Somogyi, P. (1985). Antisera to γ-aminobutyric acid. I. Production and characterization using a new model system. *Journal of Histochemistry and Cytochemistry* **33**: 229–239.

Hodnett, G.L., Crane, C.F. and Stelly, D.M. (1997). A rapid stain-clearing method for video based cytological analysis of cotton megagametophytes. *Biotechnic and Histochemistry* **72**: 16–21.

Hoffman, H. (1950). Local re-innervation in partially denervated muscle: a histo-physiological study. *Australian Journal of Experimental Biological and Medical Sciences* **28**: 383–397.

Hogg, R.M. and Simpson, R. (1975). An evaluation of solochrome cyanine R.S. as a nuclear stain similar to haematoxylin. *Medical Laboratory Technology* **32**: 301–306.

Hohmann, A., Hodgson, A.J., Skinner, J.M., Bradley, J. and Zola, H. (1988). Monoclonal alkaline phosphatase–anti-alkaline phosphatase (APAAP) complex: production of antibody, optimization of activity, and use in immunostaining. *Journal of Histochemistry and Cytochemistry* **36**: 137–143.

Holgate, C.S., Jackson, P., Cowen, P.N. and Bird, C.C. (1983). Immunogold–silver staining: a new method of immunostaining with enhanced sensitivity. *Journal of Histochemistry and Cytochemistry* **31**: 938–944.

Holmes, W. (1943). Silver staining of nerve axons in paraffin sections. *Anatomical Record* **86**: 157–187.

Holmes, W. (1947). The peripheral nerve biopsy. In Dyke, S.C. (ed.), *Recent Advances in Clinical Pathology*, pp. 402–417. London: Churchill.

Holst, M.C. and Powley, T.L. (1995). Cuprolinic Blue (quinolinic phthalocyanine) counterstaining of enteric neurons for peroxidase immunocytochemistry. *Journal of Neuroscience Methods* **62**: 121–127.

Holt, S.J. (1956). The value of fundamental studies of staining reactions in enzyme histochemistry, with reference to indoxyl methods for esterases. *Journal of Histochemistry and Cytochemistry* **4**: 541–554.

Holt, S.J. (1958). Indigogenic staining methods for esterases. In Danielli, J.F. (ed.), *General Cytochemical Methods*, Vol. 1, pp. 375–398. New York: Academic Press.

Holt, S.J. and O'Sullivan, D.G. (1958). Studies in enzyme histochemistry. I. Principles of cytochemical staining methods. *Proceedings of the Royal Society of London B* **148**: 465–480.

Holt, S.J. and Withers, R.F.J. (1952). Cytochemical localization of esterases using indoxyl derivatives. *Nature* **170**: 1012–1014.

Holt, S.J. and Withers, R.F.J. (1958). Studies in enzyme histochemistry. V. An appraisal of indigogenic reactions for esterase localization. *Proceedings of the Royal Society of London B* **148**: 520–532.

Holt, S.J., Hobbiger, E.E., Eluned, E. and Pawan, G.L.S. (1960). Preservation of integrity of rat tissues for cytochemical staining purposes. *Journal of Biophysical and Biochemical Cytology* **7**: 383–386.

Honig, M.G. and Hume, R.I. (1986). Fluorescent carbocyanine dyes allow living neurons of identified origin to be studied in long-term cultures. *Journal of Cell Biology* **103**: 171–187.

Hooghwinkel, G.J.M. and Smits, G. (1957). The specificity of the periodic acid–Schiff technique studied by a quantitative test-tube method. *Journal of Histochemistry and Cytochemistry* **5**: 120–126.

Hope, B.T., Michael, G.J., Knigge, K.M. and Vincent, S.R. (1991). Neuronal NADPH diaphorase is a nitric oxide synthase. *Proceedings of the National Academy of Sciences of the United States of America* **88**: 2811–2814.

Hopman, A.H.N., Ramaekers, F.C.S. and Speel, E.J. 1998. Rapid synthesis of biotin-, digoxigenin-, trinitrophenyl-, and fluorochrome-labelled tyramides and their application for *in situ* hybridization using CARD amplification. *Journal of Histochemistry and Cytochemistry* 46: 771–777.

Hoppert, M. (2003). *Microscopic Techniques in Biotechnology*. Weinheim: Wiley-VCH.

Hopwood, D. (1969a). Fixation of proteins by osmium tetroxide, potassium dichromate and potassium permanganate. *Histochemie* **18**: 250–260.

Hopwood, D. (1969b). Fixatives and fixation: a review. *Histochemical Journal* **1**: 323–360.

Hopwood, D. (1996). Fixation and fixatives. In Bancroft, J.D. and Stevens, A. (eds), *Theory and Practice of Histological Techniques*, pp. 23–46. Edinburgh: Churchill-Livingstone.

Hopwood, D. and Slidders, W. (1989). Tissue fixation with phenol–formaldehyde for routine histopathology. *Proceedings of the Royal Microscopical Society* **24**: A55.

Hopwood, D., Slidders, W. and Yeaman, G.R. (1989). Tissue fixation with phenol–formaldehyde for routine histopathology. *Histochemical Journal* **21**: 228–234.

Hopwood, D., Yeaman, G. and Milne, G. (1988). Differentiating the effects of microwave and heat on tissue proteins and their cross linking by formaldehyde. *Histochemical Journal* **20**: 341–346.

Horisberger, M. and Rosset, J. (1977). Colloidal gold, a useful marker for transmission and scanning electron microscopy. *Journal of Histochemistry and Cytochemistry* **25**: 295–305.

Horobin, R.W. (1980). Structure–staining relationships in histochemistry and biological staining. I. Theoretical background and a general account of correlation of histochemical staining with the chemical structure of the reagents used. *Journal of Microscopy* **119**: 345–355.

Horobin, R.W. (1982). *Histochemistry: An Explanatory Outline of Histochemistry and Biophysical Staining*. Stuttgart: Gustav Fischer.

Horobin, R.W. (1983). What the textile-dyeing literature has to offer histochemists. *Histochemical Journal* **15**: 1151–1154.

Horobin, R.W. (1988). *Understanding Histochemistry: Selection, Evaluation and Design of Biological Stains*. Chichester: Ellis Horwood.

Horobin , R.W. (2001). Uptake, distribution and accumulation of dyes and fluorescent probes within living cells: a structure–activity modelling approach. *Advances in Colour Science and Technology* **4**: 101–107.

Horobin, R.W. (2002). Biological staining: mechanisms and theory. *Biotechnic and Histochemistry* **77**: 3–13.

Horobin, R.W. (2004). Staining by numbers: a tool for understanding and assisting use of routine and special hisyopathology stains. *Journal of Histotechnology* **27**: 23–28.

Horobin, R.W. and Bancroft, J.D. (1998). *Troubleshooting Histology Stains*. Edinburgh: Churchill-Livingstone.

Horobin, R.W. and Flemming, L. (1980). Structure–staining relationships in histochemistry and biological staining. II. Mechanistic and practical aspects of the staining of elastic fibres. *Journal of Microscopy* **119**: 357–372.

Horobin, R.W. and Flemming, L. (1988). One-bath trichrome staining: investigation of a general mechanism based on a structure–staining correlation analysis. *Histochemical Journal* **20**: 23–34.

Horobin, R.W. and Goldstein, D.J. (1974). The influence of salt on the staining of tissue sections with basic dyes: an investigation into general applicability of the critical electrolyte concentration theory. *Histochemical Journal* **6**: 599–609.

Horobin, R.W. and James, N.T. (1970). The staining of elastic fibres with direct blue 152. A general hypothesis for the staining of elastic fibres. *Histochemie* **22**: 324–336.

Horobin, R.W. and Kevill-Davies, I.M. (1971a). Basic fuchsin in acid alcohol: a simplified alternative to Schiff reagent. *Stain Technology* **46**: 53–58.

Horobin, R.W. and Kevill-Davies, I.M. (1971b). A mechanistic study of the histochemical reactions between aldehydes and basic fuchsin in acid alcohol used as a simplified Schiff's reagent. *Histochemical Journal* **3**: 371–378.

Horobin, R.W. and Kiernan, J.A. (eds) (2002). *Conn's Biological Stains. A Handbook of Dyes, Stains and Fluorochromes for use in Biology and Medicine*, 10th edn. Oxford: BIOS Scientific Publications.

Horobin, R.W., Stockert, J.C. and Rashid-Doubell, F. (2006). Fluorescent cationic probes for nuclei of living cells: why are they selective? A quantitative structure–activity relations analysis. *Histochemistry and Cell Biology* **126**: 165–175.

Horobin, R.W. and Tomlinson, A. (1976). The influence of the embedding medium when staining sections for electron microscopy: the penetration of stains into plastic sections. *Journal of Microscopy* **108**: 69–78.

Horobin, R.W. and Walter, K.J. (1987). Understanding Romanowsky staining. I. The Romanowsky–Giemsa effect in blood smears. *Histochemistry* **86**: 331–336.

Hosoya, A., Hoshi, K., Sahara, N., Ninomiya, T., Akahane, S., Kawamoto, T. and Ozawa, H. (2005). Effects of fixation and decalcification on the immunohistochemical localization of bone matrix proteins in fresh-frozen bone sections. *Histochemistry and Cell Biology* **123**: 639–646.

Howard, W.B., Willhite, C.C. and Smart, R.A. (1989). Fixative evaluation and histologic appearance of embryonic rodent tissue. *Stain Technology* **64**: 1–8.

Hoyer, P.E. and Kirkeby, S. (1996). The impact of fixatives on the binding of lectins to *N*-acetyl-glucosamine residues of human syncytiotrophoblast: a quantitative histochemical study. *Journal of Histochemistry and Cytochemistry* **44**: 855–863.

Hoyer, P.E., Lyon, H., Jakobsen, P. and Andersen, A.P. (1986). Standardized methyl green–pyronin Y procedures using pure dyes. *Histochemical Journal* **18**: 90–94.

Hruba, P., Honys, D. and Tupy, J. (2005). Expression and thermotolerance of calreticulin during pollen development in tobacco. *Sexual Plant Reproduction* **18**: 143–148.

Hsu, S.-M. and Raine, L. (1981). Protein A, avidin and biotin in immunohistochemistry. *Journal of Histochemistry and Cytochemistry* **29**: 1349–1353.

Hsu, S.-M. and Soban, E. (1982). Color modification of diaminobenzidine (DAB) precipitation by metallic ions and its application for double immunocytochemistry. *Journal of Histochemistry and Cytochemistry* **30**: 1079–1082.

Hsu, S.-M., Raine, L. and Fanger, H. (1981). Use of avidin–biotin–peroxidase complex (ABC) in immunoperoxidase techniques. A comparison between ABC and unlabeled antibody (PAP) procedures. *Journal of Histochemistry and Cytochemistry* **29**: 577–580.

Hughes, R.C. (1976). *Membrane Glycoproteins.* London: Butterworths.

Hulstaert, C.E., Kalicharan, D. and Hardonk, M.J. (1983). Cytochemical demonstration of phosphatases in the rat liver by a cerium-based method in combination with osmium tetroxide and potassium ferrocyanide postfixation. *Histochemistry* **78**: 71–79.

Humason, G.L. (1979). *Animal Tissue Techniques,* 4th edn. San Francisco, CA: Freeman.

Hunger, K. (2003). *Industrial Dyes. Chemistry, Properties, Applications.* Weinheim: Wiley-VCH.

Hunt, N.C.A., Attanoos, R. and Jasani, B. (1996). High temperature antigen retrieval and loss of nuclear morphology: a comparison of microwave and autoclave techniques. *Journal of Clinical Pathology* **49**: 767–770.

Hutson, J.C., Childs, G.V. and Gardner, P.J. (1979). Considerations for establishing the validity of immunocytological studies. *Journal of Histochemistry and Cytochemistry* **27**: 1201–1202.

Hyman, J.M. and Poulding, R.H. (1961). Solochrome cyanin–iron alum for rapid staining of frozen sections. *Journal of Medical Laboratory Technology* **18**: 107.

Ichikawa, T. and Ajiki, K. 1992. Development of an *in situ* hybridization histochemistry for choline acetyltransferase mRNA with RNA probes. *Zoological Science* **9**: 305–314.

Ippolito, E., Lavelle, S. and Pedrini, V. (1981). The effect of various decalcifying agents on cartilage proteoglycans. *Stain Technology* **56**: 367–372.

Irons, R.D., Schenk, E.A. and Lee, C.K. (1977). Cytochemical methods for copper. *Archives of Pathology and Laboratory Medicine* **101**: 298–301.

Jacobs, G.F. and Liggett, S.J. (1971). An oxidation–distillation procedure for reclaiming osmium tetroxide from used fixative solutions. *Stain Technology* **46**: 207–208.

Jacot, J.L., Glover, J.P. and Robison, W.G. (1995). Improved gold chloride procedure for nerve staining in whole mounts of rat corneas. *Biotechnic and Histochemistry* **70**: 277–284.

Jain, M.K. (1982). *Handbook of Enzyme Inhibitors (1965–1977).* New York: John Wiley.

Jambor, B. (1954). Reduction of tetrazolium salt. *Nature* **173**: 774–775.

James, J. (1976). *Light Microscopic Techniques in Biology and Medicine.* The Hague: Martinus Nijhoff.

James, J. and Tas, J. (1984). *Histochemical Protein Staining Methods. (Royal Microscopical Society Microscopy Handbooks 04).* Oxford: Oxford University Press.

James, T.H. (ed.) (1977). *The Theory of the Photographic Process,* 4th edn. New York: Macmillan.

Jancso, G., Ferencsik, M., Such, G., Kiraly, K., Nagy, A. and Bujdoso, M. (1985). Morphological effects of capsaicin and its analogues in newborn and adult mammals. In Hakanson, R. and Sundler, F. (eds), *Tachykinin Antagonists,* pp. 35–44. Amsterdam: Elsevier.

Jansson, L., Ogren, S. and Lindahl, U. (1975). Macromolecular properties and end-group analysis of heparin isolated from bovine liver capsule. *Biochemical Journal* **145**: 53–62.

Jaques, L.B., Mahadoo, J. and Riley, J.F. (1977). The mast cell/heparin paradox. *Lancet* **1**: 411–413.

Jarvinen, M. and Rinne, A. (1983). The use of polyvinyl acetate glue to prevent detachment of tissue sections in immunohistochemistry. *Acta Histochemica* **72**: 751–752.

Jasani, B., Morgan, J.M. and Navabi, H. (1997). Mechanism of high temperature antigen retrieval: role of calcium chelation. *Histochemical Journal* **29**: 433.

Jasmin, G. et Bois, P. (1961). Coloration differentielle des mastocytes chez le rat. *Revue Canadienne de Biologie* **20**: 773–774.

Jeanloz, R.W. (1975). The chemistry of heparin. In Bradshaw, R.A. and Wessler, S. (eds), *Heparin: Structure, Function and Clinical Implications,* pp. 3–15. New York: Plenum Press.

Jensen, W.A. (1962). *Botanical Histochemistry.* San Francisco, CA: Freeman.

Jerome, C.A., Montanges, D.J.S. and Taylor, F.J.R. (1993). The effect of the quantitative protargol stain and Lugol's and Bouin's fixatives on cell size: a more accurate estimate of ciliate species biomass. *Journal of Eukaryotic Microbiology* **40**: 254–259.

Jessen, K.R., Thorpe, R. and Mirsky, R. (1984). Molecular identity, distribution and heterogeneity of glial fibrillary acidic protein: an immunoblotting and immunohistochemical study of Schwann cells, satellite cells, enteric glia and astrocytes. *Journal of Neurocytology* **13**: 187–200.

Jewell, S.D. and Cordial, C.R. (1996). Silver staining of nucleolar organizer regions. *Journal of Histotechnology* **19**: 241–256.

Jhaveri, S., Carman, L. and Hahm, J.-O. (1988). Visualizing anterogradely transported HRP by use of TMB histochemistry: comparison of the TMB–SNF and TMB–AHM methods. *Journal of Histochemistry and Cytochemistry* **36**: 103–105.

Johannes, M.-L. and Klessen, C. (1984). Alcian blue/PAS or PAS/alcian blue? Remarks on a classical technique used in carbohydrate histochemistry. *Histochemistry* **80**: 129–132.

Johansson, O., Virtanen, M., Hilliges, M. and Yang, Q. (1994). Histamine immunohistochemistry is superior to the conventional heparin-based staining methodology for investigations of human skin mast cells. *Histochemical Journal* **26**: 424–430.

Jones, D. (1972). Reactions of aldehydes with unsaturated fatty acids during histological fixation. *Histochemical Journal* **4**: 421–465.

Jones, E.G. and Hartman, B.K. (1978). Recent advances in neuroanatomical methodology. *Annual Review of Neuroscience* **1**: 215–296.

Jones, K.H. and Kniss, D.A. (1987). Propidium iodide as a nuclear counterstain for immunofluorescence studies on cells in culture. *Journal of Histochemistry and Cytochemistry* **35**: 123–125.

Jones, M.L. (2002). Lipids. In Bancroft, J.D. and Gamble, M. (eds), *Theory and Practice of Histological Techniques*, 5th edn. London: Churchill-Livingstone, pp. 201–230.

Jones, R.M. (ed.) (1950). *McClung's Handbook of Microscopical Technique*, 3rd edn. New York: Hoebner.

Juarranz, A., Horobin, R.W. and Proctor, G.B. (1986). Prediction of *in situ* fluorescence of histochemical reagents using a structure–staining correlation procedure. *Histochemistry* **84**: 426–431.

Junqueira, L.C.U., Bignolas, G. and Brentani, R.R. (1979). Picrosirius staining plus polarization microscopy, a specific method for collagen detection in tissue sections. *Histochemical Journal* **11**: 447–455.

Kahveci, Z., Cavusoglu, I. and Sirmali, S.A. (1997). Microwave fixation of whole fetal specimens. *Biotechnic and Histochemistry* **72**: 144–147.

Kalimo, H. and Pelliniemi, L.J. (1977). Pitfalls in the preparation of buffers for electron microscopy. *Histochemical Journal* **9**: 241–246.

Kapranos, N., Kontogeorgos, G., Frangia, K. and Kokka, E. (1997). Effect of fixation on interphase cytogenetic analysis by direct fluorescence *in situ* hybridization on cell imprints. *Biotechnic and Histochemistry* **72**: 148–151.

Kapuscinski, J. (1990). Interactions of nucleic acids with fluorescent dyes: spectral properties of condensed complexes. *Journal of Histochemistry and Cytochemistry* **98**: 1323–1329.

Kapuscinski, J. (1995). DAPI: a DNA-specific fluorescent probe. *Biotechnic and Histochemistry* **70**: 220–233.

Karaosmanoglu, T., Aygun, B., Wade, P.R. and Gershon, M.D. (1996). Regional differences in the number of neurons in the myenteric plexus of the guinea pig small intestine and colon: an evaluation of markers used to count neurons. *Anatomical Record* **244**: 470–480.

Karnovsky, M.J. (1965). A formaldehyde–glutaraldehyde fixative of high osmolality for use in electron microscopy. *Journal of Cell Biology* **27**: 137A–138A.

Karnovsky, M.J. and Fasman, G.D. (1960). A histochemical method for distinguishing between side-chain and terminal (a-acylamido) carboxyl groups of proteins. *Journal of Biophysical and Biochemical Cytology* **8**: 319–325.

Karnovsky, M.J. and Mann, M.S. (1961). The significance of the histochemical reaction for carboxyl groups of proteins in cartilage matrix. *Histochemie* **2**: 234–243.

Karnovsky, M.J. and Roots, L. (1964). A 'direct coloring' thiocholine method for cholinesterases. *Journal of Histochemistry and Cytochemistry* **12**: 219–221.

Kashiwa, H.K. and Atkinson, W.B. (1963). The applicability of a new Schiff base, glyoxal bis(2-hydroxyanil), for the cytochemical localization of ionic calcium. *Journal of Histochemistry and Cytochemistry* **11**: 258–264.

Kashiwa, H.K. and House, C.M. (1964). The glyoxal bis(2-hydroxyanil) method modified for localizing insoluble calcium salts. *Stain Technology* **39**: 359–367.

Kasten, F.H. (1960). The Chemistry of Schiff's reagent. *International Review of Cytology* **10**: 1–100.

Kasten, F.H. (1965). Loss of RNA and protein, and changes in DNA during a 30-hour cold perchloric acid extraction of cultured cells. *Stain Technology* **40**: 127–135.

Kasten, F.H. and Lala, R. (1975). The Feulgen reaction after glutaraldehyde fixation. *Stain Technology* **50**: 197–201.

Katsuyama, T. and Spicer, S.S. (1978). Histochemical differentiation of complex carbohydrates with variants of the concanavalin A–horseradish peroxidase method. *Journal of Histochemistry and Cytochemistry* **26**: 233–250.

Kaufmann, C. and Lehmann, E. (1926). Sind die in der histologischen Technik gebrauchlichen Fettdifferenzierungsmethoden spezifisch? *Virchows Archiv für pathologische Anatomie und Physiologie* **261**: 623–648.

Kawamura, K. (1986). Occurrence and release of histamine-containing granules in summer cells in adrenal glands of the frog Rana catesbeiana. *Journal of Anatomy* **148**: 111–119.

Keilin, D. and Hartree, E.F. (1938). Cytochrome oxidase. *Proceedings of the Royal Society of London B* **125**: 171–186.

Kerr, J.F.R., Wyllie, A.H. and Currie, A.R. (1972). Apoptosis: a basic biological phenomenon with wide-ranging implications in tissue kinetics. *British Journal of Cancer* **26**: 239–257.

Kiernan, J.A. (1964). Carboxylic esterases of the hypothalamus and neurohypophysis of the hedgehog. *Journal of the Royal Microscopical Society* **83**: 297–306.

Kiernan, J.A. (1974). Effects of metabolic inhibitors on vital staining with methylene blue. *Histochemistry* **40**: 51–57.

Kiernan, J.A. (1977). Recycling procedure for gold chloride used in neurohistology. *Stain Technology* **52**: 245–248.

Kiernan, J.A. (1978). Recovery of osmium tetroxide from used fixative solutions. *Journal of Microscopy* **113**: 77–82.

Kiernan, J.A. (1981). *Histological and Histochemical Methods: Theory and Practice*, 1st edn. Oxford: Pergamon Press.

Kiernan, J.A. (1984a). Chromoxane cyanine R. I. Physical and chemical properties of the dye and of some of its iron complexes. *Journal of Microscopy* **134**: 13–23.

Kiernan, J.A. (1984b). Chromoxane cyanine R. II. Staining of animal tissues by the dye and its iron complexes. *Journal of Microscopy* **134**: 25–39.

Kiernan, J.A. (1985). The action of chromium(III) in fixation of animal tissues. *Histochemical Journal* **17**: 1131–1146.

Kiernan, J.A. (1996a). Review of current silver impregnation: techniques for histological examination of skeletal muscle innervation. *Journal of Histotechnology* **19**: 257–267.

Kiernan, J.A. (1996b). Staining paraffin sections without prior removal of the wax. *Biotechnic and Histochemistry* **71**: 304–310.

Kiernan, J.A. (1996c). Vascular permeability in the peripheral autonomic and somatic nervous systems: controversial aspects and comparisons with the blood–brain barrier. *Microscopy Research and Technique* **35**: 122–136.

Kiernan, J.A. (1997). Making and using aqueous mounting media. *Microscopy Today* **97**: 16–17.

Kiernan, J.A. (2000). Formaldehyde, formalin, paraformaldehyde and glutaraldehyde: what they are and what they do. *Microscopy Today* **8**: 8–12.

Kiernan, J.A. (2001). Classification and naming of dyes, stains and fluorochromes. *Biotechnic and Histochemistry* **76**: 261–277.

Kiernan, J.A. (2002a). Suppressing autofluorescence. *Biotechnic and Histochemistry* **77**: 232.

Kiernan, J.A. (2002b). Silver staining for spirochetes in tissues: rationale, difficulties, and troubleshooting. *Laboratory Medicine* **33**, 705–708.

Kiernan, J.A. (2004). Hexazonium pararosaniline as a fixative for animal tissues. *Biotechnic and Histochemistry* **79**: 203–210.

Kiernan, J.A. (2005). Preservation and retrieval of antigens for immunohistochemistry – methods and mechanisms. Part 2. Retrieving masked antigens. *The Cutting Edge* (National Society for Histotechnology, Region IX newsletter), April 2005, pp. 5–11. Available from: http://publish.uwo.ca/~jkiernan/FixAnti2.pdf [accessed June 2007].

Kiernan, J.A. (2006). Dyes and other colorants in microtechnique and biomedical research. *Coloration Technology* **122**: 1–21.

Kiernan, J.A. (2007a). Indigogenic substrates for the detection and localization of enzymes. *Biotechnic and Histochemistry* **82**: 73–103.

Kiernan, J.A. (2007b). Histochemistry of staining methods for normal and degenerating myelin in the central and peripheral nervous systems. *Journal of Histotechnology* **30**: 87–106.

Kiernan, J.A. and Berry, M. (1975). Neuroanatomical methods. In Bradley, P.B. (ed.), *Methods in Brain Research*, pp. 1–77. London: Wiley.

Kiernan, J.A. and Stoddart, R.W. (1973). Fluorescent-labelled aprotinin: a new reagent for the histochemical detection of acid mucosubstances. *Histochemie* **34**: 77–84.

Kilpatrick, D.C. (2000). *Handbook of Animal Lectins.* Chichester: Wiley.

Kiraly, K., Lammi, M., Arokoski, J., Lapvetelainen, T., Tammi, M., Helminen, H. and Kiviranta, I. (1996a). Safranin O reduces loss of glycosaminoglycans from bovine articular cartilage during histological specimen preparation. *Histochemical Journal* **28**: 99–107.

Kiraly, K., Lapvetelainen, T., Arokoski, J., Torronen, K., Modis, L., Kiviranta, I. and Helminen, H.J. (1996b). Application of selected cationic dyes for the semiquantitative estimation of glycosaminoglycans in histological sections of articular cartilage by microspectrophotometry. *Histochemical Journal* **28**: 577–590.

Kiraly, K., Hyttinen, M.M., Lapvetelainen, T., Elo, M., Kiviranta, I., Dobai, J., Modis, L., Helminen, H.J. and Arokoski, J.P.A. (1997). Specimen preparation and quantification of collagen birefringence in unstained sections of articular cartilage using image analysis and polarizing light microscopy. *Histochemical Journal* **29**: 317–327.

Kirkeby, S. and Moe, D. (1986). Studies on the actions of glutaraldehyde, formaldehyde, and mixtures of glutaraldehyde and formaldehyde on tissue proteins. *Acta Histochemica* **79**: 115–121.

Kirkeby, S. and Blecher, S.R. (1978). Studies on the oxidizing system in Holt's medium for histochemical demonstration of esterase activity. *Acta Histochemica* **62**: 44–56.

Kishimoto, M., Ueda, K., Nakata, M., Konishi, E., Urata, Y., Tsuchihashi, Y. and Ashihara, T. (1990). Detection of the DNA strand breaks by *in situ* nick translation using non-radioactive nucleotide. *Journal of Histochemistry and Cytochemistry* **38**: 1052.

Kisilevsky, R. (2008). The amyloidoses. In Rubin, R. and Strayer, D.S. (eds), *Rubin's Pathology*, 5th edn, pp. 989–998. Philadelphia, PA: Lippincott-Raven.

Kjellstrand, P.T.T. (1977). Temperature and acid concentration in the search for optimum Feulgen hydrolysis conditions. *Journal of Histochemistry and Cytochemistry* **25**: 129–134.

Klatt, P., Schmidt, K., Uray, G. and Mayer, B. (1993). Multiple catalytic functions of brain nitric oxide synthase: biochemical characterization, cofactor-requirement, and the role of N(γ,ω)-hydroxy-L-arginine as an intermediate. *Journal of Biological Chemistry* **268**: 14781–14787.

Klaushofer, K. and Von Mayersbach, H. (1979). Freeze-substituted tissue in 5'-nucleotidase histochemistry. Comparative histochemical and biochemical investigations. *Journal of Histochemistry and Cytochemistry* **27**: 1582–1587.

Klausner, R.D. and Wolf, D.E. (1980). Selectivity of fluorescent lipid analogues for lipid domains. *Biochemistry* **19**: 6199–6203.

Kleene, S.J. and Gesteland, R.C. (1983). Dissociation of frog olfactory epithelium. *Journal of Neuroscience Methods* **9**: 173–183.

Klein, R.M. and Klein, D.T. (1970). *Research Methods in Plant Science*. Garden City, NY: American Museum of Natural History.

Klessen, C. (1974). Histochemical demonstration of thyrotropic and gonadotropic cells in the pituitary gland of the rat by the use of a lead-tetraacetate sodium bisulphite technique. *Histochemical Journal* **6**: 311–318.

Klinkner, A.M., Bugelski, P.J., Waites, C.R., Louden, C., Hart, T.K. and Kerns, W.D. (1997). A novel technique for mapping the lipid composition of atherosclerotic streaks by en face fluorescence microscopy. *Journal of Histochemistry and Cytochemistry* **45**: 743–753.

Klosen, P., Maessen, X. and Van Den Bosch De Aguilar, P. (1993). PEG embedding for immunocytochemistry: application to the analysis of immunoreactivity loss during histological processing. *Journal of Histochemistry and Cytochemistry* **41**: 455–463.

Kluver, H. and Barrera, E. (1953). A method for the combined staining of cells and fibers in the central nervous system. *Journal of Neuropathology and Experimental Neurology* **12**: 400–403.

Koch, B., Kurriger, G. and Brand, R.A. (1995). Characterization of the neurosensory elements of the feline cranial cruciate ligament. *Journal of Anatomy* **187**: 353–359.

Koelle, G.B. and Friedenwald, J.S. (1949). A histochemical method for localizing cholinesterase activity. *Proceedings of the Society for Experimental Biology and Medicine* **70**: 617–622.

Kok, L.P. and Boon, M.E. (1992). *Microwave Cookbook for Microscopists. Art and Science of Visualization*, 3rd edn. Leiden: Coulomb Press Leyden.

Kolb, B. and McClimans, J. (1986). Cryostat sectioning of Golgi–Cox tissue. *Stain Technology* **61**: 379–380.

Kooij, A., Frederiks, W.M., Gossrau, R. and Van Noorden, C.J.F. (1991). Localization of xanthine oxidase activity using the tissue protectant polyvinyl alcohol and final electron acceptor tetranitro BT. *Journal of Histochemistry and Cytochemistry* **39**: 87–93.

Koopal, S.A., Coma, M.I., Tiebosch, A.T.M.G. and Suurmeijer, A.J.H. (1998). Low-temperature heating overnight in Tris-HCl buffer pH 9 is a good alternative for antigen retrieval in formalin-fixed paraffin-embedded tissue. *Applied Immunohistochemistry* **6**: 228–233.

Kopriwa, B.M. and Leblond, C.P. (1962). Improvements in the coating technique of autoradiography. *Journal of Histochemistry and Cytochemistry* **10**: 269–284.

Korn, E.D. (1967). A chromatographic and spectrophotometric study of the products of the reaction of osmium tetroxide with unsaturated lipids. *Journal of Cell Biology* **34**: 627–638.

Kornblihtt, A.R. and Gutman, A. (1988). Molecular biology of the extracellular matrix proteins. *Biological Reviews* **63**: 465–507.

Kortenkamp, A., O'Brien, P. and Beyersmann, D. (1991). The reduction of chromate is a prerequisite of chromium binding to cell nuclei. *Carcinogenesis* **12**: 1143–1144.

Koski, J.P. and Reyes, P.F. (1986). Silver impregnation techniques for neuropathologic studies. I. Variations on Bodian's technic with a review of the theory and methods. *Journal of Histotechnology* **9**: 265–272.

Koss, L.G. and Melamed, M.R. (2006). *Koss' Diagnostic Cytology and its Histopathologic Bases*, 5th edn, Vol. 2. Philadelphia, PA: Lippincott, Williams and Wilkins.

Krajian, A.A. and Gradwohl, R.B.H. (1952). *Histopathological Technic*, 2nd edn. St Louis, MO: Mosby.

Kramer, H. and Windrum, G.M. (1955). The metachromatic staining reaction. *Journal of Histochemistry and Cytochemistry* **3**: 226–237.

Kratky, R.G., Ivey, J. and Roach, M.R. (1996). Collagen quantitation by video-microdensitometry in rabbit atherosclerosis. *Matrix Biology* **15**: 141–144.

Krikelis, H. and Smith, A. (1988). Palladium toning of silver-impregnated reticular fibers. *Stain Technology* **63**: 97–100.

Kruth, H.S. and Vaughan, M. (1980). Quantification of low density lipoprotein binding and cholesterol accumulation by single human fibroblasts using fluorescence microscopy. *Journal of Lipid Research* **21**: 123–130.

Kucharz, E.J. (1992). *The Collagens: Biochemistry and Pathophysiology*. Berlin: Springer.

Kugler, P. and Wrobel, K.-H. (1978). Meldola blue: a new electron carrier for the histochemical demonstration of dehydrogenases (SDH, LDH, G-6-PDH). *Histochemistry* **59**: 97–109.

Kuhn, K. (1987). The classical collagens: types I, II and III. In Mayne, R. and Burgeson, R.E. (eds), *Structure and Function of Collagen Types*. Orlando, FL: Academic Press.

Kumar, R.K. (1989). Immunogold–silver cytochemistry using a capillary action staining. *Journal of Histochemistry and Cytochemistry* **37**: 913–917.

Kukachka, B.F. (1977). Sectioning refractory woods for anatomical studies. *USDA Forest Service Research Note FPL-0326*. Available from: http://www.fpl.fs.fed.us/documnts/fplrn/fplrn236.pdf [accessed April 2007].

Kusakabe, M., Sakakura, T., Nishizuka, Y., Sano, M. and Matsukage, A. (1984). Polyester wax embedding and sectioning for immunohistochemistry. *Stain Technology* **59**: 127–132.

Kuypers, H.G.J.M., Catsman-Berrevoets, C.E. and Padt, R.E. (1977). Retrograde axonal transport of fluorescent substances in the rat's forebrain. *Neuroscience Letters* **6**: 127–135.

Labat-Moleur, F., Guillermet, C., Lorimier, P., Robert, C., Lantuejoul, S., Brambilla, E. and Negoescu, A. (1998). TUNEL apoptotic cell detection in tissue sections: critical evaluation and improvement. *Journal of Histochemistry and Cytochemistry* **46**: 327–334.

Lai, M., Lampert, I.A. and Lewis, P.D. (1975). The influence of fixation on staining of glycosaminoglycans in glial cells. *Histochemistry* **41**: 275–279.

Laist, J.W. (1954). *Copper, Silver and Gold. Comprehensive Inorganic Chemistry*, **2**. Princeton: van Nostrand.

Lancaster, F.E. and Lawrence, J.F. (1996). High-performance liquid chromatographic separation of carminic acid, alpha- and beta-bixin, and alpha- and beta-norbixin, and the determination of carminic acid in foods. *Journal of Chromatography A* **732**: 394–398.

Lange, M.S., Johnston, M.V., Tseng, E.E., Baumgartner, W.A. and Blue, M.E. (1999). Apoptosis detection in brain using low-magnification dark-field microscopy. *Experimental Neurology* **158**: 254–260.

Larison, K.D., BreMiller, R., Wells, K.S., Clements, I. and Haugland, R.P. (1995). Use of a new fluorogenic phosphatase substrate in immunohistochemical applications. *Journal of Histochemistry and Cytochemistry* **43**: 77–83.

Lascano, E.F. (1946). Importancia del pH en la fijacion del tejido nervioso. Creacion artificial de fijadores tipo formol-bromuro y formol-nitrato de urano de Cajal. *Archivos de la Sociedad Argentina de Anatomia Normal y Patologica* **8**: 185–194.

Lascano, E.F. and Berria, M.I. (1988). PAP labeling enhancement by osmium tetroxide–potassium ferrocyanide treatment. *Journal of Histochemistry and Cytochemistry* **36**: 697–699.

Laties, A.M., Lund, R. and Jacobowitz, D. (1967). A simplified method for the histochemical localization of cardiac catecholamine-containing nerve fibers. *Journal of Histochemistry and Cytochemistry* **15**: 535–541.

Latimer, W.M. (1952). *The Oxidation States of the Elements and their Potentials in Aqueous Solutions*, 2nd edn. Englewood Cliffs, NJ: Prentice-Hall.

Lazarow, A. and Cooperstein, S.J. (1953). Studies on the enzymatic basis for the janus green B staining reaction. *Journal of Histochemistry and Cytochemistry* **1**: 234–241.

Leblond, C.P., Glegg, R.E. and Eidinger, D. (1957). Presence of carbohydrates with free 1,2-glycol groups in sites stained by the periodic acid–Schiff technique. *Journal of Histochemistry and Cytochemistry* **5**: 445–458.

Lee, E.R., Murphy, G., El-Alfy, M., Davoli, M.A., Lamplugh, L., Docherty, A.J. and Leblond, C.P. (1999). Active gelatinase B is identified by histozymography in the cartilage resorption sites of developing long bones. *Developmental Dynamics* **190–205**: 190–205.

Lee, I., Yamagishi, N., Oboshi, K. and Yamada, H. (2004). Distribution of new methylene blue injected into the lumbosacral epidural space in cats. *Veterinary Anaesthesia and Analgesia* **31**: 190–194.

Lefkovits, I. and Pernis, P. (eds) (1979–1990) *Immunological Methods*, 4 vols. New York: Academic Press.

Leitch, A.R., Schwarzacher, T., Jackson, D. and Leitch, I.J. (1994). *In Situ Hybridization: A Practical Guide*. Oxford: BIOS Scientific Publications and Royal Microscopical Society.

Lemire, T.D. (2000). Microwave irradiated canine and feline tissues: Part 1. Morphologic evaluation. *Journal of Histotechnology* **23**: 113–120.

Lemke, C., Schwerdtieger, M., Pohlmann, I., Sammler, G. and Linss, W. (1994). A variant of a slam freezing device for electron microscopy. *Biotechnic and Histochemistry* **69**: 38–44.

Lempert-Sreter, M., Solt, V. and Lempert, K. (1963). Uber die Kondensation von Benzil mit Guanidin und *n*-butylguanidin. *Chemische Berichte* **96**: 168–173.

Leonard, J.B. and Shepardson, S.P. (1994). A comparison of heating modes in rapid fixation techniques for electron microscopy. *Journal of Histochemistry and Cytochemistry* **42**: 383–391.

Leong, A.S.Y. (1994). Fixation. In Woods, A. and Ellis, R. (eds), *Laboratory Histopathology: A Complete Reference*. Edinburgh: Churchill-Livingstone. Available from: http://home.primus.com.au/royellis/fix.htm [accessed August 2007].

Lendrum, A.C. (1947). The phloxin–tartrazine method as a general histological stain and for the demonstration of inclusion bodies. *Journal of Pathology and Bacteriology* **59**: 399–404.

Lenoir, M. (1926). Une manipulation de travaux pratiques sur la chondriome. *Revue Generale de Botanique* **38**: 720–722.

Lepault, J., Bigot, D., Studer, D. and Erk, I. (1997). Freezing of aqueous specimens: an X-ray diffraction study. *Journal of Microscopy* **187**: 158–166.

Leung, J.K., Gibbon, K.J. and Vartanian, R.K. (1996). Rapid staining method for *Helicobacter pylori* in gastric biopsies. *Journal of Histotechnology* **19**: 131.

Levanon, D. and Stein, H. (1995). Quantitative analysis of chondroitin sulphate retention by tannic acid during preparation of specimens for electron microscopy. *Histochemical Journal* **27**: 457–465.

Lever, J.D., Santer, R.M., Lu, K.-S. and Presley, R. (1977). Electron probe X-ray microanalysis of small granulated cells in rat sympathetic ganglia after sequential aldehyde and dichromate treatment. *Journal of Histochemistry and Cytochemistry* **25**: 275–279.

Levinson, J.W., Retzel, S. and McCormick, J.J. (1977). An improved acriflavine–Feulgen method. *Journal of Histochemistry and Cytochemistry* **25**: 355–358.

Lewin, L.M., Golan, R., Freidlin, P. and Shochat, L. (1999). A comparative study of spermatozoal chromatin using acridine orange staining and flow cytometry. *Comparative Biochemistry and Physiology A – Molecular and Integrative Physiology* **124**: 133–137.

Lewis, P.R. (1987). The mechanisms of positive staining. *Proceedings of the Royal Microscopical Society* **22**: 359–363.

Lhotka, J.F. (1952). Histochemical use of sodium bismuthate. *Stain Technology* **27**: 259–262.

Lhotka, J.F. (1956). On tissue argyrophilia. *Stain Technology* **31**: 185–188.

Li, C.-Y., Ziesmer, S.C. and Lazcano-Villareal, O. (1986). Use of azide and hydrogen peroxide as an inhibitor for endogenous peroxidase in the immunoperoxidase method. *Journal of Histochemistry and Cytochemistry* **35**: 1457–1460.

Liao, J.C., Ponzo, J.L. and Patel, C. (1981). Improved stability of methanolic Wright's stain with additive reagents. *Stain Technology* **56**: 251–263.

Lichtenstein, S.J. and Nettleton, G.S. (1980). Effects of fuchsin variants in aldehyde fuchsin staining. *Journal of Histochemistry and Cytochemistry* **28**: 683–688.

Liem, R.S. and Jansen, H.W. (1984). The use of chromic potassium sulphate in bone electron microscopy. *Acta Morphologica Neerlando–Scandinavica* **22**: 233–243.

Lievremont, M., Potus, J. and Guillou, B. (1982). Use of alizarin red S for histochemical staining of Ca^{2+} in the mouse; some parameters of the chemical reaction *in vitro*. *Acta Anatomica* **114**: 268–280.

Lillie, R.D. (1945). Studies on selective staining of collagen with acid anilin dyes. *Journal of Technical Methods and Bulletin of the International Association of Medical Museums* **25**: 1–47.

Lillie, R.D. (1962). The histochemical reaction of aryl amines with tissue aldehydes produced by periodic and chromic acids. *Journal of Histochemistry and Cytochemistry* **19**: 303–314.

Lillie, R.D. (1964). Histochemical acylation of hydroxyl and amino groups. Effect on the periodic acid–Schiff reaction, anionic and cationic dye and van Gieson collagen stains. *Journal of Histochemistry and Cytochemistry* **12**: 821–841.

Lillie, R.D. (1969). Mechanisms of chromation hematoxylin stains. *Histochemie* **20**: 338–354.

Lillie, R.D. (1977). *H.J. Conn's Biological Stains*, 9th edn. Baltimore, MD: Williams and Wilkins.

Lillie, R.D. and Ashburn, L.L. (1943). Supersaturated solutions of fat stains in dilute isopropanol for demonstration of acute fatty degenerations not shown by the Herxheimer technic. *Archives of Pathology* **36**: 432–435.

Lillie, R.D. and Burtner, H.J. (1953). The ferric ferricyanide reduction test in histochemistry. *Journal of Histochemistry and Cytochemistry* **1**: 87–92.

Lillie, R.D. and Donaldson, P.T. (1974). The mechanism of the ferric ferricyanide reduction reaction. *Histochemical Journal* **6**: 679–684.

Lillie, R.D. and Fullmer, H.M. (1976). *Histopathologic Technic and Practical Histochemistry*, 4th edn. New York: McGraw-Hill.

Lillie, R.D., Henderson, R. and Gutierrez, A. (1968a). The diazosafranin method: control of nitrite concentration and refinements in specificity. *Stain Technology* **43**: 311–313.

Lillie, R.D., Pizzolato, P. and Donaldson, P.T. (1968b). Hematoxylin substitutes: a survey of mordant dyes tested and consideration of the relation of their structure to performance as nuclear stains. *Stain Technology* **51**: 25–41.

Lillie, R.D., Pizzolato, P., Dessauer, H.C. and Donaldson, P.T. (1971). Histochemical reactions at tissue arginine sites with alkaline solutions of α-naphthoquinone-4-sodium sulfonate and other *o*-quinones and oxidized *o*-diphenols. *Journal of Histochemistry and Cytochemistry* **19**: 487–497.

Lillie, R.D., Pizzolato, P. and Donaldson, P.T. (1976). Nuclear stains with soluble metachrome metal mordant lake dyes. The effect of chemical endgroup blocking reactions and the artificial introduction of acid groups into tissues. *Histochemistry* **49**: 23–35.

Lindner, L.E. (1993). Improvements in the silver-staining technique for nucleolar organizer regions (AgNOR). *Journal of Histochemistry and Cytochemistry* **41**: 439–445.

Lindvall, O. and Bjorklund, A. (1974). The glyoxylic fluorescence histochemical method: a detailed account of the methodology for the visualization of central catecholamine neurons. *Histochemistry* **39**: 97–127.

Lison, L. (1955). Staining differences in cell nuclei. *Quarterly Journal of Microscopical Science* **96**: 227–237.

Litwin, J.A. (1985). Light microscopic histochemistry on plastic sections. *Progress in Histochemistry and Cytochemistry* **16**: 1–84.

Liu, C.-C., Sherrard, D.J., Maloney, N.A. and Howard, G.A. (1987). Reactivation of bone acid phosphatase and its significance in bone histomorphometry. *Journal of Histochemistry and Cytochemistry* **35**: 1355–1363.

Liu, Y.L., Gu, Q. and Cynader, M.S. (1993). An improved staining technique for cytochrome-c oxidase. *Journal of Neuroscience Methods* **49**,: 181–184.

Llewellyn, B.D. (1974). Mordant blue 3: a readily available substitute for hematoxylin in the routine hematoxylin and eosin stain. *Stain Technology* **49**: 347–349.

Llewellyn, B.D. (1978). Improved nuclear staining with mordant blue 3 as a hematoxylin substitute. *Stain Technology* **53**: 73–77.

Llewellyn, B.D. (2005). Hematoxylin and hematein. Available from: http://stainsfile.info/StainsFile/dyes/75290.htm [accessed April 2007].

Llewellyn-Smith, I.J., Pilowsky, P. and Minson, J.B. (1993). The tungstate-stabilized tetramethylbenzidine reaction for light and electron microscopic immunocytochemistry and for revealing biocytin-filled neurons. *Journal of Neuroscience Methods* **46**: 27–40.

Loach, P.A. (1976). Oxidation–reduction potentials, absorbance bands and molar absorbance of compounds used in biochemical studies. In Fasman, G.D. (ed.), *Handbook of Biochemistry and Molecular Biology. Physical and Chemical Data*, Vol. 1, pp. 122–130. Cleveland, Ohio: CRC Press.

Loberg, E.M. and Torvik, A. (1992). Neuronal uptake of plasma proteins in brain contusions: an immunohistochemical study. *Acta Neuropathologica* **84**: 234–237.

Locke, F.S. (1895). Towards the ideal circulating fluid for the isolated frog's heart. *Journal of Physiology* **18**: 232–233.

Login, G.R. and Dvorak, A.M. (1993). A review of rapid microwave fixation technology: its expanding niche in morphologic studies. *Scanning* **15**: 58–66.

Lojda, Z. (1979). The histochemical demonstration of peptidases by natural substrates. *Histochemistry* **62**: 305–323.

Lojda, Z. and Malis, F. (1972). Histochemical demonstration of enterokinase. *Histochemie* **32**: 23–39.

Lojda, Z., Gossrau, R. and Schiebler, T.H. (1979). *Enzyme Histochemistry. A Laboratory Manual*. Berlin: Springer-Verlag.

Longin, A., Souchier, C., Ffrench, M. and Bryon, P.A. (1993). Comparison of anti-fading agents used in fluorescence microscopy: image analysis and laser confocal microscopy study. *Journal of Histochemistry and Cytochemistry* **41**: 1833–1840.

Loren, I., Bjorklund, A., Falck, B. and Lindvall, O. (1976). An improved histofluorescence procedure for freeze-dried paraffin-embedded tissue based on combined formaldehyde–glyoxylic acid perfusion with high magnesium content and acid pH. *Histochemistry* **49**: 177–192.

Loren, I., Bjorklund, A., Falck, B. and Lindvall, O. (1980). The aluminum–formaldehyde (ALFA) histofluorescence method for improved visualization of catecholamines and indoleamines. 1. A detailed account of the methodology for central nervous tissue using paraffin, cryostat or vibratome sections. *Journal of Neuroscience Methods* **2**: 277–300.

Low, F.N. and McClugage, S.G. (1994). Microdissection by ultrasonication: application to early chick embryos. *Biotechnic and Histochemistry* **69**: 136–147.

Lu, Q.L. and Partridge, T.A. (1998). A new blocking method for application of murine monoclonal antibody to mouse tissue sections. *Journal of Histochemistry and Cytochemistry* **46**: 977–983.

Lu, W.X., Chen, H.Y. and Wolf, M.E. (1996). A ribonuclease-resistant method of *in situ* hybridization histochemistry in rat brain tissue. *Journal of Neuroscience Methods* **65**: 69–76.

Lucassen, P.J., Chung, W.C.J., Vermeulen, J.P., Vanlookeren, M., Vandierendonck, C.J.H. and Swaab, D.F. (1995). Microwave-enhanced *in situ* end-labeling of fragmented DNA: parametric studies in relation to postmortem delay and fixation of rat and human brain. *Journal of Histochemistry and Cytochemistry* **43**: 1163–1171.

Lulai, E.C. and Morgan, W.C. (1992). Histochemical probing of potato periderm with neutral red: a sensitive cytofluorochrome for the hydrophobic domain of suberin. *Biotechnic and Histochemistry* **67**: 185–195.

Luna, L.G. (1968). *Manual of Histologic Staining Methods of the Armed Forces Institute of Pathology*, 3rd edn. New York: McGraw-Hill.

Lundqvist, M., Arnberg, H., Candell, J., Malmgren, M., Wilander, E., Grimelius, L. and Oberg, K. (1990). Silver stains for identification of neuroendocrine cells. A study of the chemical background. *Histochemical Journal* **38**: 615–623.

Lunn, G. and Sansone, E.B. (1990). *Destruction of Hazardous Chemicals in the Laboratory*. New York: Wiley Interscience.

Luppa, H. and Andrä, J. (1983). The histochemistry of carboxyl ester hydrolases: problems and possibilities. *Histochemical Journal* **15**: 111–137.

Luther, P.W. and Bloch, R.J. (1989). Formaldehyde-amine fixatives for immunocytochemistry of cultured *Xenopus* myocytes. *Journal of Histochemistry and Cytochemistry* **37**: 75–82.

Lycette, R.M., Danforth, W.F., Koppel, J.L. and Olwin, J.H. (1970). The binding of luxol fast blue ARN by various biological lipids. *Stain Technology* **45**: 155–160.

Lyman, W.J., Reehl, W.F. and Rosenblatt, D.H. (eds) (1982). *Handbook of Chemical Property Estimation Methods*. New York: McGraw-Hill.

Lynch, G., Smith, R.L., Mensah, P. and Cotman, C. (1973). Tracing the dentate gyrus mossy fiber system with horseradish peroxidase histochemistry. *Experimental Neurology* **68**: 167–173.

Lynch, M.J. (1965). Staining reticulin with gold. *Stain Technology* **40**: 19–25.

Lynn, J.A., Whitaker, B.P., Hladik, C.L., Robinson, R.J., Joie, J.B., Stigliano, W.W. and Carson, F.L. (1994). Zinc isopropyl alcoholic unbuffered formalin as a postfixative for routine surgical pathology specimens. *Journal of Histotechnology* **17**: 105–109.

Lyon, H. (1991). *Theory and Strategy in Histochemistry. A Guide to the Selection and Understanding of Techniques.* Berlin: Springer-Verlag.

Lyon, H.O. (2002). Dye purity and dye standardization for biological staining. *Biotechnic and Histochemistry* **77**: 57–80.

Lyon, H.O., Deleenheer, A.P., Horobin, R.W., Lambert, W.E., Schulte, E.K.W., Vanliedekerke, B. and Wittekind, D.H. (1994). Standardization of reagents and methods used in cytological and histological practice with emphasis on dyes, stains and chromogenic reagents. *Histochemical Journal* **26**: 533–544.

Lyon, H., Jakobsen, P., Hoyer, P. and Andersen, A.P. (1987). An investigation of new commercial samples of methyl green and pyronine Y. *Histochemical Journal* **19**: 381–384.

Lyon, H., Schulte, E. and Hoyer, P.E. (1989). The correlation between uptake of methyl green and Feulgen staining intensity of cell nuclei. An image analysis study. *Histochemical Journal* **21**: 508–513.

MacCallum, D.K. (1973). Positivity Schiff reactivity of aortic elastin without prior HIO_4 oxidation: influence of maturity and a suggested source of the aldehyde. *Stain Technology* **48**: 117–122.

Maeda, I., Imai, H., Arai, R., Tago, M., Nagai, T., Sakamoto, T., Kitahama, K., Onteniente, B. and Kimura, H. (1987). An improved coupled peroxidatic oxidation method of MAO histochemistry for neuroanatomical research at light and electron microscopic levels. *Cellular and Molecular Biology* **33**: 1–11.

Magrassi, L. and Graziadei, P.P.C. (1995). Cell death in the olfactory epithelium. *Anatomy and Embryology* **192**: 77–87.

Maillet, M. (1963). Le reactif au tetraoxyde d'osmium–iodure du zinc. *Zeitschrift für mikroskopische–anatomische Forschung* **76**: 397–425.

Mainwaring, W.I.P., Parish, J.H., Pickering, J.D. and Mann, N.H. (1982). *Nucleic Acid Biochemistry and Molecular Biology.* Oxford: Blackwell.

Maisch, J.M. (1885). On the adulteration of saffron. *Analyst* **10**: 200–203.

Makela, O. (1957). Studies in haemagglutinins of Leguminosae seeds. *Acta Medicinae Experimentalis et Biologiae Fenniae* **35(Suppl. 11)**: 1–133.

Malinin, G. (1977). Stable sudanophilia of 'bound' lipids in tissue culture cells is a staining artifact. *Journal of Histochemistry and Cytochemistry* **25**: 155–156.

Malinin, G. (1980). The *in situ* determination of melting–solidification points of lipid inclusions in fixed cultured cells. *Journal of Histochemistry and Cytochemistry* **28**: 708–709.

Malkusch, W., Rehn, B. and Bruch, J. 1995. Advantages of sirius red staining for quantitative morphometric collagen measurements in lungs. *Experimental Lung Research* **21**: 67–77.

Mallory, F.B. (1905). A contribution to the classification of tumors. *Journal of Medical Research* **13**: 113–136.

Malm, M. (1962). *p*-Toluenesulphonic acid as a fixative. *Quarterly Journal of Microscopical Science* **103**: 163–171.

Malmgren, H. and Sylven, B. (1955). On the chemistry of the thiocholine method of Koelle. *Journal of Histochemistry and Cytochemistry* **3**: 441–448.

Maneta-Peyret, L., Compere, P., Moreau, P., Goffinet, G. and Cassagne, C. (1999). Immunocytochemistry of lipids: chemical fixatives have dramatic effects on the preservation of tissue lipids. *Histochemical Journal* **31**: 541–547.

Mann, G. (1902). *Physiological Histology. Methods and Theory.* Oxford: Clarendon Press.

Marchi, V. (1892). Sur l'origine et le cours des pedoncles cerebellaux et sur leurs rapports avec les autres centres nerveux. *Archives Italiennes de Biologie* **17**: 190–201.

Marcos, R., Rocha, E. and Monteiro, R.A.F. (2001). Strategies to maximize adhesion of thick sections of the brown trout liver for stereological purposes. *Journal of Histotechnology* **24**: 37–42.

Marletta, M.A., Yoon, P.S., Iyengar, R., Leaf, C.D. and Wishnok, J.S. (1988). Macrophage oxidation of L-arginine to nitrite and nitrate: nitric oxide is an intermediate. *Biochemistry* **27**: 8706–8711.

Marshall, P.N. (1977). Thin layer chromatography of Sudan dyes. *Journal of Chromatography* **136**: 353–357.

Marshall, P.N. (1978). Romanowsky-type stains in haematology. *Histochemical Journal* **10**: 1–29.

Marshall, P.N. and Horobin, R.W. (1972a). The chemical nature of the gallocyanin–chrome alum staining complex. *Stain Technology* **47**: 155–161.

Marshall, P.N. and Horobin, R.W. (1972b). The oxidation products of haematoxylin and their role in biological staining. *Histochemical Journal* **4**: 493–503.

Marshall, P.N. and Horobin, R.W. (1973). The mechanism of action of 'mordant' dyes – a study using preformed metal complexes. *Histochemie* **35**: 361–371.

Marshall, P.N. and Horobin, R.W. (1974). A simple assay procedure for mixtures of hematoxylin and hematein. *Stain Technology* **49**: 137–142.

Martin, S.J., Reutelingsperger, C.P.M. and Green, D.R. (1996). Annexin V: a specific probe for apoptotic cells. In Cotter, T.G. and Martin, S.J. (eds), *Techniques in Apoptosis*, pp. 107–119. London: Portland Press.

Martinez-Lage, P. and Munoz, D.G. (1997). Prevalence and disease associations of argyrophilic grains of Braak. *Journal of Neuropathology and Experimental Neurology* **56**: 157–164.

Mason, D.Y. and Biberfeld, P. (1980). Technical aspects of lymphoma immunohistology. *Journal of Histochemistry and Cytochemistry* **28**: 731–745.

Mason, J.T. and O'Leary, T.J. (1991). Effects of formaldehyde fixation on protein secondary structure: a calorimetric and infrared spectroscopic investigation. *Journal of Histochemistry and Cytochemistry* **39**: 225–229.

Mason, S.F. (1956). *Main Currents of Scientific Thought. A History of the Sciences*. London: Routledge and Kegan Paul.

Masson, P. (1911). Le safran en technique histologique. *Comptes Rendus de la Societe de Biologie* **70**: 573–574.

Masson, P. (1929). Some histological methods. Trichrome stainings and their preliminary techniques. *Journal of Technical Methods and Bulletin of the International Association of Medical Museums* **12**: 75–90.

Mattioda, G., Metivier, B. and Guette, J.P. (1983). What you can do with glyoxal. *Chemtech* **13**: 478–481.

Matyas, J.R., Benediktsson, H. and Rattner, J.B. (1995). Tissue transfer technique for transferring animal tissues onto membrane substrates for rapid histological evaluation. *Journal of Histotechnology* **18**: 307–313.

Mauro, A., Germano, I., Giaccone, G., Giordana, M.T. and Schiffer, D. (1985). 1-Naphthol basic dye (1-NBD). An alternative to diaminobenzidine (DAB) in immunoperoxidase techniques. *Histochemistry* **83**: 97–102.

Maxwell, M.H. (1988). Osmium tetroxide: an historical appreciation. *Proceedings of the Royal Microscopical Society* **23**: 229–232.

Mayall, B.H. and Gledhill, B.L. (1977). The Fifth Engineering Foundation Conference on Automatic Cytology. *Journal of Histochemistry and Cytochemistry* **25**: 479–952.

Mayne, R. and Burgeson, R.E. (1987). *Structure and Function of Collagen Types*. Orlando, FL: Academic Press.

Mays, E.T., Feldhoff, R.C. and Nettleton, G.S. (1984). Determination of protein loss during aqueous and phase partition fixation using formalin and glutaraldehyde. *Journal of Histochemistry and Cytochemistry* **32**: 1107–1112.

Mazurkiewicz, J.E., Hossler, F.E. and Barrnett, R.J. (1978). Cytochemical demonstration of sodium, potassium adenosine triphosphatase by a hemepeptide derivative of ouabain. *Journal of Histochemistry and Cytochemistry* **26**: 1042–1052.

McAuliffe, C.A. (ed.) (1977). *The Chemistry of Mercury*. London: Macmillan.

McAuliffe, W.G. and Nettleton, G.S. (1984). Phase partition fixation for electron microscopy. *Journal of Histochemistry and Cytochemistry* **32**: 913.

McGadey, J. (1970). A tetrazolium method for non-specific alkaline phosphatase. *Histochemie* **23**: 180–184.

McIsaac, G. and Kiernan, J.A. (1974.). Complete staining of neuromuscular innervation with bromoindigo and silver. *Stain Technology* **49**: 211–214.

McKinney, B. and Grubb, C. (1965). Non-specificity of thioflavine-T as an amyloid stain. *Nature* **205**: 1023–1024.

McKay, R.B. (1962). An investigation of the anomalous staining of chromatin by the acid dyes, methyl blue and aniline blue. *Quarterly Journal of Microscopical Science* **103**: 519–530.

McLean, I.W. and Nakane, P.K. (1974). Periodate–lysine–paraformaldehyde fixative. A new fixative for immunoelectron microscopy. *Journal of Histochemistry and Cytochemistry* **22**: 1077–1083.

McManus, J.F.A. and Mowry, R.W. (1960). *Staining Methods. Histologic and Histochemical*. New York: P.B. Hoeber.

McMillan, P.J., Engen, P.C., Dalgleish, A. and McMillan, J. (1983). Improvement of the butyl methacrylate–paraffin embedment. *Stain Technology* **58**: 125–130.

McNulty, J.M., Kambour, M.J. and Smith, A.A. (2004). Use of an improved zirconyl hematoxylin stain in the diagnosis of Barrett's esophagus. *Journal of Cellular and Molecular Medicine* **8**: 382–387.

Mehes, G., Kalman, E. and Pajor, L. (1993). *In situ* fluorescent visualization of nucleolar organizer region-associated proteins with a thiol reagent. *Journal of Histochemistry and Cytochemistry* **41**: 1413–1417.

Meloan, S.N., Valentine, L.S. and Puchtler, H. (1971). On the structure of carminic acid and carmine. *Histochemie* **27**: 87–95.

Mendelson, D., Tas, J. and James, J. (1983). Cuprolinic blue: a specific dye for single-stranded RNA in the presence of magnesium chloride. II. Practical applications for light microscopy. *Histochemical Journal* **15**: 1113–1121.

Mengel, M., Werner, M. and Von Wasielewski, R. (1999). Concentration dependent and adverse effects in immunohistochemistry using the tyramine amplification technique. *Histochemical Journal* **31**: 195–200.

Mera, S.L. and Davies, J.D. (1984). Differential Congo red staining: the effects of pH, non-aqueous solvents and the substrate. *Histochemical Journal* **16**: 195–210.

Merchan-Perez, A., Gilloyzaga, P., Bartolome, M.V., Remezal, M., Fernandez, P. and Rodriguez, T. (1999). Decalcification by ascorbic acid for immuno- and affinohistochemical techniques on the inner ear. *Histochemistry and Cell Biology* **112**: 125–130.

Merchenthaler, I., Stankovics, J. and Gallyas, F. (1989). A highly sensitive one-step method for silver intensification of the nickel–diaminobenzidine endproduct of peroxidase reaction. *Journal of Histochemistry and Cytochemistry* **37**: 1563–1565.

Merritt, A.J., Jones, L.S. and Potten, C.S. (1996). Apoptosis in murine intestinal crypts. In Cotter, T.G. and Martin, S.J. (eds), *Techniques in Apoptosis*, pp. 269–299. London: Portland Press.

Messier, B. and Leblond, C.P. (1960). Cell proliferation and migration as revealed by radioautography after injection of thymidine-H3 into male rats and mice. *American Journal of Anatomy* **106**: 247–285.

Mesulam, M.-M. (1978). Tetramethyl benzidine for horseradish peroxidase neurohistochemistry: a non-carcinogenic blue reaction-product with superior sensitivity for visualizing neural afferents and efferents. *Journal of Histochemistry and Cytochemistry* **26**: 106–117.

Mesulam, M.-M. and Rosene, D.L. (1977). Differential sensitivity between blue and brown reaction procedures for HRP neurohistochemistry. *Neuroscience Letters* **5**: 7–14.

Mesulam, M.-M. and Rosene, D.L. (1979). Sensitivity in horseradish peroxidase neurohistochemistry: a comparative and quantitative study of nine methods. *Journal of Histochemistry and Cytochemistry* **27**: 763–773.

Miklossy, J. and Van der Loos, H. (1987). Cholesterol ester crystals in polarized light show hways in the human brain. *Brain Research* **426**: 377–380.

Miklossy, J. and Van der Loos, H. (1991). The long-distance effects of brain lesions: visualization of myelinated pathways in the human brain using polarizing and fluorescence microscopy. *Journal of Neuropathology and Experimental Neurology* **50**: 1–15.

Miller, R.T. and Kubier, P. (1997). Blocking of endogenous avidin-binding activity in immunohistochemistry – the use of egg whites. *Applied Immunohistochemistry* **5**: 63–66.

Miller, R.T., Kubier, P., Reynolds, B., Henry, T. and Turnbow, H. (1999). Blocking of endogenous avidin-binding activity in immunohistochemistry – the use of skim milk as an economical and effective substitute for commercial biotin solutions. *Applied Immunohistochemistry and Molecular Morphology* **7**: 63–65.

Minard, B.J. and Cawley, L.P. (1978). Use of horseradish peroxidase to block nonspecific enzyme uptake in immunoperoxidase microscopy. *Journal of Histochemistry and Cytochemistry* **26**: 685–687.

Mir, M.M., Fazili, K.M. and Qasim, M.A. (1992). Chemical modification of buried lysine residues of bovine serum albumin and its influence on protein conformation and bilirubin binding. *Biochimica et Biophysica Acta* **1119**: 261–267.

Mitchell, B.S., Dhami, D. and Schumacher, U. (1992). *In situ* hybridisation: a review of methodologies and applications in the biomedical sciences. *Medical Laboratory Science* **49**: 107–118.

Moller, W. and Moller, G. (1994). Chemical dehydration for rapid paraffin embedding. *Biotechnic and Histochemistry* **69**: 289–290.

Molnar, J. (1952). The use of rhodizonate in enzymatic histochemistry. *Stain Technology* **27**: 221–222.

Monroe, C.W. and Frommer, J. (1967). Neutral red-fast green FCF, a single stain for mammalian tissues. *Stain Technology* **42**: 262–264.

Monsan, P., Puzo, G. and Marzarguil, H. (1975). Étude du mécanisme d'établissement des liaisons glutaraldéhyde–protéines. *Biochimie* **57**: 1281–1292.

Montero, C., Segura, D.I. and Gutierrez, M. (1991). Blockade of the antigen-antibody reaction using benzil condensation with the guanidyl residue of arginine. *Histochemical Journal* **23**: 125–131.

Montes, G.S. and Junqueira, L.C.U. (1991). The use of the picrosirius-polarization method for the study of the biopathology of collagen. *Memorias Instituto Oswaldo Cruz (Rio de Janeiro)* **86**: 1–11.

Moore, K.L., Graham, M.A. and Barr, M.L. (1953). The detection of chromosomal sex in hermaphrodites from a skin biopsy. *Surgery, Gynecology and Obstetrics* **96**: 641–648.

Moos, T. and Mollgard, K. (1993). A sensitive post-DAB enhancement technique for demonstration of iron in the central nervous system. *Histochemistry* **99**: 471–475.

Morales, A., Schwint, A.E. and Itoiz, M.E. (1996). Nucleolar organizer regions in a model of cell hyperactivity and regression. *Biocell* **20**: 251–258.

Moreno, L.M.G., Cimadevilla, J.M., Pardo, H.G., Zahonero, M.C. and Arias, J.L. (1997). NOR activity in hippocampal areas during the postnatal development and ageing. *Mechanisms in Ageing and Development* **97**: 173–181.

Moreton, R.B. (1981). Electron-probe X-ray microanalysis: techniques and applications in biology. *Biological Reviews* **56**: 409–461.

Mori, B. and Bellani, L.M. (1996). Differential staining for cellulosic and modified plant cell walls. *Biotechnic and Histochemistry* **71**: 71–72.

Mori, S., Sternberger, N.H, Herman, N.M. and Sternberger, L.A. (1991). Leakage and neuronal uptake of serum protein in aged and Alzheimer brains: a postmortem phenomenon with antemortem etiology. *Laboratory Investigation* **64**: 345–351.

Mori, S., Sternberger, N.H., Herman, M.M. and Sternberger, L.A. (1992). Variability of laminin immunoreactivity in human autopsy brain. *Histochemistry* **97**: 237–241.

Morris, C.M., Candy, J.M., Oakley, A.E., Bloxham, C.A. and Edwardson, J.A. (1992). Histochemical distribution of non-haem iron in the human brain. *Acta Anatomica* **144**: 235–257.

Morris, J.H., Hudson, A.R. and Weddell, G. (1972). A study of degeneration and regeneration in the divided rat sciatic nerve based on electron microscopy. IV. Changes in fascicular microtopography, perineurium and endoneurial fibroblasts. *Zeitschrift fur Zellforschung* **124**: 165–203.

Morris, S.M., Stone, P.J., Rosenkrans, W.A., Calore, J.D., Albright, J.T. and Franzenblau, C. (1978). Palladium chloride as a stain for elastin at the ultrastructural level. *Journal of Histochemistry and Cytochemistry* **26**: 635–644.

Morrison, R.T. and Boyd, R.N. (1992). *Organic Chemistry*, 6th edn. Engelwood Cliffs, NJ: Prentice-Hall.

Morstyn, G., Pyke, K., Gardner, J., Ashcroft, R., Defazio, A. and Bhathal, P. (1986). Immunohistochemical identification of proliferating cells in organ culture using bromodeoxyuridine and a monoclonal antibody. *Journal of Histochemistry and Cytochemistry* **34**: 697–701.

Morthland, F.W., De Bruyn, P.P.H. and Smith, N.H. (1954). Spectrophotometric studies on the interaction of nucleic acids with aminoacridines and other basic dyes. *Experimental Cell Research* **7**: 201–214.

Morton, D. (1978). A comparison of iron histochemical methods for use on glycol methacrylate embedded tissues. *Stain Technology* **53**: 217–223.

Motherby, H., Marcy, T., Hecker, M., Ross, B., Nadjari, B., Auer, H., Muller, K.M., Haussinger, D., Strauer, B.E. and Bocking, A. (1998). Static DNA cytometry as a diagnostic aid in effusion cytology I. DNA aneuploidy for identification and differentiation of primary and secondary tumors of the serous membranes. *Analytical and Quantitative Cytology and Histology* **20**: 153–161.

Movat, H.Z. (1955). Demonstration of all connective tissue elements in a single section. *Archives of Pathology* **60**: 289–295.

Mowry, R.W. (1978). Aldehyde fuchsin staining, direct or after oxidation: problems and remedies, with special reference to human pancreatic B cells, pituitaries and elastic fibers. *Stain Technology* **53**: 141–154.

Mowry, R.W. and Emmel, V.M. (1977). The production of aldehyde fuchsin depends on the pararosaniline (C.I. No. 42500) content of basic fuchsins which is sometimes negligible and is sometimes mislabeled. *Journal of Histochemistry and Cytochemistry* **25**: 239.

Mpoke, S.S. and Wolfe, J. (1997). Differential staining of apoptotic nuclei in living cells: application to macronuclear elimination in Tetrahymena. *Journal of Histochemistry and Cytochemistry* **45**: 675–683.

Mrini, A., Moukhles, H., Jacomy, H., Bosler, O. and Doucet, G. (1995). Efficient immunodetection of various protein antigens in glutaraldehyde-fixed brain tissue. *Journal of Histochemistry and Cytochemistry* **43**: 1285–1291.

Mugnaini, E. and Dahl, A.L. (1983). Zinc–aldehyde fixation for light-microscopic immunocytochemistry of nervous tissues. *Journal of Histochemistry and Cytochemistry* **31**: 1435–1438.

Müller, T. (1989). Paraffin sections of nervous tissue supravitally stained with methylene blue: a new, reliable and simple fixation technique. *Stain Technology* **64**: 93–96.

Muller, A., Bogge, H. and Diemann, E. (2003). Structure of a cavity-encapsulated nanodrop of water. *Inorganic Chemistry Communications* **6**: 523–524.

Muller, T. (1992). Light-microscopic demonstration of methylene blue accumulation sites in mouse brain after supravital staining. *Acta Anatomica* **144**: 39–44.

Muller, W. and Firsching, R. (1991). Demonstration of elastic fibres with reagents for detection of magnesium. *Journal of Anatomy* **175**: 195–202.

Müller-Walz, R. and Zimmermann, H.W. (1987). Uber Romanowsky–Farbstoffe und den Romanowsky–Giemsa-Effekt. 4. Mitteilung: Bindung von Azur B an DNA. *Histochemistry* **87**: 157–172.

Mullink, H., Walboomers, J.M.M., Tadema, T.M., Jansen, D.J. and Meijer, C.J.L.M. (1989). Combined immuno- and non-radioactive hybridocytochemistry on cells and tissue sections: influence of fixation, enzyme pretreatment, and choice of chromogen on detection of antigen and DNA sequences. *Journal of Histochemistry and Cytochemistry* **37**: 603–609.

Munoz, D.G. (1999). Stains for the differential diagnosis of degenerative dementias. *Biotechnic and Histochemistry* **74**: 311–333.

Muralt, A. von (1943). Die sekundare Thiochromfluorescenz des peripheren Nerven und ihre Beziehung zu Bethes Polarizationsbild. *Pflugers Archiv für gesamte Physiologie* **247**: 1–10.

Murgatroyd, L.B. (1976). The preparation of thin sections from glycol methacrylate embedded tissue using a standard rotary microtome. *Medical Laboratory Sciences* **33**: 67–71.

Murray, G.I. and Ewen, S.W.B. (1992). A new fluorescence method for alkaline phosphatase histochemistry. *Journal of Histochemistry and Cytochemistry* **40**: 1971–1974.

Murray, G.I., Burke, M.D. and Ewen, S.W.B. (1986). Glutathione localization by a novel *o*-phthalaldehyde histofluorescence method. *Histochemical Journal* **18**: 434–440.

Murray, G.I., Burke, M.D. and Ewen, S.W.B. (1989). Enzyme histochemistry on freeze-dried, resin-embedded tissue. *Journal of Histochemistry and Cytochemistry* **37**: 643–652.

Murray, R.G.E., Doetsch, R.N. and Robinow, C.F. (1994). Determinative and cytological light microscopy. In Gerhardt, P., Murray, R.G.E., Wood, W.A. and Krieg, N.R. (eds), *Methods for General and Molecular Bacteriology*, pp. 21–41. Washington, DC: American Society for Microbiology.

Musto, L. (1981). Improved iron–hematoxylin stain for elastic fibers. *Stain Technology* **56**: 185–187.

Nairn, R.C. (1976). *Fluorescent Protein Tracing*, 4th edn. London: Churchill-Livingstone.

Nakae, Y. and Stoward, P.J. (1997). Effects of tissue protectants on the kinetics of lactate dehydrogenase in cells. *Journal of Histochemistry and Cytochemistry* **45**: 1417–1425.

Nakamura, T., Sakai, T. and Hotchi, M. (1995). Histochemical demonstration of DNA double strand breaks by *in situ* 3'-tailing reaction in apoptotic endometrium. *Biotechnic and Histochemistry* **70**: 33–39.

Nakao, K. and Angrist, A.A. (1968). A histochemical demonstration of aldehyde in elastin. *American Journal of Clinical Pathology* **49**: 65–67.

Nakos, G. and Gossrau, R. (1994). When NADPH diaphorase (NADPHd) works in the presence of formaldehyde, the enzyme appears to visualize selectively cells with constitutive nitric oxide synthase (NOS). *Acta Histochemica* **96**: 335–343.

Namimatsu, S., Ghazizadeh, M. and Sugisaki, Y. (2005). Reversing the effects of formalin fixation with citraconic anhydride and heat: a universal antigen retrieval method. *Journal of Histochemistry and Cytochemistry* **53**: 3–11.

Naoumenko, J. and Feigin, I. (1961). A modification for paraffin sections of the Cajal gold-sublimate stain for astrocytes. *Journal of Neuropathology and Experimental Neurology* **20**: 602–604.

Nath, J. and Johnson, K.L. (1998). Fluorescence *in situ* hybridization (FISH): DNA probe production and hybridization criteria. *Biotechnic and Histochemistry* **73**: 6–22.

Nath, J. and Johnson, K.L. (2000). A review of fluorescence *in situ* hybridization (FISH): current status and future prospects. *Biotechnic and Histochemistry* **75**: 54–78.

Nathan, P.W. and Smith, M.C. (1955). Long descending tracts in man. I. Review of present knowledge. *Brain* **78**: 248–303.

Nathan, P.W., Smith, M. and Deacon, P. (1996). Vestibulospinal, reticulospinal and descending propriospinal nerve fibres in man. *Brain* **119**: 1809–1833.

National Toxicology Program (1978). 13-Week subchronic toxicity studies of Direct Blue 6, Direct Black 38, and Direct Brown 95 dyes. *NTP Study Reports*. Available from: http://ntp.niehs.nih.gov/ntpweb/index.cfm?objectid= 070449A0-B27D-012E-6D351A85CED41949 [accessed January 2007].

Nauta, W.J.H. and Ebbesson, S.O.B. (eds) (1970). *Contemporary Research Methods in Neuroanatomy*. Berlin: Springer.

Nauta, W.J.H. and Gygax, P.A. (1954). Silver impregnation of degenerating axons in the central nervous system: a modified technic. *Stain Technology* **29**: 91–93.

Nedzel, G.A. (1951). Intranuclear birefringent inclusions, an artifact occurring in paraffin sections. *Quarterly Journal of Microscopical Science* **92**: 343–346.

Negoescu, A., Lorimier, P., Labat-Moleur, F., Drouet, C., Robert, C., Guillermet, C., Brambilla, C. and Brambilla, E. (1996). *In situ* apoptotic cell labeling by the TUNEL method: improvement and evaluation on cell preparations. *Journal of Histochemistry and Cytochemistry* **44**: 958–968.

Negri, C., Donzelli, M., Bernardi, R., Rossi, L., Burkle, A. and Scovassi, A.I. (1997). Multiparametric staining to identify apoptotic human cells. *Experimental Cell Research* **234**: 174–177.

Neiss, W.F. (1984). Electron staining of the cell surface coat by osmium–low ferrocyanide. *Histochemistry* **80**: 231–242.

Nelson, J.R. (2000). Physics of impregnation. *Microscopy Today* **8**: 24.

Nettleton, G.S. (1982). The role of paraldehyde in the rapid preparation of aldehyde fuchsin. *Journal of Histochemistry and Cytochemistry* **30**: 175–178.

Nettleton, G.S. and Carpenter, A.M. (1977). Studies on the mechanism of the periodic acid–Schiff histochemical reaction for glycogen using infrared spectroscopy and model chemical compounds. *Stain Technology* **52**: 63–77.

Nettleton, G.S. and McAuliffe, W.G. (1986). A histological comparison of phase-partition fixation with fixation in aqueous solutions. *Journal of Histochemistry and Cytochemistry* **34**: 795–800.

Neumann, M. and Gabel, D. (2002). Simple method for reduction of autofluorescence in fluorescence microscopy. *Journal of Histochemistry and Cytochemistry* **50**: 437–439.

Newman, G.R., Jasani, B. and Williams, E.D. (1982). The preservation of ultrastructure and antigenicity. *Journal of Microscopy* **127**: RP5–RP6.

Newman, S.B., Borysko, E. and Swerdlow, M. (1949). New sectioning techniques for light and electron microscopy. *Science* **110**,: 66–68.

Nguyen-Legros, J., Bizot, J., Bolesse, M. and Pulicani, J.-P. (1980). 'Noir de diaminobenzidine': une nouvelle methode histochimique de revelation du fer exogene. *Histochemistry* **66**: 239–244.

Nicholson, M.L. and Monkhouse, W.S. (1985). Cholesterol retention in tissue sections: an assessment of different techniques. *Journal of Anatomy* **140**: 538.

Nicolet, B.H. and Shinn, L.A. (1939). The action of periodic acid on α-amino alcohols. *Journal of the American Chemical Society* **61**: 1615.

Nicolson, G.L. (1974). The interactions of lectins with animal cell surfaces. *International Review of Cytology* **39**: 89–190.

Nielsen, L.F., Moe, D., Kirkeby, S. and Garbasch, C. (1998). Sirius red and acid fuchsin staining mechanisms. *Biotechnic and Histochemistry* **73**: 71–77.

Nielson, A.J. and Griffith, W.P. (1978). Tissue fixation and staining with osmium tetroxide: the role of phenolic compounds. *Journal of Histochemistry and Cytochemistry* **26**: 138–140.

Nielson, A.J. and Griffith, W.P. (1979). Tissue fixation by osmium tetroxide. A possible role for proteins. *Journal of Histochemistry and Cytochemistry* **27**: 997–999.

Niendorf, A., Dietel, M., Arps, H. and Childs, G.V. (1988). A novel method to demonstrate parathyroid hormone binding on unfixed living target cells in culture. *Journal of Histochemistry and Cytochemistry* **36**: 307–309.

Nilsson, M., Hellstrom, S. and Albiin, N. (1991). Decalcification by perfusion: a new method for rapid softening of temporal bones. *Histology and Histopathology* **6**: 415–420.

Noller, C.R. (1965). *Chemistry of Organic Compounds*, 3rd edn. Philadelphia, PA: Saunders.

Norton, W.T., Korey, S.R. and Brotz, M. (1962). Histochemical demonstration of unsaturated lipids by a bromine–silver method. *Journal of Histochemistry and Cytochemistry* **10**: 83–88.

Notani, G.W., Parsons, J.A. and Erlandsen, S.L. (1979). Versatility of *Staphylococcus aureus* protein A in immunocytochemistry. Use in unlabeled antibody enzyme systems and fluorescent methods. *Journal of Histochemistry and Cytochemistry* **27**: 1438–1444.

Nuehring, L.P., Steffens, W.L. and Rowland, G.N. (1991). Comparison of ruthenium hexammine trichloride method to other methods of chemical fixation for preservation of avian physial cartilage. *Histochemical Journal* **23**: 201–214.

Nygaard, O.F. and Potter, B.L. (1959). Effect of X-radiation on DNA metabolism in various tissues of the rat. 1. Incorporation of C14-thymidine into DNA during the first 24 hours postirradiation. *Radiation Research* **10**: 462–476.

Ohnishi, T., Amamoto, K. and Terayama, H. (1973). Polysaccharides associated with chromosomes and their behaviour in the cell cycle. *Histochemie* **35**: 1–10.

Oliver, C., Lewis, P.R. and Stoward, P.J. (1991). Esterases. In Stoward, P.J. and Pearse, A.G.E. (eds), *Histochemistry, Theoretical and Applied*, Vol. 3, pp. 219–239. Edinburgh: Churchill-Livingstone.

Olkowski, Z.L. and Manocha, S.L. (1973). Muscle spindle. In Bourne, G.H. (ed.), *The Structure and Function of Muscle*, Vol. 2, pp. 365–482. New York: Academic Press.

Ollett, W.S. (1951). Further observations on the Gram–Twort stain. *Journal of Pathology and Bacteriology* **63**: 166.

Ornstein, L., Mautner, W., Davis, B.J. and Tamura, R. (1957). New horizons in fluorescence microscopy. *Journal of the Mount Sinai Hospital* **24**: 1066–1078.

Osterberg, R. (1974). Metal ion–protein interactions in solution. In Sigel, H. (ed.), *Metal Ions in Biological Systems*, Vol. 3, pp. 45–88. New York: Marcel Dekker.

Overend, W.G. and Stacey, M. (1949). Mechanism of the Feulgen nucleal reaction. *Nature* **163**: 538–540.

Page, K.M. (1965). A stain for myelin using solochrome cyanin. *Journal of Medical Laboratory Technology* **22**: 224–225.

Paladino, G. (1890). D'un nouveau procede pour les recherches microscopiques du systeme nerveux central. *Archives Italiennes de Biologie* **13**: 484–486.

Paljarvi, L., Garcia, J.H. and Kalimo, H. (1979). The efficiency of aldehyde fixation for electron microscopy: stabilization of rat brain tissue to withstand osmotic stress. *Histochemical Journal* **11**: 267–276.

Panicker, J.N., Shenoy, K.T. and Augustine, J. (1996). A cytological study of hepatitis B surface antigen localization using orcein staining in hepatocellular carcinoma. *Indian Journal of Medical Research* **104**: 374–376.

Panula, P., Happola, O., Airaksinen, M.S., Auvinen, S. and Virkamaki, A. (1988). Carbodiimide as a tissue fixative in histamine immunohistochemistry and its application in developmental neurobiology. *Journal of Histochemistry and Cytochemistry* **36**: 259–269.

Papadimitriou, J.M., Van Duijn, P., Brederoo, P. and Streefkerk, J.G. (1976). A new method for the cytochemical demonstration of peroxidase for light, fluorescence and electron microscopy. *Journal of Histochemistry and Cytochemistry* **24**: 82–90.

Pardue, S., Zimmerman, A.L. and Morrison-Bogorad, M. (1994). Selective postmortem degradation of inducible heat shock protein 70 (hsp70) mRNAs in rat brain. *Cellular and Molecular Neurobiology* **14**: 341–357.

Park, C.M., Reid, P.E., Owen, D.A., Dunn, W.L. and Volz, D. (1987). Histochemical procedures for the simultaneous visualization of neutral sugars and either sialic acid and its *O*-acyl variants or *O*-sulphate ester. II. Methods based upon the periodic acid–phenylhydrazine–Schiff reaction. *Histochemical Journal* **19**: 257–263.

Parmley, R.T., Spicer, S.S. and Alvarez, C.J. (1978). Ultrastructural localization of nonheme cellular iron with ferrocyanide. *Journal of Histochemistry and Cytochemistry* **26**: 729–741.

Pasteels, J.L. and Herlant, M. (1962). Notions nouvelles sur la cytologie de l'antehypophyse chez le rat. *Zeitschrift für Zellforschung* **56**: 20–39.

Pastore, J.N., Clampett, C., Miller, J., Porter, K. and Miller, D. (1995). A rapid immunoenzyme double labeling technique using EPOS reagents. *Journal of Histotechnology* **18**: 35–39.

Pauling, L. (1970). *General Chemistry*, 3rd edn. San Francisco, CA: Freeman.

Pearse, A.G.E. (1968a). Common cytochemical and ultrastructural characteristics of cells producing polypeptide hormones (the APUD series) and their relevance to thyroid and ultimobranchial C-cells and calcitonin. *Proceedings of the Royal Society of London B* **170**: 71–80.

Pearse, A.G.E. (1968b,1972). *Histochemistry, Theoretical and Applied*, 3rd edn, 2 vols. Edinburgh: Churchill-Livingstone.

Pearse, A.G.E. and Polak, J. (1975). Bifunctional reagents as vapour- and liquid-phase fixatives for immunohistochemistry. *Histochemical Journal* **7**: 179–186.

Pearse, A.G.E. and Stoward, P.J. (1980,1985,1991). *Histochemistry, Theoretical and Applied*, 4th edn, Vols 1–3. Edinburgh: Churchill-Livingstone.

Pelletier, M. and Vitale, M.L. (1994). Filipin vs enzymatic localization of cholesterol in guinea pig, mink, and mallard duck testicular cells. *Journal of Histochemistry and Cytochemistry* **42**: 1539–1554.

Penfield, W. (1927). The mechanism of cicatricial contraction in the brain. *Brain* **50**: 499–517.

Penfield, W. and Cone, W.V. (1950). Neuroglia and microglia (the metallic methods). In Jones, R.M. (ed.), *McClung's Handbook of Microscopical Technique*, pp. 399–431. New York: Hoeber.

Penney, D.P. and Powers, J.M. (1995). Report from the Biological Stain Commission Laboratory. Light green SF yellowish. *Biotechnic and Histochemistry* **70**: 217.

Penney, D.P., Powers, J.M., Frank, M. and Churukian, C. (2002). Analysis and testing of biological stains – the Biological Stain Commission procedures. *Biotechnic and Histochemistry* **77**: 237–275.

Pepler, W.J. and Pearse, A.G.E. (1957). The histochemistry of the esterases of the rat brain, with special reference to those of the hypothalamic nuclei. *Journal of Neurochemistry* **1**: 193–202.

Perrin, D.D. and Dempsey, B. (1974). *Buffers for pH and Metal Ion Control*. London: Chapman and Hall.

Peters, A. (1955a). Experiments on the mechanism of silver staining. I. Impregnation. *Quarterly Journal of Microscopical Science* **96**: 84–102.

Peters, A. (1955b). Experiments on the mechanism of silver staining. II. Development. *Quarterly Journal of Microscopical Science* **96**: 103–115.

Peters, A. (1955c). Experiments on the mechanism of silver staining. III. Electron microscope studies. *Quarterly Journal of Microscopical Science* **96**: 317–322.

Peters, A. (1981). The Golgi-electron microscope technique. In Johnson, J.E. (ed.), *Current Trends in Morphological Techniques*, Vol. 1, pp. 187–212. Boca Raton, FL: CRC Press.

Peters, A., Palay, S.L. and Webster, H.D.F. (1991). *The Fine Structure of the Nervous System*, 3rd edn. New York: Oxford University Press.

Petithory, J.C., Ardoin, F., Ash, L.R., Vandemeulebroucke, E., Galeazzi, G., Dufour, M. and Paugam, A. (1997). Microscopic diagnosis of blood parasites following a cytoconcentration technique. *American Journal of Tropical Medicine and Hygiene* **57**: 637–642.

Pfüller, U., Franz, H. and Preiss, A. (1977). Sudan black B: chemical studies and histochemistry of the blue main component. *Histochemistry* **54**: 237–250.

Phend, K.D., Rustioni, A. and Weinberg, R.J. (1995). An osmium-free method of Epon embedment that preserves both ultrastructure and antigenicity for post-embedding immunocytochemistry. *Journal of Histochemistry and Cytochemistry* **43**: 283–292.

Phillips, L.L., Autilio-Gambetti, L. and Lasek, R.J. (1983). Bodian's silver method reveals molecular variation in the evolution of neurofilament proteins. *Brain Research* **278**: 219–223.

Pickering, J.G., Ford, C.M. and Chow, L.H. (1996). Evidence for rapid accumulation and persistently disordered architecture of fibrillar collagen in human coronary restenosis lesions. *American Journal of Cardiology* **78**: 633–637.

Pignal, F., Maurice, M. and Feldmann, G. (1982). Immunoperoxidase localization of albumin and fibrinogen in rat liver fixed by perfusion or immersion: effect of saponin on the intracellular penetration of labeled antibodies. *Journal of Histochemistry and Cytochemistry* **30**: 1004–1014.

Pileri, S.A., Roncador, G., Ceccarelli, C., Piccioli, M., Briskomatis, A., Sabattini, E., Ascani, S., Santini, D., Piccaluga, P.P., Leone, O., Damiani, S., Ercolessi, C., Sandri, F., Pieri, F., Leoncini, L. and Falini, B. (1997). Antigen retrieval techniques in immunohistochemistry: comparison of different methods. *Journal of Pathology* **183**: 116–123.

Pirila, E., Maisi, P., Salo, T., Kolvunen, E. and Sorsa, T. (2001). *In vivo* localization of gelatinases (MMP-2 and -9) by *in situ* zymography with a selective gelatinase inhibitor. *Biochemical and Biophysical Research Communications* **287**: 766–774.

Platt, J.L. and Michael, A.F. (1983). Retardation of fading and enhancement of intensity of immunofluorescence by *p*-phenylenediamine. *Journal of Histochemistry and Cytochemistry* **31**: 840–842.

Ploton, D., Menager, M., Jeannesson, P., Himber, G., Pigeon, F. and Adner, J.J. (1986). Improvement in the staining and in the visualization of the argyrophilic proteins of the nucleolar organizer region at the optical level. *Histochemical Journal* **18**: 5–14.

Plumel, M. (1948). Tampon au cacodylate de sodium. *Bulletin de la Société de Chimie Biologique* **30**: 129–130.

Pochhammer, C., Dietsch, P. and Siegmund, P.R. (1979). Histochemical detection of carbonic anhydrase with dimethylaminonaphthalene-5-sulfonamide. *Journal of Histochemistry and Cytochemistry* **27**: 1103–1107.

Podolsky, D.K. (1985). Oligosaccharide structures of human colonic mucin. *Journal of Biological Chemistry* **260**: 8262–8271.

Polak, J.M. and McGee, J. O'D. (1998). *In Situ Hybridization. Principles and Practice*, 2nd edn. Oxford: Oxford University Press.

Polak, J.M. and Van Noorden, S. (1997). *Introduction to Immunocytochemistry*, 2nd edn. *Royal Microscopical Society Microscopy Handbooks*, Vol. 37. Oxford: BIOS Scientific Publications.

Polak, J.M. and Varndell, I.M. (eds) (1984). *Immunolabelling for Electron Microscopy*. Amsterdam: Elsevier.

Polak, M. (1948). Sobre la importancia del bromuro de amonio de la solucion fijadora de Cajal en la impregnacion argentica del tejido nervioso. *Archivos de la Sociedad Argentina de Anatomia Normal y Patologica* **10**: 224–234.

Policard, A., Bessis, M. and Bricka, M. (1952). La fixation des cellules isolees observee au contraste de phase et au microscope electronique. I. Action des differents fixateurs. *Bulletin de Microscopie Appliquée (2e Serie)* **2**: 29–42.

Pollock, J.S., Forstermann, U., Tracey, W.R. and Nakane, M. (1995). Nitric oxide synthase isozymes antibodies. *Histochemical Journal* **27**: 738–744.

Ponder, B.A. and Wilkinson, M.M. (1981). Inhibition of endogenous tissue alkaline phosphatase with the use of alkaline phosphatase conjugates in immunohistochemistry. *Journal of Histochemistry and Cytochemistry* **29**: 981–984.

Popescu, A. and Doyle, R.J. (1996). The Gram stain after more than a century. *Biotechnic and Histochemistry* **71**: 145–151.

Pouradier, J. (1977). Properties of gelatin in relation to its use in the preparation of photographic emulsions. In James, T.H. (ed.), *The Theory of the Photographic Process*, pp. 67–76. New York: Macmillan.

Prento, P. (1978). Rapid dehydration-clearing with 2,2-dimethoxypropane for paraffin embedding. *Journal of Histochemistry and Cytochemistry* **26**: 865–867.

Prento, P. (1980). The effect of histochemical methylation on the phosphate groups of nucleic acids: interpretation of the absence of nuclear basophilia. *Histochemical Journal* **12**: 661–668.

Prento, P. (1993). Van Gieson's picrofuchsin: the staining mechanisms for collagen and cytoplasm, and an examination of the dye diffusion rate model of differential staining. *Histochemistry* **99**: 163–174.

Prento, P. (1995). Glutaraldehyde for electron microscopy: a practical investigation of commercial glutaraldehydes and glutaraldehyde-storage conditions. *Histochemical Journal* **27**: 906–913.

Prento, P. (2001). A contribution to the theory of biological staining based on the principles for structural organization of biological macromolecules. *Biotechnic and Histochemistry* **76**: 137–161.

Presnell, J.K. and Schreibman, M.P. (1997). *Humason's Animal Tissue Techniques*, 5th edn. Baltimore, MD: Johns Hopkins University Press.

Proctor, G.B. and Horobin, R.W. (1983). The aging of Gomori's aldehyde-fuchsin: the nature of the chemical changes and the chemical structures of the coloured components. *Histochemistry* **77**: 255–267.

Proctor, G.B. and Horobin, R.W. (1988). Chemical structures and staining mechanisms of Weigert's resorcin-fuchsin and related elastic fiber stains. *Stain Technology* **63**: 101–111.

Puchtler, H. (1958). Significance of the iron hematoxylin method of Heidenhain. *Journal of Histochemistry and Cytochemistry* **6**: 401–402.

Puchtler, H. and Isler, H. (1958). The effect of phosphomolybdic acid on the stainability of connective tissues by various dyes. *Journal of Histochemistry and Cytochemistry* **6**: 265–270.

Puchtler, H. and Sweat, F. (1964a). Effect of phosphomolybdic acid on the binding of Sudan black B. *Histochemie* **4**: 20–23.

Puchtler, H. and Sweat, F. (1964b). Histochemical specificity of staining methods for connective tissue fibers: resorcin–fuchsin and van Gieson's picro-fuchsin. *Histochemie* **4**: 24–34.

Puchtler, H. and Waldrop, F.S. (1978). Silver impregnation methods for reticular fibers and reticulin: a reinvestigation of their origins and specificity. *Histochemistry* **57**: 177–187.

Puchtler, H. and Waldrop, F.S. (1979). On the mechanism of Verhoeff's elastica stain: a convenient stain for myelin sheaths. *Histochemistry* **62**: 233–247.

Puchtler, H., Sweat, F. and Kuhns, J.G. (1964). On the binding of direct cotton dyes by amyloid. *Journal of Histochemistry and Cytochemistry* **12**: 900–907.

Puchtler, H., Waldrop, F.S. and Valentine, L.S. (1973). Polarization microscopic studies of connective tissue stained with picro-sirius red FBA. *Beitrag fur Pathologie* **150**: 174–187.

Puchtler, H., Meloan, S.N. and Waldrop, F.S. (1988). Are picro-dye reactions for collagen quantitative? Chemical and histochemical considerations. *Histochemistry* **88**: 243–256.

Puchtler, H., Waldrop, F.S., Conner, H.M. and Terry, M.S. (1968). Carnoy fixation: practical and theoretical considerations. *Histochemie* **16**: 361–371.

Puchtler, H., Waldrop, F.S., Meloan, S.N., Terry, M.S. and Connor, H.M. (1970). Methacarn (methanol-Carnoy) fixation. Practical and theoretical considerations. *Histochemie* **21**: 97–116.

Purves, D., Voyvodic, J.T., Magrassi, L. and Yawo, H. (1987). Nerve terminal remodeling visualized in living mice by repeated examination of the same neuron. *Science* **238**: 1122–1126.

Qu, Z.Q., Andersen, J.L. and Zhou, S. (1997). Visualisation of capillaries in human skeletal muscle. *Histochemistry and Cell Biology* **107**: 169–174.

Quinn, B. and Graybiel, A.M. (1996). A differentiated silver intensification procedure for the peroxidase–diaminobenzidine reaction. *Journal of Histochemistry and Cytochemistry* **44**: 71–74.

Quintarelli, G., Scott, J.E. and Dellovo, M.C. (1964a). The chemical and histochemical properties of alcian blue. II. Dye binding by tissue polyanions. *Histochemie* **4**: 86–98.

Quintarelli, G., Scott, J.E. and Dellovo, M.C. (1964b). The chemical and histochemical properties of alcian blue. III. Chemical blocking and unblocking. *Histochemie* **4**: 99–112.

Quintero-Hunter, I., Grier, H. and Muscato, M. (1991). Enhancement of histological detail using metanil yellow as counterstain in periodic acid Schiff's hematoxylin staining of glycol methacrylate tissue sections. *Biotechnic and Histochemistry* **66**: 169–172.

Raap, A.K. (1983). Studies on the phenazine methosulphate–tetrazolium salt capture reaction in NAD(P)$^+$-dependent dehydrogenase cytochemistry. III. The role of superoxide in tetrazolium reduction. *Histochemical Journal* **15**: 977–986.

Raap, A.K. and Van Duijn, P. (1983a). Studies on the phenazine methosulphate–tetrazolium salt capture reaction in NAD(P)P$^+$-dependent dehydrogenase cytochemistry. II. A novel hypothesis for the mode of action of PMS and a study of the properties of reduced PMS. *Histochemical Journal* **15**: 881–893.

Raap, A.K., Van Hoof, G.R.M. and Van Duijn, P. (1983b). Studies on the phenazine methosulphate–tetrazolium salt capture reactioin in NAD(P)$^+$-dependent dehydrogenase cytochemistry. I. Localization artefacts caused by the escape of reduced coenzyme during cytochemical reactions for NAD(P)$^+$-dependent dehydrogenases. *Histochemical Journal* **15**: 861–879.

Ralis, H.M., Beesley, R.A. and Ralis, Z.A. (1973). *Techniques in Neurohistology*. London: Butterworths.

Ramon Moliner, E. (1970). The Golgi–Cox technique. In Nauta, W.J.H. and Ebbesson, S.O.B. (eds), *Contemporary Research Methods in Neuroanatomy*, pp. 32–55. Berlin: Springer.

Ranki, A., Reitamo, S., Konittinen, Y.T. and Hayry, P. (1980). Histochemical identification of human T lymphocytes from paraffin sections. *Journal of Histochemistry and Cytochemistry* **28**: 704–707.

Raymond, W.A. and Leong, A.S.Y. (1989). Nucleolar organizer regions relate to growth fractions in human breast carcinoma. *Human Pathology* **20**: 741–746.

Rashid, F. and Horobin, R.W. (1991). Accumulation of fluorescent non-cationic probes in mitochondria of cultured cells: observations, a proposed mechanism, and some implications. *Journal of Microscopy* **163**: 233–241.

Rashid, F., Horobin, R.W. and Williams, M.A. (1991). Predicting the behaviour and selectivity of fluorescent probes for lysosomes and related structures by means of structure–activity models. *Histochemical Journal* **23**: 450–459.

Reid, L. and Clamp, J.R. (1978). The biochemical and histochemical nomenclature of mucus. *British Medical Bulletin* **34**: 5–8.

Reid, P.E. and Owen, D.A. (1988). Some comments on the mechanism of the periodic acid–Schiff–Alcian blue method. *Histochemical Journal* **20**: 651–654.

Reid, P.E., Culling, C.F.A., Dunn, W.L., Clay, M.G. and Ramey, C.W. (1978). A correlative chemical and histochemical study of the *O*-acetylated sialic acids of human colonic epithelial glycoproteins in formalin fixed paraffin embedded tissues. *Journal of Histochemistry and Cytochemistry* **26**: 1033–1041.

Reid, P.E., Dunn, W.L., Ramey, C.W., Coret, E., Trueman, L. and Clay, M.G. (1984a). Histochemical identification of side chain substituted *O*-acylated sialic acids: the PAT-KOH-Bh-PAS and the PAPT-KOH-Bh-PAS procedures. *Histochemical Journal* **16**: 623–639.

Reid, P.E., Dunn, W.L., Ramey, C.W., Coret, E., Trueman, L. and Clay, M.G. (1984b). Histochemical studies of the mechanism of the periodic acid–phenylhydrazine–Schiff (PAPS) procedure. *Histochemical Journal* **16**: 641–649.

Reid, P.E., Volz, D., Park, C.M., Owen, D.A. and Dunn, W.L. (1987). Methods for the identification of side chain *O*-acyl substituted sialic acids and for the simultaneous visualization of sialic acid, its side chain *O*-acyl variants and *O*-sulphate ester. *Histochemical Journal* **19**: 396–398.

Reid, P.E., Volz, D., Cho, K.Y. and Owen, D.A. (1988). A new method for the histochemical demonstration of *O*-acyl sugars in human colonic epithelial glycoproteins. *Histochemical Journal* **20**: 510–518.

Reid, P.E., Iagallo, M., Nehr, S., Jankunis, M., Morrow, L. and Trueman, L. (1993). Mechanism of connective tissue techniques. 1. The effect of dye concentration and staining time on anionic dye procedures. *Histochemical Journal* **25**: 821–829.

Reinecke, M. and Walther, C. (1978). Aspects of turnover and biogenesis of synaptic vesicles at locust neuromuscular junctions as revealed by zinc iodide–osmium tetroxide (ZIO) reacting with intravesicular SH-groups. *Journal of Cell Biology* **78**: 839–855.

Reiner, A. and Gamlin, P. (1980). On noncarcinogenic chromogens for horseradish peroxidase. *Journal of Histochemistry and Cytochemistry* **28**: 187–189.

Reusche, E. (1991). Silver staining of senile plaques and neurofibrillary tangles in paraffin sections: a simple and effective method. *Pathology Research and Practice* **187**: 1045–1049.

Richardson, K.C. (1969). The fine structure of autonomic nerves after vital staining with methylene blue. *Anatomical Record* **164**: 359–378.

Ricard-Blum, S., Dublet, B. and van der Rest, M. (2000). *Unconventional Collagens: Types VI, VII, VIII, IX, X, XII, XIV, XVI and XIX*. Oxford: Oxford University Press.

Rieck, G.D. (1967). *Tungsten and its Compounds*. Oxford: Pergamon.

Ringer, S. (1893). The influence of carbonic acid dissolved in saline solutions on the ventricle of the frog's heart. *Journal of Physiology* **14**: 125–130.

Ripellino, J.A., Klinger, M.M., Margolis, R.U. and Margolis, R.K. (1985). The hyaluronic acid binding region as a specific probe for the localization of hyaluronic acid in tissue sections. *Journal of Histochemistry and Cytochemistry* **33**: 1060–1066.

Rittman, B.R. and Mackenzie, I.C. (1983). Effects of histological processing on lectin binding patterns in oral mucosa and skin. *Histochemical Journal* **15**: 467–474.

Roberts, G.P. (1977). Histochemical detection of sialic acid residues using periodate oxidation. *Histochemical Journal* **9**: 97–102.

Robinow, C. and Kellenberger, E. (1994). The bacterial nucleoid revisited. *Microbiological Reviews* **58**: 211–232.

Robinson, J.M. and Karnovsky, M.J. (1983). Ultrastructural localization of several phosphatases with cerium. *Journal of Histochemistry and Cytochemistry* **31**: 1197–1208.

Robinson, M.M. (1987). Fixation and immunofluorescent analysis of creatine kinase isozymes in embryonic skeletal muscle. *Journal of Histochemistry and Cytochemistry* **35**: 717–722.

Robinson, P.C. and Bradbury, S. (1992). *Qualitative Polarized-Light Microscopy*. Microscopy Handbooks, **09**. Oxford: Oxford University Press and Royal Microscopical Society.

Rodrigo, J., Nava, B.E. and Pedrosa, J. (1970). Study of vegetative innervation in the oesophagus. I. Perivascular endings. *Trabajos del Instituto Cajal de Investigaciones Biologicas* **62**: 39–65.

Rodriguez, L.A. (1955). Experiments on the histologic locus of the hematoencephalic barrier. *Journal of Comparative Neurology* **102**: 27–45.

Roe, R., Corfield, A.P. and Williamson, R.C.N. (1989). Sialic acid in colonic mucin: an evaluation of modified PAS reactions in single and combination histochemical procedures. *Histochemical Journal* **21**: 216–222.

Rohlich, P. (1956). Demonstration of acetylcholinesterase on motor end-plates after embedding in polyethylene glycol. *Nature* **178**: 1398.

Rommanyi, G., Deak, G. and Fischer, J. (1975). Aldehyde–bisulphite–toluidine blue (ABT) staining as a topo-optical reaction for demonstration of linear order of vicinal OH groups in biological structures. *Histochemistry* **43**: 333–348.

Roque, A.L., Jaferay, N.A. and Coulter, P. (1965). A stain for the histochemical demonstration of nucleic acids. *Experimental and Molecular Pathology* **4**: 266–274.

Ros Barcelo, A., Munoz, R. and Sabater, F. (1989). Activated charcoal as an adsorbent of oxidized 3,3'-diaminobenzidine in peroxidase histochemistry. *Stain Technology* **64**: 97–98.

Rosen, A.D. (1981). End-point determination in EDTA decalcification using ammonium oxalate. *Stain Technology* **56**: 48–49.

Rosenthal, S.I., Puchtler, H. and Sweat, F. (1965). Paper chromatography of dyes. *Archives of Pathology* **80**: 190–196.

Rosenwald, A., Reusche, E., Ogomori, K. and Teichert, H.M. (1993). Comparison of silver stainings and immunohistology for the detection of neurofibrillary tangles and extracellular cerebral amyloid in paraffin sections. *Acta Neuropathologica* **86**: 182–186.

Rostgaard, J., Qvortrup, K. and Poulsen, S.S. (1993). Improvements in the technique of vascular perfusion-fixation employing a fluorocarbon-containing perfusate and a peristaltic pump controlled by pressure feedback. *Journal of Microscopy* **172**: 137–151.

Roth, J. (1982). Applications of immunocolloids in light microscopy. Preparation of protein A–silver and protein A–gold complexes and their application for localization of single and multiple antigens in paraffin sections. *Journal of Histochemistry and Cytochemistry* **30**: 691–696.

Roth, J., Bendayan, M. and Orci, L. (1978a). Ultrastructural localization of intracellular antigens by the use of protein A–gold complex. *Journal of Histochemistry and Cytochemistry* **26**: 1074–1081.

Roth, J., Binder, M. and Gerhard, U.J. (1978b). Conjugation of lectins with fluorochromes: an approach to histochemical double labeling of carbohydrate components. *Histochemistry* **56**: 265–273.

Rowlands, D.C., Crocker, J. and Ayres, J.G. (1990). Silver staining of nucleolar organizer region associated proteins using polyethylene glycol as the protective colloidal developer. *Histochemical Journal* **22**: 555–559.

Rubbi, C.P., Qiu, J. and Rickwood, D. (1994). An investigation into the use of protein cross-linking agents as cell fixatives for confocal microscopy. *European Journal of Histochemistry* **38**: 269–280.

Ruijgrok, J.M., Boon, M.E., Feirabend, H.K.P. and Ploeger, S. (1993). Does microwave irradiation have other than thermal effects on glutaraldehyde crosslinking of collagen. *European Journal of Morphology* **31**: 290–297.

Rungby, J., Kassem, M., Eriksen, E.F. and Danscher, G. (1993). The von Kossa reaction for calcium deposits: silver lactate staining increases sensitivity and reduces background. *Histochemical Journal* **25**: 446–451.

Rutenberg, A.M., Rosales, C.L. and Bennett, J.M. (1965). An improved method for the demonstration of leukocyte alkaline phosphatase activity in clinical application. *Journal of Laboratory and Clinical Medicine* **65**: 698–705.

Ruzin, S.E. (1999). *Plant Microtechnique and Microscopy*. Oxford: Oxford University Press.

Rye, D.B., Saper, C.B. and Wainer, B.H. (1984). Stabilization of the tetramethylbenzidine (TMB) reaction product: application for retrograde and anterograde tracing, and combination with immunohistochemistry. *Journal of Histochemistry and Cytochemistry* **32**: 1145–1153.

Sabatini, D.D., Bensch, K. and Barrnett, R.J. (1963). Cytochemistry and electron microscopy. The preservation of cellular ultrastructure and enzymatic activity by aldehyde fixation. *Journal of Cell Biology* **17**: 19–58.

Sakai, W.S. (1973). Simple method for differential staining of paraffin embedded plant material using toluidine blue O. *Stain Technology* **48**: 247–249.

Sakanaka, M., Magari, S., Shibasaki, T., Shinoda, K. and Kohno, J. (1988). A reliable method combining horseradish peroxidase with immuno-α-galactosidase staining. *Journal of Histochemistry and Cytochemistry* **36**: 1091–1096.

Salthouse, T.N. (1962). Luxol fast blue ARN: a new solvent azo dye, with improved staining qualities for myelin and phospholipids. *Stain Technology* **37**: 313–316.

Salthouse, T.N. (1963). Reversal of solubility characteristics of 'Luxol' dye–phospholipid complexes. *Nature* **199**: 821.

Sambrook, J., Fritsch, E.F. and Maniatis, T. (1989). *Molecular Cloning: A Laboratory Manual*, 2nd edn. Cold Spring Harbor, NY: Cold Spring Harbor Laboratory Press.

Samuel, D.M. (1944). The use of an agar gel in the sectioning of mammalian eggs. *Journal of Anatomy* **78**: 173–175.

Samuel, E.P. (1953a). Gold toning. *Stain Technology* **28**: 225–229.

Samuel, E.P. (1953b). The mechanism of silver staining. *Journal of Anatomy* **87**: 278–287.

Sanderson, C. (1997). Entering the realm of mineralized bone processing: a review of the literature and techniques. *Journal of Histotechnology* **20**: 259–266.

Sanderson, C., Radley, K. and Mayton, L. (1995). Ethylenediaminetetraacetic acid in ammonium hydroxide for reducing decalcification time. *Biotechnic and Histochemistry* **70**: 12–18.

Sanderson, J.B. (1994). *Biological Microtechnique. Microscopy Handbooks*, **28**. Oxford: BIOS Scientific Publications and Royal Microscopical Society.

Sanger, J.W. (1975). Intracellular localization of actin with fluorescently labelled heavy meromyosin. *Cell and Tissue Research* **161**: 431–444.

Santini, M. (ed.) (1975). *Golgi Centennial Symposium: Perspectives in Neurobiology*. New York: Raven Press.

Sanwicki, E., Hauser, T.R., Stanley, T.W. and Elbert, W. (1961). The 3-methyl-benzothiazolone hydrazone test. *Analytical Chemistry* **33**: 93–96.

Sato, Y., Akimoto, Y., Kawakami, H., Hirano, H. and Endo, T. (2001). Location of sialoglycoconjugates containing Siaa2-3Gal and Siaa2-6Gal groups in the rat hippocampus and the effect of aging on their expression. *Journal of Histochemistry and Cytochemistry* **49**: 1311–1319.

Satoh, T. and Hosokawa, M. (1998). The mammalian carboxylesterases: from molecules to functions. *Annual Review of Pharmacology and Toxicology* **38**: 257–288.

Saxena, P.N. (1957). Formalin–chloride fixation to improve silver impregnation of the Golgi apparatus. *Stain Technology* **32**: 203–208.

Sayk, J. (1954). Ergebnisse neuer liquor-cytologischer Untersuchungen mit den Sedimentierkammer-Verfahren. *Ärztliche Wochenschrift* **9**: 1042–1046.

Scalet, M., Crivellato, E. and Mallardi, F. (1989). Demonstration of phenolic compounds in plant tissues by an osmium–iodide postfixation procedure. *Stain Technology* **64**: 273–280.

Scarselli, V. (1961). Histochemical demonstration of aldehydes by *p*-phenylenediamine. *Nature* **190**: 1206–1207.

Schabadasch, A. (1930). Untersuchungen zur Methodik der Methylenblaufarbung des vegetativen Nervensystems. *Zeitschrift für Zellforschung* **10**: 221–243.

Schichnes, D., Nemson, J.A. and Ruzin, S.E. (2005). Microwave protocols for plant and animal tissues. *Microscopy Today* **13**: 50–53. Available from: http://www.microscopy-today.com/cgi-bin/MTWWWListingSQL.pl [accessed April 2007].

Schimmelschmidt, K., Hoffmann, H. and Baier, E. (1963). Polycondensation dyes. A new principle for the preparation of wash-fast cotton dyeings. *Angewandte Chemie – International Edition in English* **2**: 30–31.

Schmidt, R. and Moenke-Blankenburg, L. (1986). Modern physical methods for analysing elements and structures in histochemistry. *Acta Histochemica* **80**: 205–213.

Schnell, S.A., Staines, W.A. and Wessendorf, M.W. (1999). Reduction of lipofuscin-like autofluorescence in fluorescently labeled tissue. *Journal of Histochemistry and Cytochemistry* **47**: 719–730.

Schook, P. (1980). The effective osmotic pressure of the fixative for transmission and scanning electron microscopy. *Acta Morphologica Neerlando-Scandinavica* **18**: 31–45.

Schrijver, I.A., Melief, M.J., Vanmeurs, M., Companjen, A.R. and Laman, J.D. (2000). Pararosaniline fixation for detection of co-stimulatory molecules, cytokines, and specific antibody. *Journal of Histochemistry and Cytochemistry* **48**: 95–103.

Schroder, M. (1980). Osmium tetraoxide *cis* hydroxylation of unsaturated substrates. *Chemical Reviews* **80**: 187–213.

Schubert, M. and Hamerman, D. (1956). Metachromasia: chemical theory and histochemical use. *Journal of Histochemistry and Cytochemistry* **4**: 159–189.

Schulte, E.K.W. (1994). Improving biological dyes and stains: quality testing versus standardization. *Biotechnic and Histochemistry* **69**: 7–17.

Schulte, E.K.W. and Fink, D.K. (1995). Hematoxylin staining in quantitative DNA cytometry: an image analysis study. *Analytical Cellular Pathology* **9**: 257–268.

Schulte, E.K.W. and Wittekind, D.H. (1989). Standardized thionin–eosin Y: a quick stain for cytology. *Stain Technology* **64**: 255–256.

Schulz-Harder, B. and Graf Von Keyserlingk, D. (1988). Comparison of brain ribonucleases of rabbit, guinea pig, rat, mouse and gerbil. *Histochemistry* **88**: 587–594.

Schwarz, A. and Futerman, A.H. (1997). Determination of the localization of gangliosides using anti-ganglioside antibodies: Comparison of fixation methods. *Journal of Histochemistry and Cytochemistry* **45**: 611–618.

Scopsi, L. and Larsson, L.-I. (1986). Bodian's silver impregnation of endocrine cells. A tentative explanation to the staining mechanism. *Histochemistry* **86**: 59–62.

Scott, J.E. (1967). On the mechanism of the methyl green–pyronin stain for nucleic acids. *Histochemie* **9**: 30–47.

Scott, J.E. (1970). Critical electrolyte concentration (CEC) effects in interactions between acid glycosaminoglycans and organic cations and polycations. In Balazs, E.A. (ed.), *Chemistry and Molecular Biology of the Extracellular Matrix*, Vol. 2, pp. 1105–1119. London: Academic Press.

Scott, J.E. (1972a). Histochemistry of alcian blue. II. The structure of alcian blue 8GX. *Histochemie* **30**: 215–234.

Scott, J.E. (1972b). Histochemistry of alcian blue. III. The molecular biological basis of staining by alcian blue 8GX and analogous phthalocyanins. *Histochemie* **32**: 191–212.

Scott, J.E. (1974). The Feulgen reaction in polyvinyl alcohol or polyethylene glycol solution. 'Fixation' by excluded volume. *Journal of Histochemistry and Cytochemistry* **22**: 833–835.

Scott, J.E. and Dorling, J. (1969). Periodate oxidation of acid polysaccharides. III. A PAS method for chondroitin sulphates and other glycosamino-glycuronans. *Histochemie* **19**: 295–301.

Scott, J.E. and Harbinson, R.J. (1969). Periodate oxidation of acid polysaccharides. II. Rates of oxidation of uronic acids in polyuronides and acid mucopolysaccharides. *Histochemie* **19**: 155–161.

Scott, J.E., Quintarelli, G. and Dellovo, M.C. (1964). The chemical and histochemical properties of alcian blue. I. The mechanism of alcian blue staining. *Histochemie* **4**: 73–85.

Sechrist, J.W. (1969). Neurocytogenesis. I. Neurofibrils, neurofilaments and the terminal mitotic cycle. *American Journal of Anatomy* **124**: 117–134.

Segade, L.A.G. (1987). Pyrocatechol as a stabilizing agent for *o*-tolidine and *o*-dianisidine: a sensitive new method for HRP. *Journal fur Hirnforschung* **28**,: 331–340.

Segura, D.I., Montero, C. and Gutierrez, M. (1994). Diacetyl for blocking the histochemical reaction for arginine. *Biotechnic and Histochemistry* **69**: 1–6.

Seidler, E. (1979). Zum Mechanismus der Tetrazoliumsalzreduktion und Wirkungsweise des Phenazinmethosulphates. *Acta Histochemica* **65**: 209–218.

Seidler, E. (1980). New nitro-monotetrazolium salts and their use in histochemistry. *Histochemical Journal* **12**: 619–630.

Selye, H. (1965). *The Mast Cells*. Washington, DC: Butterworths.

Sen, S. (1992). Programmed cell death: concept, mechanism and control. *Biological Reviews* **67**: 287–319.

Serbedzija, G.N., Burgan, S., Fraser, S.E. and Bronner-Fraser, M. (1991). Vital dye labelling demonstrates a sacral neural crest contribution to the enteric nervous system of chick and mouse embryos. *Development* **111**: 857–866.

Seveus, L., Vaisala, M., Hemmila, I., Kojola, H., Roomans, G.M. and Soini, E. (1994). Use of fluorescent europium chelates as labels in microscopy allows glutaraldehyde fixation and permanent mounting and leads to reduced autofluorescence and good long-term stability. *Microscopy Research and Technique* **28**: 149–154.

Shannon, W.A. (1981). Light and electron microscopy cytochemistry of monoamine oxidase and other amine oxidative enzymes. In Johnson, J.E. (ed.), *Current Trends in Morphological Techniques*, Vol. 3, pp. 193–242. Boca Raton, FL: CRC Press.

Sharif, N.A. (ed.) (1993). *Molecular Imaging in Neuroscience. A Practical Approach*. Oxford: Oxford University Press.

Sharon, N. and Lis, H. (2003). *Lectins*, 2nd edn. Dordrecht: Kluwer.

Shea, S.M. (1971). Lanthanum staining of the surface coat of cells. Its enhancement by the use of fixatives containing alcian blue. *Journal of Cell Biology* **51**: 611–620.

Shelley, W.B. (1970). Sodium rhodizonate staining of the keratogenous zone of the hair follicle and lingual papilla. *Histochemie* **22**: 169–176.

Shi, S.-R., Key, M.E. and Kalra, K.L. (1991). Antigen retrieval in formalin-fixed, paraffin-embedded tissue: an enhancement method for immunohistochemical staining based on microwave oven heating of tissue sections. *Journal of Histochemistry and Cytochemistry* **39**: 741–748.

Shi, S.-R., Chaiwun, B., Cote, R.J. and Taylor, C.R. (1993). Antigen retrieval technique utilizing citrate buffer or urea solution for immunocytochemical demonstration of androgen receptor in formalin-fixed paraffin sections. *Journal of Histochemistry and Cytochemistry* **41**: 1599–1604.

Shi, S.-R., Chaiwun, B., Young, L., Imam, A., Cote, R.J. and Taylor, C.R. (1994). Antigen retrieval using pH 3.5 glycine–HCl buffer or urea solution for immunohistochemical localization of Ki-67. *Biotechnic and Histochemistry* **69**: 213–218.

Shi, S.R., Imam, S.A., Young, L., Cote, R.J. and Taylor, C.R. (1995). Antigen retrieval histochemistry under the influence of pH using monoclonal antibodies. *Journal of Histochemistry and Cytochemistry* **43**: 193–201.

Shi, S.R., Cote, R.J., Yang, C., Chen, C., Xu, H.J., Benedict, W.F. and Taylor, C.R. (1996). Development of an optimal protocol for antigen retrieval: a 'test battery' approach exemplified with reference to the staining of retinoblastoma protein (pRB) in formalin-fixed paraffin sections. *Journal of Pathology* **179**: 347–352.

Shi, S.R., Liu, C. and Taylor, C.R. (2007). Standardization of immunohistochemistry for formalin-fixed, paraffin-embedded tissue sections based on the antigen-retrieval technique: from experiments to hypothesis. *Journal of Histochemistry and Cytochemistry* **55**: 105–109.

Shibata, K., Fujita, S., Takahashi, H., Yamaguchi, A. and Koji, T. (2000). Assessment of decalcifying protocols for detection of specific RNA by non-radioactive *in situ* hybridization in calcified tissues. *Histochemistry and Cell Biology* **113**: 153–159.

Shore, J. (ed.) (2002a). *Colorants and Auxiliaries: Organic Chemistry and Application Properties.* 2nd edn, Vol. 1 (*Colorants*). Bradford: Society of Dyers and Colourists.

Shore, J. (2002b). Fluorescent brightening agents. In *Colorants and Auxiliaries: Organic Chemistry and Application Properties.* 2nd edn, Vol. 2 (*Auxiliaries*), pp. 760–812. Bradford: Society of Dyers and Colourists.

Shotton, D.E. (ed.) (1993). *Electronic Light Microscopy: The Principles and Practice of Video-enhanced Contrast, Digital Intensified Fluorescence, and Confocal Scanning Light Microscopy.* New York: Wiley-Liss.

Silbert, J.E., Kleinman, H.K. and Silbert, C.K. (1975). Heparins and heparin-like substances of cells. In Bradshaw, R.A. and Wessler, S. (eds), *Heparin* (*Advances in Experimental Biology and Medicine*), pp. 51–60. New York: Plenum Press.

Silveira, S.R. and Hadler, W.A. (1978). Catalases and peroxidases detection techniques suitable to discriminate these enzymes. *Acta Histochemica* **63**: 1–10.

Silverman, J. (1999). D-Limonene – a serviceable and safe routine clearing agent. *Microscopy Today* **7**: 18.

Silverman, M.S. and Tootell, R.B.H. (1987). Modified technique for cytochrome oxidase histochemistry: increased staining intensity and compatibility with 2-deoxyglucose autoradiography. *Journal of Neuroscience Methods* **19**: 1–10.

Sims, D.E. and Horne, M.M. (1994). Non-aqueous fixative preserves macromolecules on the endothelial cell surface: an *in situ* study. *European Journal of Morphology* **31**: 251–255.

Sinicropi, D.V., Hoke, V.B. and McIlwain, D.L. (1989). Isolation of motoneuron cell bodies from spinal cord stored at −70°C in ethylene glycol. *Analytical Biochemistry* **180**: 286–290.

Slater, M. (1989). Adherence of LR White sections to glass slides for silver enhancement of immunogold labeling. *Stain Technology* **64**: 297–299.

Slayter, E.M. and Slayter, H.S. (1992). *Light and Electron Microscopy.* Cambridge: Cambridge University Press.

Sloop, G.D., Roa, J.C., Delgado, A.G., Balart, J.T., Hines, M.O. and Hill, J.M. (1999). Histologic sectioning produces TUNEL reactivity – a potential cause of false-positive staining. *Archives of Pathology and Laboratory Medicine* **123**: 529–532.

Smith, C.W. and Hollers, J.C. (1970). The pattern of binding of fluorescein-labeled concanavalin A to the motile lymphocyte. *Journal of Reticuloendothelial Society* **8**: 458–464.

Smith, I.C., Carson, B.L. and Ferguson, T.L. (1978). *Trace Metals in the Environment*, Vol 4. (*Palladium and Osmium*). Ann Arbor, MI: Ann Arbor Science Publishers.

Smith, M.B. and March, J. (2007). *March's Advanced Organic Chemistry*, 6th edn. New York: Wiley.

Smithson, K.G., MacVicar, B.A. and Hatton, G.I. (1983). Polyethylene glycol embedding: a technique compatible with immunocytochemistry, enzyme histochemistry, histofluorescence and intracellular staining. *Journal of Neuroscience Methods* **7**: 27–41.

Sneed, M.C. and Brasted, R.C. (1955). The lanthanide series. In *Comprehensive Inorganic Chemistry*, Vol. 4. Ch. 6. Princeton, NJ: van Nostrand.

Sobell, H.M., Tsai, C.C., Jain, S.C. and Gilbert, S.G. (1977). Visualization of drug–nucleic acid interactions at atomic resolution. III. Unifying structural concepts in understanding drug–DNA interactions and their broader implications in understanding protein–DNA interactions. *Journal of Molecular Biology* **144**: 333–365.

Society of Dyers and Colourists. (1971–1996). *Colour Index International*, 4th revision of 3rd edn. Vols 1–9 (1971–1992); CD-ROM Version 2 with additions to 1996 print edn. Bradford: Society of Dyers and Colourists.

Sofroniew, M.V. and Schrell, U. (1982). Long-term storage and repeated use of diluted antisera in glass staining jars for increased sensitivity, reproducibility, and convenience of single- and two-color light microscopic immunocytochemistry. *Journal of Histochemistry and Cytochemistry* **30**: 504–511.

Soini, E., Pelliniemi, L.J., Hemmila, I.A., Mukkala, V.M., Kankare, J.J. and Frojdman, K. (1988). Lanthanide chelates as new fluorochrome labels for cytochemistry. *Journal of Histochemistry and Cytochemistry* **36**: 1449–1551.

Soldani, C., Scovassi, A.I., Canosi, U., Bramucci, E., Ardissino, D. and Arbustini, E. (2005). Multicolor fluorescence technique to detect apoptotic cells in advanced coronary atherosclerotic plaques. *European Journal of Histochemistry* **49**: 47–52.

Sollenberger, P.Y. and Martin, R.B. (1968). Carbon–nitrogen and nitrogen–nitrogen double bond condensation reactions. In Patai, S. (ed.), *The Chemistry of the Amino Group*, pp. 349–406. London: Wiley Interscience.

Somogyi, P. and Takagi, H. (1982). A note on the use of picric acid–paraformaldehyde–glutaraldehyde fixative for correlated light and electron microscopic immunocytochemistry. *Neuroscience* **7**: 1779–1783.

Sorvari, T.E. and Lauren, P.A. (1973). The effect of various fixation procedures on the digestibility of sialomucins with neuraminidase. *Histochemical Journal* **5**: 405–512.

Sorvari, T.E. and Stoward, P.J. (1970). Some investigations of the mechanism of the so-called 'methylation' reactions used in mucosubstance histochemistry. *Histochemie* **24**: 106–119.

Spacek, J. (1989). Dynamics of the Golgi method: a time-lapse study of the early stages of impregnation in single sections. *Journal of Neurocytology* **18**: 27–38.

Sparrow, J.R. (1980). Immunohistochemical study of the blood–brain barrier. Production of an artifact. *Journal of Histochemistry and Cytochemistry* **26**: 570–572.

Spessert, R., Wohlgemuth, C., Reuss, S. and Layes, E. (1994). NADPH-diaphorase activity of nitric oxide synthase in the olfactory bulb: co-factor specificity and characterization regarding the interrelation to NO formation. *Journal of Histochemistry and Cytochemistry* **42**: 569–575.

Spessert, R. and Claassen, C. (1998). Histochemical differentiation between nitric oxide synthase-related and -unrelated diaphorase activity in the rat olfactory bulb. *Histochemical Journal* **30**: 41–50.

Spicer, S.S. and Lillie, R.D. (1961). Histochemical identification of basic proteins with Biebrich scarlet at alkaline pH. *Stain Technology* **36**: 365–370.

Spicer, S.S. and Schulte, B.A. (1992). Diversity of cell glycoconjugates shown histochemically: a perspective. *Journal of Histochemistry and Cytochemistry* **40**: 1–38.

Spicer, S.S. and Warren, L. (1960). The histochemistry of sialic acid containing mucoproteins. *Journal of Histochemistry and Cytochemistry* **8**: 135–137.

Spicer, S.S., Naegele, J.R. and Schulte, B.A. (1996). Differentiation of glycoconjugates localized to sensory terminals and selected sites in brain. *Journal of Comparative Neurology* **365**: 217–231.

Staines, W.A., Meister, B., Melander, T., Nagy, J.I. and Hokfelt, T. (1988). Three-color immunofluorescence histochemistry allowing triple labeling within a single section. *Journal of Histochemistry and Cytochemistry* **36**: 145–151.

Starzak, M. and Mathlouthi, M. (2003). Cluster composition of liquid water derived from laser-Raman spectra and molecular simulation data. *Food Chemistry* **82**: 3–22.

Steedman, H.F. (1960). *Section Cutting in Microscopy*. Oxford: Blackwell.

Stefanini, M., De Martino, C. and Zamboni, L. (1967). Fixation of ejaculated spermatozoa for electron microscopy. *Nature* **216**: 173–174.

Stefanovic, B.D., Ristanovic, D., Trpinac, D., Dordeviccamba, V., Lackovic, V., Bumbasirevic, V., Obradovic, M., Basic, R. and Cetkovic, M. (1998). The acidophilic nature of neuronal Golgi impregnation. *Acta Histochemica* **100**: 217–227.

Stelmack, B.M. and Kiernan, J.A. (1977). Effects of triiodothyronine on the normal and regenerating facial nerve of the rat. *Acta Neuropathologica* **40**: 151–155.

Sternberger, L.A. and Sternberger, N.H. (1986). The unlabeled antibody method: comparison of peroxidase–antiperoxidase with avidin–biotin complex by a new mathod of quantification. *Journal of Histochemistry and Cytochemistry* **34**: 599–605.

Stoddart, R.W. (1984). *The Biosynthesis of Polysaccharides*. London: Croom Helm.

Stoddart, R.W. and Kiernan, J.A. (1973). Aprotinin, a carbohydrate-binding protein. *Histochemie* **34**: 275–280.

Stoddart, R.W. and Kiernan, J.A. (1973). Histochemical detection of the α-D-arabinopyranoside configuration using fluorescent-labelled concanavalin A. *Histochemie* **33**: 87–94.

Stoward, P.J. and Burns, J. (1971). Studies in fluorescence histochemistry. VII. The mechanism of the complex reactions that may take place between protein carboxyl groups and hot mixtures of acetic anhydride and pyridine in the acetic anhydride–salicylhydrazide–zinc (or fluorescent ketone) method for localizing protein C-terminal carboxyl groups. *Histochemical Journal* **3**: 127–141.

Stoward, P.J. and Pearse, A.G.E. (1991). *Histochemistry, Theoretical and Applied*, 4th edn, Vol. 3. (*Enzyme Histochemistry*). Edinburgh: Churchill-Livingstone.

Strangeways, T.S.P. and Canti, R.G. (1927). The living cell *in vitro* as shown by dark-ground illumination and the changes induced in cells by fixing reagents. *Quarterly Journal of Microscopical Science* **71**: 1–14 (and Plates 1–5).

Straus, W. (1964). Factors affecting the cytochemical reaction of peroxidase with benzidine and the stability of the blue reaction product. *Journal of Histochemistry and Cytochemistry* **12**: 462–469.

Streefkerk, J.G. and Van Der Ploeg, M. (1974). The effect of methanol on granulocyte and horseradish peroxidase quantitatively studied in a film model system. *Histochemistry* **40**: 105–111.

Streit, P. and Reubi, C. (1977). A new and sensitive staining method for axonally transported horseradish peroxidase (HRP) in the pigeon visual system. *Brain Research* **126**: 530–537.

Streit, W.J. (1990). An improved staining method for rat microglial cells using the lectin from *Griffonia simplicifolia* (GSAI-B4). *Journal of Histochemistry and Cytochemistry* **38**: 1683–1686.

Strich, S.J. (1968). Notes on the Marchi method of staining degenerating myelin in the peripheral and central nervous system. *Journal of Neurology Neurosurgery and Psychiatry* **31**: 110–114.

Sumi, Y., Inoue, T., Muraki, T. and Suzuki, T. (1983a). A highly sensitive chelator for metal staining, bromopyridylazo-diethylaminophenol. *Stain Technology* **58**: 325–328.

Sumi, Y., Inoue, T., Muraki, T. and Suzuki, T. (1983b). The staining properties of pyridylazophenol analogs in histochemical staining of a metal. *Histochemistry* **77**: 1–7.

Sumi, Y., Ito, M.T., Yoshida, M. and Akama, Y. (1999). Highly sensitive chelating agents for histochemical staining of rare earth metals. *Histochemistry and Cell Biology* **112**: 179–182.

Sumner, B.E.H. (1965). A histochemical study of aldehyde–fuchsin staining. *Journal of the Royal Microscopical Society* **84**: 329–338.

Sumner, B.E.H. (1988). *Basic Histochemistry*. Chichester: Wiley.

Sun, A., Nguyen, X.V. and Bing, B. (2002). Comparative analysis of an improved thioflavin-S stain, Gallyas silver stain, and immunohistochemistry for neurofibrillary tangle demonstration on the same sections. *Journal of Histochemistry and Cytochemistry* **50**: 463–472.

Suurmeijer, A.J.H., van der Wijk, J., van Veldhuisen, D.J., Yang, F.S. and Cole, G.M. (1999). Fractin immunostaining for the detection of apoptotic cells and apoptotic bodies in formalin-fixed and paraffin-embedded tissue. *Laboratory Investigation* **79**: 619–620.

Swaab, D.F., Pool, C.W. and Van Leeuwen, F.W. (1977). Can specificity ever be proved in immunocytochemical staining? *Journal of Histochemistry and Cytochemistry* **25**: 388–390.

Swan, M.A. (1999). Improved ultrastructural preservation: a role for osmoprotection during cellular fixation. *Microscopy and Analysis* **37**: 23–25.

Swank, L. and Davenport, H.A. (1935). Chlorate–osmic–formalin method for degenerating myelin. *Stain Technology* **10**: 87–90.

Swash, M. and Fox, K.P. (1972). Techniques for the demonstration of human muscle spindle innervation in neuromuscular disease. *Journal of the Neurological Sciences* **15**: 291–302.

Switzer, R.C. (2000). Application of silver degeneration stains for neurotoxicity testing. *Toxicologic Pathology* **28**: 70–83.

Taatjes, D.J., Roth, J., Peumans, W. and Goldstein, I.J. (1988). Elderberry bark lectin–gold techniques for the detection of Neu5Ac(α2,6)Gal/GalNAc sequences: applications and limitations. *Histochemical Journal* **20**: 478–490.

Tago, H., Kimura, H. and Maeda, T. (1986). Visualization of detailed acetylcholinesterase fiber and neuron staining in rat brain by a sensitive histochemical procedure. *Journal of Histochemistry and Cytochemistry* **34**: 1431–1438.

Tanaka, C., Itokawa, Y. and Tanaka, S. (1973). The axoplasmic transport of thiamine in rat sciatic nerve. *Journal of Histochemistry and Cytochemistry* **21**: 81–86.

Tanaka, J., Mishiro, K., Watanabe, J. and Kanamura, S. (1995). Visualization of acetylcholine in the mouse brain by a combination of immunohistochemistry with ionic fixation. *Acta histochemica et cytochemica* **28**: 231–237.

Tandler, C.J. (1980). Dithiocarbamylation in histochemistry: carbon disulfide as a reagent for the visualization of primary amino groups with the light and electron microscope. *Journal of Histochemistry and Cytochemistry* **28**: 499–506.

Tarantilis, P.A., Polissiou, M. and Manfait, M. (1994). Separation of picrocrocin, *cis-trans*-crocins and safranal of saffron using high performance liquid chromatography with photodiode-array detection. *Journal of Chromatography A* **664**: 55–61.

Tas, J. (1977). The alcian blue and combined alcian blue–safranin O staining of glycosaminoglycans studied in a model system and in mast cells. *Histochemical Journal* **9**: 205–230.

Tas, J., Mendelson, D. and Noorden, C.J.F. (1983). Cuprolinic blue: a specific dye for single-stranded RNA in the presence of magnesium chloride. I. Fundamental aspects. *Histochemical Journal* **15**: 801–804.

Tatton, N.A. and Kish, S.J. (1997). *In situ* detection of apoptotic nuclei in the substantia nigra compacta of 1-methyl-4-phenyl-1,2,3,6-tetrahydropyridine-treated mice using terminal deoxynucleotidyl transferase labelling and acridine orange staining. *Neuroscience* **77**: 1037–1048.

Taylor, C.R., Shi, S.R., Chen, C., Young, L., Yang, C. and Cote, R.J. (1996a). Comparative study of antigen retrieval heating methods: microwave, microwave and pressure cooker, autoclave, and steamer. *Biotechnic and Histochemistry* **71**: 263–270.

Taylor, C.R., Shi, S.R. and Cote, R.J. (1996b). Antigen retrieval for immunohistochemistry – status and need for greater standardization. *Applied Immunohistochemistry* **4**: 144–166.

Taylor, K.B. (1961). The influence of molecular structure of oxazine and thiazine dyes on their metachromatic properties. *Stain Technology* **26**: 73–83.

Tekola, P., Baak, J.P.A., Belien, J.A.M. and Brugghe, J. (1994). Highly sensitive, specific, and stable new fluorescent DNA stains for confocal laser microscopy and image processing of normal paraffin sections. *Cytometry* **17**: 191–195.

Terner, J.Y. and Hayes, E.R. (1961). Histochemistry of plasmalogens. *Stain Technology* **36**: 265–278.

Terracio, L. and Schwabe, K.G. (1981). Freezing and drying of biological tissues for electron microscopy. *Journal of Histochemistry and Cytochemistry* **29**: 1021–1028.

Tewari, J.P., Sehgal, S.S. and Malhotra, S.K. (1982). Microanalysis of the reaction product in Karnovsky and Roots histo-chemical localization of acetylcholinesterase. *Journal of Histochemistry and Cytochemistry* **30**: 436–440.

Thibodeau, T.R., Shah, I.A., Mukherjee, R. and Hosking, M.B. (1997). Economical spray-coating of histologic slides with poly-L-lysine. *Journal of Histotechnology* **20**: 369–370.

Thiry, M. (1995). Ultrastructural detection of nucleic acids by immunocytology. In Morel, G. (ed.), *Visualization of Nucleic Acids*, pp. 111–135. Boca Raton, FL: CRC Press.

Thorball, N. and Tranum-Jensen, J. (1983). Vascular reactions to perfusion fixation. *Journal of Microscopy* **129**: 123–139.

Thorstensen, T.C. (1969). *Practical Leather Technology*. New York: van Nostrand-Reinhold.

Titford, M. (2001). Comparison of historic Grubler dyes with modern counterparts. *Biotechnic and Histochemistry* **76**: 23–30.

Titford, M. (2002). Save that dye! *Microscopy Today* **10**: 31–34.

Tomasi, V.H. and Rovasio, R.A. (1997). Softening of plant specimens (Equisetaceae) to improve the preparation of paraffin sections. *Biotechnic and Histochemistry* **72**: 209–212.

Tournier, I., Bernuau, D., Poliard, A., Schoevaert, D. and Feldmann, G. (1987). Detection of albumin mRNAs in rat liver by *in situ* hybridization: usefulness of paraffin embedding and comparison of various fixation procedures. *Journal of Histochemistry and Cytochemistry* **35**: 453–459.

Tramezzani, J.H., Chiocchio, S. and Wassermann, G.F. (1964). A technique for light and electron microscopic identifica-tion of adrenalin- and noradrenalin-storing cells. *Journal of Histochemistry and Cytochemistry* **12**: 890–899.

Tranzer, J.P. and Richards, J.G. (1976). Ultrastructural cytochemistry of biogenic amines in nervous tissue: methodologic improvements. *Journal of Histochemistry and Cytochemistry* **24**: 1178–1193.

Trigoso, C.I. and Stockert, J.C. (1995). Fluorescence of the natural dye saffron: selective reaction with eosinophil leuco-cyte granules. *Histochemistry and Cell Biology* **104**: 75–77.

Troyer, D.L., Cash, W.C., Provo-Klimek, J. and Kennedy, A.G. (2002). A novel method for preparing histology slides with-out a microtome. *Anatomia, Histologia, Embryologia* **31**: 129–131.

Tsuji, S. (1974). On the chemical basis of the thiocholine methods for demonstration of acetylcholinesterase activities. *Histochemistry* **42**: 99–110.

Tsuji, S. and Alameddine, H.S. (1981). Silicotungstic acid for cytochemical localization of water soluble substance(s) of cholinergic motor nerve terminal. *Histochemistry* **73**: 33–37.

Tsuji, S. and Larabi, Y. (1983). A modification of the thiocholine–ferricyanide method of Karnovsky and Roots for local-ization of acetylcholinesterase activity without interference by Koelle's copper thiocholine iodide precipitate. *Histochemistry* **78**: 317–323.

Tsuji, S., Alameddine, H.S., Nakanishi, S. and Ohoka, T. (1983). Molybdic and tungstic heteropolyanions for 'ionic fixa-tion' of acetylcholine in cholinergic motor nerve terminals. *Histochemistry* **77**: 51–66.

Tsutsumi, Y. and Kamoshida, S. (2003). Pitfalls and caveats in histochemically demonstrating apoptosis. *Acta Histochemica et Cytochemica* **36**: 271–280.

Tull, A.G. (1972). Hardening of gelatin by direct oxidation. In Cox, R.J. (ed.), *Photographic Gelatin*, pp. 127–134. London: Academic Press.

Tyler, N.K. and Burns, M.S. (1991). Comparison of lectin reactivity in vessel beds of the rat eye. *Current Eye Research* **10**: 801–810.

Uehara, F., Ohba, N., Nakashima, Y., Yanagita, T., Ozawa, M. and Muramatsu, T. (1993). A fixative suitable for insitu hybridization histochemistry. *Journal of Histochemistry and Cytochemistry* **41**: 947–953.

Urase, K., Fujita, E., Miho, Y., Kouroku, Y., Mukasa, T., Yagi, Y., Momoi, M.Y. and Momoi, T. (1998). Detection of activated caspase-3 (CPP32) in the vertebrate nervous system during development by a cleavage site-directed antiserum. *Developmental Brain Research* **111**: 77–87.

Urieli-Shoval, S., Meek, R.L., Hanson, R.H., Ferguson, M., Gordon, D. and Benditt, E.P. (1992). Preservation of RNA for *in situ* hybridization: Carnoy's versus formaldehyde fixation. *Journal of Histochemistry and Cytochemistry* **40**: 1879–1885.

Valdez, B.C., Henning, D., Le, T.V. and Busch, H. (1995). Specific aspartic acid-rich sequences are responsible for silver staining of nucleolar proteins. *Biochemical and Biophysical Research Communications* **207**: 485–491.

Vallet, P.G., Guntern, R., Hof, P.R., Golaz, J., Delacourte, A., Robakis, N.K. and Bouras, C. (1992). A comparative study of histological and immunohistochemical methods for neurofibrillary tangles and senile plaques in Alzheimer's dis-ease. *Acta Neuropathologica* **83**: 170–178.

Valnes, K. and Brandtzaeg, P. (1985). Retardation of immunofluorescence fading during microscopy. *Journal of Histochemistry and Cytochemistry* **33**: 755–761.

Van Damme, E.J.M., Peumans, W.J., Pusztai, A. and Bardocz, S. (1998). *Handbook of Plant Lectins. Properties and Biomedical Applications*. Chichester: Wiley.

Vandenbergh, B.A.I., Swartzendruber, D.C., Bosvandergeest, A., Hoogstraate, J.J., Schrijvers, A.H.G.J., Bodde, H.E., Junginger, H.E. and Bouwstra, J.A. (1997). Development of an optimal protocol for the ultrastructural examination of skin by transmission electron microscopy. *Journal of Microscopy* **187**: 125–133.

Van den Munckhof, R.J.M. (1996). *In situ* heterogeneity of peroxisomal oxidase activities: an update. *Histochemical Journal* **28**: 401–429.

Van Den Pol, A.N. (1984). Colloidal gold and biotin–avidin conjugates as ultrastructural markers for neural antigens. *Quarterly Journal of Experimental Physiology* **69**,: 1–33.

Van der Loos, C. (1999). *Immunoenzyme Multiple Staining Methods*. Oxford: BIOS Scientific Publications.

Van der Loos, C., Das, P.K. and Houthoff, H.-J. (1987). An immunoenzyme triple staining method using both polyclonal and monoclonal antibodies from the same species. Application of combined direct, indirect, and avidin–biotin complex (ABC) technique. *Journal of Histochemistry and Cytochemistry* **35**: 1199–1204.

Vandesande, F. (1979). A critical review of immunocytochemical methods for light microscopy. *Journal of Neuroscience Methods* **1**: 3–23.

Van Duijn, P. (1956). A histochemical specific thionine–SO$_2$ reagent and its use in a bi-color method for deoxyribonucleic acid and periodic acid–Schiff positive substances. *Journal of Histochemistry and Cytochemistry* **4**: 55–63.

Van Gijlswijk, R.P.M., Wiegant, J., Raap, A.K. and Tanke, H.J. (1996). Improved localization of fluorescent tyramides for fluorescence *in situ* hybridization using dextran sulfate and polyvinyl alcohol. *Journal of Histochemistry and Cytochemistry* **44**: 389–392.

Van Gijlswijk, R.P.M., Zijlmans, H.J.M.A.A., Wiegant, J., Bobrow, M.N., Erickson, T.J., Adler, K.E., Tanke, H.J. and Raap, A.K. (1997). Fluorochrome-labeled tyramides: use in immunocytochemistry and fluorescence *in situ* hybridization. *Journal of Histochemistry and Cytochemistry* **45**: 375–382.

Van Goor, H., Gerrits, P.O. and Hardonk, M.J. (1989). Enzyme histochemical demonstration of alkaline phosphatase activity in plastic-embedded tissues using a Gomori-based cerium–DAB technique. *Journal of Histochemistry and Cytochemistry* **37**: 399–403.

Van Noorden, C.J.F. and Butcher, R.W. (1984). Histochemical localization of NADP-dependent dehydrogenase activity with four different tetrazolium salts. *Journal of Histochemistry and Cytochemistry* **32**: 998–1004.

Van Noorden, C.J.F. and Frederiks, W.M. (1992). *Enzyme Histochemistry: A Laboratory Manual of Current Methods*. *Microscopy Handbooks*, **26**. Oxford: Oxford University Press and Royal Microscopical Society.

Van Noorden, C.J.F. and Frederiks, W.M. (1993). Cerium methods for light and electron microscopical histochemistry: review. *Journal of Microscopy* **171**: 3–16.

Van Noorden, C.J.F. and Frederiks, W.M. (2002). Metabolic mapping by enzyme histochemistry. In Kiernan, J.A. and Mason, I. (eds), *Microscopy and Histology for Molecular Biologists: A User's Guide*, pp. 277–311. London: Portland Press.

Van Noorden, C.J.F. and Tas, J. (1982). The role of exogenous electron carriers in NAD(P)-dependent dehydrogenase cytochemistry studied *in vitro* and with a model system of polyacrylamide films. *Journal of Histochemistry and Cytochemistry* **30**: 12–20.

Van Wyk, J.H. (1993). Histological techniques to improve testing of pulpal response of teeth to filling material. *Biotechnic and Histochemistry* **68**: 290–301.

Varki, A., Cummings, R., Esko, J., Freeze, H., Hart, G. and Marth, J. (eds) (1999). *Essentials of Glycobiology*. Cold Spring Harbor, NY: Cold Spring Harbor Laboratory Press.

Vartanian, R.K., Leung, J.K., Davis, J.E., Kim, Y.B. and Owen, D.A. (1998). A novel alcian yellow–toluidine blue (Leung) stain for *Helicobacter* species: comparison with standard stains, a cost-effectiveness analysis, and supplemental utilities. *Modern Pathology* **11**: 72–78.

Vaughn, J.E. and Pease, D.C. (1967). Electron microscopy of classically stained astrocytes. *Journal of Comparative Neurology* **131**: 143–154.

Vaughn, K.C. (ed.) (1987). *CRC Handbook of Plant Cytochemistry* (2 vols). Boca Raton, FL: CRC Press.

Vdovenko, A.A. and Williams, J.E. (2000). Blastocystis hominis: neutral red supravital staining and its application to *in vitro* drug sensitivity testing. *Parasitology Research* **86**: 573–581.

Velican, C. and Velican, D. (1970). Structural heterogeneity of basement membranes and reticular fibres. *Acta Anatomica* **77**: 540–559.

Velican, C. and Velican, D. (1972). Silver impregnation techniques for the histochemical analysis of basement membranes and reticular fiber networks. In Glick, D. and Rosenblaum, R.M. (eds), *Techniques of Biochemical and Biophysical Morphology*, Vol. 1, pp. 143–190. New York: Wiley.

Venkataraman, K. (1952–1978). *The Chemistry of Synthetic Dyes. Vols I–VIII*. New York: Academic Press.

Vermeer, B.J., Van Gent, C.M., De Bruijn, W.C. and Boonders, T. (1978). The effect of digitonin-containing fixatives on the retention of free cholesterol and cholesterol esters. *Histochemical Journal* **10**: 287–298.

Vial, J. and Porter, K.R. (1975). Scanning microscopy of dissociated cells. *Journal of Cell Biology* **67**: 345–360.

Vidal, B. de C. (1978). The use of the fluorescent probe 8-anilinonaphthalene sulfate (ANS) for collagen and elastin histochemistry. *Journal of Histochemistry and Cytochemistry* **26**: 196–201.

Voet,, D., Voet, J.G. and Pratt, C.W. (2006). *Fundamentals of Biochemistry*, 2nd edn. Hoboken, NJ: Wiley.

Vohringer, P., Nindl, G., Aich, B., Kortje, K.H. and Rahmann, H. (1995). Comparative methodological investigations on the cytochemical localization of calcium in brain and inner ear of cichlid fish. *Microscopy Research and Technique* **31**: 317–325.

Volpon, L. and Lancelin, J.M. (2000). Solution NMR structures of the polyene macrolide antibiotic filipin III. *FEBS Letters* **478**: 137–140.

Volz, D., Reid, P.E., Park, C.M., Owen, D.A., Dunn, W.L. and Ramey, C.W. (1986). Can 'mild' periodate oxidation be used for the specific histochemical identification of sialic acid residues? *Histochemical Journal* **18**: 579–582.

Volz, D., Reid, P.E., Park, C.M., Owen, D.A. and Dunn, W.L. (1987). A new method for the selective periodate oxidation of total tissue sialic acids. *Histochemical Journal* **19**: 311–318.

von Bohlen und Halbach, O. and Kiernan, J.A. (1999). Diaminobenzidine induces fluorescence in nervous tissue and provides intrinsic counterstaining of sections prepared for peroxidase histochemistry. *Biotechnic and Histochemistry* **74**: 236–243.

von Bohlen und Halbach, O. and Kiernan, J.A. (2000). Double-staining with DAB reaction products and fluorescence immunohistochemistry – can we trust the results? *Abstracts of European Neuroscience Association Meeting, Brighton, June 2000*. Oxford: Blackwell/European Neuroscience Association.

Walker, J.F. (1964). *Formaldehyde*, 3rd edn. New York: Reinhold.

Waring, D.R. and Hallas, G. (eds) (1990). *The Chemistry and Application of Dyes*. New York: Plenum Press.

Warthin, A.S. and Starry, A.C. (1920). A more rapid and improved method of demonstrating spirochetes in tissues. *American Journal of Syphilis, Gonorrhea and Venereal Diseases* **4**: 97–102.

Waterman, H.C. (1934). Preliminary notes on chromic fixation in alcoholic media. *Stain Technology* **9**: 23–31.

Waters, S.E. and Butcher, R.G. (1980). Studies on the Gomori acid phosphatase reaction: the preparation of the incubaton medium. *Histochemical Journal* **12**: 191–200.

Waters, W.A. (1958). Mechanisms of oxidation by compounds of chromium and manganese. *Quarterly Reviews* **12**: 277–300.

Watson, J. (2005). Prestaining with nuclear fast red as a blocking reaction to clean up reticulum stains and intensify fiber staining. *Journal of Histotechnology* **28**: 99–104.

Watson, J.D. and Crick, F.H.C. (1953). Molecular structure of nucleic acids. A structure for deoxyribose nucleic acid. *Nature* **171**: 737–738.

Watson, S.J. and Barchas, J.D. (1977). Catecholamine histofluorescence using cryostat sectioning and glyoxylic acid in unperfused frozen brain: a detailed description of the technique. *Histochemical Journal* **9**: 183–195.

Watson, S.J. and Ellison, J.P. (1976). Cryostat technique for central nervous system histofluorescence. *Histochemistry* **50**: 119–127.

Wattenberg, L.W. and Leong, J.L. (1960). Effects of coenzyme Q10 and menadione on succinic dehydrogenase activity as measured by tetrazolium salt reduction. *Journal of Histochemistry and Cytochemistry* **8**: 296–303.

Weber, P., Harrison, F.W. and Hof, L. (1975). The histochemical application of dansylhydrazine as a fluorescent labeling reagent for sialic acids in glycoconjugates. *Histochemistry* **45**: 271–277.

Wedrychowski, A., Ward, W.S., Schmidt, W.N. and Hnilica, L.S. (1985). Chromium-induced cross-linking of nuclear proteins and DNA. *Journal of Biological Chemistry* **260**: 7150–7155.

Weinberg, R.J. and Van Eyck, S.L. (1991). A tetramethylbenzidine/tungstate reaction for horseradish peroxidase histochemistry. *Journal of Histochemistry and Cytochemistry* **39**: 1143–1148.

Weir, E.E., Pretlow, T.G., Itts, A. and Williams, E.E. (1974). Destruction of endogenous peroxidase activity in order to locate antigens by peroxidase-labeled antibodies. *Journal of Histochemistry and Cytochemistry* **22**: 51–54.

Weisblum, B. and De Haseth, P.L. (1972). Quinacrine: a chromosome stain specific for deoxyadenylate–deoxythymidylate-rich regions in DNA. *Proceedings of the National Academy of Sciences of the United States of America* **69**: 629–632.

Werner, M., von Wasielewski, R. and Komminoth, P. (1996). Antigen retrieval, signal amplification and intensification in immunohistochemistry. *Histochemistry and Cell Biology* **105**: 253–260.

White, D.L., Mazurkiewicz, J.E. and Barrnett, R.J. (1979). A chemical mechanism for staining by osmium tetroxide–ferrocyanide mixtures. *Journal of Histochemistry and Cytochemistry* **27**: 1084–1091.

White, E.H. and Woodcock, D.J. (1968). Cleavage of the carbon–nitrogen bond. In Patai, S. (ed.), *The Chemistry of the Amino Group*, pp. 407–497. London: Wiley Interscience.

White, R., Hu, F. and Roman, N.A. (1983). False dopa reaction in studies of mammalian tyrosinase: some characteristics and precautions. *Stain Technology* **58**: 13–19.

Whitmore, F.C. (1921). *Organic Compounds of Mercury*. New York: Chemical Catalog Company.

Whittaker, P. (1995). Polarized light microscopy in biomedical research. *Microscopy and Analysis* **44**: 15–17.

Whittaker, P., Kloner, R.A., Boughner, D.R. and Pickering, J.G. (1994). Quantitative assessment of myocardial collagen with picrosirius red staining and circularly polarized light. *Basic Research in Cardiology* **89**: 397–410.

Whyte, A., Loke, Y.W. and Stoddart, R.W. (1978). Saccharide distribution in human trophoblast demonstrated using fluorescein-labelled lectins. *Histochemical Journal* **10**: 417–423.

Wigglesworth, V.B. (1952). The role of iron in histological staining. *Quarterly Journal of Microscopical Science* **93**: 105–118.

Wigglesworth, V.B. (1957). The use of osmium tetroxide in the fixation and staining of tissue. *Proceedings of the Royal Society B* **147**: 185–199.

Wigglesworth, V.B. (1988). Histological staining of lipids for the light and electron microscope. *Biological Reviews* **63**: 417–431.

Williams, G. and Jackson, D.S. (1956). Two organic fixatives for acid mucopolysaccharides. *Stain Technology* **31**: 189–191.

Williams, R.M. and Atalla, R.H. (1981). Interactions of Group II cations and borate anions with nonionic saccharides. Studies on model polyols. In Brant, D.A. (ed.), *Solution Properties of Polysaccharides (ACS Symposium Series 150)*, Vol. 2, pp. 317–330. Washington, DC: American Chemical Society.

Willinger, M. and Schachner, M. (1980). GM1 ganglioside as a marker for neuronal differentiation in mouse cerebellum. *Developmental Biology* **74**: 101–117.

Willingham, M.C. (1983). An alternative fixation-processing method for preembedding ultrastructural immunocytochemistry of cytoplasmic antigens: the GBS (glutaraldehyde–borohydride–saponin) procedure. *Journal of Histochemistry and Cytochemistry* **31**: 791–798.

Willingham, M.C. (1999). Cytochemical methods for the detection of apoptosis. *Journal of Histochemistry and Cytochemistry* **47**: 1101–1109.

Wingate, R. (2002). Digital and confocal photomicrography. In Kiernan, J.A. and Mason, I. (eds), *Microscopy and Histology for Molecular Biologists*, pp. 23–50. London: Portland Press.

Willis, R.J. and Kratzing, C.C. (1974). The chemistry of the silver precipitation method used for the histochemical localization of ascorbic acid. *Stain Technology* **49**: 381–386.

Winkelmann, R.K. (1960). *Nerve Endings in Normal and Pathologic Skin*. Springfield, IL: Thomas.

Winkelmann, R.K. and Schmit, R.W. (1957). A simple silver method for nerve axoplasm. *Proceedings of Staff Meetings of the Mayo Clinic* **32**: 217–222.

Wittekind, D.H. (1983). On the nature of Romanowsky–Giemsa staining and its significance for cytochemistry and histochemistry: an overall review. *Histochemical Journal* **15**: 1029–1047.

Wittekind, D.H. (2002). Romanowsky–Giemsa stains. In Horobin, R.W. and Kiernan, J.A. (eds), *Conn's Biological Stains. A Handbook of Dyes, Stains and Fluorochromes for use in Biology and Medicine*, 10th edn, pp. 303–312. Oxford: BIOS Scientific Publications.

Wittekind, D.H. and Kretschmer, V. (1987). On the nature of Romanowsky–Giemsa staining and the Romanowsky–Giemsa effect. II. A revised Romanowsky–Giemsa staining procedure. *Histochemical Journal* **19**: 399–401.

Wittekind, D., Schulte, E., Schmidt, G. and Frank, G. (1991). The standard Romanowsky–Giemsa stain in histology. *Biotechnic and Histochemistry* **66**: 282–295.

Wöhlrab, F. and Gossrau, R. (1991). *Katalytische Enzymhistochemie. Grundlagen und Methoden für die Electronenmikroskopie*. Berlin: Gustav Fischer.

Wöhlrab, F., Seidler, E. and Kunze, D.K. (1979). *Histo- und Zytochemie dehydrierender Enzyme. Grundlagen und Problematik*. Leipzig: Barth.

Wolff, J. and Covelli, I. (1969). Factors in the iodination of histidine in proteins. *European Journal of Biochemistry* **9**: 371–377.

Wollin, A. and Jaques, L.B. (1973). Metachromasia: an explanation of the colour change produced in dyes by heparin and other substances. *Thrombosis Research* **2**: 377–382.

Wolman, M. (1971). A fluorescent histochemical technique for gamma-aminobutyric acid. *Histochemie* **28**: 118–130.

Wolman, M. and Bubis, J.J. (1965). The cause of the green polarization colour of amyloid stained with Congo red. *Histochemie* **4**: 351–356.

Wolters, G.H.J., Pasma, A., Konijnendijk, W. and Bouman, P.R. (1979). Evaluation of the glyoxal-bis-(2-hydroxyanil)-method for staining of calcium in model gelatin films and pancreatic islets. *Histochemistry* **62**: 137–151.

Wong-Riley, M.T.T. (1989). Cytochrome oxidase: an endogenous marker for neuron activity. *Trends in Neurosciences* **12**: 94–101.

Wouterlood, F.G., Nederlof, J. and Paniry, S. (1983). Chemical reduction of silver chromate: a procedure for electron microscopical analysis of Golgi-impregnated neurons. *Journal of Neuroscience Methods* **7**: 235–308.

Wreford, N.G.M., Singhaniyam, W. and Smith, G.C. (1982). Microspectrofluorometric characterization of the fluorescent derivatives of biogenic amines produced by aqueous aldehyde (Faglu) fixation. *Histochemical Journal* **14**: 491–505.

Wu, M. and Kiernan, J.A. (2001). A new method for surface staining large slices of fixed brain, using a copper phthalocyanine dye. *Biotechnic and Histochemistry* **76**: 253–255.

Wyllie, A.H., Kerr, J.F.R. and Currie, A.R. (1980). Cell death: the significance of apoptosis. *International Review of Cytology* **68**: 251–306.

Wynnchuk, M. (1992). Minimizing artifacts in tissue processing: part 1. Importance of softening agents. *Journal of Histotechnology* **15**: 321–323.

Wynnchuk, M. (1993). Minimizing artifacts in tissue processing: part 2. Theory of tissue processing. *Journal of Histotechnology* **16**: 71–73.

Xi, K. and Burnett, P.A. (1997). Staining paraffin embedded sections of scald of barley before paraffin removal. *Biotechnic and Histochemistry* **72**: 173–177.

Yack, J.E. (1993). Janus green B as a rapid, vital stain for peripheral nerves and chordotonal organs in insects. *Journal of Neuroscience Methods* **49**: 17–22.

Yamabayashi, S. (1987). Periodic acid–Schiff–alcian blue: a method for the differential staining of glycoproteins. *Histochemical Journal* **19**: 565–571.

Yamadori, I., Yoshino, T., Kondo, E., Cao, L., Akagi, T., Matsuo, Y. and Minowada, J. (1998). Comparison of two methods of staining apoptotic cells of leukemia cell lines: terminal deoxynucleotidyl transferase and DNA polymerase I reactions. *Journal of Histochemistry and Cytochemistry* **46**: 85–90.

Yamashita, S. (2007). Heat-induced antigen retrieval: mechanisms and application to histochemistry. *Progress in Histochemistry and Cytochemistry* **41**: 141–200.

Yamashita, S. and Okada, Y. (2005a). Application of heat-induced antigen retrieval to aldehyde-fixed fresh frozen sections. *Journal of Histochemistry and Cytochemistry* **53**: 1321–1432.

Yamashita, S. and Okada, Y. (2005b). Mechanisms of heat-induced antigen retrieval: analyses *in vitro* employing SDS-PAGE and immunohistochemistry. *Journal of Histochemistry and Cytochemistry* **53**: 12–21.

Yan, P., Seelentag, W., Bachmann, A. and Bosman, F.T. (2007). An agarose matrix facilitated sectioning of tissue microarray blocks. *Journal of Histochemistry and Cytochemistry* **55**: 21–24.

Yi, C.F., Gosiewska, A., Burtis, D. and Geesin, J. (2001). Incorporation of fluorescent enzyme substrates in agarose gel for *in situ* zymography. *Analytical Biochemistry* **291**: 27–33.

Yu, Y. and Chapman, C.M. (2003). Masson trichrome stain: postfixation substitutes. *Journal of Histotechnology* **26**: 131–134.

Zacks, S.I. (1973). *The Motor Endplate*, 2nd edn. Huntington, NY: Krieger.

Zagon, I.S., Vavra, J. and Steele, I. (1970). Microprobe analysis of protargol stain deposition in two protozoa. *Journal of Histochemistry and Cytochemistry* **18**: 559–564.

Zamboni, L. and De Martino, C. (1967). Buffered picric acid–formaldehyde: a new, rapid fixative for electron microscopy. *Journal of Cell Biology* **35**: 148A.

Zbaeren, J., Solenthaler, M., Schaper, M., Zbaeren-Colbourn, D. and Haeberli, A. (2004). A new fixative allowing accurate immunostaining of kappa and lambda immunoglobulin light chain expressing B cells without antigen retrieval in paraffin-embedded tissue. *Journal of Histotechnology* **27**: 87–92.

Zhang, P.J., Wang, H.Q., Wrona, E.L. and Cheney, R.T. (1998). Effects of tissue fixatives on antigen preservation for immunohistochemistry: a comparative study of microwave antigen retrieval on Lillie fixative and neutral buffered formalin. *Journal of Histotechnology* **21**: 101–106.

Zhou, D.-S. and Komuro, T. (1995). Ultrastructure of the zinc iodide–osmic acid stained cells in guinea pig small intestine. *Journal of Anatomy* **187**: 481–485.

Zhu, L.J., Perlaky, L., Henning, D. and Valdez, B.C. (1997). Cloning and characterization of a new silver-stainable protein SSP29, a member of the LRR family. *Biochemistry and Molecular Biology International* **42**: 927–935.

Ziomek, C.A., Lepire, M.L. and Torres, I. (1990). A highly fluorescent simultaneous azo dye technique for demonstration of nonspecific alkaline phosphatase activity. *Journal of Histochemistry and Cytochemistry* **3**: 437–442.

Zirkle, C. (1928). The effect of hydrogen-ion concentration upon the fixation image of various salts of chromium. *Protoplasma* **4**: 201–227.

Zirkle, C. (1933). Cytological fixation with the lower fatty acids their compounds and derivatives. *Protoplasma* **18**: 90–111.

Zollinger, H. (2003). *Color Chemistry. Synthesis, Properties and Applications of Organic Dyes and Pigments*, 3rd edn. Weinheim: Wiley-VCH.

Zollinger, H. (1994). *Diazo Chemistry*, Vol. 1. (*Aromatic and Heteroaromatic Compounds*). Weinheim: VCH Verlag.

Zuniga, A.A., Olano, C. and Bigger, C. (1994). Simplified dehydration and clearing of sponges and corals. *Journal of Histotechnology* **17**: 55–57.

Zurita, F., Jimenez, R., Burgos, M. and Delaguardia, R.D. (1998). Sequential silver staining and *in situ* hybridization reveal a direct association between rDNA levels and the expression of nucleolar organizing regions: a hypothesis for NOR structure and function. *Journal of Cell Science* **111**: 1433–1439.

Glossary

Many terms are defined in the text. For these, consult the index. The following list includes a variety of chemical and histological terms with which some readers may be unfamiliar. Chapter 19 includes a glossary of terms used in immunohistochemistry.

Acetal. Compound formed by condensation of one molecule of an aldehyde with two molecules of an alcohol to give the structure:

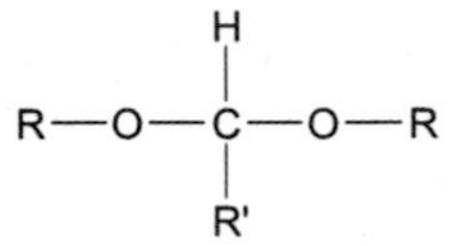

$$R-O-\underset{\underset{\textstyle R'}{|}}{\overset{\overset{\textstyle H}{|}}{C}}-O-R$$

in which R, R′ are carbon atoms of alkyl or aryl groups.

Adduct. Compound formed by combination of two others without the loss of any atoms. Often used when the precise structure of the addition compound is uncertain, or when one of the components is a reagent used for analytical purposes.

Albumen. The principal protein of egg white. The penultimate **e** distinguishes it from the **albumins**.

Albumin. A type of protein that is soluble in water and precipitated by high concentrations of salts (e.g. saturation with $(NH_4)_2SO_4$). Examples are serum albumin and egg albumen. *Compare with* **globulin**.

Anion, Anionic. An anion is a negatively charged atom or molecule, which would be attracted to the positive electrode (anode) in electrophoresis.

Aprotic solvent. A polar solvent that does not contain an ionizable hydrogen atom. Its molecules cluster around (solvate) cations, but leave anions relatively unimpeded, so that the latter will be more reactive than when dissolved in an ordinary (protic) polar solvent. Examples are dimethylsulphoxide and *N,N*-dimethylformamide.

Astrocyte. A neuroglial cell with numerous cytoplasmic processes, some of which form end-feet on capillary blood vessels.

Axon. That cytoplasmic process of a neuron that is specialized for the conduction of trains of impulses, usually away from the cell body.

Canonical forms. The different structures that exist, at instants in time, of an organic compound in which resonance occurs. In writing canonical structures, only bonds and sites of electric charge may be varied; the positions of the atoms may not be changed.

Cation, Cationic. A cation is a positively charged atom or molecule, which would be attracted to the negative electrode (cathode) in electrolysis or electrophoresis.

Caudal. Towards the tail of an animal. Used mainly to refer to relative positions along the axis of the central nervous system.

Chromatin. The material in the nucleus of a cell (excluding the nucleolus) that is stained by cationic dyes and by some dye–metal complexes such as aluminium–haematein. Consists of the DNA and nucleoprotein (histone) of the chromosomes.

Colloid. A substance composed of either large molecules (macromolecules) or large aggregates of smaller molecules, dispersed in a liquid medium. The sizes (diameters or comparable average dimensions) of the particles range from 1 to 500 nm. Individual suspended particles as small as 1 nm can be detected with visible light, but the distinction between one or two particles (**resolution**) cannot be made if the size and separation are less than 200 nm.

Common ion effect. The tendency of a salt to become less soluble when the concentration of one of its ions in a solution greatly exceeds that of the other ion.

Condensation. Combination of two molecules with elimination of a compound of low molecular weight such as water.

Delocalized π-electrons. Electrons that are shared by more than two atoms and cannot therefore be said to form part of any individual covalent bond. π-electrons are associated with double or triple bonds, and with resonant structures such as aromatic rings.

Dendrites. Processes of a neuron specialized for receiving synaptic connections and conducting graded changes of membrane potential towards the cell body. Dendrites are usually multiple and shorter than the axon, and their most prominent cytoskeletal organelles are microtubules rather than neurofilaments.

Dialysis. (a) Passage of small, but not large, molecules through a membrane. (b) A technique for the purification or concentration of solutions of proteins or other macromolecular substances, using tubing that is permeable only to smaller molecules.

Dimer. A molecule formed by the union of two molecules of the same compound.

Enantiomers. Isomers whose three-dimensional structures are mirror images of one another.

Eukaryotic cell. A cell in which the DNA is associated with histone and contained in a membrane-bound nucleus, as in animals, plants, fungi and protozoans.

Furanose. A sugar whose ring structure consists of four carbon atoms and one oxygen atom, so that it could be thought of as a derivative of furan:

Gel. A colloidal solution with a semi-solid consistency due to extensive hydrogen bonding between the suspended macromolecules and the 'solvent', which is usually water.

Gel filtration. A technique whereby molecules of different size are separated by virtue of their entry or non-entry into the pores contained in beads of a suitably designed polymer. Usually, the polymer is packed in a chromatography column and a solution containing the substances to be separated is applied at the top. When the column is eluted with a suitable solvent, the larger molecules are released first and the smaller molecules later.

Glia, glial. See **neuroglia**.

Globulin. A protein that is insoluble in pure water but soluble at neutral pH in dilute aqueous solutions of simple salts (such as chloride or sulphate of sodium, potassium or ammonium). Globulins are precipitated by half-saturation with $(NH_4)_2SO_4$. Examples include the **immunoglobulins** (Chapter 19) and many other animal and plant proteins.

Glycocalyx. The carbohydrate-containing material present on the outer surfaces of all cells.

Haem. The non-protein portion of the haemoglobin molecule. Often used more generally for iron–porphyrin prosthetic groups of proteins, such as occur in many enzymes and cytochromes.

Haematin. A pigment formed when haemoglobin is degraded in acid conditions. Also known as acid haematin. Do not confuse it with haematein (Chapter 5).

Haemopoietic tissue. Tissue such as red bone marrow in which the cells of the blood are produced.

Hemiacetal. Compound formed by condensation of one molecule of an aldehyde with one molecule of an alcohol to give the structure:

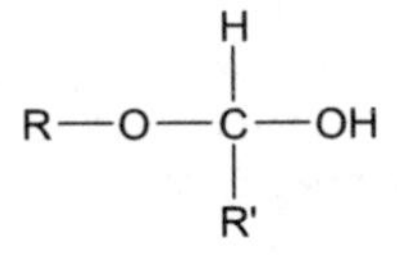

$$R-O-\overset{\displaystyle H}{\underset{\displaystyle R'}{C}}-OH$$

in which R, R′ are carbon atoms of alkyl or aryl groups. The hemiacetal configuration occurs in the ring structures of sugars.

Homoiothermic (also **homeothermic**). Maintaining a constant body temperature; warm-blooded. Mammals and birds are homoiothermic.

Hydrophilic. Describes substances that attract water: water molecules are able to come into intimate contact with a hydrophilic compound because the latter contains oxygen or nitrogen atoms with which hydrogen bonds can be formed. Hydrophilic compounds are also **polar**.

Hydrophobic. Describes substances that repel water: a hydrophobic compound has few or no atoms capable of forming hydrogen bonds, and it is typically **non-polar**.

Hydroxyalkylation. Addition of an aldehyde or ketone to an aromatic ring.

Hypertonic. Having a higher osmotic pressure than blood or extracellular fluid.

Hypotonic. Having a lower osmotic pressure than blood or extracellular fluid.

Imide. A compound in which the two bonds of the NH radical are joined to acyl groups, to give the structure:

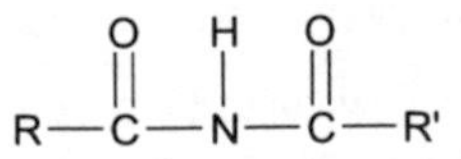

$$R-\overset{\displaystyle O}{\underset{}{\overset{\|}{C}}}-\overset{\displaystyle H}{\underset{}{N}}-\overset{\displaystyle O}{\underset{}{\overset{\|}{C}}}-R'$$

Imine. A compound containing the configuration:

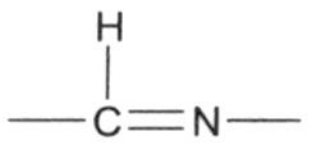

$$-\overset{\overset{\displaystyle H}{|}}{C}=N-$$

Such compounds are also known as **azomethines**, **anils**, or **Schiff's bases**. The term 'imino' is sometimes applied (though not in this book) to the >NH group of secondary amines.

Isomers. Compounds with the same molecular formulae but different structures.

Isotonic. Having the same osmotic pressure as blood or extracellular fluid.

Ketal. A compound formed by condensation of a ketone with an alcohol, to give the structure:

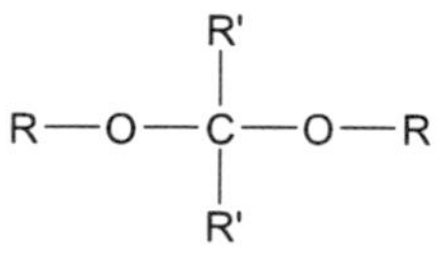

$$R-O-\overset{\overset{\displaystyle R'}{|}}{\underset{\underset{\displaystyle R'}{|}}{C}}-O-R$$

Le Chatelier's principle. When a constraint is applied to any system in equilibrium, the system will always react in a direction that tends to counteract the applied constraint. For chemical equilibria, the constraint may be a change in concentration of a reactant, or a change of temperature, etc. The law of mass action and the common ion effect are examples of this principle.

Lipofuscin. A yellow or light brown autofluorescent pigment containing lipids and proteins, found as granules within the cytoplasm of cells, especially in old animals. Thought to be the indigestible remains of phagocytosed material.

Metabolite. Any substance participating in a chemical reaction in a living organism.

Monoamine oxidase. An enzyme that catalyses the oxidative degradation of biogenic monoamines such as noradrenaline and serotonin (Chapters 16 and 17).

Myelin. The sheath surrounding many of the axons of the central and peripheral nervous systems of vertebrate animals. It contains numerous proteins and lipids and is formed from the plasmalemmae of the neuroglial cells that ensheath the axon. The myelin is trophically dependent upon the axon; it disintegrates and is phagocytosed if the axon is separated from its neuronal cell body.

Neuroglia. Cells intimately associated with neurons in the central and peripheral nervous systems. Neuroglial cell types include the myelin forming cells: Schwann cells of peripheral nerves and oligodendrocytes in the central nervous system. Other types are astrocytes, microglial cells, satellite cells of ganglia, and non-neuronal cells in the nervous systems of invertebrate animals. The word is commonly shortened to **glia**.

Neurohypophysis. The portion of the pituitary gland (hypophysis) derived from the central nervous system. Comprises the median eminence of the ventral surface of the brain, and the stalk and posterior lobe of the gland. These regions contain cystine-rich neurosecretory material.

Neuropil. Tissue within the nervous system consisting of axons and dendrites, with numerous synapses but without neuronal cell bodies or tracts of myelinated axons.

Neurosecretion. The production of a substance by a neuron for release into the blood. The word is sometimes also applied to neurons whose axons terminate upon endocrine cells. (Neurons of the latter type do not usually contain classical neurosecretory material with a high content of cystine.)

Non-polar solvent. A hydrophobic liquid, not miscible with water, such as benzene or carbon tetrachloride. A molecule is non-polar because its electrons are symmetrically distributed.

Notochord. An embryonic structure that occupies the position of the future vertebral column; also present in the adult forms of chordates such as the amphioxus that do not have vertebrae.

Nucleoside. A molecule of ribose or deoxyribose joined at position 1′ to a purine or pyrimidine base.

Nucleotide. A molecule of ribose or deoxyribose joined at position 1′ to a purine or pyrimidine base and at position 3′ or 5′ to a phosphate group. A single unit of a DNA or RNA sequence (Chapter 10).

Oligodendrocyte. A neuroglial cell with few cytoplasmic processes; responsible for formation of myelin sheaths in the central nervous system.

Oligonucleotide. A short sequence of nucleotides, typically 10 to 50 base pairs in length.

Periodontal membrane. The connective tissue that anchors a tooth into its bony socket.

Plasmalemma. The membrane forming the outside surface of a cell. Also called the cell membrane. Not to be confused with the cell wall in plants, which is external to the plasmalemma.

Poikilotherms. Organisms that live at the same temperature as their environments (all organisms other than mammals and birds).

Polar solvent. A liquid miscible with water and capable of dissolving ionized substances. A molecule is polar because its molecules are dipoles: the electrons are unevenly distributed, so that one end of the molecule is relatively electropositive and the other end relatively electronegative. The electronegative atom is most frequently oxygen or nitrogen.

Polynucleotide. A strand of DNA or RNA composed of a large number of nucleotides.

Prokaryotic cell. A cell whose DNA is not contained in a membrane-bound nucleus, as in archaea and bacteria.

Pyranose. A sugar whose ring structure consists of five carbon atoms and one oxygen atom, so that it can be thought of as a derivative of the hypothetical substance pyran:

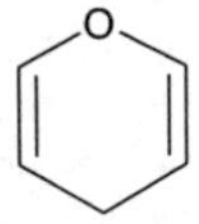

Quinhydrone. The darkly coloured substance formed when hydroquinone is half-oxidized to quinone; formed by hydrogen bonding of hydroquinone to p-quinone:

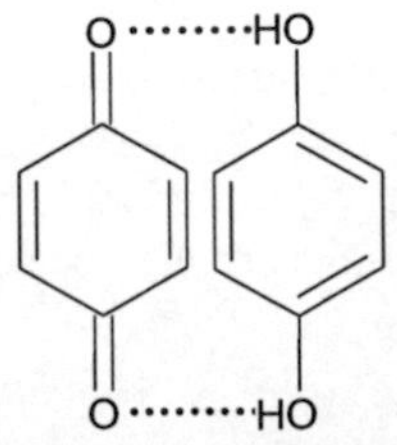

Reserpine. A drug that releases biogenic monoamines from the cells in which they are stored. The cells are thereby depleted of amines.

Resolution. The shortest distance that visibly separates two different points. For an ideal light microscope with an apochromatic oil immersion objective of high numerical aperture this is about 200 nm (0.2 μm). In routine work there is blurring of detail in areas less than 1 μm across, though strongly and specifically stained smaller objects such as bacteria may nevertheless be identifiable. Ultraviolet microscopy (expensive because now seldom used) and confocal microscopy (expensive equipment and supplies) provide resolution to 100 nm. The electron microscope (expensive equipment that needs expensive servicing) provides resolution to the level of macromolecules (1 nm) but is poorly suited to the collection of histochemical data.

Ribosome. A granule in the cytoplasm, containing much RNA, which is the site of translation from messenger RNAs to proteins. Ribosomes are attached to membranes of rough endoplasmic reticulum and occur also as spherical aggregates (polyribosomes). The structural RNA of ribosomes (rRNA) accounts for the cytoplasmic basophilia of neurons and other cells that synthesize large amounts of protein.

Rostral. Towards the beak or nose of an animal. Mainly applied to levels of the axis of the central nervous system.

Salting out. Precipitation of an ionic compound (such as a dye) by adding an excess of one of its ions to the solution. Also applied to precipitation of protein by addition of an inorganic salt to its solution (*see* **albumin, globulin**).

Sol. A colloidal dispersion of an inorganic substance, such as gold, ferric hydroxide or sulphur, in a 'solvent', which is usually water. Unlike a gel, a sol is a mobile liquid. The particles suspended in a sol are charged; the balancing opposite charge is carried by the solvent molecules surrounding each particle.

Sulphoamino. The radical

$$-\overset{\overset{\text{H}}{|}}{\text{N}}-\text{SO}_3\text{H}$$

Tunicates. A subphylum of the Chordata, also known as Urochordata, including the ascidians or sea squirts. Only the larval form has a notochord. The adult animal is tubular and is covered externally by a 'test' (exoskeleton) composed of cellulose.

Vital staining. The application of dyes to living cells. With **intravital staining**, the dye is administered to the whole animal or plant. With **supravital** (or supervital) staining, freshly excised tissue is treated with a dye solution. Vital staining cannot be obtained when the tissue is dead, but the distinction between dead and alive varies with the technique. Fluorescent compounds used as vital stains are often called **probes** for the organelles or other intracellular domains in which they lodge.

Wallerian degeneration. The fragmentation and eventual disappearance of axons and their myelin sheaths following severance of the axon or destruction of its neuronal cell body.

Zwitterionic. A zwitterion is a molecule that has both positively and negatively charged groups. All amino acids are zwitterionic, as are many useful buffers such as HEPES (Chapter 20). Dye molecules are zwitterionic if they have the potential to be anions or cations, depending on the pH of the solution.

Index

Reagents are indexed under the most significant parts of their names. Thus, sodium borohydride is Borohydride, sodium. Where a chemical name begins with a number or Greek letter, this is omitted, as are such prefixes as *bis*- *o*-, *p*- and *N*-. To find 5-hydroxytryptamine, look for Hydroxytryptamine; for *N*-ethylmaleimide, see Ethylmaleimide. Dyes are indexed under their trivial names, Colour Index application names and C.I. numbers.

HISTOLOGICAL AND HISTOCHEMICAL METHODS

Fourth edition

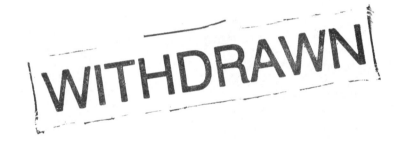

HISTOLOGICAL AND HISTOCHEMICAL METHODS
Theory and Practice

Fourth edition

J. A. Kiernan

Department of Anatomy and Cell Biology, The University of Western Ontario, London, Ontario, Canada

Scion

Fourth edition © Scion Publishing Ltd, 2008
First published 2008, reprinted 2009, 2010, 2011, 2012

ISBN 978 1 904842 42 2

First edition published 1981 (Oxford: Pergamon Press)
Second edition published 1990 (Oxford: Pergamon Press)
Third edition published 1999 (Oxford: Butterworth Heinemann)

A CIP catalogue record for this book is available from the British Library.

Scion Publishing Limited
The Old Hayloft, Vantage Business Park, Bloxham Road, Banbury,
Oxfordshire OX16 9UX
www.scionpublishing.com

Important Note from the Publisher

The information contained within this book was obtained by Scion Publishing
Limited from sources believed by us to be reliable. However, while every effort has
been made to ensure its accuracy, no responsibility for loss or injury whatsoever
occasioned to any person acting or refraining from action as a result of information
contained herein can be accepted by the authors or publishers.

Typeset by Phoenix Photosetting, Chatham, Kent, UK
Printed and Bound by TJ International Ltd, Padstow, UK